Newsweek

ENCYCLOPEDIA
OF
FAMILY HEALTH
AND FITNESS

Newsweek

ENCYCLOPEDIA OF FAMILY HEALTH AND FITNESS

KENNETH ANDERSON

Richard J. Wagman, M.D., F.A.C.P.

Medical Consultant

In Association with the Editors of
NEWSWEEK BOOKS

Herbert A. Gilbert, Managing Editor

NEWSWEEK BOOKS
New York

Printed in the United States of America.

First Edition 1980

Library of Congress Cataloging in Publication Data
Anderson, Kenneth N
Newsweek encyclopedia of family health and fitness.
Includes index.
1. Medicine, Popular. 2. Health. I. Wagman,
Richard J., 1932–   II. Newsweek, inc. III. Title.
RC81.A548   616'.024   79-3539
ISBN 0-88225-292-5

Editorial Staff

Herbert A. Gilbert, Managing Editor

Elaine Golt Gongora, Art Director and Designer
Eva Galan, Copy Editor
Elaine Andrews, Copy Editor
Alex Orr, Artist

Alvin Garfin, Publisher

ACKNOWLEDGMENTS

The author and editors of the NEWSWEEK ENCYCLOPEDIA OF FAMILY HEALTH AND FITNESS *wish to acknowledge the contributions of information and advice from the following individuals and organizations:*

Harold Federman, M.D.
American Cancer Society, Inc.
American Council for Healthful Living
American Heart Association, Inc.
American Medical Association
American Optometric Association
American Osteopathic Association
American Podiatry Association
American Public Health Association
The Arthritis Foundation
Federation of American Societies for Experimental Biology
Food and Drug Administration
Montefiore Hospital & Medical Center
National Association of Community Health Centers, Inc.
National Association of Home Health Agencies
National Cancer Institute
National Association for Health Services Research
National Center for Health Statistics
National Council for Homemaker—Home Health Aide Services, Inc.
National Council on Alcoholism

National Dairy Council
The National Foundation—March of Dimes
National Heart, Lung, and Blood Institute
National Institute for Occupational Safety and Health
National Institute of Arthritis, Metabolism, and Digestive Diseases
National Institute of Dental Research
National Institute of Mental Health
National Institute of Neurological and Communicative Disorders and Stroke
National Institute on Aging
National Institute on Alcohol Abuse and Alcoholism
National Society to Prevent Blindness
New York Hospital—Cornell Medical Center
Pharmaceutical Manufacturers Association
President's Council on Physical Fitness
Surgeon General, United States Air Force
United Cerebral Palsy Associations
United States Consumer Product Safety Commission
United States Department of Agriculture
United States Department of Health and Human Services
United States Public Health Service
Visiting Nurses Association of New Haven

CONTENTS

CONTENTS

FOREWORD

The maintenance of good health and the early detection of disease require that each of us be familiar with the basic facts of anatomy and physiology, the body functions, and the early signs and symptoms of illness.

Written specifically from the patient's point of view, the *Newsweek Encyclopedia of Family Health and Fitness* offers comprehensive, carefully researched medical information for the 1980's, including the most recent advances and findings, in concise, clear, and readable language.

Expertly prepared by the author and editors of *Newsweek Books*, the encyclopedia is designed to enable readers to be informed patients, capable of communicating effectively with their doctors and participating in their own and their families' health program and treatment. The author and editors of this health encyclopedia are ever mindful of the uniqueness of every human being and the consensus of the medical community that proper diagnosis and treatment is an individual matter requiring close cooperation between patient and physician.

Medically authoritative and easy to consult, this book describes the body's normal operation, explains what can go wrong and how to distinguish between signs and symptoms of a serious illness and those of a minor disorder.

In addition to basic anatomical and physiological descriptions, the book contains responsible self-help information about health, nutrition, and weight control and physical fitness. Although all the major diseases are thoroughly described, the encyclopedia will likely be consulted most frequently for the so-called minor or nuisance ailments—headaches, hemorrhoids, low back pain—ailments that rarely disable but cause aches and pains and a loss of a feeling of well-being. Other features offer advice on how to choose a doctor and little-known ways to reduce your own medical and hospital costs.

The complex world of medicine and health care is all here.

The reader need only consult the detailed table of contents and the extensive index. Most of the chapters contain an alphabetized glossary of medical terms encountered but rarely understood precisely. The question and answer sections included in many chapters enable readers to evaluate their own symptoms and formulate questions for their physicians.

This is not a book for casual reading. It is a serious, reliable reference work that presents the risks and dangers to good health and suggests ways of modifying and adapting one's lifestyle in order to live a long and healthy life.

This book, with its sensible advice on self-care and preventive medicine, will please advocates of consumer medicine.

Because of its well-balanced approach to health and medical care, this encyclopedia may well be described as the most essential book for the family library.

E. L. Wynder, M.D., President
American Health Foundation

HOW TO FIND A DOCTOR

First, a bit of advice for everybody concerned about his health: don't wait until you have a medical emergency to learn how to find a qualified doctor. Before you finish reading this chapter you should know how to locate a doctor in your home neighborhood or while traveling in a strange community.

Ideally, you should be well acquainted with one or more doctors who have examined you on more than one occasion and have immediate access to your medical records, which will include pertinent information that might be helpful in an emergency. The records should include some details of surgery or previous hospitalization, a list of medications you take regularly, data concerning your allergies to drugs or other substances, past diseases and inoculations, the basic condition of your heart and lungs, results of laboratory tests, and so on.

Ideally, also, you should have some acquaintance with your local hospital or medical clinic facilities, and local ambulance and paramedical services. You don't have to wait until a relative or friend is sick to visit a hospital. Many hospitals welcome volunteers who are willing to spend part of their spare time helping with the nonmedical needs of patients, such as distributing reading materials to those confined to beds.

If you happen to be one of those persons who have a phobia about hospitals, you should at least know the address and telephone number of a hospital near your home. Almost everybody in our modern society can expect to be a hospital patient at least once. Because people today tend to live longer, they are increasingly likely to make multiple trips to hospitals for the very lifesaving treatments and techniques that make longer life possible—heart pacemaker implants, intensive care facilities for heart attack victims, rehabilitative surgery for survivors of accidents, organ transplants, etc.

Generally speaking, we are relatively healthy people today, despite some deficiencies in health care delivery systems. There are striking variations in health care quality among various western nations and in different regions of individual countries. Some European nations, for example, may claim slightly better records than the United States in certain categories, such as infant mortality rates or the longevity of the male population. But those countries do not have America's great disparities of subpopulations with varied economic, cultural, and ethnic backgrounds—factors which account in part for differences in health care performance. In America, states which claim the lowest infant mortality rates, such as Utah, also have the smallest population of blacks, who account for much more than a fair share of infant mortality cases.

How Many Doctors Are There?

Canada and the United States have approximately the same proportion of physicians per population, about one doctor for every 565 persons, although the precise figure may vary from year to year. By comparison, the U.S.S.R. claims one physician for each 307 persons. On the other hand, the Upper Volta has about one doctor for every 93,000 persons, and Honduras has one doctor for every 3,300 members of the population, one nurse for each 10,000 citizens, and one dentist per 20,000 persons.

The United States has more dentists and psychiatrists than any country in the world. In the U.S. there is roughly one dentist for every 2,000 persons, but they are not evenly distributed—people in the Middle Atlantic states have twice as many dentists per 1,000 persons as residents of southeastern states. Like dentists, the availability of psychiatrists and other doctors depends upon what part of America you are in when you need one. Most psychiatrists are concentrated in cities, such

as New York City. Twice as many physicians practice in cities as in rural areas, on a per population basis, but suburbs have four times as many physicians per 1,000 population as the inner cities.

A person who begins a search for medical advice or treatment with little or no prior knowledge of who's who or who's where in the world of medicine would have little difficulty in becoming confused. In the first place, not all doctors are actually physicians. One dictionary of abbreviations lists more than 50 different professions, in addition to medicine and dentistry, in which the practitioners are allowed to identify themselves as doctors.

A medical specialty group once hired a public relations man who held a Doctor of Philosophy degree in journalism. As a "doctor" associated with a medical association, he was often prodded for free medical advice at parties and other gatherings. To each inquiry, he politely and accurately replied, "I'm sorry I can't help you with that particular problem. It's not in my specialty." Fortunately, very few bothered to ask the next obvious question, "Just what is your specialty?"

The more than five million persons actively involved in health care in the U.S. include more than 860,000 nurses, 365,000 physicians, and 112,000 dentists. The precise numbers are not too important because they change almost daily as new classes graduate, foreign graduates join the ranks, older doctors and nurses retire or change from private practice to teaching or administrative jobs, and so on. Perhaps the reason you may never see the same exact figures for the population of doctors or other health personnel twice is that there are many ways of calculating the available number of doctors. Some totals include only licensed Doctors of Medicine, or M.D.'s, while other totals include physicians who are D.O.'s, or Doctors of Osteopathy (also known as Osteopathic Physicians). Some total numbers of M.D.'s include only nonfederal physicians involved in direct patient care, who may or may not be in general practice or be members of a hospital staff. Of a total of nearly 380,000 M.D.'s in a recent year, excluding M.D.'s with temporary foreign addresses, only 204,000 actually were in direct patient care with an office-based practice. The rest were inactive, working for the government, in research, or involved in such activities as teaching or hospital staffing.

So while there are plenty of licensed physicians about, only about half the total number of doctors are involved in what was once known as "private practice." Thus, if you take a shot in the dark and call just any physician for an appointment or an emergency, there's a 50 percent chance that the doctor will not be prepared or equipped to handle your case because he will not have an office that offers primary patient care.

Of the active office-based physicians in patient care, about half are specialists, reducing further the chances of getting a general practice physician by randomly sampling the physicians in a typical community. More than 10 percent of all active physicians surveyed in a recent study by The Department of Health and Human Services were specialists in psychiatry and neurology. A nearly equivalent percentage were specialists in pathology or radiology. Thousands more were specialists in skin diseases, plastic surgery, ophthalmology, otolaryngology, or other specific areas of medical practice which might not

be the answer to your particular needs for advice or treatment.

In fact, of a total of 330,000 active physicians covered in the federal study, only 205,000 had an office-based practice, and of that number, only 51,000 doctors were engaged in general practice. While all physicians have the same general training in anatomy, physiology, and other basic medical subjects, and although they spend periods of internship handling emergency child delivery situations, broken arms, and heart attacks, an experienced ophthalmologist or radiologist may not have the best qualifications for handling an emergency beyond his own medical specialty.

Also, despite the good intentions of the author of the Hippocratic Oath, any doctor today who tries to play the role of the Good Samaritan by treating a problem beyond his own medical responsibilities faces the risk of a malpractice lawsuit if his voluntary efforts to save a life or limb have less than perfect results.

Physicians and most other health professionals must be licensed by the state in which they perform their services. Medical doctors, osteopathic physicians, dentists, optometrists, practical and registered nurses, podiatrists, and veterinarians are required to have licenses in the states in which they practice their profession. If a physician is licensed in one state, he cannot legally practice in another state without obtaining a license in the second state, also. However, temporary state licenses may be granted to out-of-state physicians who are taking special training in a hospital.

State licensing requirements for other health professionals vary from state to state. Most states license chiropractors, nursing home administrators, and psychologists. Fewer than half the states license midwives, medical technologists, opticians, and audiologists.

What It Takes To Become a Medical Practitioner

In order to be a licensed M.D., a person must complete an approved program in medical college. The requirements for admission to medical colleges and their curriculums vary somewhat, but the programs must be approved by a joint committee of the American Medical Association and the Association of American Medical Colleges for accreditation in the U.S. Admission requirements usually include at least three years of premedical college courses, with emphasis on biology, chemistry, and physics. Preference generally is given to students who have acquired at least a baccalaureate degree in one of the major subject areas. The student also must pass a standard Medical College Admissions Test.

Most medical colleges have a four-year program of training, with two years devoted to basic courses in human anatomy, embryology, pharmacology, and related subjects, and the last two years spent in practical application of the background knowledge in so-called clinical courses, working with doctors in hospitals. Some schools cover the same subjects in an accelerated program that allows completion of medical college in three years. Some schools also offer a combined pre-med and medical college curriculum, leading to an M.D. degree within six years rather than the traditional eight.

However, all medical college students must pass a series of National Board examinations designed to test their abilities at the end of various stages of their medical education.

After completing medical college, at which time the M.D. degree is awarded, a physician enters another stage of training that starts with a period of one year of internship in a hospital. After completing internship, a physician usually spends an additional two to five years at a hospital as a resident. The residency program leads eventually to certification as a specialist in one of about 50 primary or subspecialty fields of medicine.

The complete program of training for a specialist in some areas of medicine can require 14 years of intensive study beyond high school. If a doctor also spends two or more years in military service, he (or she) could easily be from 30 to 35 years of age before starting an office practice.

There are some 20 primary medical specialties. Even the area of Family Practice is now considered a medical specialty that may require special training. A doctor who completes his specialty training may apply for certification before a board of examiners who will review his background and residency work in the area of expertise. The applicant will be given oral and written tests relating to the specialty, and in some cases there may be an additional requirement of actual practice in the specialty before the doctor will be "board certified" in that subject. However, the physician can practice a specialty without being board certified.

A doctor does not have to have an M.D. degree to be a physician. Osteopathic physicians who have a D.O. degree, for Doctor of Osteopathy, receive the same basic medical education as M.D. physicians, but they get additional training in osteopathy. Osteopathic physicians define their approach to treatment as a system of medical practice based on the theory that "disease is due chiefly to mechanical derangement in tissues, placing emphasis on restoration of structural integrity by manipulation of the parts. The uses of medicines, surgery, proper diet, psychotherapy, and other measures are included in osteopathy."

Like M.D.'s, the D.O.'s are persons who entered medical college, or more precisely an osteopathic college, after completing a pre-med program of college courses. After four years of medical training, including special osteopathy courses, they undergo additional training as hospital interns and may then enter residency training that will lead to certification by a specialty board. For most run-of-the-mill diseases and injuries, the average patient can expect the same type of therapy from either an M.D. or D.O. doctor. In most communities D.O.'s enjoy the same practice privileges as M.D.'s. A clinic or group practice may have both M.D.'s and D.O.'s on the staff. In recent years the trend has been toward a complete merger of the two types of medical practice.

Most doctors of osteopathy practice in Pennsylvania, Ohio, Michigan, Missouri, and Texas, although, like doctors of medicine, they are licensed in practice in every state of the U.S.

Chiropractors are still another type of medical practitioner found in nearly any community of the U.S., although most members of the group are located in New England and the North Central states. Chiropractic, as the method of treatment is known, is based on a theory that most diseases of the human body are caused by subluxation, or misalignment of the bones. The chiropractor treats the disease by manipulating the bones.

Although medical doctors have not ac-cepted the concepts of chiropractors, certain techniques of orthopedic surgery appear to follow chiropractic reasoning in some disorders involving the vertebral column. For example, compression of a nerve root by misalignment of vertebrae could be the cause of pain and loss of function of a body part served by the nerve. A chiropractor would try to provide relief by manipulating the vertebrae; a medical doctor would try to relieve the condition with drugs and surgery.

Chiropractors are allowed to use X-rays in making a diagnosis of faulty alignment of bones. But since they are not physicians they are not permitted to dispense prescription drugs. Nor are they permitted to perform surgery. Their course of treatments may include physiotherapy and diet planning.

A chiropractor generally has had at least two years of college-level training, followed by four years of instruction in a medical school specializing in chiropractic. He has a degree of Doctor of Chiropractic, or D.C., and is authorized to be addressed as "doctor." He must be licensed by the state in order to practice chiropractic.

There are several other nonphysician types of doctors who use methods of treatment not entirely accepted by the medical establishment. They include homeopaths, whose therapies are based on a theory that disease can be treated by drugs which can produce the same disease symptoms in healthy persons; naturopaths, who believe diseases can be treated by drugless techniques utilizing light, air, water, and special foods; naprapaths, who treat bodily ills with steam or water baths; and a variety of other therapists who may use acupuncture, herbs, or religion to treat human ills. The therapies offered by nonphysician practitioners apparently help some of the people some of the time, since they are accepted by state licensing boards and have enjoyed a continuing popularity among patients who also have access to the services of physicians.

Whatever Happened To the Old Family Doctor?

Once upon a time people tended to live for several generations in the same community. Each family usually had a family doctor who may have attended local schools with the parents or grandparents, and who later delivered their children and grandchildren. He often was an old personal friend and neighbor as well as a physician, and there was no doubt as to who should be summoned in an emergency or for treatment of a chronic illness.

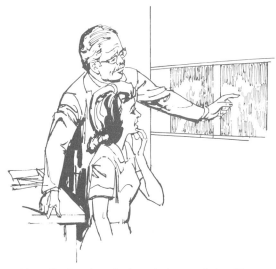

No matter how busy he is, a doctor usually is willing to take time to explain to a patient the nature of the person's health and the results that might be expected from the treatment recommended. Because X-ray films used in doctor's offices today are almost immediately available, a patient can have a doctor's explanation for a common problem such as heartburn supported by X-ray evidence within a few minutes.

Finding a doctor today for most patients may not be as simple as it once was, however, because American families often move from one part of the nation to another—an average of one move every five years, according to one survey—which means that they must find new and possibly different medical resources at frequent intervals. Doctors themselves tend to move about a bit, occasionally leaving a practice to teach or retire, or to seek better job opportunities and living conditions in a different community. The physician may be replaced by a young doctor who has just completed a tour of military service or a hospital residency in a specialty such as pediatrics or internal medicine.

Ways to Contact a Physician

For a person who has moved to a new area, or who has lived in a community for a long period of time but never before felt the need for professional medical care, there are several ways to go about establishing contact with a physician. One of the easiest approaches, obviously, is to use the telephone directory. Most telephone directory yellow pages list doctors according to their specialties, which is helpful for making an appointment with a specialist in child psychiatry or ophthalmology, for example. Many doctors include in their telephone directory listing some information about their specialty, such as "Practice Limited to Allergy" or "Practice Limited to Rheumatology." The listing also may state "Hours by Appointment" or "By Appointment Only," indicating it would not be wise to drop by the office for an examination just because you happened to be in the neighborhood.

Telephone directories may contain a number you can call if you need emergency medical care and are unable to reach your regular doctor. The emergency telephone service usually is sponsored by the local county medical society.

The county or state medical society also can be a source of information regarding doctors who might be available to serve you on a regular basis. The telephone number of the medical society or association usually is listed in the white pages of the telephone directory under "Medical Society of...." If you call the local medical society, tell them where you live and what sort of doctor you need for general family health care or special health problems. The medical society will offer the names, addresses, and telephone numbers of several possible physicians with offices in your general area. Don't expect the medical society to recommend one doctor in preference to others, however.

If you want to learn something about a doctor's credentials, there are a couple of sources you can tap, usually without going through a medical society office. One is the *American Medical Directory*, published by the American Medical Association at rather frequent intervals. The directory lists every M.D. in America, including those in government service or overseas on temporary assignment, regardless of whether or not they may be members of the A.M.A. This multiple-volume directory lists doctors in alphabetical order, last name first, and by geographic location. If you want to learn something about the background of a doctor when you have only his name, you can find his geographic listing in the alphabetical portion of the directory. The geographic volumes provide such information as the name of the medical school from which the doctor graduated, the year in which he was licensed, his specialty, type of prac-

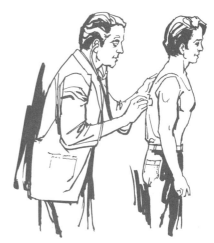

The doctor-patient relationship often is improved when the patient gets a thorough physical examination before the onset of illness. The information obtained about the health of a patient when he is in a healthy condition becomes a better benchmark for measuring the seriousness of a future injury or illness. A doctor often finds it difficult to judge the normal health of a person who waits until he is desperately sick before seeking medical care.

tice, and membership in specialty organizations.

The information in the *American Medical Directory* is presented in coded form, but the codes are rather easy to decipher. Each volume contains several pages of material explaining the code system, which probably is necessary to condense the professional profiles of several hundred thousand physicians into a few bound volumes.

A typical listing in the directory might read as follows in one of the geographic volumes under New York, New York: STURDLEY, Samuel S. 1438 E. 55 St. 10017 #024-01 L50 OBG, PD +85 *020. To translate this code, you would look through the code explanations in the front of the volume and find that Dr. Samuel S. Sturdley of the above listed business address graduated from Harvard University Medical School in Boston (#024-01) and was licensed to practice in 1950 (L50). The code, +85, means he has been certified by the American Board of Surgery. OBG, PD are abbreviations for Obstetrics & Gynecology (OBG) and Pediatrics (PD), which are his main areas of patient care. The code, *020, means that Dr. Sturdley's type of medical practice is direct patient care.

A first-year resident would be identified by the code, *011, under the category of type of practice. The code, *012, indicates the physician is in advanced resident training for a specialty. Doctors who are engaged in administrative activities in a hospital or health agency are identified by the code, *030, at the end of their listing, while doctors primarily involved in teaching at medical schools or other educational institutions have the code, *040.

Physicians who have teaching responsibilities often spend part of their time in direct patient care, so the fact that a doctor is a member of a medical college or nursing school faculty would not necessarily mean that the physician would not be available as a personal doctor during non-teaching hours. However, doctors employed in administrative tasks or who are retired or otherwise inactive—those inactive doctors being identified by codes from *071 to *075—probably would not be anxious to handle your case.

Medical college codes in the *American Medical Directory* begin with "0" for medical schools in the U.S. and Canada. They range from 001-02 for the University of Alabama School of Medicine in Birmingham to 068-01 for the University of Saskatchewan College of Medicine in Saskatoon.

Graduates of foreign medical colleges are identified with medical education numbers that start with 118-01 for the Faculty of Medicine, Kabul University, in Afghanistan, and run to 965-01 for the University of Zambia School of Medicine in Lusaka, Zambia. Graduates of institutions not listed as medical schools by the A.M.A. are assigned the medical education code number of 200.

If you plan to move in the near future to another part of the country, you may want to borrow a copy of the directory to obtain the names and addresses of physicians to contact after you reach your new home. This information might be more practical for a person moving to a small community such as Clarendon Hills, Illinois, which would have a dozen or so doctors to choose from, rather than Chicago, a few miles away, which has so many physicians that their names fill nearly 60 pages of the directory.

One helpful innovation for female patients who prefer to have a woman doctor is the publication in 1979 by the American Medical Association of a special volume of the *American Medical Directory* devoted to names, addresses, and medical background data of all the women doctors in America.

A second good source of information about the doctor who may become responsible for your health care is the *Directory of Medical Specialists*, which is published by Marquis-Who's Who. This directory provides more details about the background of each doctor listed than does the *American Medical Directory*, although it lists only physicians who are certified members of various specialty boards. If you are merely seeking information about a local GP who has not taken the additional training that leads to specialty certification, you probably will not find him listed in the *Directory of Medical Specialists*.

But a doctor who is listed in the directory is allowed to provide a considerable amount of background information about his or her training, including the names and dates of the medical college attended and of the hospitals where the doctor interned and did resident training, plus the names of schools and courses involved in postgraduate education, military service, current hospital affiliation, and so on. The information about hospital affiliation can be important if a patient wants a doctor with hospital privileges.

Whereas the coded information in the *American Medical Directory* generally packs all the highlights of a doctor's background into one line, the information in the *Directory of Medical Specialists* may be abbreviated but not coded, and may often run to 20 to 30 lines. Instead of showing that a John Doe graduated from Columbia University College of Physicians and Surgeons in New York in 1949 as "035-01-49" in the A.M.A. directory, the Marquis version presents the same information as "MD Colum (P&S) 49," which makes for easier reading for a layman checking a doctor's background.

Some information in the *Directory of Medical Specialists* may not be essential to a prospective patient. For example, the biographical information showing that the doctor once was a "Visiting Fel (Primate Biology Lab) Yale 48," or was a major in the Medical Corps of the Army of the U.S. from 1942 to 1946, won't much interest a patient seeking treatment for gallstones or a hiatus hernia.

Some doctors in telephone and other directories may list initials after their M.D. or D.O. The initials usually refer to their certification as members of specialty organizations, such as AAP for American Academy of Pediatrics or FAAFP for Fellow American Academy of Family Practice. But there is one set of initials following a doctor's name that has nothing to do with medical specialties; the initials "PC" mean simply that the doctor's practice is a Professional Corporation.

When To Call the Doctor

In an emergency or when a doctor is needed suddenly because of illness during a trip, a good source of names and numbers is the local medical society. The first doctor you call, or even the second or third, may not be available immediately. If the doctor's wife or office assistant understands the nature of your illness or injury, he or she often can be of help in locating another suitable physician faster than a layman can.

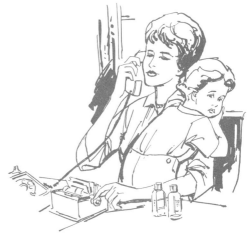

A new mother often has concerns about the health of a child for a number of reasons, including the fact that a baby is unable to communicate clearly about the cause of its distress. Small children normally have physiological functions that are somewhat different from those of adults, such as a normally rapid pulse, which can confuse a new parent. A telephone call to a doctor who has the child's medical records available can help ease such anxieties.

Most doctors have somewhat unpredictable office and hospital schedules because of constant interruptions by emergencies, child deliveries, surgery with unexpected complications, and so on. Even house calls today are not so rare that a doctor might not be away from his office because of one or more house calls.

Regarding the house call controversy, most doctors prefer that the patient visit the office because it is no longer feasible to carry a complete medical armamentarium in a little black bag, as in the "good old days" of doctoring. A modern medical office may be part of a group practice or clinic equipped like a minihospital to handle myriad diagnostic procedures, from X-rays and electrocardiograms to blood tests and eye tests. The chances of finding the cause and cure of a medical problem are immensely greater if it is possible for the patient to go to the doctor, rather than vice versa.

When a physician is called, there are certain bits of information that should be presented to the doctor, his nurse, or secretary right away. The caller should explain who the patient is and should give the address and telephone number of the patient. If the doctor's office has medical records of previous visits or calls, that information can be pulled from the files for reference. If the doctor has not examined the patient previously or cannot respond at the moment, information about the location of the patient will help the doctor to find the patient later.

The person calling the doctor's office should be prepared to describe the nature of the illness or injury. The doctor or one of his assistants may want to know whether the patient has pain and where the pain is located. Additional information would cover such symptoms as breathing difficulty, loss of consciousness, mental confusion, bleeding, swelling, lumps, skin rash, coughing, vomiting, diarrhea, or other signs.

If it is necessary for the doctor to make a house call, explicit instructions should be provided so the doctor doesn't have to waste time exploring a strange neighborhood. If the doctor can't come immediately, the phone line should be kept free so the doctor's office can check back. A doctor often cannot contact an ill or injured person because the patient's line is busy with calls to friends and relatives.

In many emergencies the best move is to take the patient directly to the emergency room of the nearest hospital. If the patient cannot be moved easily, call a private ambulance service or the police or fire department. The emergencies justifying such action include chest pain, abdominal pain, severe burns, suspected poisoning, convulsions, hemorrhage, or broken bones. If the situation is truly serious, the patient should go to a hospital where proper attention can be given to the medical problem. If the doctors on duty decide that the problem does not warrant hospitalization, the patient can always be sent home.

A medical problem that is not an emergency should be handled by making an appointment during a doctor's regular office hours.

If the purpose of a phone call is to obtain information or ask a question, the caller should leave word with the nurse or secretary and suggest that the doctor return the call at his convenience. The doctor may not have immediate access to the answers and may need some time to find the correct information based on the patient's medical records.

Many doctors develop a phobia about

patients who make "false alarm" calls, or who call about trivial matters during busy office hours or while he may be trying to enjoy dinner with his family. For that reason, many doctors depend upon telephone answering services and unlisted numbers for their home telephones. The answering service will keep in touch with the doctor and relay urgent calls. No doctor knowingly ignores a medical emergency, but to make his services available to any or all patients on a fair and equal basis, he must budget his time carefully and keep his lines of communication open.

Emergency or urgent calls to doctors are warranted when the patient's symptoms, such as abdominal or chest pains, are too severe to be endured any longer. Another reason for an urgent call to a doctor might be the result of symptoms that persist for a number of days for no easily identifiable cause, such as nose bleeds that occur for no apparent reason. Still another problem that could be considered serious enough to warrant an urgent call to a doctor is a symptom that occurs repeatedly for no easily determined cause—for example, digestive distress that recurs despite efforts to avoid possible causes such as overindulgence.

Accidents that result in severe or uncontrolled bleeding or in unconsciousness should be considered medical emergencies. So are accidents that result in signs of broken bones, or any condition marked by signs of shock such as pale, cold skin, sweating, and a weak pulse, with or without loss of consciousness. Persistent severe vomiting, serious or extensive burns, suddenly lost or blurred vision, and sudden mental changes marked by confusion, grogginess, or agitation are other conditions that should prompt one to find a doctor as quickly as possible.

Practitioners of Holistic Medicine

There are many medical conditions that seem to defy scientific diagnosis and prognosis. Careful studies have shown that the remission or recurrence of cancer and other diseases can be related to anxiety and stress. A woman may experience a heart attack when she is forced to sell her home and move to a distant city, or she may suffer a flare-up of arthritis about the time a grown child marries and leaves home.

A new type of medical technique, not generally accepted by the established medical profession and not always practiced by licensed physicians, has evolved in recent years with the goal of trying to treat such health problems. Popularly known as holistic medicine, this innovative kind of therapy blends a modern knowledge of human anatomy and physiology with some of the ancient Oriental mind-control methods such as yoga, meditation, and breath control. The idea is not entirely new because some promoters of homeopathic medicine once used similar methods of treating disease, utilizing natural cures and placebo effects to produce relief of symptoms without actually administering a medication to the patient.

However, the concept of holistic medicine, including the argument that a patient can exercise voluntary control over his involuntary nervous system, has been made more believable by certain demonstrations. For example, biofeedback devices have shown that an individual can indeed regulate his blood pressure, heart beat, and other body functions simply by exercising mind control over his organs. Furthermore, it has been found in recent years that there may be more than one nervous system pathway between the mind and the body. Yogis and Zen masters use entirely different methods of entering a trance-like state in which their bodies are not affected by such stimuli as lights, sounds, or sudden changes in temperature. The yoga type of trance enables the individual to be unaware of the world around him, while the Zen master is fully aware of what is going on around him but he is able to maintain a meditative state without being distracted.

Medical doctors have found that patients under hypnosis may or may not experience pain when told that a needle will be jabbed into their flesh, depending upon whether they are told how they will react. Studies of this phenomenon have resulted in the discovery that when a patient anticipates the feeling of pain, a certain chemical that seems to be associated with pain suddenly appears in the bloodstream. But when the patient believes there will be no pain from a needle, the chemical does not appear in the bloodstream. The body also produces a chemical that

helps to suppress pain, a substance called endorphin—a term derived from the words *endogenous* and *morphine,* suggesting a self-produced narcotic—when the mind has instructions to reduce or eliminate the feeling of pain.

In addition to the traditional types of medical doctors, the practitioners of holistic medicine, and chiropractors, there are healers who use herbs, diets, acupuncture, and religious faith to relieve the signs and symptoms of disease. In most cases, the patient has wide freedom of choice in the type of medical practitioner he or she prefers for the treatment of a health problem. In most areas, local laws prohibit only the use of techniques or substances that have proved to be dangerous or ineffective. Often the laws are unnecessary because a doctor or other type of healer who fails to help a patient solve a health problem will find that the patient goes looking for another doctor.

GLOSSARY

HOW TO FIND A DOCTOR

The alphabetized list of entries below consists of special terms and definitions relating to general health care that the reader should know something about before seeking the services of a physician. Words in italics refer to other entries in this Glossary.

allopathy A system of therapeutics based on the belief that a disease can be cured by the administration of medicines that produce effects different from those caused by the disease. The term "allopathic physician" sometimes is applied erroneously to M.D.'s.

American Board of Medical Specialties A nonprofit organization of more than 20 medical specialty groups that helps establish qualification standards for physicians who enter training toward *certification* as a practitioner in one of the recognized medical specialties.

A.M.A. An abbreviation for the American Medical Association.

A.N.A. American Nurses Association.

anesthesiology The administration of anesthetics or other drugs that produce a loss of sensation or consciousness during surgical, obstetrical, or medical procedures. The anesthesiologist, a doctor or nurse certified to handle this responsibility, may be in charge of heart-lung machines or other life-support systems in an operating room.

A.O.A. Abbreviation for the American Osteopathic Association.

audiology The diagnosis and treatment of hearing problems. An audiologist may operate equipment used to test a patient's ability to evaluate sounds of various frequencies and intensities.

baccalaureate A term used to identify a level of education equivalent to the degrees of Bachelor of Science or Bachelor of Arts. Many training programs for nurses, technologists, and therapists who work with doctors are baccalaureate programs.

certification A process whereby a nongovernmental agency or association grants recognition to an individual who has achieved demonstrated competence in an area of health care.

clinical laboratory The name of the laboratory used by the doctor for performing tests on blood, urine, and other body substances. It may be located in a hospital, clinic, or group practice facility, or the laboratory may be an independent facility in another community to which blood or other samples are sent for testing. Hospitals also may have an anatomical laboratory for examining tissues of patients.

closed staff A term used to describe hospitals where only doctors whose applications have been approved by the hospital board of trustees, or a similar governing body, can admit and care for patients. If a doctor does not have staff membership at a closed-staff hospital, his patients may be admitted for treatment at one of the open-staff hospitals that accept the patients of any licensed physician. Most American hospitals are closed-staff facilities.

colon and rectal surgery A medical specialty for doctors who perform surgical correction of disorders of the colon and rectum.

consulting physician A doctor who is allowed to consult with hospital staff doctors but is not permitted to admit his own patients to the hospital. He is usually a specialist in a branch of medicine.

courtesy staff Doctors who are allowed to use a hospital only occasionally on behalf of a patient.

cultists A term sometimes used by members of the medical establishment to identify health practitioners who do not accept the principles of scientific medicine. M.D. or D.O. physicians usually have little or no contact with members of medical cults who promote unproved remedies, such as fad diets that often provide no benefits and can delay the start of effective therapies.

cytology The study of body fluids to detect changes in tissues such as abnormal cells that might indicate the onset of cancer. Technologists who handle such studies for doctors are called cytotechnologists.

dental hygienist A technician who assists a *dentist* in preventive care of a patient's teeth. While there are no special education requirements for a dental assistant, a dental hygienist must complete two years of formal education and training and be licensed by the state.

dentist A doctor who specializes in the diagnosis and treatment of disorders involving the teeth and related structures of the mouth and jaws. A person must have at least two years of college, and preferably a college degree, and pass a dental aptitude test to be accepted as a dental college student. Dental college training lasts four years, the first two years of which include the same courses taken by medical college students and special courses relating to the anatomy and physiology of mouth and jaw tissues. These special courses are emphasized in the last two years of dental college. Dentists are not required to serve periods as interns or residents unless they enter a specialty such as root canal therapy.

denturist Another name for dental laboratory technician, a person who works in the manufacture of artificial teeth, including caps, crowns, and dentures.

diplomate A title which may be equivalent in meaning to a board-certified medical specialist.

In some organizations the title may indicate that the doctor is a member of the board that certifies other doctors as specialists.

dispensary A section of a hospital that provides outpatient care for persons whose illness or injury is not serious enough to require overnight hospitalization. The dispensary may or may not be a part of the emergency room of a hospital.

EEG An abbreviation for electroencephalogram, which means simply a recording of brain waves. The doctor may need an EEG for accurate diagnosis of possible brain damage in a patient. An EEG is made by placing the electrodes of an electroencephalograph on the patient's head, and usually it is a painless procedure.

EKG or ECG Abbreviation for electrocardiogram, or a recording by an electrocardiograph of electrical impulses produced by the heart muscle. Many doctors have an EKG made as part of a routine medical examination in order to detect possible subtle changes in heart function.

equivalency A term sometimes used by medical personnel when deciding which of several similar drugs might be used for treating a disease. Drugs that contain the same type and amount of an active substance may be called chemically equivalent. Biologically equivalent drugs are medicines that are likely to be absorbed and excreted by the patient at the same rate. Clinically equivalent drugs are medicines that have the same effect in curing or controlling a medical problem.

ethical drugs A term used by medical personnel to describe medicines that can be obtained only with a doctor's prescription. *Nonprescription drugs*, also known as proprietary or over-the-counter drugs, are not called unethical drugs. Ethical drugs are so named because they are not promoted to the general public but may be intensively promoted to physicians.

exit The word usually is used to identify a doorway to the outside, but the medical profession uses "exit" to mean that patients have a free choice of physicians in clinics, *health maintenance organizations*, or similar health care facilities. The exit principle gives patients some control over the medical profession by rejecting doctors who fail to give quality care.

extended care facility A section of a hospital or nursing home that provides special long-term health care for patients who are able to handle most of their daily living needs but because of a moderate illness are unable to be released for care at home.

faith healers Medical practitioners who use the power of religious faith or belief to treat a disease or disorder.

family planning service Family planning is a nice way of saying birth control. Many health care agencies offer a family planning service or facility.

family practice A medical specialty for physicians who must pass a special examination and be certified by the American Board of Family Practice.

fee-for-service A system of paying a doctor for each service or procedure provided the patient. The fees usually are adjusted according to the time required and the difficulty of the service or procedure. Some doctors use a sliding fee scale which permits a variation in the amount charged a patient according to his financial ability to pay the bill. Other doctors may use a relative value scale to set the fee according to an index number that reflects the complexity of the procedure or treatment; the index number is then multiplied by a dollar figure to calculate the fee charged.

foreign medical graduates Graduates of medical schools other than those located in the U.S. and Canada. FMG's, as they are sometimes identified by the medical profession, are allowed to serve as interns or residents in U.S. hospitals if they pass a special examination designed to test their competency.

formulary The list of drugs used by the medical staff of a hospital or clinic. The drugs usually are listed according to their generic, or chemical, names, rather than by brand names.

free clinic A community or neighborhood health care center that provides patient care with a staff of volunteer health professionals who charge a token fee or no fee at all. Free clinics may be located in old store fronts of poor neighborhoods where patients are generally transients or members of minority groups.

generic drugs Drugs identified by their chemical or medical names rather than by brand or proprietary names.

group practice Generally, a group practice is an association of three or more doctors who share facilities and income according to an agreed plan. A group practice may provide single-specialty care, general practice care, or multispecialty care. A group practice often permits doctors to provide more sophisticated diagnostic and treatment facilities and equipment than any of the doctors could acquire on his own.

health department A state, county, or city government agency that collects data, called vital statistics, regarding births, deaths, and certain diseases. A public health department also is responsible for controlling contagious diseases, supervising the quality of drinking water and the sanitation of food stores and restaurants, promoting maternal and child health education, and providing laboratory facilities relating to public health situations.

health maintenance organization Abbreviated HMO, a health maintenance organization offers the services of a multispecialty group practice on a prepaid basis. Each patient enrolling in an HMO program pays a fixed fee regardless of the amount of patient care he or she needs or receives. An HMO may or may not be affiliated with a hospital.

home care Care of a patient in his own home by doctors, nurses, therapists, or other health professionals. Home care programs may be organized by or supervised by a hospital or nursing home to provide long-term health care for patients who are able to cope with living in their own homes despite being disabled by chronic disease or injury.

home health aides A term sometimes used to identify physical therapists or other specialized health professionals who work with public health nurses, such as members of the Visiting Nurses Association, in caring for patients confined to their homes.

house staff A term used to identify interns and residents who are doctors working at a hospital to receive additional training. The term sometimes is used to distinguish the interns and residents from the doctors who are regularly and continuously employed by the hospital.

indemnity A word used by health insurance organizations to mean a benefit paid to a patient for a claim or loss covered by the insurance policy. A claim is defined as a request for payment or a demand for a benefit provided by terms of the insurance policy.

inpatient A patient who is, at least temporarily, a resident of a hospital, nursing home, facility for the mentally retarded, or a similar institution. A patient who resides at home but reports to a hospital, clinic, or similar facility for treatment during the day is called an outpatient.

intensive care unit A ward or section of a hospital that is set aside for the intensive nursing care of patients with serious infectious diseases or other types of severe illness. An intensive care unit sometimes is identified by the initials ICU. Heart attack patients usually are treated in a separate section that is identified as a coronary care unit (CCU).

internal medicine A medical specialty that generally provides treatment of diseases that do not require surgery. These can include allergies, diseases of the heart and blood vessels, respiratory diseases, and problems of the digestive tract. There also are subspecialties

within the field of internal medicine; for example, an internal medicine specialist may treat primarily cardiovascular diseases.

A specialist in internal medicine sometimes is called an internist, which is not the same as a hospital intern.

layman or layperson An individual who is not a health professional such as a physician. Although patients are usually laypersons, laypersons also may have health care responsibilities in supervising medical and hospital activities through government agencies or as members of a hospital board of trustees.

major medical A term often used to identify a type of health insurance designed to provide coverage for major illnesses and surgical procedures by paying for all expenses not covered by conventional policies such as Blue Cross/Blue Shield.

Medicaid A word commonly used to identify the terms of a 1965 U.S. Social Security amendment known officially as Title XIX: Grants to the States for Medical Assistance Payments. It is a federal-state matching funds program to provide at least a portion of needed health care to persons on public assistance or to medically indigent families not on welfare. The services available and amount of funding vary according to individual state plans.

Medicare A U.S. Social Security program that provides health insurance for the aged. Medicare is administered in two parts. Part A provides basic protection against the costs of hospital and post-hospital services, including up to 90 days of inpatient hospital care during any single illness, plus home health care and outpatient hospital diagnostic services. Part B is a voluntary insurance program financed by contributions from Social Security recipients and the federal government to pay for physician services and home health care not covered by Part A.

nonprescription drugs Medicines such as aspirin that are advertised to the public and are available without a doctor's prescription.

nonprofit hospital A hospital that may be operated by a religious or community group to provide hospital services where such services might not be available otherwise. Alternatives are city, county, or state-operated hospitals, or proprietary hospitals, which may be owned by one or more physicians and operated primarily for the benefit of the patients of the doctor-owners.

ophthalmology A medical specialty for physicians whose practice is limited primarily to medical and surgical treatment of eye problems. To be certified as an ophthalmologist, a person must have an M.D. degree and a license to practice, plus at least four full years of graduate training in ophthalmology, covering such subjects as nutrition and metabolism of the eye and physiologic optics, and must have passed both written and oral examinations.

An optometrist, who has the degree of O.D., for Doctor of Optometry, must have attended a college of optometry for three to four years after attending college for at least two years, and must be licensed to examine eyes for vision problems and related abnormalities, and to prescribe and fit eyeglasses.

An optician fits and grinds eye glasses and contact lenses prescribed by an ophthalmologist. Opticians usually are high school graduates who have completed about five years of on-the-job training.

An orthoptist, who must have a college degree plus at least one year of special training, assists ophthalmologists in correcting visual problems, such as crossed eyes, with exercises and similar techniques.

O-T-C drugs Over-the-counter drugs, or non-prescription medications, sometimes identified as "customer choice" drugs.

peer review A review of the quality of health care provided patients that involves supervision of a physician's work by fellow physicians.

physiatrist A medical doctor who specializes in the treatment and rehabilitation of disabled or physically handicapped persons. A physical therapist assists a physiatrist in the practice of what is called physical medicine.

radiology A medical specialty for physicians who use radiant energy, such as X-rays and radioactive isotopes, to diagnose and treat diseases.

referral When one doctor sends a patient to another doctor who may have special qualifications needed for treating a medical problem. The doctor receiving the referral usually is a specialist in another field of medicine.

thoracic surgeon A doctor who specializes in surgical treatment of diseases of the lungs, esophagus, and related organs.

tissue committee A group of senior hospital staff physicians who check the performance of surgeons by examining specimens of tissue removed during surgery.

urologist A physician who specializes in the diagnosis and treatment, including surgery, of diseases of the urinary tract. A urologist also treats problems of the genital tract of male patients.

visiting nurses A home care nursing service provided by voluntary agencies—Visiting Nurses Association or Visiting Nurse Service—to assist physicians with bedside care of patients and to make available health supervision, education, and counseling. The nurses, who have special training in public health, often are assisted by specialized therapists.

QUESTIONS AND ANSWERS
DOCTORS

Q: *Is the old family doctor a vanishing breed?*

A: If you refer to the old family doctor who traveled by horse and buggy and carried all his medicines and equipment in a little black bag, he has become a part of the nostalgic past. As devoted to the care of the sick and injured as was that old family doctor, however, he would be as out of place in today's world of medicine as a horse and buggy would be on an interstate highway.

The tools and medicines he carried in his bag usually were the best a doctor could find in those days. But some of the medicines were compounded in his office from herbs and opiates and alcohol—their purpose might often be to make the patient comfortable while nature did the healing. There were no "wonder drugs" such as antibiotics or synthetic hormones in that little black bag.

There still are thousands of family doctors available, but they usually call themselves primary-care physicians. Most of them are better educated, better trained, and better equipped than the old family doctor. And if you were really ill, you would want the care of the new breed of doctors rather than the vanishing breed.

Q: *Is it true that young doctors seldom become general practitioners?*

A: To put the situation in a proper perspective, we probably should define the term "general practitioners." There are general or family practitioners who have become a sort of minority with respect to the total number of licensed physicians, yet they account for more than 40 percent of all visits to physicians in the U.S. By that fact alone, they form the major primary-care category of doctors.

Now, in addition to general or family practi-

tioners, there are several primary-care specialties. These include specialists in internal medicine, who handle nearly all of the basic medical problems that are nonsurgical (and some that are), such as heart disease, high blood pressure, diabetes, and so on. Another primary-care specialty is pediatrics, the category of "baby doctors" who handle the health care of youngsters from infancy to the beginning of adult years. The obstetrician-gynecologist, who treats the diseases of women and delivers babies, is a primary-care physician. The primary-care specialists often double as general practitioners or "family doctors," even though they have taken special post-graduate training in their specialties. And they handle about 30 percent of all visits to doctors' offices.

To conclude a long answer to a short question, the proportion of medical school graduates entering the primary-care specialties increased from about 35 percent to 45 percent between the 1960s and the 1970s. Although the primary-care specialties attract less than half of all young doctors, those combined specialties, including family practice specialists, account for more than 70 percent of all patient visits.

Q: *Don't doctors in big cities make house calls any more?*

A: Some doctors still make house calls at any time, and most doctors will make house calls when they seem to be the most feasible way to examine or treat a patient who is unable to travel to a doctor's office or clinic. Most patients who make appointments to see a doctor have had the occasional experience of spending more time in the waiting room than expected, because the doctor had to interrupt his schedule in order to make a call outside the office.

If a doctor makes a house call that was not

really necessary, it may mean that a number of other patients are delayed in obtaining their fair share of the doctor's daily schedule of office hours. That is just one reason why a doctor may seem reluctant to make a house call unless there is an urgent medical problem.

Another reason is that a modern doctor's office may be equipped with the latest and finest equipment and medications for diagnosing and treating most of the basic medical problems he will encounter during the day. He can't simply pack up all his gear and tote it from door to door like a saddlebag doctor of the Old West, and he may not be able to provide the best in scientific medical care without his office gear. So, any patient in the city, as well as in the country, probably can find a doctor who will make a house call, but the chances are that a patient will not be able to get the quality of care available at the doctor's office.

Q: *Why is it so difficult for a young college student to get into medical school?*
A: In some ways it should be easier to get into medical school today than it was during the past couple of decades, providing the student is properly qualified. In the 1950s, for example, there were about 85 medical schools in the U.S.

with an enrollment of nearly 30,000 students. In the 1970s the number of medical schools had increased to more than 120, and the total enrollment had grown to about 55,000 students. The total number of medical school graduates per year nearly doubled during that period, from more than 6,000 to around 12,000.

But getting accepted as a freshman medical school student probably is just as competitive as ever. It's unlikely that any candidate will be accepted for one of the approximately 15,000 openings each year without at least a bachelor's degree and top grades in the biological and other sciences. Now, during a typical year in the U.S., there are nearly 1,000,000 bachelor's degrees awarded and about 300,000 higher college degrees. Around 60,000 degrees are awarded each year in the biological sciences, plus a similar number of degrees, including master's and doctorates, in chemistry and the health sciences. Without going any further into the statistical odds, you probably can visualize what any hopeful medical school candidate must compete with, in addition to getting a high score on the national screening examinations for prospective medical school applicants. Yet, every year many thousands of students make the grade and begin a successful career in the field of medicine.

2

THE SKIN

When you visit a doctor's office for a physical examination, the doctor may extend his hand to greet you. But in touching your own hand, the doctor may be doing something more important than merely showing that he is friendly. A doctor who is good at his business of correctly diagnosing the state of your health must be something of a detective. And by touching your hand for a moment he usually can pick up a few clues that will help in outlining the picture of your physical condition.

Is your hand warm or cold to the touch of another person? Is the skin soft or rough? Does your hand feel moist or dry? How firm is your grasp of another's hand? All these quick impressions during the moment of a handshake can be quite revealing to a physician, who probably has held the hands of thousands of different individuals since he entered medical school. Through years of study and practice, a doctor develops a special sensitivity for vital clues that the skin itself may display.

You may have thought of your skin as some sort of leathery sheath designed by nature to help hold the body's organs in place, or as a somewhat soft shell intended to protect your body from the hostile environment of the world outside. If so, you were partly correct. One purpose of your skin is to provide a protective shield around sensitive body tissues. And the skin does help to hold internal organs in place.

But the skin itself is a vital organ—and a relatively large one. The skin of the average adult human weighs approximately six pounds, making it as heavy as the brain and liver combined. The total surface of your skin, from scalp to sole, covers an area of nearly 22 square feet. As an indicator of how physiologically active the skin is, this organ uses about one-third of the total volume of blood flowing through the circulatory system.

If you could examine one square inch of your skin under a microscope, you would find almost 15 feet of tiny blood vessels. That same square inch of skin might also contain more than 70 feet of nerves, plus hundreds of assorted nerve endings. Since your skin represents a boundary between your body tissues and the rest of the world, the nerve endings have an important responsibility in alerting the body to changes in the environment. Some nerve endings detect the pressure of objects you come in contact with, others can detect temperature changes, and still others are pain sensors.

While certain nerve endings in the skin are designed to alert the brain and central nervous system to various contacts with the environment, which may or may not be threats to your well-being, the skin also contains numerous nerve endings that help the body react to the environment. One nerve ending, for example, may signal a sweat gland to secrete fluid in order to cool the skin's surface when the air surrounding the body is uncomfortably warm. Another nerve ending, in response to cold or fear, may trigger a tiny muscle beneath the surface of the skin to contract, producing a tiny bump commonly known as "gooseflesh."

Skin Signs Your Doctor Looks For

Because your skin—far from being a lifeless shell—is richly endowed with vital connections to other organ systems of your body, it's almost impossible to conceal certain health problems from an examining physician. Many diseases within the body will quite literally surface through the skin, producing signs or symptoms that are health clues. In a similar manner, the skin also mirrors certain emotions. Your skin may display signs of fear, anger, or embarrassment by changing color, or you might perspire, even in a cool room, as a result of some personal concern. The so-called lie detectors used to determine whether or not a person responds truthfully to questions depend upon physiological reactions that can be

detected through the skin. It's not surprising, therefore, that a doctor may begin a physical examination by carefully studying the patient's skin.

A doctor's examination of the skin usually is conducted in a piecemeal manner, starting with the scalp and working downward to the toes. In most cases, the patient's body will not be entirely uncovered at any one time. And unless a doctor mentions the purpose of his survey of skin surfaces, a patient may not even be aware that a search for subtle signs of injury or disease is under way.

The doctor will look for bruises, bumps, lumps, the degree of oiliness, excessive sweating, and so on. Any significant variation from the broad spectrum of what is considered normal skin appearance could be one piece of a jigsaw puzzle. When combined with other bits of the puzzle taken from other phases of the examination, the skin's signs will help complete a rather accurate picture of the state of one's health.

By touching certain skin areas with his fingers or the palms of his hands—a technique called palpation—the doctor can occasionally detect health signs that would be missed if he depended only upon evidence that he could see. One area of skin, for example, might be noticeably warmer or cooler than a neighboring surface. A particular point on the skin could be painfully tender to the touch. Or a lump that might be a small tumor could be concealed beneath a flat skin surface.

When you have learned more about your own skin—what's normal and what's not—you will be better equipped to monitor the state of your own health. You should take a minute or two before or after bathing to examine the surfaces of your own skin. If the skin appears to be normal, you can feel somewhat assured that your health is average or better, at least as far as skin signs are concerned. On the other hand, if you discover a suspicious sore, a lump, or an area of fiery discoloration, you might want to bring the matter to the attention of a doctor. However, a lump or lesion could be nothing more serious than a paper cut or a mosquito bite, a type of bodily insult that for most individuals could be controlled by some item in the family medicine chest.

Aspects of a Healthy Skin

Before you try to interpret the meaning of some of the more common skin signs of health, it would be wise to consider what you can expect in the way of an ordinary piece of healthy human skin.

Although human skin is composed of three basic layers of tissue cells—epidermis, dermis, and subcutaneous tissue—there are wide variations in the structure of skin samples from different areas of the body. The skin of the eyelids, for example, is very thin, measuring only about 1/50th of an inch in thickness. The skin on the palms of the hands is nearly 1/3rd of an inch in thickness, a difference of nearly 16 times the thickness of the eyelid's skin. Skin on the palms of the hands has a very thick layer of epidermis, but the palms have no hair follicles or sebaceous, or oil, glands. The skin of the scalp has a thin layer of epidermis, but it contains numerous hair follicles and sebaceous glands. Skin on the back opposite the chest area generally contains a thin layer of epidermis but a very deep layer of dermis.

Some skin areas contain a profusion of nerve endings, but in other parts of the body nerve endings are few and far between. The fingertips of humans are espe-

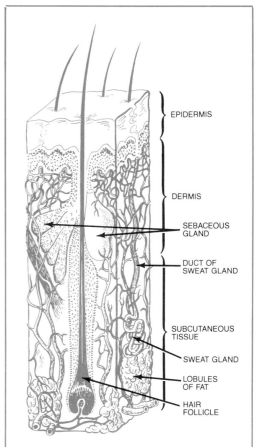

Human skin is composed of a series of layers of cells. The epidermis, or outer covering of the skin, is itself composed of several layers. The outermost layer of dead horny cells gradually wears away as new cells are pushed up from an inner layer of epidermal cells. Beneath the epidermis is the dermis, a thicker layer of connective tissue, nerves, blood vessels, and ducts for sweat and oil glands. Beneath the dermis is the subcutaneous layer of fatty tissue that provides a cushion and support function.

cially rich in nerve endings that are sensitive to pressure or tactile sensation. You can test yourself in this matter by closing your eyes and touching your fingertip in several different places with a sharp object such as a pin or the end of a pen or pencil. Usually, you can tell quite accurately the exact point on the finger-tip's skin where the pressure was applied even though you can't see the place touched. But let someone touch several different areas on your back with the same pin or pen, and chances are you will not be able to locate the precise point of contact. You may even miss by an inch or more because nerve endings designed to detect tactile sensations are not as thickly distributed in the skin of the back.

Even the texture of the skin can vary in different body areas. While the surface of the skin generally appears smooth to the naked eye, a closer examination under a microscope will show a series of uneven hills and valleys that by comparison might make a mountain range seem flat. Skin textures can change quickly over an area as small as one's hand or a single finger, with hair follicles on one side and the indi-vidually distinctive pattern of fingerprints on the other.

The skin of children is soft and flexible,

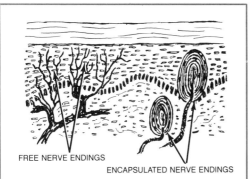

FREE NERVE ENDINGS

ENCAPSULATED NERVE ENDINGS

The skin is richly supplied with free and encap-sulated nerve endings that detect pain, heat, cold, pressure, stretching, and other contacts between the body and the environment.

and more elastic than in older individuals. Find a loose bit of skin on a child and pull it away from the body, then let it snap back to its original position. Try the same test on the skin of an adult who is middle-aged or older; the skin will return to its normal position much more slowly.

The Skin's Outer Layer

The epidermis, or outer layer of the skin, has been described as similar to the bark of a tree. However, the human epidermis is more remarkable than tree bark in that it is constantly changing. The outermost layer of skin cells of the epidermis that you see today probably will be gone to-morrow or the next day, to be replaced by another outermost layer. You really won't notice the difference from one day to the next because the outermost layer of skin is about 30 skin cells in thickness. And the cells are dead. They are flat, shrunken hulks of skin cells that have been pushed upward from layers of living tissue far-ther beneath the surface.

A skin cell of the epidermis has a life span of about three to four weeks. When a new epidermal cell is born, it pushes out-ward against the older cells. The outer layer of your skin is thus constantly re-newing itself. As the epidermal cells move outward they gradually change into horny, scale-like bits of tissue that are soaked off or rubbed off when they reach the outer surface. Depending upon the thickness of the skin, it takes about a month for a new epidermal cell to flake off or wash off the body after pushing about 30 other cells ahead of it. Therefore, it can be said that we have a completely new skin every month and a new skin sur-face every day.

The dead skin cells of the epidermis

form a superficial layer sometimes called the stratum corneum, or horny layer. The tough, horny quality of the skin cells is due mainly to a substance known as keratin, which can be produced quickly and in quantity by the living cells of the epidermis when there is unusual pressure on the skin. An especially thick layer of horny skin tissue can accumulate on skin areas exposed to friction and pressure. A callus on the foot or hand is an example of keratin buildup. Medical studies have shown that repeated scratching of the skin can cause an increased production of keratin and a thicker epidermis in the area scratched.

Although the stratum corneum of the epidermis is composed of dead, horny skin cells, that part of the skin is sensitive to changes in temperature and humidity. In cold, dry weather, water may be drawn out of the horny layer, resulting in a condition commonly called *chapping.* The skin surface may look dry and scaly. During bathing, however, the horny layer may absorb great quantities of moisture and acquire for a brief period a swollen, wrinkled appearance.

Repeated washing with soap and water, while helpful in achieving cleanliness, can actually have a damaging effect on the outermost skin layer and weaken its protective function. Some grease-cutting solvents not only remove protective fatty tissues from deeper layers of the skin, but they also damage the ability of the epidermis to hold water. It is water rather than grease that makes the outer layer of the skin soft and pliable. The purpose of skin oils is to form emulsions that help hold water in the skin so it will not evaporate quickly. Skin oils also help to lubricate the skin but will not soften the cells' horny substance in the absence of water.

Generally, the sloughing off of dead skin cells each day is nature's own way of cleaning the body surface. Stains caused by dirt, paint, or other substances that do not penetrate into deeper layers of the skin are eventually shed from the outside of the body much as a snake sheds its skin at regular intervals. The main difference is that we shed our outer skin every day in the form of billions of microscopic cells, rather than in one continuous sheath.

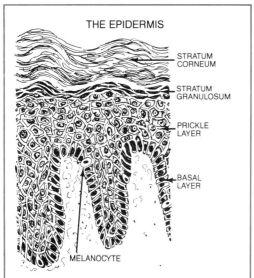

THE EPIDERMIS

STRATUM CORNEUM

STRATUM GRANULOSUM

PRICKLE LAYER

BASAL LAYER

MELANOCYTE

Close-up drawing of a cross-section of the epidermis shows it is composed of several layers. The stratum corneum is made of dead, horny skin cells. The stratum granulosum is a transitional layer of living cells being pushed upward into the stratum corneum. The prickle layer contains cells that are arranged in a criss-cross pattern to form a fibrous net that gives the skin strength. The basal layer is composed of the "mother cells" that produce the other cells of the epidermis. Melanocytes are the source of the pigment that gives a person skin coloring.

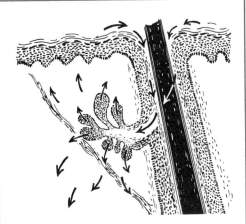

THE ROUTE OF PENETRATION INTO NORMAL SKIN

The skin serves as a barrier against invasion of the body by foreign substances, such as bacteria or poisons. But disease organisms and toxic chemicals can penetrate the skin by following the openings around hair shafts and through oil glands into tissues beneath the skin.

on a hot, dry day, the answer in part is that cholesterol is deposited in your skin by nature as a moisture flow barrier.

The skin is not a perfect barrier against any or all substances in the environment. Foreign substances that cannot break through the multiple layers of dead cells in the stratum corneum sometimes penetrate the skin through such tiny openings as the hair follicles, the microscopic tubes that extend deeply into the skin to hold the hair roots. Foreign substances also can penetrate the skin through openings of oil glands. Chemicals that are fat soluble are easily absorbed through oil glands or hair follicles. In fact, if a foreign substance were to be passed through the skin deliberately—for example, a medication to be administered through the skin—the most effective site would be a skin area covered with hair follicles and oil glands. Sweat glands, on the other hand, do not

Somewhere beneath the horny layer of the epidermis is a membrane that serves as an additional barrier against the invasion of microbes, water, and many other substances that might penetrate the stratum corneum's 30 or so layers of dead skin cells. The barrier membrane also helps prevent the loss of moisture to the outside from tissues, vital organs, and fluids deep within the body. Control of moisture flow both into and out of the body through the skin barrier also is influenced by a substance that is found in many common foods but which can be manufactured by many tissues within the human body. That substance is cholesterol. If you have ever wondered why your body doesn't become completely waterlogged while swimming, or why your body fluids don't evaporate

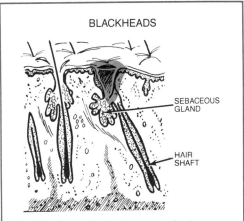

BLACKHEADS

SEBACEOUS GLAND

HAIR SHAFT

Blackheads result when the ducts of sebaceous, or oil, glands in the skin become blocked. The oil and cellular debris plug turns black because of exposure to air.

seem to be effective routes for penetration of the skin's defenses.

Skin thickness, particularly thickness of the horny layer, is a factor in the permeability of the skin. The palms of the hands and soles of the feet seldom become sites for skin allergies because the offending substance generally is unable to penetrate the many layers of skin cells. Any break in the skin, such as a wound or ulceration, however, permits an inflammation or infection to spread quickly through areas in which the epidermis has been damaged.

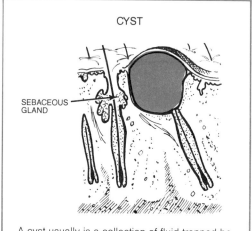

A cyst usually is a collection of fluid trapped beneath the skin, often because of an obstruction in a duct near the skin surface.

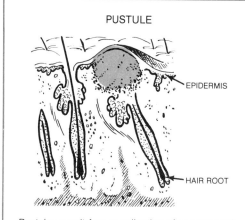

Pustules result from a collection of pus trapped under the skin, often occurring from a bacterial infection at the site of a hair follicle.

arm to "turn blue," the natural pink coloration will return if the arm is placed in an atmosphere of nearly pure oxygen. Testing the permeability of the skin could be a dangerous game for an untrained person. But the evidence that the human bloodstream can absorb oxygen through the skin supports the generations-old idea that people can breathe through their skins.

Special Skin Tissues: The Hair and Nails

Some fat-soluble vitamins, such as vitamins A and D, will penetrate the skin. Certain hormones will permeate the skin. In fact, breast enlargement and menstrual irregularities have resulted from application of female sex hormones to the skin. Some gases also pass directly through the skin. Medical scientists have demonstrated that if normal blood flow to an arm is interrupted by a tourniquet, causing the

Before describing the skin layers beneath the epidermis, some mention should be made of a couple of skin structures that are closely related to the horny layer of dead skin cells on the outside of the epidermis. They are the hair and nails, which are specialized types of skin tissue. Hair follicles form during fetal life, several months before birth, as tiny invaginations, or downward growths, of the layers of the skin. The hair itself then grows outward from the bottom of the follicle. After birth, hair follicles no longer develop in the epidermis. Thus, it might be said that all the true hair you will ever have is what you were born with. Hair follicles that are lost by disease or injury are not replaced by nature.

Just as the skin varies in size and texture over different parts of the body, hair ranges from soft, nearly invisible filaments on the forehead to short, stiff eyelashes and long, flexible shafts on the scalp. Hair usually can be found in one form or another on every skin surface of the body, with the exception of the palms of the hands and soles of the feet.

Hair grows in a manner similar to that of the horny layer of the epidermis. At the base of each follicle is a root, which may be located deep in the subcutaneous layer of the skin. New cells are being formed continuously at the root, with each new generation of hair cells pushing the previous generation outward. The hair cells develop in the pattern of tightly formed columns or shafts which extend beyond the top of the hair follicles. Some hair shafts grow at an average rate of about 1/10th of an inch per week, growing faster during warm summer months and slower during cold winter periods.

When examined under a microscope, a shaft of curly hair appears in cross-section to be relatively flat, and a shaft of straight hair is round or oval-shaped. The outer surface of a hair shaft, when magnified, appears to be a carpet of tiny, overlapping scales. An inner layer of hair cells contains the pigment that gives the hair shaft its color. The white hair of an older person lacks the pigment, but the loss of color does not necessarily mean the hair shaft has less vitality.

One of the fastest growing tissues of the human body, hair has a remarkable ability to regenerate as long as the portion of the root that produces new cells is not damaged. Even repeated plucking of shafts of hair will not destroy a hair root unless the matrix cells which produce new hair cells are removed along with the hair shaft.

However, most of your body hair does not grow at its rapid pace all the time. After a continuous period of growth, lasting perhaps a number of years, an individual hair follicle may shut down for a rest period. The hair shaft in the follicle may remain until it falls out or is pushed out by a new hair that develops in the follicle after the rest period has ended.

With some 100,000 hair follicles in your scalp, you probably will not be aware that a particular hair is no longer growing, even though you may notice the loss of several strands of hair each day. Each hair follicle seems to function quite independently of the other follicles in the area. Under normal conditions only a small percentage of the total hair follicles take a rest at the same time. With the exceptions of balding and certain diseases, new hair shafts are produced at about the same rate that old hairs are lost because of the follicle rest periods.

In the case of balding, the hair follicles take a sort of permanent rest. The follicle sheds its last strand of hair and shrivels away, losing its powers of regeneration. There are factors such as heredity and male sex hormones that affect balding patterns in men. The tendency to become bald is inherited from a grandfather, with the mother (the daughter of the grandfather) providing the genetic link that determines the balding pattern of men in the following generation. Male sex hormones affect scalp hair in men as well as the growth of facial hair in beards and mustaches, pubic hair of the genital area, and axillary hair in the armpits.

Men who were castrated at an early age do not develop the body hair associated with normal sexual maturity, such as facial and pubic hair, although they may have a normal growth of scalp hair. Interestingly, however, if castrated males are administered male sex hormones, pubic and facial hair develop. If they have inherited the genes for baldness, they may suddenly develop baldness after receiving injections of male sex hormones.

Facial hair may appear in women after they have reached their menopausal stage of life, as a result of changes in sex hormone levels.

Like the skin itself, the hair can reveal certain clues about the health of an individual. During periods of illness, your hair may become thinner, develop split strands, slow down its normal growth rate, and generally become more difficult to manage. Barbers and beauticians frequently notice changes in the health of hair when the body is experiencing a systemic disease. A doctor making a careful examination of the skin also may find certain health signs in the condition of one's hair.

Fingernails and toenails, as well as hair strands, are rich in keratin, the horny material found in the dead cells of the outer layer of the epidermis. But the horny cells of the nails are packed together much more tightly and under normal circumstances do not flake off or soak off like horny cells of the stratum corneum. The nails grow more slowly than hair; the new cells push the older cells steadily outward at a rate of about one inch every eight months. In some older cultures it was

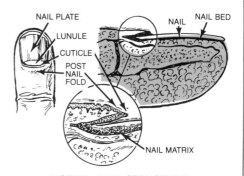

NORMAL NAIL STRUCTURE

Finger and toenails are similar in structure and growth to hairs. They grow slowly outward from a broad follicle-like source in the epidermis but run generally parallel to the skin surface. The illustration shows how closely the nail is to the underlying bone.

fashionable to let the fingernails grow to great lengths as a symbol of wealth and power—the possessor of long fingernails obviously did not have to work with his or her hands.

Fingernails have little importance in modern civilization, however, and the slower growing toenails are even less useful. Anatomically, nails develop from an invagination of the epidermis, in a sort of follicle similar to a hair follicle. The horny cells of the nail are produced from a thin layer separating the epidermis from the underlying skin layer, or dermis. The layer that becomes nail tissue, known technically as the stratum lucidum, rests upon a modified part of the dermis that is the nail bed. The epidermis grows over the base of the nail.

The nail material is essentially colorless but may appear pink or white depending upon the way in which light is reflected from surfaces beneath the nail. Where the nail bed is richly endowed with tiny blood vessels, for example, the nail may appear to be pink. In the area of the lunula, or half-moon, near the base of the nail, the color is whitish to lightly pink because the underlying tissue contains keratin-producing cells which reflect white light. By squeezing a finger along both sides of the fingernail, you can change the color from pink to white as the pressure interrupts blood flow through the capillaries in the nail bed. Except for the free edge of the nail plate, where it overlays the tip of a finger or toe, the nail is surrounded by a thin layer of tissue called a nail fold, which actually is a fold of skin. In addition, a fine rim of horny material, known as the cuticle, underlies the skin fold at the bottom of the half-moon. The cuticle and nail folds occasionally become sites for bacterial invasion of the skin. These sites may become especially vulnerable to disease organisms if the nail folds are damaged by careless manicuring practices.

When a doctor examines the skin, he frequently inspects the nails because they can provide many clues to the true state of a person's health. Nails may thicken or grow rapidly, for example, as a result of nail biting or repeated injury at work or play. Some diseases, on the other hand, may retard the normal growth rate or alter the form of the nails. While nails that are thin, brittle, or easily split do not necessarily indicate that the owner is in poor health, such effects might suggest that the doctor look closer at other sources of diagnostic information. Nails may be in poor condition because of inadequate nutrition or as a result of aging, or both. As one grows older, tiny ridges may begin to appear in the surface of the nail plate; these ridges may eventually grow into more prominent lines that run from the cuticle to the free edge of the nail. Such ridges may be normal for an older person, but in some cases they might help explain to the doctor the possible cause of other signs or symptoms of ill health in a patient. A ridge or groove running the length of the nail plate on a single finger or toe would suggest that some injury may have occurred to the cell-forming root of the nail. If the ridge or groove extends over only a portion of the nail plate, a doctor could guess rather accurately when the accident occurred. Most kinds of temporary damage to nails, including hematomas or "blood blisters" that develop beneath a nail, gradually vanish as the nail grows outward at the normal rate of about 1/8th of an inch per month.

Lines that run across the width of the nail plate can suggest specific health problems. A severe infection or heart disease can interrupt normal nail formation, leaving depressed or thin areas across the nail plates. Since nail plate formation is a low-priority item among vital bodily functions, the human body's resources during periods of life-threatening disease are directed mainly toward the business of restoring good health, and while nails may continue to grow during such periods, their growth generally will be slow and inefficient. If white lines appear across the base of the nails, an examining doctor might well suspect the presence of a liver or kidney ailment and order laboratory tests.

Skin Color

Skin color is determined primarily by the presence of a black pigment, called melanin, in the epidermis. The function of melanin in the skin cells seems to be to protect the skin against the ultraviolet rays of the sun. Ultraviolet rays cause sunburn and skin cancer, conditions that occur less frequently in skin that is darkly pigmented. Melanin in turn is produced by special cells in the epidermis called melanocytes. Most people, regardless of skin color, have approximately the same number of melanocytes in their skin. But dark-skinned humans have melanocytes that are larger and more active in producing melanin.

Albinos, or people with no skin color, and those whose normal skin has lost pigment—a condition called vitiligo—also have the usual amount of melanocytes in their epidermis. In those individuals, however, the melanocytes simply do not produce the pigment that accounts for skin color. Freckles generally appear in skin areas that otherwise lack melanocytes. Melanocytes are most likely to be found around hair follicles, and the most active pigment-producing cells usually are located in skin surfaces that normally get the most exposure to sunlight. Too much exposure to ultraviolet light can cause a loss of pigmentation; the melanin molecules become oxidized and colorless. This effect is most often seen in hair that becomes bleached or lighter in color after prolonged exposure to sunlight.

Melanocytes are related at the embryonic stage of life to nerve cells, and they retain some of their characteristics long after they have drifted away from the rest of the nervous system and imbedded themselves in the skin. Activity of the nervous system and certain hormones can affect melanin production, regardless of the amount of exposure to sunlight. Exposure to certain chemicals also can alter skin coloration. As a result of the neural-hormon-al relationships with melanocytes, the doctor examining a patient's skin often can find clues to hidden health problems. A rather wide assortment of diseases involving the brain and central nervous system may be marked by skin that becomes darker without exposure to ultraviolet rays. Removal of the adrenal glands may be followed by increased melanin production in the epidermis, while administration of certain hormone drugs will cause the skin to lighten again. Ingestion of female sex hormones can cause a darkening of the skin around the nipples, and administration of male sex hormones to a castrated man will permit his skin to tan normally in sunlight—an effect that does not occur without the use of such sex hormones.

In addition to melanin, blood contributes to normal skin color. A doctor may find that a skin that has become lighter or darker than usual can be a useful clue in determining that a circulatory problem has developed. A poor blood supply system or lack of hemoglobin in the red blood cells, for example, could affect a person's skin color.

Distinctive Skin Patterns: Our Fingerprints

The epidermis fits quite snugly atop the dermis, or "true skin," with the help of millions of tiny cone-shaped projections that protrude from the top of the dermis. The tiny projections are called papillae. The bottom layer of the epidermis is covered with millions of dimple-like pits, one for each papilla. The papillae frequently contain special nerve endings, such as receptors that are sensitive to pressure or to cold. By protruding deeply into the epidermis, the papillae can carry the nerve endings much closer to the outer surface of the skin than might be possible otherwise. Although the papillae are well scattered around the body, they are most numerous in skin areas that are most likely to be exposed to the environment. Nerve endings that are sensitive to the tactile sensation, or the sense of touch, for example, are heavily concentrated in the fingertips.

Papillae in the skin of the hands and feet tend to occur in parallel rows, which result in ridges of epidermis on the palms and soles. The ridges in turn form the distinctive patterns of our fingerprints. It has been estimated that an average palmprint will contain about 300 such ridges from the fingertips to the wrist area. Some medical scientists who have made a careful study of the details of human anatomy claim that there is a precise ratio between the width of a ridge on a person's skin and the height of that person when he or she is seated. A detective presumably could therefore estimate the height of an individual by measuring one of the person's fingerprints.

There are approximately 100 different characteristics of an individual fingerprint that can vary from one person to the next. For practical purposes, police departments need no more than a dozen of these characteristics for identification of an individual. Even with only a dozen characteristics known for 10 fingers, the chances of another person turning up with exactly the same set of fingerprint patterns is a virtual impossibility.

The Skin's Inner Layer

Below the cell layers that are next to the epidermis is the main body of the corium, or dermis. Examined under a microscope, the corium appears to be a densely packed complex of nerve cells, blood vessels, lymph vessels, muscle fibers, connective tissue fibers, oil glands, sweat glands, hair follicles, and cells of stored fat.

Blood flow through the skin can be altered up or down automatically according to the needs of the body to conserve heat or get rid of excess heat. The heat of the body is produced by "burning" calories of energy. Under ideal conditions, the body produces just the right amount of heat needed to maintain normal body temperature of about 98.6 degrees Fahrenheit, or 37 degrees Celsius. But for most people, contacts with the outside world are seldom ideal as far as normal human body needs are concerned. When the temperature surrounding the body is too warm, or when a person burns calories too rapidly during physical exercise, or both, the body's excess warmth is carried to the skin via the blood system so the heat can be radiated through the skin. At such times, the arteries carrying blood to the skin may dilate, or expand, allowing as much as two or three quarts of blood per minute to circulate just beneath the surface of the skin.

Under conditions of a cold environment or lack of bodily activity, on the other hand, the body may need to conserve warmth, and it will do so by constricting the flow of blood to the skin. Instead of two or three quarts of blood flow per minute through the skin, the flow might be reduced to as little as one or two ounces of blood per minute for the entire skin surface of the body. In situations of extreme cold exposure, blood flow to the skin may be so severely restricted that the tissues fail to receive enough warmth and nutrition to function normally, and skin surfaces may become frozen or permanently damaged.

Blood flow supplies the energy and nutrients needed by skin tissues. Under normal conditions, the skin cells get adequate nourishment. The blood circulation through the dermis and the underlying layer of subcutaneous tissue is more than 20 times the amount required by the skin cells for normal activity. Blood flow to the skin can be interrupted temporarily, for from a few minutes to as much as an hour, without serious damage. A rebound effect increases the flow to a far greater than normal level to make up for any loss of nutrients after the blood flow is restored.

The lymph system of the skin is part of the blood circulatory system, and like that system its vessels form a network. The lymph fluid that flows in the system bathes the tissue cells of the skin with nutrients and collects their waste products. A lymph capillary extends into each papilla of the dermis; a loop of blood system capillary also extends into each papilla. Through an interchange of fluids, some substances carried to the skin by the blood system capillaries are returned from the skin via the lymph vessels. The lymph system eventually drains into veins, and the dissolved substances start over again as part of the blood. Near the surface of the skin, blood and lymph systems work side by side.

Fatty Deposits Children are more likely than adults to have deposits of fat in the skin. As most individuals grow older, they lose the fatty deposits of the skin. At the same time, the elastic fibers of connective tissue in the skin lose their resilience. A result of those changes is the appearance of wrinkles in the skin of older individuals. Fatty tissue also may be lost from skin deposits when a person reduces his or her food intake. When a person goes on a

crash diet or must undergo starvation, fat that has been deposited under the skin usually is the first fat to be absorbed by the body for use as fuel. Conversely, when a person gains body weight by consuming more calories than required by the body for normal functioning, the fat is likely to appear first in storage cells under the surface of the skin.

Sweat Glands Sweat glands begin to appear in the human skin at a very early stage—several months before birth. Sweat glands eventually appear on nearly all skin surfaces, with the lips being one of a very few exceptions. The body usually has a total of somewhere around two million sweat glands. Most of them are

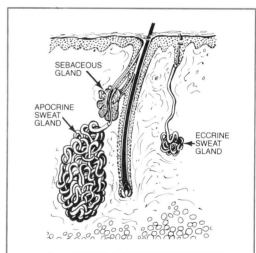

GLANDULAR APPENDAGES OF THE EPIDERMIS

The deeper layers of the epidermis contain oil, or sebaceous, glands as well as two kinds of sweat glands. Apocrine sweat glands occur mainly in the armpits and genital areas; eccrine sweat glands are the main source of sweat produced when the weather is hot and humid.

concentrated in such unlikely places as the palms of the hands, the soles of the feet, the forehead, and the axillae, or armpits.

There are two kinds of sweat glands. True sweat glands are known technically as eccrine glands. A second kind, the apocrine glands, appear during the fertile years of human life and usually are of more interest to an examining physician than to the apocrine glands' owner, who generally is not aware of their existence.

Eccrine sweat glands do not store the fluid known as sweat, but the glands can produce enormous amounts of perspiration on very short notice after the body has been exposed to high temperatures or vigorous bodily activity. Sweat is essentially a very dilute salt solution. It is pro-duced by the eccrine sweat glands on the command of a heat-regulating center in the brain. When released on the body surface, the perspiration, or sweat, evaporates quickly or gradually, depending upon the humidity of the environment. The effect of sweat evaporation is to cool the body surface. It is not unusual on a warm day for an individual to lose more than a quart of sweat.

Perspiration also can result from emotional stress. Some individuals experience profuse sweating, especially from eccrine glands in the forehead, after eating spicy foods.

The apocrine glands produce a milky kind of perspiration in very tiny amounts during periods of stress, such as fear or

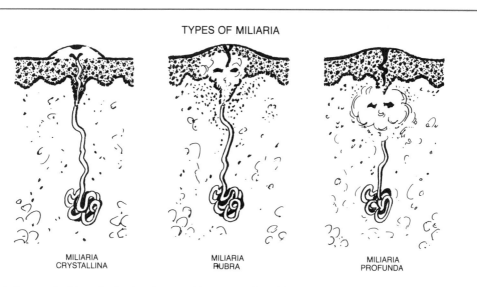

TYPES OF MILIARIA

MILIARIA
CRYSTALLINA

MILIARIA
RUBRA

MILIARIA
PROFUNDA

Miliaria is a medical term for heat rash caused by a blocked outlet from a sweat gland in the skin. In its most simple form, miliaria crystallina, sweat accumulates in tiny blisters at the top of the epidermis. A sweat gland obstruction deeper in the skin causes sweat to spread into the skin instead of onto the surface. The result, miliaria rubra, is prickly heat inflam-mation with itching and a reddish rash. When sweat is blocked deep in the subcutaneous tissues there usually is acute and severe discomfort with possible damage to the tissues beneath the skin. A person suffering from this condition, miliaria profunda, may not be able to tolerate heat or exercise and needs to be in a cool, dry environment.

anger. The apocrine glands are found mainly in the skin areas of the armpits, the anal-genital region, around the mammary nipples, and occasionally on the eyelids. The apocrine sweat glands function only after the start of puberty, or sexual maturity, and their activity declines with menopause in females and a comparable period of the male life span.

Most individuals are not aware that there are two different forms of perspiration. One reason is that when apocrine sweat glands produce their form of perspiration the eccrine glands also become active. Another is that the eccrine glands yield such comparatively generous amounts of sweat that apocrine secretions are rarely noticed.

Doctors frequently take an interest in apocrine sweat glands because they can be the source of such medical problems as infections and inflammations. Apocrine glands are more numerous in women than in men, and perhaps for that reason apocrine gland problems are more common among females. Some doctors feel that certain types of apocrine gland infections are a result of careless shaving of the hair in the armpits or use of underarm ointments or chemicals.

One kind of apocrine gland that most individuals are better acquainted with is a modified apocrine gland located in the ear canals. These apocrine glands secrete a substance that doctors call cerumen but most people call ear wax.

Effects of Stress and Allergies A famous physician, Sir William Osler, wrote that "the skin is the mirror of the soul. When the soul weeps, so does the skin." Doctor Osler's comment was intended to illustrate that the skin, like the heart and the digestive system, frequently responds to emotional stress. But the manner in which some individuals react to psychological pressures can be reflected in skin effects that may prove as baffling to the examining doctor as to the patient. An example is the appearance of a type of skin disorder known as hives. Little white to pinkish bumps called papules may appear on the skin like myriad insect bites. The cause of the rash might be the same kind of anxiety that produces sweating in another individual.

The skin is so closely associated with other body systems and functions that an ailment's fiery rash might be due to a food allergy, a reaction to a medicine, contact with an industrial chemical, or a disease organism. As in a case of anxiety-caused hives, an examining doctor must be a sort of medical detective to evaluate all the various possible causes and come up with an accurate diagnosis. Even the best-trained and most experienced physicians occasionally find a set of signs and symptoms that defy diagnosis.

When your own body is involved, however, you do have some advantages over a doctor examining you for the first time. First, you know better than the doctor about your general well-being, whether you feel sick or in good health. Second, you are acquainted with your own health history and that of your family, so you should have a fairly good idea of your own allergies, past illnesses and injuries, whether members of your family died of stroke or heart disease, etc. Third, you probably are aware of recent contacts with foods, insects, chemicals, people who had similar signs or symptoms of illness, and so on. For example, you may experience headaches or dizziness at work, on the way to work, or at home, but when you go to a doctor's office for a checkup,

SUNBURN

EPIDERMIS

CORIUM

MALPIGHIAN
LAYER

MELANIN
GRANULES

DERMIS

When the skin is exposed to the sun's ultraviolet rays, the skin may react by producing melanin pigment granules as a protection against damage by the sun's radiation. The melanin granules cause the skin to appear darker. Too much sunlight causes a dilation or swelling of the blood vessels in the skin layer beneath the epidermis, as in the middle illustration. The dilated blood vessels give the skin the reddish coloration associated with sunburn. If the skin is allowed to adapt gradually to exposure to ultraviolet light, the corium layer becomes thick and dark with melanin, as in the illustration at right, so that damage to tissues below the epidermis is less likely to occur than it would if the exposure were sudden.

you suddenly feel fine. An examining doctor might be led to believe that your illness is psychosomatic or that you are a malingerer. But if the signs and symptoms return when you go back home or back to work, you might well suspect that the problem is caused by a substance in your work or home environment. You may find the offending substance and remove it from your home or place of work, just as you would eliminate from your diet a food item that made you ill.

Some skin ailments fit into this general rule-of-thumb for diagnosing disorders that affect your own body. With a bit of do-it-yourself detective work you frequently can associate a skin rash with perhaps wearing a garment that has been treated with a dye or cleaning chemical known to cause an allergic reaction, with a recent outing to an area infested with insects, with use of a new brand of rug cleaner, and so on. Some skin disorders can be treated with simple home remedies; others may require immediate professional medical attention.

GLOSSARY
THE SKIN

The following alphabetized entries provide some guidelines to help you determine possible causes and cures for abnormalities you notice on your own skin. Words in italics appear elsewhere in this Glossary as entries.

abrasion A wound affecting mainly the epidermis, and sometimes only the outer layers of the epidermis—for example, a skinned elbow or skinned knee. The wound can extend deeply into the dermis, or corium, and become filled with a blood clot which later forms a *scab.*

Clean the abrasion thoroughly of all foreign material. Irrigation may be adequate for removing dirt and bacteria, but scrubbing the wound area may be necessary. Dirt or other matter that can't be absorbed by surrounding tissues may form an unwanted tattoo when the wound heals, in addition to possibly harboring infectious disease organisms.

If protected from infection by a sterile bandage, an abrasion usually heals itself by regenerating epidermal cells over the exposed area. When the wound surface becomes covered with new layers of epidermis, the scab usually sloughs off. Topical ointments or gauze moistened with salt water may be applied to the wound area to help the healing process. The new skin layer might be sensitive to sunlight for several months and should be protected during sunbathing or other periods of prolonged exposure to the sun's rays.

abscess A collection of pus within a defined area. An abscess of the skin, sometimes called a *pustule,* can be at the surface or deep in the skin layers. An area of abscess may or may not show redness, but it usually is painful, especially when pressure is applied.

An abscess should be treated by a doctor because of the danger of the infection spreading throughout the body. If untreated, an abscess usually increases in size until it ruptures and drains.

acne A common skin condition afflicting mostly young men and women and marked by an assortment of blackheads (comedones), whiteheads (small closed cysts), and pustules. Some experts believe acne may be several different diseases rather than one skin ailment with several different manifestations. Acne affects individuals in various ways. For some persons, acne is primarily a cosmetic problem involving the appearance of a few blackheads. For others, it is an increasingly serious problem marked by painful *lesions* and *pustules* that cover not only the face but the neck and the trunk as far down as the waistline. Acne sometimes can be triggered or aggravated by exposure to heat and humidity typical of a tropical environment.

Acne usually involves the sebaceous, or oil, glands of the skin. During childhood the sebaceous glands are fairly dormant, but they increase in size and activity at the start of puberty, apparently as a result of sex hormone influences. As the oil from the glands is pushed to the surface of the skin, it undergoes chemical changes that result in the dark pigmentation at the opening of the gland that warrants the name, blackhead. Occasionally the oil becomes trapped under the skin, as in a closed comedone or blackhead; the blocked oil duct may rupture into surrounding tissues, producing an inflammation of the skin. The condition can be aggravated further by an invasion of the affected area by bacteria.

There is some evidence that acne tends to "run in the family," that is, persons whose mothers and/or fathers experienced acne problems are most likely to become acne patients. In unusually severe cases of acne, the disorder may involve the apocrine glands of the armpits and anal-genital region, as well as the face, neck, and scalp.

The effects of acne frequently diminish after puberty, and many individuals, particularly those whose skin is naturally dark, find relief from acne by exposing their skin to sunlight. However, the sunbathing treatment is not universally effective. It is less helpful to persons with light skin and hair color. Some young people find that sunbathing only exacerbates their acne problems.

A number of creams, lotions, powders, gels, and similar products are available without a prescription from drug counters; such products generally are helpful for mild cases when the medication is used sparingly and temporarily, at least until it can be determined whether the products are beneficial or harmful. In treating acne, each individual's skin may seem to be as different from the next person's as their fingerprints differ; a medication that helps one case of acne might aggravate the skin condition of another. Products that contain sulfur, resorcinol, and salicylic acid are generally regarded as safe for most mild cases of acne. Regular washing of the face with ordinary soap and water helps mild cases by removing excess oil, dead skin cells, and skin bacteria. Most commonly available treatments produce some drying, scaling, and degerming of the skin surface, but they do little to eliminate closed comedones and inflamed cysts.

Treatment of acne by a physician may extend to the use of antibiotics, prescription of contraceptive pills for female patients, vitamin therapy, diets eliminating fatty foods, application of hot medicated compresses, skin-irritating treatments, and cryosurgery, which involves freezing and causes the skin to peel.

acne rosacea A skin disease marked by a flushed appearance around the nose and surrounding facial areas. Acne rosacea usually appears around middle age, but it can develop during a person's twenties, and it eventually may become permanent. The skin of the nose particularly may become thick and red with prominent veins, and occasionally pustules will form.

Treatment usually is the same as that applied for common acne, that is, topical medications, antibiotics, hot medicated compresses, exposure to sunlight, and temporary hormone therapy. Elimination of certain foods from the diet, such as coffee, alcohol, highly seasoned and extremely hot or cold foods, may be tested on a trial basis to determine whether a particular food causes flareups of the condition.

actinic keratosis A type of skin tumor caused by exposure to sunlight; sometimes called senile keratosis. The tumors have nothing to do with being senile but are more likely to occur on the skin of older persons for the simple reason that they have had more years of exposure to the actinic, or ultraviolet, rays of the sun. Farmers and sailors, who work in the sunlight, are likely candidates for this skin disorder, and so are people who live and work in "sun belt" regions. Blondes and redheads are more susceptible to actinic tumors than dark-haired individuals.

Actinic tumors may first appear as reddish scales in small areas of the skin. The spot gradually becomes elevated and acquires a grayish, hornlike peak. Tumors of this type that appear on the face, scalp, or hands are not likely to become the kind of cancer that metastasizes, or spreads through the bloodstream to other body areas. But actinic keratoses that appear on a mucuous membrane, such as the lip, can metastasize and should be removed by a surgeon as soon as possible.

Actinic keratoses are usually treated by application of a medicine such as 5-fluorouracil, obtained by a doctor's prescription. The sun-caused skin tumors can be avoided somewhat by regular use of sunscreen chemicals and by wearing a hat when venturing into the sunlight for a prolonged period.

adenoma, sebaceous An overgrowth of a sebaceous gland. A condition commonly found on the aging skin of an older person, particularly on the facial skin.

albinism A genetic disorder in which there is no pigment, or color, of the skin. The skin of albinos, persons suffering from albinism, contains the skin cells involved in the manufacture of skin pigments, but the cells do not produce the pigment factor, melanin, that colors human skin.

alopecia The loss of hair or thinning of hair due to illness or other factors. The loss may be temporary or permanent. One form of alopecia, known as alopecia cachectica, is associated with malnutrition. A more common form of the disorder, alopecia areata, is marked by the sudden loss of scalp hair in small patches; in some cases it affects the hair of the entire body.

Depending upon the cause of hair loss, treatment may include avoiding exposure of the hair to sunlight and chemicals used to straighten or wave the hair, or the injection of steroid hormones. Alopecia may occur after childbirth, and it also can be caused by wearing pony-tail hairstyles.

angioma A nonmalignant type of tumor involving blood vessels, usually capillaries; sometimes identified as a birthmark or strawberry mark on the skin. Some kinds of angiomas are fully developed at birth, others do not develop until after birth. An angioma may enlarge after birth, or remain the same size.

The treatment of angiomas usually depends upon the type, size, location, and other factors. The so-called strawberry angioma, one of the most common forms of the disorder, usually disappears without treatment during childhood and is rarely seen in adults. The port-wine stain type of angioma usually does not disappear spontaneously but frequently is treated cosmetically, that is, by applying a cream that masks the coloration of the angioma. A small angioma occasionally may be removed surgically.

Two types of angiomas may occur in older individuals. Spider or starburst angiomas can appear as a central red spot with blood vessels radiating from it. A spider angioma may occur after a sunburn or, less commonly, as a sign of liver cirrhosis; a variation called venous stars may be associated with increased blood pressure in a vein. The small, bright red cherry angiomas usually appear on the trunk of the body of an individual after middle age. They are not harmful and are removed only for cosmetic reasons.

atopic dermatitis A chronic and recurrent kind of eczema, marked by itching, irritation, and inflammation of skin areas. The disease often is mistakenly diagnosed as an allergy. The ailment may first appear at birth, then disappear during the child's preschool years. Or it may continue throughout childhood and seem to disappear after the individual becomes an adult.

Persons who suffer from atopic dermatitis have skin that is extremely sensitive to any stimulus that might trigger an itching spasm, including such diverse things as wool fibers, ordinary soap, cold temperatures, and high humidity. The skin becomes dry, thick, and scaley. The condition is aggravated, particularly in children, by rubbing and scratching, which in turn encourage the development of infections. Vaccination for smallpox or exposure to persons infected with herpes simplex, or cold sore, may make an atopic dermatitis patient critically ill.

Treatment of atopic dermatitis may include careful bathing with mild soaps followed by application of moisture-trapping skin oils, avoiding wool and other fabric materials that cause itching, staying out of overheated rooms, and keeping the fingernails clipped short. A doctor may prescribe the use of steroid-hormone creams or less expensive bland creams such as zinc oxide or petrolatum, injections of steroid hormones, and, when individually effective, antihistamine-type medications.

basal cell epithelioma A common type of skin cancer, occurring most frequently in persons over the age of 40. It is a slow-growing tumor, with dilated capillaries, that may appear translucent. This kind of tumor tends to develop in skin areas with a heavy concentration of oil glands and repeated exposure to actinic rays of the sun. Basal cell epitheliomas sometimes are likened to icebergs because only the tip of a large tumor may appear at the surface of the skin. The danger of such skin tumors is that the underlying portion may invade neighboring soft tissues or bones around the ears or eyes.

Treatment of a basal cell epithelioma usually requires surgical removal of the tumor or the use of radiation or chemical therapy to slowly destroy the growth.

blastomycosis A type of fungus infection marked by the appearance of a *chancre*like lesion on the skin. The appearance of a lesion is followed by enlargement of the lymph nodes in the area and a general feeling of being mildly sick. A blastomycosis lesion may gradually enlarge, discharge pus, and leave a thick scar if untreated. Treatment usually requires hospitalization while powerful drugs are administered intravenously. The human body does not develop an immunity to the fungus infection, which usually continues to spread across the skin until it is destroyed.

blister A collection of fluid under the skin that results from irritation of the skin tissues. A burn, irritating chemical, or pressure are among the causes. The fluid in a common water blister is lymph that has leaked from the injured cells. When blood vessels beneath the skin are broken, the fluid may be a mixture of lymph and blood.

The skin over a blister should not be broken unless pressure from the blister produces severe pain. If unbroken, the blister can be covered with a mild antiseptic and protective dressing. Once the skin is broken, the injury should be treated as a wound.

candidiasis A disease, also known as *moniliasis,* caused by a yeastlike fungus that grows in moist, warm areas of the body. It frequently affects the skin around the margins of the fingernails and can cause a deformed appearance in the nail plate.

carbuncle A bacterial infection involving the hair follicles. The infection usually occurs deep in the skin tissues, and a number of adjacent hair follicles can be affected. Carbuncles are most likely to occur on the back of the neck, and they can be very painful. Treatment usually consists of antibiotics and, when necessary, surgical incision to drain the lesion.

cellulitis An acute inflammation of the subcutaneous tissues of the skin, usually caused by streptococcus or staphyococcus types of bacteria. The surface of the skin appears to be discolored by a dusky red or purple area that is tender. The site of the infection usually feels warmer than surrounding skin regions. Cellulitis generally is treated by the application of antibiotics.

Erysipelas is a form of cellulitis. Another variation of the disease is caused by a bacterium called *Hemophilus influenzae;* it affects mainly infants and young children, and usually requires hospitalization for effective treatment by antibiotics.

chancre A skin lesion that usually appears as an eroded papule, or sore that originally was raised above the skin surface. The border of a chancre frequently is raised and firm. The chancre generally is painless, but lymph glands in the area may be enlarged and hard. A chancre usually is associated with a syphilis infection and frequently is found in the genital area. However, it also can occur anywhere the disease organism can find a tiny break in the skin surface, and it may be found on the face or fingers.

A venereal chancre usually will heal completely in four to six weeks, even without treatment. However, disappearance of the lesion can be misleading because the disease organism, a spirochete, merely has spread beneath the surface of the skin to attack more vital organs. Treatment usually consists of injections of large doses of penicillin; other antibiotics are employed for patients who are allergic to penicillin.

chancroid A lesion similar to a chancre but usually more inflamed and painful. Several chancroid sores may occur in the same area, usually in the genital region, and like the venereal chancre they are usually associated with sexual contact with an infected person. A chancroid may appear within three to five days after exposure. A venereal chancroid is caused by an organism called *Haemophilus ducreyi*, and treatment involves application of sulfa drugs or antibiotics. A chancroid is not the same as a chancre, but it is not unusual for a person to be infected by the two organisms, which produce the different types of skin lesions at the same time.

chicken pox A viral childhood disease, also known as *varicella*, that occurs rarely in adults. It produces distinct skin markings about two weeks after exposure to an infected person. The skin signs include tiny red patches, about the size of a pinhead, which appear on the trunk and soon spread to the face and sometimes the hands and feet. Blisters of clear fluid then appear in the tiny sores. The clear fluid next becomes yellowish, and the skin lesions finally become covered with a brown crust which gradually flakes off as healing progresses. The disease generally is mild, but it can become complicated by secondary infections due to picking of the crusts or scratching of the skin lesions.

chigger bites A disorder caused by the larvae of chigger mites burrowing into the skin. The mites normally live in grass, shrubs, or grain stems and attach themselves to humans who enter their domain for picnicking, golfing, hunting, or crop harvesting. After finding a host, the larvae usually move over the skin until they are stopped by the pressure of a belt or other tightly fitted item of clothing. There they burrow into the skin until they find a capillary and gorge themselves on blood. The larvae eventually fall off, but while burrowing and feeding they cause a severe itching sensation and may raise nodules on the skin surface. The itching can continue for days or weeks after the mites have dropped off the body. Occasionally, bits of insect bodies remain in the skin, a factor that extends the period of irritation.

Chigger infestation can be controlled somewhat by wearing clothing that fits tightly at the wrists, ankles, and neckline, and by applying an insect repellent around the wrists and ankles. Sulfur-containing repellents reportedly are most effective. After contact with chigger larvae, wash the skin carefully with soap and lather, and do not rinse the lather off for at least ten minutes. After bathing the skin, apply an anti-itching preparation. Persons who are particularly sensitive to chigger bites and are required to work in areas infested by the mites can sometimes obtain protection by sensitization injections prepared from bodies of the insects.

chilblains A kind of skin inflammation caused by exposure to cold. The affected skin areas, usually on the feet, hands, ears, and nose, develop a burning and itching sensation. The skin becomes mottled, swollen, and dark red. The cause apparently is due to poor circulation of the blood near the skin, a somewhat natural reaction of the temperature-regulating center of the body to extreme cold.

Preventive measures include use of warm protective clothing during winter months, avoiding prolonged exposure to cold or chilling environments outside and inside, and efforts to improve circulation of blood in the extremities by massage and exercise. Inflamed skin areas should be treated with tincture of iodine or zinc oxide.

cold sore Also known as fever blister or *herpes simplex*, a cold sore is a sore or blister caused by the herpes simplex virus. On close examination the sore usually appears as a cluster of tiny blisters or painful swellings on the skin of a mucous membrane area, such as the lips. The sores also may infect genital areas or the outer tissues of the eyes. The watery blisters generally rupture after a few days and are replaced by a crust as the lesion heals.

There is no simple way to prevent outbreaks of cold sores. They usually are associated with severe colds, but other causes can be exposure to sunlight, emotional upsets, and allergies. A number of nonprescription medications, some of which contain zinc oxide or calamine lotion, are available to relieve the symptoms of cold sores.

contact dermatitis A type of skin inflammation that follows exposure to an irritating substance. If the skin has acquired a sensitivity to a particular substance by repeated exposure over a prolonged period of time, a severe case of contact dermatitis can be produced by a very small concentration of the offending substance. Contact dermatitis usually is marked by redness, an itching sensation, scaling of the skin, and in severe cases by eruptions of fluid-filled vesicles on the skin surface. Exposed skin areas, such as the face and hands, are the most common sites of contact dermatitis. However, many cases of dermatitis are caused by sensitivity to dyes and materials used in the manufacture of shoes, socks, and underwear that therefore affect skin areas not usually exposed to the environment.

Sources of substances causing contact dermatitis include plants, among them chrysanthemums as well as poison ivy; fruits and vegetables, from oranges to onions; evergreen trees; kerosene and turpentine; drugs and detergents; numerous household products such as waxes and polishes, hair sprays, dyes, tonics, deodorants, and antiperspirants. It may be difficult to pinpoint the exact substance or source of a substance producing an individual contact dermatitis reaction because the signs and symptoms may not appear for many hours after exposure. Some allergic reactions do not appear until several days after exposure. One kind of contact dermatitis involves a substance contained in an antiseptic soap, but the effects do not occur until after the skin washed with the soap is exposed to sunlight or ultraviolet light.

Except for avoiding a substance that causes contact dermatitis, there is little that can be done to relieve the problem. Cold, wet compresses, soaking in salt water, and certain creams and lotions containing calamine may of-fer temporary relief. In severe cases, a doctor may prescribe the use of steroid hormones and medications to control secondary infections.

corns Cone-shaped growths of the horny layer of the epidermis usually found on the toes or other areas where the skin is subjected to repeated friction and pressure. Hard corns occur on surface areas and usually have rounded, burnished tops as a result of rubbing against an external surface such as a shoe. Soft corns usually occur between the toes and are moist and grayish in appearance. Corns develop as a natural epidermal reaction intended to protect more delicate tissues beneath the skin surface; the skin generally is thickest over areas that get the most "wear" in contact with the environment. A corn is simply an abnormally thick layer of epidermis and is usually associated with the wearing of poorly fitted shoes.

Corns usually can be removed with ointments or other medications that help dissolve the mass of horny tissue. Because of the danger of infection, extreme caution should be used in trimming or removing corns. In a complicated case, corn removal should be handled by an orthopedic surgeon or a podiatrist.

creeping eruption A name applied to a skin disorder caused by the burrowing of a parasite such as the hookworm. A small papule or blister-like eruption appears on the skin where the larvae enter the body. The point of entry usually is on the buttocks, the feet, or hands, where the body has been in contact with an infested patch of ground such as a beach or children's sandpile. As the larvae burrow through the skin they leave a thin, red, raised line that wanders along the surface. The line can advance by as much as an inch a day, producing inflammation and itching. The disorder may become complicated by secondary infections and eruptions of the skin.

Despite the distinctive signs of larvae activity, doctors sometimes have difficulty in tracking the culprit, especially after it has been active for some time. It may not be in the area of inflammation and may not even be at the end of a burrow where it could be destroyed by cryosurgery, that is, through the application of dry ice or liquid nitrogen. An alternative therapeutic measure is the application of a drug called thiabendazole.

depigmenting agents Chemicals that inhibit the formation of melanin pigment in the skin cells. An example is monobenzyl ether hydroquinone, which can be used for cosmetic purposes to lighten skin areas that are overly enriched with melanin. Certain chemicals used in industry have a similar effect, causing accidental loss of pigmentation.

dermatitis An inflammation of the skin. It may be marked by redness, itching, the formation of small blisters called vesicles, oozing or discharge of fluids at the skin surface, crusting and scaling, or a combination of these effects. Dermatitis may be acute, as in the effects of close contact with poison ivy, or chronic, as in the condition commonly called *eczema*. See also *nummular dermatitis; pityriasis; schistosomal dermatitis; seborrheic dermatitis; stasis dermatitis.*

dermatosis Any disease of the skin.

DLE (discoid lupus erythematosus) A disease marked by scaling eruptions of the skin of the face, scalp, ears, chest, and arms. The condition may begin as a small red patch of skin following a minor injury to the area or a sunburn. The abnormal red skin patch, a disc of erythematous skin as the name of the ailment suggests, may gradually spread along a border of scaling skin cells. The person affected by the disease may appear to be in normal health except for the highly pigmented and scarring skin tissue. However, laboratory tests frequently indicate a variety of abnormal results, including the presence of a blood factor found in cases of arthritis.

Therapy may include the use of antimalarial

drugs and steroid hormones. When exposure to sunlight appears to aggravate the condition, treatment usually involves the application of sunscreens on the skin plus the use of clothing that protects exposed skin areas. Cosmetics are available to mask disfiguring scars caused by the disorder, and wigs not only cover *alopecia* (hair loss) but protect the scalp from excessive sunlight.

ecthyma An ulcer or skin erosion resulting from the highly contagious children's disease, *impetigo*. The skin surrounding the ulcer may be inflamed. Treatment is by application of antibiotic ointments or antibiotics administered by mouth or injection in order to approach the problem from inside the skin surface.

eczema A chronic form of dermatitis. See *atopic dermatitis.*

epithelioma See *basal cell epithelioma.*

erysipelas A form of bacterial *cellulitis*, involving an inflammation of the subcutaneous tissues. This painful disease produces a red, patchy inflammation, usually on the face, and causes fever, headache, and vomiting in the patient. Erysipelas is caused by a form of streptococcus bacteria and is treatable with penicillin or other kinds of antibiotics.

erysipeloid An erysipelas type of bacterial skin inflammation observed on the hands of people who work with fresh meat and fish. A form of *contact dermatitis.*

erythema A term used to describe a variety of disorders marked by a vivid red discoloration of the skin surface, due to dilation of the capillaries in the papillae of the dermis. In some cases the erythema may appear in uneven patches, as spots resembling bruises, or as nodules or papules. The erythema effect frequently is caused by a reaction to a drug or medicine, but it also can be precipitated by a viral or bacterial infection, or in older people by a malignant growth in a deep organ.

One variation, erythema nodosum, has been

associated with scarlet fever, tuberculosis, tonsilitis, and fungus infections. The redness is accompanied by chills, fever, and inflamed nodules. Tender painful lesions up to an inch or more in diameter may appear around the joints. Relief usually is provided by bed rest, analgesics, and treatment of the infection responsible for the erythema.

Another variation, erythema multiforme, also may appear as a reaction to a virus or bacteria. The lesions appear as expanding circles of redness which gradually clear in the center, after which new lesions form, creating a bull's-eye pattern. Erythema multiforme can represent a very severe illness; the mouth, eyes, anal-genital region, and vital internal organs may become involved if early medical treatment is not given. Untreated, the disorder can be fatal. A person showing signs of erythema multiforme may be hospitalized for therapy including steroid hormones, antibiotics, and other medications.

erythsama A superficial bacterial infection of the skin, usually occurring in tropical and subtropical climates. The brownish scaling patches sometimes appear to be a fungal infection. There is little or no inflammation associated with the infection, which responds easily to antibiotics.

exanthema A term referring to a skin eruption. The skin eruptions of measles and chicken pox are called exanthemas.

folliculitis An inflammation of the hair follicles. The inflammation may be due to an ingrown hair, without bacterial involvement, or the folliculitis may be caused by a bactcrial infection.

frostbite A term used to describe the effect of extreme cold on skin tissues. The skin may appear white and numb after exposure to cold temperatures, and after rewarming the skin usually will become red and feel uncomfortable. Rapid rewarming in bath water at a temperature of around 105 degrees Fahrenheit for 20 to 30 minutes is the recommended treatment for frostbite. Blistering or ulceration in the rewarmed skin areas may be a sign of tissue damage that requires professional medical attention to prevent gangrene.

fungal infections Inflammation of the horny layer of the skin by any of several kinds of microsocopic plants. The effects can range from slight scaling, breaks in the skin between the toes, or reddish discoloration to blisters and oozing eruptions of the skin. Examples include athlete's foot, *blastomycosis*, and *ringworm infection*.

furuncles Acute inflammation of hair follicles. The problem usually begins deeper in the skin layers than *folliculitis*. Furuncles frequently become boils, accompanied by pain and tenderness, and eventually erupting and draining. A common home remedy for furuncles is "hot packing" the boil with hot, wet compresses. However, if new furuncles appear nearby, professional medical attention may be required to control spreading bacterial infection.

German measles A viral infection marked by the appearance of round pink spots on the skin. The spots may be so closely packed that they appear like a generalized *erythema*. The spots first appear on the head but spread over the trunk within the first day or so. The infection's effects last only a few days, and the disease generally causes no permanent harm to the patient. However, the virus can cause birth defects in the fetus of a pregnant woman who acquires the disease during the first three months of pregnancy. German measles also is known as *rubella*.

granuloma A term referring to a kind of skin inflammation. A common form is granuloma inguinale, marked by a series of ulcers that spread over the lower abdomen and buttocks, including the anal-genital region. The disease responds to antibiotic therapy. Other types of granulomas may appear on the face or the legs as a result of an infection apparently induced by shaving.

ground itch A common name for *hookworm disease.*

hemangioma A variation of the term *angioma.*

herpes simplex The technical name for the virus that causes *cold sores,* or fever blisters. One of the most infectious skin diseases affecting humans, the herpes lesions can occur on any skin surface of the body. A herpes infection in the area of the eye can have serious consequences because of possible damage to the sensitive membranes of the eyeball. A type of herpes simplex is associated with a vaginal infection linked to cancer of the cervix, but it is not the same strain of herpes that causes cold sores.

Spirits of camphor and other medications are available for relieving symptoms of herpes lesions, but no generally effective preventive measure has been found. Some physicians have tried repeated inoculations with small-pox vaccine as a therapy to reduce the recurrent appearance of herpes simplex blisters, but the results have been inconclusive.

herpes zoster This disease also is known as shingles, zoster, or varicella. It is caused by the same kind of virus that is responsible for chicken pox; some medical scientists believe the virus simply becomes dormant in one's body after a chicken pox infection, and reappears later in life in the form of shingles.

The skin signs of herpes zoster include the development of groups of small blisters with a base of reddened skin. The rash usually appears on one side of the trunk and forms a pattern which follows the route of a branch of the central nervous system. In older persons, particularly aging individuals with debilitating diseases, the inflammation of the herpes outbreak can be associated with severe pain. Whereas the symptoms of a herpes zoster attack in an otherwise normal child may last only a few days or weeks, the effects in an older person can continue for months or years.

When herpes zoster attacks an aging individual, the physician may find the sign of shingles a clue to a possible hidden case of *lymphoma,* a type of cancer, or some other serious disease. A zoster infection in the area of the eye can be especially hazardous because of the possibility of damage to sensitive tissues of the eyeball.

Treatment for infections of herpes zoster generally is limited to aspirin or other medications to relieve pain and fever, antihistamines to relieve the itching sensation of the skin eruptions, and application of calamine lotion to increase the rate of drying of the lesions. Local skin infections resulting from the lesions can be treated with hot saltwater compresses or antibiotic ointments. In more severe cases, the doctor may prescribe more potent pain killers and steroid hormones for relief of the neuralgia that may accompany shingles.

hirsutism A term meaning abnormally heavy or active hair growth, usually due to an alteration in function of the hair follicles. The opposite type of hair follicle malfunction, hereditary *alopecia,* is manifested by the failure to grow hair.

histiocytoma A small, hard, button-like lesion on the skin. The lesion, technically a tumor, frequently appears at the site of an earlier insect bite. A histiocytoma rarely becomes a malignant growth.

hives A rash of localized swellings on the skin, appearing usually as white or pink eruptions against a background of redness. The papules or lesions can be small or large. They may cover a small skin surface or an entire area of the body such as the face or trunk. The hives, also known by their medical name of *urticaria,* cause a pronounced itching sensation that may persist for a few hours or a few days. The typical outbreak of hives is more annoying than serious, but some individuals may experience dizziness, fainting, and a drop in blood pressure along with the skin eruptions. These are signs of anaphylactoid shock, a condition that requires immediate medical attention.

Hives can be triggered in various individuals

by certain medications and foods, extreme heat or cold, or even physical exercise. If the condition continues for more than a few days, a doctor should be consulted.

Chronic urticaria can be caused by the same agents that produce the acute hives described above. The problem of chronic hives sometimes can be solved by eliminating all nonessential medicines that may be used by the individual and eliminating in round-robin fashion the foods that could be the culprits. If the afflicted person can live on sweetened tea for two days, the hives should subside if a regularly eaten food is involved. Then food items in the usual diet can be added one at a time to determine if the hives recur. If a food or medicine does not appear to be a cause, a doctor may suggest tests for possible parasites in the digestive tract or factors in the home or working environment. Treatment by antihistamines is frequently helpful.

hookworm disease An ailment, sometimes known as ground itch, caused by larvae that burrow through the skin to reach the bloodstream of humans and other animals. The larvae most often work through the skin of the foot, producing a raised lesion or eruption at the point of entry. The lesion may be accompanied by a rash and swelling of the ankle as the hookworm larvae work their way through the skin. Once in the bloodstream, the larvae travel through the body to reach the intestinal tract. They deposit eggs in feces which may reach the soil and hatch into another generation of hookworm larvae.

If untreated, a hookworm infestation of the body can be quite damaging to the digestive tract and other internal organs, and it can cause death. The hookworm larvae can be removed from the body by administering certain potent medications, such as tetrachlorethylene. But preventive measures are a better alternative. They include wearing shoes in tropical and subtropical regions where the hookworm thrives, and making sure that feces are deposited in a place other than the surface of the

soil. For reasons known only to nature, the hookworm larvae seem unable to move more than about 12 inches vertically and thus can be trapped in deep latrines.

hyperpigmentation A skin condition marked by excess pigmentation. The cause can be as varied as the use of antimalarial drugs, physical injury, the jaundice of liver disease, oral contraceptive pills, and pregnancy. These can produce a chloasmic pigmentation, or irregularly sized, light-brown patches, on the face.

icthyosis A disorder sometimes called "fish skin" disease because of a buildup of dry, scaly skin cells. The condition is attributed to the failure of the horny layer of skin to shed the outer dead cells with the result that the horny layer simply thickens. Icthyosis usually is hereditary and may appear during infancy, but it does not affect the baby's health. The disease occurs in several forms and may end spontaneously or continue through the life of the individual. Patients do not experience an itching sensation because of the skin condition. Treatment consists of warm baths to help soften the skin and soak off the excess horny layer cells, and the use of creams or oils to counteract the drying effect of the disorder.

impetigo A highly contagious skin infection that usually is caused by a streptococcus bacteria, which may later damage the kidneys. Infants and young children are likely targets of the disease, although older individuals also can be infected. The skin becomes covered in affected areas by raised vesicles of fluid, or pus, which may last only briefly and are followed by formation of a crust. In severe cases there may be ulceration of the skin. Treatment requires the use of antibiotics. Care must be taken to insure that secondary infections do not complicate the problem.

insect bites Most insect bites, or stings, produce some degree of local swelling, redness, pain, and itching at the site. The signs and symptoms of insect bites or stings will vary according to the sensitivity of the individual and the species of insect responsible for the attack. The bite of a millipede, for example, is characterized in most cases by an intense burning and itching sensation lasting from one hour to perhaps as long as 24 hours. Stings by hymenoptera—bees, wasps, yellow jackets—may result in a painful swelling and in some instances damage to vital organ systems. The sting victim might experience difficult breathing, a drop in blood pressure, and general collapse, all signs of an extremely serious condition known as anaphylactic shock.

First aid for victims of insect stings should be directed toward protecting the victim's general physical condition if there are signs or symptoms of fainting, shock, abdominal pains, breathing difficulty, or general swelling of the observable body tissues. In such cases the most important thing that can be done is to rush the individual to the nearest hospital emergency room or doctor's office. Time is very important in protecting an insect sting victim from anaphylactic shock, a condition that may be a possibly fatal allergic reaction to insect venom.

Emergency treatment for less severe reactions to insect stings includes, in the case of honey bee stings, removal of the stinger and attached sac of venom, which usually is left behind in the wound. The stinger and venom sac should be carefully pried loose with a sharp, pointed knife blade, avoiding any pressure on the sac that could squeeze more venom into the sting wound. The venom of hymenoptera is similar to that of certain poisonous snakes. Any bits of insect bodies, other than a honeybee stinger, left in the skin surface usually can be removed with adhesive cellophane tape.

Minor bites and stings generally can be controlled by application of ice, which helps reduce the chemical activity of the venom and retards its rate of absorption by the body tissues. Care should be exercised in the use of ice; too much cold on the bite could result in frostbite. Discomfort caused by minor bites and stings can be relieved by the use of antihistamines and aspirin. Over-the-counter medications and prescription drugs intended for insect stings and bites are available.

People who are sensitive to insect venom usually are advised to carry antihistamines and epinephrine preparations that can be used quickly after an insect sting. Joggers, hikers, picnickers, and others likely to encounter insects should be cautious about wearing brightly colored garments or perfumes, scented hair sprays, or deodorants that might attract these nearsighted stinging insects.

intertrigo A medical term used to indicate the inflammation of skin surfaces produced by chafing. In addition to the friction of opposing skin surfaces rubbing against each other, the warmth of the body and presence of moisture can contribute to the redness, abrasion, and maceration of intertrigo. Obesity and hot, humid weather generally aggravate the condition. Symptoms include burning and itching. If early treatment is not started, the disorder can become complicated by fungal or bacterial infection. Intertrigo can develop on almost any skin area that rubs against another skin surface such as the toes, the genital region, the armpits, etc.

Compresses, dusting powders, and, in serious cases, steroid hormones are used to treat this condition. Intertrigo sometimes can be prevented by wearing loose clothing and by using dusting powders on surfaces of skin that tend to rub together.

itching The sensation, known by the medical term pruritus, is caused by irritating stimuli on the skin that apparently affect nerve endings located in the papillae under the epidermis. Just as some individuals have a greater tolerance for pain than others, some people seem able to tolerate skin irritations that would trigger in other persons the urge to scratch the irritated skin area. Severe itching sensations graduate into a type of burning pain, demonstrating a relationship between pain and itching. There also is ample evidence that pain killers will stop itching sensations.

Itching may be caused by drug or food allergies, in addition to irritating agents on the skin surface. Itching also may be the first sign of a number of physical changes and illnesses, ranging from pregnancy and menopause to diabetes, Hodgkin's disease, ailments of the liver or kidneys, and certain kinds of cancer.

Treatments for itching are almost as varied as the causes, and may include soaking the skin in warm, wet starch or oatmeal, taking antihistamine tablets, applying preparations that contain menthol and camphor, and the administration of steroid hormones or other prescription drugs.

jaundice A discoloration or *hyperpigmentation* of the skin due to an accumulation of bile pigments in the bloodstream. The bile pigment produces a yellow coloration to the skin and to the normally white areas of the eyes, with the depth of color depending upon the concentration of bile pigments in the blood. The yellowish skin tint of jaundice may first be noticed when the skin is exposed to sunlight; it is not as easily visible in artificial light. The bile pigment, known by the medical name of bilirubin, is a by-product of the breakdown of old red blood cells. It ordinarily goes through physiological processes ending in excretion, but it tends to accumulate in the blood as a result of liver ailments such as hepatitis and of gallstones. To eliminate the problem of jaundiced skin, the doctor must treat the cause, which usually involves the liver and/or gallbladder.

jellyfish stings Stings produced by contact with the tentacles of saltwater marine animals, such as the Portuguese man-of-war, can result in severe pain and itching of the affected skin area. Severe reactions similar to those associated with wasp and bee stings can occur in persons sensitive to jellyfish toxin. The Portuguese man-of-war usually inhabits ocean waters of tropical and subtropical climates, such as Florida coastal waters, but it may be carried onto beaches or beyond its normal home area by storms or swift sea currents.

Jellyfish stings should be washed with generous amounts of fresh water, if available, or salt water if fresh water is not available. The stingers, called nematocysts, left in the skin by a jellyfish tentacle should be carefully removed. Antihistamines and analgesics should help relieve the symptoms. If a serious reaction threatens, a doctor should be consulted.

jockstrap itch An inflammation affecting the skin areas in the anal-genital region and including the inner thigh surfaces. Only one side of the body is affected in most cases, but both sides can become involved. The original fungal infection may be complicated by the invasion of bacteria, yeast, or other irritants. The medical term for jockstrap itch is tinea.

Treatment usually includes topical antifungal medicine or griseofulvin. Doctors frequently recommend that jockstrap itch patients avoid wearing tight clothing and that affected areas be bathed carefully, with all the soap rinsed away and the skin dried completely.

junction nevus A medical term sometimes used to identify a pigmented mole. The growth usually is widely rooted in the corium, or dermis, layer of the skin and is often associated with hair follicles. Nevi, the plural of nevus, are of some concern to doctors because they may suddenly develop into malignant tumors.

keloid A common type of nonmalignant skin tumor that may be an overgrowth of a scar. A typical keloid is elevated above the surrounding skin surface, is reddish in coloration, and is firm and smooth. Keloids sometimes are mistaken for scar tissue, but scars normally flatten out as a lesion heals. A keloid may be accompanied by tenderness and an itching or burning sensation. Keloids cannot be surgically removed but large, unsightly ones may be shrunken by X-ray therapy.

keratin A tough protein substance manufactured by cells of the epidermis. The horny layer of the epidermis, as well as the hair and nails, contain a large proportion of keratin. The hard keratin of hair cells can be softened with water and certain chemicals so the hair may be reshaped, as when a woman's hair is set in a new coiffure by a beautician.

keratosis A type of lesion that involves a tumor of the skin. Keratoses most often appear in persons over the age of 40, although certain kinds may occur in childhood. One kind of keratosis, *seborrheic keratosis*, commonly occurs on the head or neck as a large drop of wax, becoming larger, darker, and more raised as time passes. The affected person eventually becomes concerned because the growth is a cosmetic problem, marring physical appearance, or because it may interfere with hair combing. Seborrheic keratosis generally poses no serious health threat and can be removed surgically under a local anesthetic.

Actinic keratoses are reddish, scaly lesions that rise above the skin surface with a gray horny top. They are commonly found on the skin of older persons who are frequently exposed to sunlight; many have dry, aging, wrinkled skin of the type sometimes described as "sailor's skin" or "farmer's skin." A similar type of keratosis is sometimes found on the lips of cigarette or pipe smokers, in which case the cause is irritation from the heat of burning tobacco. But sunlight also can be a factor. A keratosis of the lip requires surgical excision and biopsy because of the chance the growth may be malignant. Actinic keratoses on other body areas seldom become malignant and can be removed by application of chemotherapy.

larva migrans A medical term for the skin ailment more commonly known as *creeping eruption,* caused by a parasite carried in dog and cat feces.

LE (lupus erythematosus) An abbreviation for a group of diseases marked by red scaly patches on the skin. One form, *DLE (discoid lupus erythematosus),* seems to affect only the skin and responds well to treatment. A more serious form of the disease group, *SLE (systemic lupus erythematosus),* has similar skin effects, but the systemic form can also involve vital organ systems such as the blood or kidneys.

leishmaniasis A disease caused by a protozoa that enters the skin through the bite of a species of tropical fly. The bite may be marked by only a pigmented spot or in more serious cases by a skin ulcer sometimes called an Oriental sore. The ulcer may take from 2 to 12 months to heal and can leave a sunken scar. The disease can be acquired in warm climate areas of Europe and Asia as well as in Africa and Latin America.

leprosy Sometimes called Hansen's disease, leprosy is one of the oldest and most common chronic skin diseases in the world. It is a moderately infectious disease transmitted from one human to another. A bacteria is the disease agent. The first signs of the disease may be a reddening of skin areas, particularly on the legs, at the same time that a nasal obstruction, accompanied by nosebleeds, develops. Ulcers and tubercular nodules gradually appear on the skin and the mucous membranes. As the nervous system becomes involved, the patient usually feels a tingling sensation along with weakness and numbness.

Although the disease can be disabling, death rarely results directly from an infection of leprosy. While the disease usually is acquired in tropical or subtropical countries, the nearly 10 million known cases of leprosy have been found in such varied parts of the world as the United States, Russia, Korea, Japan, Romania, Portugal, and Spain.

lesion A rather well defined area of abnormal skin tissue caused by an injury or infection.

lichen planus A skin disease that usually involves the mucous membranes of the mouth as well as the skin surface. Signs of the disease begin with the appearance of shiny flat-topped eruptions along the wrists and arms. The eruptions may occur simultaneously on the mucous membranes, on the skin of the trunk, and on the genitals. The lesions usually itch and new lesions then develop along the scratch marks.

Treatment of lichen planus may include administration of steroid hormone drugs and exposure to warm sunlight. The lesions of the mucous membranes may require additional special therapy, and the person afflicted usually must avoid the use of tobacco and hot or irritating foods and beverages. The mouth lesions can persist for months or years, with the danger of eventually developing into a form of cancer.

lymphoma A form of malignant disease involving the lymphatic system of the body. Generally, lymphoma diseases do not involve the skin, but one type, known technically as a T-cell lymphoma, begins with skin disorders which may range from *dermatitis* to *alopecia,* or include tumors and ulcerations of the skin. Treatment usually is by radiation or chemotherapy.

macules A medical term used to indicate circumscribed color variations of the skin, such as red spots. Flat moles and freckles are other examples of macules on the skin.

measles A highly infectious viral disease marked by skin signs that include small bluish-white lesions called Koplik spots in the mouth. The Koplik spots eventually may appear to merge or run together. They are followed shortly by a rash of red pimples that begin around the hairline and then spread over the body. The skin develops a burning itch. As the rash and accompanying fever, nasal discharge, and other symptoms subside, the rash turns into brownish scales that are shed from the skin. See also *German measles.*

melanocytes Skin cells that produce the dark melanin pigment which gives skin and hair its coloration.

melanoma A type of tumor that may develop from a pigmented mole. A melanoma can become a serious malignancy of the sort that spreads to other parts of the body. Pigmented growths on the feet and other body areas where they are subject to rubbing or other irritating factors seem most likely to change from benign to malignant tumors.

melanosis A medical term used to describe abnormal skin coloration, which may be natural or due to a medical problem. The darkened skin that results from exposure to sunlight is a form of melanosis, and so is the appearance of dark skin on the face or around the nipples of a woman during pregnancy. Melanosis also may occur as an indication of Addison's disease or *pellagra.*

melasma A form of melanosis resulting in a skin coloration over a particular area of the body. It is usually due to the use of cosmetics or oral contraceptive pills or because of pregnancy.

miliaria A skin disorder involving obstruction of the sweat glands. One form, miliaria rubra, results in severe itching and the appearance of tiny red swellings about the sweat glands. The disorder appears particularly in a hot environment where release of perspiration from the blocked sweat duct would help relieve the heat effects. One method of treatment is to keep the patient in a cool room with low humidity. Miliaria rubra also is known by the common name of prickly heat.

Sometimes, as a result of severe dermatitis from a drug reaction, the sweat glands may become permanently damaged. Persons with permanently damaged sweat glands may have difficulty in tolerating sweat-producing conditions, such as physical exercise or living in a warm, humid climate. When sweat glands are blocked but functioning, the sweat usually is forced into tissues beneath the skin surface. The condition is relieved by a cool, dry environment. See illustration page 33.

mole The common name for a skin growth or tumor which usually is pigmented. Mole is a word derived from the old Anglo-Saxon language and means literally "a spot," which is how a mole may first appear on the skin. Some moles are present at birth. Others develop during childhood and disappear in late adult years. Some moles involve hair shafts but others may be hairless. A mole may develop in the nail matrix, causing a darkly pigmented section of a fingernail or toenail.

A mole generally is harmless, except for cosmetic aspects, but any change in a mole—such as sudden enlargement, a change in coloration in or around the base, loss of hair from the mole, or bleeding or ulceration—can be signs that the mole is evolving from a harmless colored skin growth into a dangerous cancer. Any sudden change in a mole's condition, therefore, should be checked by a doctor.

moniliasis A type of skin inflammation caused by a yeast-like fungus that is most likely to appear in warm, moist body areas. The organism responsible for moniliasis normally lives in the digestive tract of humans, but it may appear in such areas as the mouth or vagina after antibiotic therapy for other health problems. Moniliasis of the mouth of a child causes a disease condition known as thrush. A moniliasis inflammation of the hands may appear if the hands are frequently immersed in warm water. The condition is also known as *candidiasis*.

Therapy for moniliasis includes application of gentian violet, antibiotic creams and lotions, and, in some cases, steroid hormone medications.

morphea A skin disorder, also known as localized *scleroderma*, marked by the appearance of *plaques* of hardened dead skin cells. The plaques may form lines of white markings that persist for months or even years. The disease may appear after an injury and may or may not involve tissues beneath the skin. Steroid hormone injections are sometimes effective in relieving the condition.

mycosis fungoides A type of *lymphoma* tumor that first appears on the skin as reddish dry patches and may eventually spread to the lymphatic system and internal organs. The lesions may appear and disappear for no apparent reason, and might be mistaken for signs of *psoriasis*. When the disorder shows definite signs of being a lymphoma, treatment may include the use of steroid hormones, radiation, or cancer chemotherapy.

myxedema A thyroid gland disorder with signs and symptoms involving the skin, including loss of hair, sweat gland failure, and thickening of the skin about the nose.

nail bed A thin layer of tissue beneath the nail plate that contributes the pinkish coloration observed beneath the plate.

nail matrix A layer of cells at the root of a fingernail or toenail. The matrix generates the horny *keratin* substance which grows outward from the root as the nail plate.

nevus A medical term for an abnormal skin growth, usually applied to the pigmented lesion commonly called a *mole*.

nummular dermatitis A chronic, recurrent type of dermatitis that usually occurs in small circular patches on the trunk, arms, and legs. It may be marked by severe itching. The disease is most likely to afflict men in their middle years. It may be complicated by secondary infections due to bacteria.

Treatment for the nummular dermatitis condition may involve steroid hormone therapy, exposure of the affected skin areas to sunlight or ultraviolet lamp light, and antihistamines. Antibiotics may be prescribed for secondary infections.

otitis externa A medical term sometimes used to indicate a skin infection or inflammation that involves the outer surfaces of the ear.

oxyuriasis Pinworm infection that actually involves the gastrointestinal tract but frequently causes itching of the skin around the anus.

paddie foot A common term for a skin condition caused by prolonged immersion of the feet in water in a tropical region. The horny layer of epidermis becomes macerated and may slough off, exposing the inner layers of skin to infections of fungi and bacteria.

papule A small raised lesion on the skin. A *wart* is one example of a papule. Others are the skin eruptions associated with *psoriasis*.

patch test A test used by doctors to determine whether a person is sensitive to a particular substance. A patch of cloth or paper is impregnated with a small amount of the substance and placed next to the skin for a short period of time. If the skin under the test material becomes red and inflamed, the examining physician usually assumes that the patient is sensitive or allergic to the substance.

pediculosis A skin condition caused by lice, which infest body areas covered with hair and attach their eggs, or nits, firmly to the hair shafts. The nits frequently are the most visible clue to the presence of lice since the insects usually conceal themselves in the seams of clothing. Pediculosis is seldom encountered in areas where modern hygiene techniques are followed, but the lice can be acquired in places with poor sanitation. Lice are destroyed by careful application of lotions and creams. A common name for body lice is cooties.

pellagra A vitamin deficiency disease with signs and symptoms that involve the skin. The skin of pellagra sufferers can become thick and red, especially on the hands and arms, although the legs, trunk, and neck also may be involved. The skin may become cracked and acquire secondary infections. Since lack of niacin in the diet is responsible for pellagra, a diet rich in sources of niacin, part of the vitamin B complex, often is prescribed to correct the deficiency.

pemphigus A group of skin diseases which have in common the appearance of watery blisters. One form of the disease occurs among infants with *impetigo* or congenital syphilis. A type of pemphigus that occurs in adults can be very serious if not treated in the early stages. The skin and areas of mucous membrane erode or slough off under slight pressure such as rubbing the affected surface. The eroded skin becomes vulnerable to secondary infections. When the membranes of the mouth are affected, eating becomes difficult, and the patient may suffer from malnutrition in addition to the immediate effects of the disease. The condition usually responds well to therapy involving the use of steroid hormones.

pernio A medical term for *chilblains*.

photosensitivity A skin condition that causes severe reactions to sunlight or artificial ultraviolet light. Dark-skinnned, black-haired individuals generally are less sensitive to sunlight than blue-eyed blondes and redheads. However, skin color does not always protect against photoallergic effects that can be caused by sunlight or ultraviolet light on certain chemicals in cosmetics and medicines. Sulfa drugs, for example, may cause a photoallergic reaction in patients who use them; chemicals used in certain antiseptic soaps also have been known to cause photoallergic reactions when skin washed with the soaps was later exposed to sunlight. Persons who are photosensitive should wear protective clothing and use sunscreen creams or lotions on skin areas exposed to sunlight for prolonged periods.

pigment The natural human skin pigment is melanin, a black substance produced by cells called *melanocytes* located in the epidermis. People who are dark-skinned usually have the same number of melanocytes as fair-skinned individuals, but the melanocytes in the skins of darkly pigmented persons are larger and provide more protection against prolonged exposure to sunlight.

pilosebaceous A medical term meaning simply an oil gland that is associated with a hair follicle. The term is sometimes used to explain how certain substances can enter the body through the skin barrier. The answer is that they get beneath the epidermis by sneaking through the hair follicles and their attached sebaceous, or oil, glands.

pinworm A small worm that infests the digestive tract but can cause an itching sensation in the region of the anus. The medical term for pinworm infection is *oxyuriasis*.

pityriasis A form of dermatitis that usually involves the trunk of the body, although it may extend to the arms and legs. The eruptions, apparently caused by a viral infection, begin as a single oval papule with a salmon-colored center and scaly border. The original lesion, sometimes called a mother plaque, is followed within a week or two by numerous small papules of the same kind. The disease requires no special treatment in most cases since it runs its course over a period of a month or two. Symptoms are usually mild except for effects of inflammation and itching. Steroid hormones may be administered for severe cases, and recovery seems to be aided by exposure of the lesions to sunlight.

plantar warts Skin growths usually found on the sole or heel of the foot. The warts are painful because of pressure that results from walking. Plantar warts usually do not appear as raised lesions, and they are likely to be surrounded by callus, thick layers of horny epidermal skin cells.

Plantar warts can be removed by surgical excision or the application of corrosive medications that dissolve the growths. Pain from the warts can be relieved by wearing pads that prevent undue pressure on the affected areas. Plantar warts are contagious and are apparently spread by a virus; family members, military personnel, and others who share communal living facilities risk acquiring plantar warts from a member of the group who suffers from the viral infection.

plaques Skin lesions that form patches on the surface of the epidermis, usually after several smaller eruptions in the same area have merged. Plaques may cover an area of an inch or more in diameter and usually are slightly raised and scaly.

poison ivy reaction A kind of contact *dermatitis* caused by exposure to a substance, urushiol, present in the leaves and other parts of poison ivy, poison oak, and poison sumac. The chemical produced by the plants binds with skin cells to produce a rash of watery blisters, accompanied by a burning, itching sensation. The skin effects may not appear immediately and sometimes are delayed for up to a week after contact. Direct contact with plant surfaces is not needed to acquire the poison ivy reaction; humans can develop the symptoms by petting animals that have rubbed against leaves of the plants or by inhaling smoke from burning poison ivy or poison oak plants.

One can become sensitive by repeated exposure to the chemical produced by this family of plants so that the symptoms become increasingly severe with each contact.

The best treatment, of course, is to avoid the plant materials or wear protective clothing when around poison oak, poison ivy, or poison sumac. In case of accidental contact with poison ivy or similar plants, the skin surfaces should be washed immediately with a strong soap and water to remove the plant resin causing the reaction. The plant substance also can be neutralized with a mixture of two percent ferric chloride in alcohol. If any of the plant materials have been eaten, as happens occasionally by children "playing house," the emergency therapy should be the same as if a poison had been ingested: induce vomiting and dilute the stomach contents with salt water, milk, or another neutralizing fluid.

pompholyx A medical term of Greek origin meaning bubbles, used to describe the watery blisters that appear on the skin and usually only on the hands. The blisters resemble those of poison ivy reaction, but there may be little or no irritation when the eruptions appear. The attacks usually are associated with excessive sweating of the palms during warm, humid weather or periods of nervous tension. The eruptions are self-limiting and may last for several weeks. Pompholyx eruptions may occur on the fingers as well as the hands; they sometimes appear on the feet as well.

pruritis A Latin word that means simply an *itching* effect, which may be due to a variety of causes ranging from dermatitis, a worm infestation, or a systemic disease such as diabetes mellitus.

psoriasis A rather common skin disease that may appear at any time of life but is most common among adults. It usually begins around the elbows and knees, the scalp and ears, or the trunk, and it spreads to other body surfaces. The first eruptions may appear as tiny red spots which merge to form a patch of reddish skin with a distinctive margin that separates the coloration from the normal skin surrounding it. When the eruptions heal they tend to leave reddish or brownish red stains on the skin. In one form, psoriasis results in thick silver-white skin scales; when the scales are dislodged from the skin, tiny bleeding points appear where the scales were. When psoriasis invades the skin of the palms or soles, the disease causes deep fissures that can disable the patient. The nails also may become involved in the disease. In some cases the patient experiences symptoms of rheumatoid arthritis with effects on the joints that increase or subside according to the course of the skin ailment.

A wide range of therapies are available for the treatment of psoriasis, which is fortunate since no general remedy seems to be equally effective for all patients. Some cases of psoriasis, for example, improve with exposure to sunlight, while other cases are aggravated by sunbathing. Daily baths and shampoos with special bath oils and soaps are helpful in removing scales. White petrolatum or other emollients or creams applied to the affected areas may relieve itching. Other therapies include coal tar applications, steroid hormones, methotrexate, and a psoralen compound used in conjunction with exposure to long-wave ultraviolet light.

purpura A disease caused by the escape of red blood cells from the capillaries that produces a skin effect resembling a bruise. In some cases the skin discoloration may be a stippled brownish-red. Purpura frequently is a sign of a blood system disorder or, when accompanied by fever, an indication that the individual has an acute infection such as Rocky Mountain spotted fever.

pustule A small swelling on the skin that contains pus. See illustration page 26.

pyoderma An inflammation of the subcutaneous tissues of the skin. The condition frequently results from bacterial invasion of a skin area

that originally was affected by a form of dermatitis.

Raynaud's disease A circulatory ailment involving the arteries of the fingers or toes. The skin may turn white or bluish because of the impaired circulation, and the fingers or toes become numb. The effect usually is triggered by exposure to cold or by tobacco smoking, or both. Treatment is by drug therapy.

ringworm infection A fungal infection of the skin marked by a dull red inflammation with dry scaling. The fungus may affect only one hand or one foot at first, but it soon spreads to the thighs, lower trunk, or other body areas if not controlled properly in the early stages. Poor hygiene habits, warm temperatures, and high humidity encourage spread of the fungus. Ringworm gets its name from the resulting pattern of ring-shaped lesions. Ringworm infections of the hands and feet may easily spread to the nails, causing thick, distorted nail plates.

Effective control of ringworm is possible with the use of griseofulvin. Dusting powders and certain creams and ointments are available for preventing recurrence of ringworm. Whitfield's ointment is a commonly available remedy for ringworm.

rosacea A skin disorder, sometimes identified as *acne rosacea*, marked by flushing and occasionally the appearance of *pustules* and thickened red skin about the nose, forehead, and cheeks. Since the flareups of redness can be triggered by the use of alcoholic beverages, the condition sometimes is called by the common name of whiskey nose.

roseola An infectious disease affecting small children, usually characterized by eruptions on the skin of small red spots similar to those associated with *measles*. The skin eruptions are accompanied by fever, although the fever symptoms usually subside as the eruptions develop. The skin eruptions generally appear on the trunk of the body and last only a few days. Although sometimes confused with measles, roseola is not accompanied by the bluish-white Koplik spots in the mouth that distinguish a measles infection.

rubella Another name for *German measles*. Like *roseola*, the disease is marked by the appearance of small red spots on the trunk and the absence of Koplik spots. However, the reddish macules usually begin on the head and spread over the trunk, whereas roseola spots rarely appear on the head or the extremities.

rubeola The medical name for *measles*. Rubeola measles usually appear first on the forehead and behind the ears, then spread over the face, trunk, arms, and legs. The disease also is marked by fever, running nose, Koplik spots inside the mouth, and eye ailments that may include conjunctivitis and photophobia, or extreme sensitivity to light.

sarcoidosis A disease that can involve the lungs, heart, or nervous system with manifestations that include skin nodules and inflammation. The disfiguring skin lesions associated with the disease are sometimes identified as sarcoids. The skin lesions usually subside within a couple of weeks after therapy for the underlying infection has begun. Steroid hormones generally are used to control the effects of sarcoidosis.

scab A plug of dried clotted blood and cellular debris of the skin that fills the opening of a wound at the start of the healing of an injury that involves a break in the skin. The lower or deeper portion of the clotted blood and cell debris is absorbed by the tissues while new skin layers and scar tissue bridge the gap across the wound. After the scar matures, the scab is sloughed off.

scabies A highly contagious parasitic skin disease caused by a tiny insect sometimes called an itchmite. The itchmite, more properly identified as *Sarcoptes scabiei*, burrows under the skin and lays its eggs. The eggs hatch into larvae that continue the reproductive cycle under the skin until they are destroyed. The human host suffers from severe itching, particularly during the night, and eventually develops secondary infections from scratching. Signs of scabies are short, straight burrow marks in the skin near areas of inflammation; the marks usually occur around the wrists, fingers, or elbows, but also may be found in such places as the buttocks or genitals, or the breasts of women. The scabies mites may be removed by applying medications available with a doctor's prescription.

scar A skin covering of connective tissue fibers produced by the skin cells to protect a healing wound. The connective tissue fibers usually are produced randomly at first under the scab, but the scar fibers become organized in a pattern something like a woven fabric as the scar matures. Layers of epidermis and dermis eventually spread across the wound beneath the scar to complete the healing process.

scarlet fever An infectious disease with symptoms of nausea, high fever, sore throat, headache, and a rash of tiny, bright red spots on the skin. Children under the age of 12 are most likely to develop the bacterial infection, which also goes by the name of scarlatina. The scarlet rash frequently begins around the neck or chest, then spreads over most of the rest of the body. The rash lasts only a few days and is followed more than a week later by scaling and peeling of the skin. While complications are infrequent, the patient must be guarded against damage to the heart, kidneys, and other organs.

Treatment is based mainly on the use of antibiotics and careful nursing for the patient, who usually is required to remain in bed for three weeks or longer.

schistosomal dermatitis A skin rash acquired by bathing in lakes or ponds contaminated with the species of schistosomal flukes that infect some animals and birds. A brief itching sensation may be experienced as the flukes burrow into the skin. About 12 hours later, severely itching lesions appear on the affected skin area; the lesions are usually surrounded by a small region of inflammation. Watery blisters appear for several days, then disappear except for small spots marking the sites of eruption.

Schistosomal dermatitis, also known as swimmer's itch, can be prevented by avoiding shallow waters in which the schistosomes are more likely to thrive and by drying the skin immediately after leaving the water. Application of anti-itching medications helps to relieve symptoms of the infestation.

scleroderma Another term for *morphea*, a disease marked by the appearance of plaques of hardened skin.

scurvy A vitamin deficiency disease with symptoms that include bleeding beneath the skin. The disorder, caused by a lack of vitamin C in the diet, also is marked by bleeding, spongy gums and a feeling of extreme weakness. Loss of blood under the skin presents an appearance like that of *purpura*.

seawater itch A skin eruption similar in some respects to swimmer's itch, or *schistosomal dermatitis*, except that the effect occurs after swimming in salt water whereas the schistosomal disorder affects only fresh water swimmers. Seawater itch appears as hives or insect bites on skin areas usually covered by a swim suit rather than on exposed skin. Treatment consists simply of applying medications to relieve the itching sensation.

seborrheic dermatitis A disorder characterized by a reddish scaling eruption which may involve the scalp, the ears, the armpits, and the skin folds of the genital region. A mild form of the disorder is ordinary dandruff. In severe cases, however, there can be fissuring of the skin and secondary infections.

A number of nonprescription medications are available for relieving the symptoms of seborrheic dermatitis; creams and shampoos to treat the condition frequently contain sulfur and salicylic acid. For serious cases a doctor may prescribe a steroid hormone preparation.

Special medications are needed also for secondary infections and for protecting fissured skin areas.

seborrheic keratosis A common form of noncancerous skin tumor that usually appears on the head, neck, or trunk of the body. A seborrheic keratosis growth can begin as a waxy white plaque, but it tends to become larger and darker over a period of months or years. The color of established growths of this type can range from yellow to black. Except when they present cosmetic problems, such as developing on the face, or become raised far enough above the skin surface to become irritated from friction, seborrheic keratoses present no serious problems. They can be removed surgically but will leave small scars.

shingles A common term for *herpes zoster*.

SLE (systemic lupus erythematosus) A serious disease that may affect the circulatory system, the kidneys, or other organs of the body while at the same time causing a rather distinctive skin rash in most cases. The skin symptoms, which tend to indicate the seriousness of the disease, may range from a red to a dusky brown coloration, sometimes producing a "butterfly" image on the face, with one "wing" on either side of the nose. During periods of severe attacks, the skin may develop watery blisters or purpuralike bleeding, and small hemorrhages may occur under the nails, with ulceration of the fingers. SLE's skin symptoms are easily aggravated by exposure to sunlight and certain drug reactions. Pregnancy can result in exacerbation of the symptoms.

Treatment for SLE includes bed rest, protection from direct sunlight, analgesics to control arthritic symptoms, antimalarial drugs, and steroid hormones.

smallpox A once common but now rare viral disease with skin effects that include blisters, pustules that rupture easily, and yellowish-brown scabs that fall off over an extended shedding period. Smallpox, or *variola*, can be highly contagious since the virus causing the disease is present in the nose and throat of patients, in the blisters and scabs that form on the skin, and in bodily excretions.

The onset of the disease is marked by high fever, nausea, headaches, chills, and muscle pains. The skin signs do not appear for three or four days and then only as small red pimples on the face and wrists. However, the pimples quickly spread over other body areas, become blisters filled with pus, and eventually turn into a dark, dry crust that falls off. Pitted scars, called pockmarks, identify the points on the skin surface where the blisters first appeared. The patient usually must spend at least one month in confinement while the disease runs its course; the time span from pimples to pockmarks is at least four weeks.

Complications can include bronchopneumonia and damage to the eyes and ears. Vaccination that protects against smallpox has been available since the 18th century, which is why the disease is now rare. Vaccination administered even after the start of the disease can help control some effects of the infection.

sporotrichosis A fungal disease that tends to affect farmers and other outdoor workers who contract the infection after an injury that breaks the skin. A chancre-like sore develops at the point of injury, and sometimes nodules appear in a line along a branch of the lymphatic system draining the infection site. The infection usually is treated with a potassium iodide medication.

stasis dermatitis A skin disorder characterized by red, scaling, itching skin on the inner surfaces of the lower portion of the legs. Stasis dermatitis reflects the health condition of the circulatory system. The cause is a failure of the leg veins to function normally, and the skin problem tends to occur in individuals with thrombophlebitis or varicose veins. After the skin disorder subsides, the circulatory problem is treated by surgery, support hose, or other methods. In the meantime, the skin areas are quite sensitive to *contact dermatitis* and drug reactions.

steroid acne An acnelike rash that appears on the skin as a drug reaction to steroid hormones. Similar skin eruptions are produced in various individuals by a wide assortment of medications ranging from antibiotics to aspirin. See also *acne*.

synovial cyst A blister filled with fluid originally secreted from a joint lining, such as the lining of a finger joint. The fluid pushes to the skin surface and fills a sac, which is the cyst.

syphilis A venereal disease caused by a microscopic organism called a spirochete, because of its spiral shape. Although the disease organism can cause devastating health effects to vital internal organ systems, most of the early signs and symptoms of syphilis are found in skin lesions. One of the first signs, for example, is the *chancre*, a hard eroded lesion that appears on the penis about two to ten weeks after sexual contact with an infected person. A similar lesion develops in the vagina but is less noticeable except to an examining doctor. Chancres can appear on other body surfaces, such as the lips.

Some six weeks or more after the appearance of a chancre, secondary syphilis signs can be found on skin surfaces, ranging from eroded mucous patches in the mouth or vagina to patches of alopecia, or hair loss, on the sides of the head. Other signs are hard, scaly, raised lesions on the hands and feet; white, moist, wart-like growths in the anal-genital area; and a measles-like rash on the trunk of the body.

Treatment involves injection of large doses of penicillin, or other antibiotics if the patient is allergic to penicillin.

thrush A form of the skin fungus disease, *moniliasis*, which sometimes invades the mouth of infants.

tinea A type of fungus that invades the skins of humans, for example, *Tinea capitis*, which causes *ringworm infection* of the scalp.

trench foot A disease caused by prolonged exposure of the feet to temperatures near the freezing point. Wet stockings and tightly fitted shoes or boots contribute to the condition, which is marked by a feeling of cold and numbness. Extreme sensitivity to cold conditions and circulatory problems in the lower extremities develop later. Trench foot was so named because the disorder was encountered frequently by combat soldiers of past wars. The hazard still threatens hunters and other outdoor enthusiasts who are likely to be exposed to cold temperature.

tropical acne A form of *acne* generally peculiar to persons in warm, humid climates. The acne lesions may suddenly erupt explosively over the face, neck, chest, and back, frequently affecting persons who had never before had acne. The lesions of tropical acne usually are more extensive and inflamed than in other forms of acne.

tropical wet foot Another term for *paddie foot*, a disorder characterized by thick macerated skin on the soles of feet that have been immersed in warm tropical waters for prolonged periods.

tumor A mass of abnormal tissue which serves no useful function to the supporting body of tissue. A tumor may be benign or harmless, or it can be malignant, as in the case of a cancer that spreads to the surrounding tissues.

ulcer An open sore in the surface of the skin (or other membrane) that may invade and erode underlying tissues. An ulcer of the skin can be started by a number of different kinds of bodily insults, ranging from injury or burns to insect bites or bacterial infections.

urticaria A medical term used to describe *hives* or a similar type of localized tissue swelling, or small raised lesions on the skin surface. Urticaria pigmentosa is an unusual kind of swelling on the skin caused by an injury that affects mastocyte cells, which contain large amounts of histamine. Even a mild pressure such as rubbing can release histamine from the mastocyte cells of a person whose skin is sensitive to this kind of stimulus.

varicella The medical term for *chicken pox*.

variola A term the doctor may use when referring to *smallpox*.

verruca The medical term for *wart*. A medical notation of "verruca plana juvenilis" may be translated as "the child has warts on his skin."

vesicle A small watery skin blister such as the kind caused by *cold sores* or sunburn.

vitiligo A skin disorder marked by the loss of melanin pigment. The pigment-forming melanocytes remain in the skin, but they quit producing melanin with the result that oval or irregular patches of depigmented skin appear. The disorder not unusually affects persons who are members of the same families. It is mainly of cosmetic concern except in cases where it might be a sign of a thyroid disorder, pernicious anemia, diabetes, or Addison's disease.

Treatment involves the use of psoralen drugs, which make the skin darken under ultraviolet light, followed by exposure to sunlight or ultraviolet lamp light. An alternative is the use of cosmetics to mask contrasting skin color borders.

wart A common type of generally harmless skin tumor caused by a virus. Warts vary in appearance from small, dry, grayish, raised lesions to small, flat, brown spots on the face, or large, moist, white skin tumors in the anal-genital region. Treatment alternatives include freezing the warts with liquid nitrogen, surgery under local anesthesia, salicylic acid plasters that help soak off the warts, or the use of other medications that tend to dissolve the warts so they can be lifted out of the skin.

wen A sebaceous cyst on the skin.

wheals Small superficial skin blisters such as those produced by insect bites or hives.

winter itch A type of *dermatitis* that occurs rather commonly in the skin of older persons during cold weather, usually as a result of drying out of the skin. Remedies that help relieve the symptoms include the skin oils and creams that help the skin hold moisture. In severe cases a doctor may prescribe steroid hormones.

Wood's light A special kind of ultraviolet lamp used by doctors in diagnosing certain kinds of skin disorders. The species of fungus that causes ringworm, for example, will produce a brilliant green fluorescence under a Wood's light apparatus, while the bacteria that causes erythasma symptoms produce a coral red fluorescence under the same light.

xanthelasma Soft xanthoma-type plaques that develop in the skin of the eyelids and beneath the eyes. The cholesterol plaques frequently are a sign of fat metabolism or cardiovascular health problems.

xanthoma A raised skin lesion, usually yellowish in color, caused by an accumulation of cholesterol under the skin.

zoster Short for *herpes zoster*, or shingles, a skin eruption caused by the same virus that produces the symptoms of chicken pox.

QUESTIONS AND ANSWERS

THE SKIN

Q: *Is it true that shaving makes a man's beard grow faster?*
A: No. The hair shafts that appear above the surface of the skin are composed of lifeless cells. Nothing you do to a dead hair shaft will alter its growth pattern as long as the hair-forming cells at the root are not disturbed.

Q: *Will taking vitamin E improve hair growth on the scalp?*
A: There is little evidence that any vitamin will have a significant influence on hair growth. In certain cases of malnutrition, hair loss or fragile scalp hairs may be observed, but the cause is due to a protein deficiency rather than to a vitamin lack.

Q: *I have heard stories about people whose hair turned white overnight because of a frightening experience. Is this possible?*
A: Hair color is produced by melanin-forming cells beneath the skin as the hair shaft grows outward from the root at a rate of about 1/25th of an inch (1/3rd of a millimeter) a day. Most of the visible hair on one's head, therefore, received its coloring matter some weeks or months ago, and only the use of a bleaching chemical could turn dark hair white in less than one day.

Q: *Is dark hair healthier than gray hair?*
A: No. The color of one's hair is not related to the health of the hair.

Q: *I lost a fingernail in an accident recently. Will it grow again?*
A: If the cells that form the nail plate were not damaged, a new fingernail should grow over the nail bed in about three or four months, depending in part on the season of the year.

Q: *What difference does the season make in how fast hair or nails will grow?*

A: Hair and nails grow more rapidly during the summer and at a slower rate during the winter months.

Q: *How long does it take for a woman to grow hair that is waist length or longer?*
A: At an average growth rate of 1/25th of an inch a day, it would take 20 years or more to produce waist length hair.

Q: *Will eyebrow hairs grow back if they are plucked?*
A: If the matrix cells in the root of the follicle aren't destroyed, normal hair will reform in the eyebrows.

Q: *Do dark-skinned people ever develop skin cancers?*
A: Dark-skinned people can develop cancers of the skin, but they are rare. The melanin pigment of the skin cells that is responsible for the dark coloration protects the skin cells against ultraviolet rays of the sun. The ultraviolet light from the sun is a primary cause of skin cancers.

Q: *What is the "seven-year-itch"?*
A: The seven-year-itch is a popular name for scabies, a disease caused by a mite that burrows under the skin to lay eggs that hatch into more mites. The disease is fairly contagious and easily transmitted from one person to another. The scabies infection probably got its popular name from the fact that once scabies becomes established in a family or other group of persons living together, who reinfect each other with mites, it can take quite a long while to finally eliminate the disease.

Q: *I have acquired several brown spots on my hands in recent years. A friend calls them liver spots. Are they a sign of liver disease?*

A: The so-called liver spots have nothing to do with your liver. They are caused by years of exposure to the wind and sun, and are quite similar to the pigment accumulations in the skin that we call freckles.

Q: *Are there any exercises that will get rid of skin wrinkles?*
A: Wrinkles of the skin are caused by tissue changes between the major muscle groups and the outer layers of skin, such as loss of fat deposits and degeneration of elastic connective tissues—effects that cannot be reversed by exercising the muscles.

Q: *What causes hangnails and what can be done to stop them from developing?*
A: Hangnails actually involve the skinfolds alongside a nail and are a result of drying and cracking of the skin in that area. The hangnail usually is noticed while manicuring the nails or after a minor injury to the fingernail area. The use of creams and oils that help moisten the skin surface, carefully manicuring the nail to avoid tearing the skinfolds, and wearing rubber gloves while the hands are in dishwater will help prevent hangnails.

Q: *Are there any dishwashing detergents that will make my skin smooth and soft?*
A: Since most detergents are designed to dissolve dirt and grease, it's unlikely that the same harsh chemicals would improve the skin texture.

Q: *My hair sometimes has a greenish tint after I've been swimming in motel pools. Is the green color from chlorine that has been added to the water in the pool?*
A: The green coloring you notice in your hair after swimming probably is the result of an interaction involving the chlorine in swimming pool water and a chemical sometimes added to prevent the growth of algae. The algae-killing chemical frequently contains a copper compound that reacts with chlorine to produce a green deposit. It usually is more noticeable on blonde or other light-colored hair. One solution to the problem is to wear a bathing cap when swimming in a pool that has been treated with algae-control chemicals.

Q: *I get red marks under the rings on my fingers. Does this mean I am allergic to the rings?*
A: Some people are allergic to nickel, a metal sometimes used in rings. The reaction is a form of contact dermatitis. Another possibility is that any uneven surfaces inside the ring may catch and hold bits of soap that could produce the skin irritation. Try removing the rings before putting your hands in soapy water, and check the areas on the inner surfaces of the rings, especially where there may be open spaces under stone settings, for bits of accumulated soap.

Q: *Are there any foods or beverages that are likely to cause an outbreak of acne?*
A: Whether a particular food item or beverage will aggravate acne is pretty much an individual reaction. Some people believe that chocolate, nuts, or other foods can aggravate a case of acne, while others claim such food items have no effect on acne. If you suspect a certain food might cause an acne problem, you can make your own test by eliminating that food item in all forms for several weeks. Then resume eating that food and see if there is a sudden flareup of acne. The results are not "proof positive" that a food item aggravates acne, but it's a good indicator of a possible relationship.

Q: *Some years ago I had my girl friend's name tattooed on my arm. I married another girl and now my wife wants the tattoo removed. Can the tattoo be removed by a laser beam?*
A: Lasers have been used to remove tattoos, but there are several "catches" to consider. One is that laser treatment for tattoo removal is more effective for small tattoos than large ones, since only a small skin area can be treated at one time. Another catch is that the service is available only at a few specialized institutions. Also, you need to be referred by a physician who feels the laser treatment is the most appropriate method of removing your

particular tattoo. There is little about the procedure that is magic: the pigment of the tattoo absorbs the energy of the laser beam, burning out the tattooed skin cells. After the burned skin area heals, a scar replaces the tattoo. Other methods of tattoo removal may involve surgery, dermabrasion, and the use of chemicals that cause the pigment to fade or to be altered by irritation of the surrounding skin cells.

Q: *How does dermabrasion work?*
A: Dermabrasion, which is used for reducing or removing acne scars as well as for altering tattoo pigments, removes the outer layers of skin with a rapidly revolving brush. The skin is anesthetized, sometimes by freezing the surface, before the brush is applied. The brush literally planes off the surface of the skin. The procedure causes the thinner skin layer that is left to swell and produce crusts which drop off a week or two later. A new skin surface develops during the following weeks. The new skin may or may not retain any of the disfiguring scars, pits, pigments, or other features that warranted dermabrasion in the first place, but generally those abnormal features are less noticeable than before. The new skin surface must be protected against sunburn and other irritants for several months after dermabrasion.

Q: *Does electrolysis remove unwanted hair permanently?*
A: If the electrolysis procedure destroys all of the hair-forming cells at the root of the hair shaft, electrolysis is required only once. Frequently, however, a few remaining hair root cells are left to produce a new hair shaft, in which case the electrolysis treatment may have to be repeated.

Q: *Are there any medications that will remove cigarette stains from the fingers?*
A: Some home remedies that have been recommended include vinegar and lemon juice, which may have a mild bleaching effect. The tobacco stains usually involve only the outer layers of epidermis, and those skin cells normally will be shed within a couple of weeks, anyway, if you

are not in a hurry to get rid of the stains. Meanwhile, if you must smoke, make sure the cigarette tobacco doesn't come in contact with your skin.

Q: *If I scratch the skin of my arm with a pin or pencil point, a raised red mark appears along the scratch. Is this normal?*
A: The effect, sometimes called "skin writing," or dermographism, is unusual but not abnormal. Some people simply have skin that is extremely sensitive to pressure; the reason is unknown. The condition may be temporary or last a lifetime. The only symptom that may be troublesome is itching, which tends to develop with welts, or red marks, caused by tight-fitting clothing items such as garters, belts, bra straps, etc.

Q: *How long should it take to get a good suntan?*
A: There is no rule of thumb that would be true for all people in all parts of the world during all seasons; sunlight generally is more intense later in the summer season than at the start of summer, and blondes and redheads usually are more sensitive to sunlight. But for general guidelines, on the first day early in the summer season expose the front and back side of the body for 15 to 20 minutes per side. Repeat the exposure the next day, adding about 5 to 10 minutes for each side. On the third day, add a few more minutes of sun exposure to each side. By the fourth day the first signs of a suntan should appear. After the first week of gradually increasing exposure to sunlight, you should have enough of a start in order to be protected from serious sunburn during further sunbathing.

Q: *How can you get rid of a suntan in a hurry?*
A: You can mask a suntan with cosmetics that lighten the skin coloration while the natural tan gradually fades away (and you avoid further exposure to sunlight). But there is no safe and simple way to quickly bleach all the melanin pigment from your epidermis.

Q: *How do sunscreens work?*

A: Sunscreen preparations contain chemicals that absorb certain portions of the ultraviolet light spectrum, thereby preventing those burning rays from reaching the skin. None of the commercially available sunscreens, however, provides complete protection from the effects of sunlight, and most of the preparations must be replaced on the skin after intervals of a few hours since they are easily washed off during swimming, or by perspiration, or by rubbing against clothing, chairs, and so on.

3

THE HEAD AND NECK

While a doctor takes your hand in greeting, and makes a few quick mental notes about the temperature, texture, and other characteristics of the skin he is touching, he also will be looking into your face. Nothing unusual about that, you say, since most people meet on a face-to-face basis.

However, an experienced doctor can pick up quite a few health clues during a brief moment of looking at your face. A person suffering from parkinsonism, for example, will probably have a different sort of facial expression, sometimes described as an immobile stare, from a patient with hyperthyroidism, whose retracted eyelids might produce a startled expression.

Hopefully, you will smile at the doctor, and the appearance of your mouth and teeth can add a few more bits of information about your general physical condition. In addition, the posture of the head and neck, plus the myriad details about the skin and hair on the head and neck, should contribute quite an assortment of health data for an alert doctor. Healthy skin, healthy hair, sound teeth, and other signs

of a good physical condition are as important as signs and symptoms of a physical ailment to the doctor trying to size up a patient's general health. For the doctor, all this business of collecting health clues is just part of his job. He must be a sort of medical Sherlock Holmes who observes a skin lesion here, an old scar there, a swollen eyelid, a strange way of holding the head at an angle, and possibly additional factors that will help his diagnosis, before the actual examination and discussion of a health problem begins.

Your head, and particularly your face, can disclose quite a lot of information about your general health. In the chapter about the skin, you learned about various signs and symptoms of diseases involving organ systems deep in the body which made their presence known with itching, redness, eruptions, or other manifestations on the outside of the body. In a similar manner, a remarkable number of systemic ailments may be discovered first by the ways in which they affect the eyes, ears, nose, throat, and mouth, or other areas of the head and neck.

When the doctor examines the head and

neck closely, he usually will inspect the face for any deformities. He may ask that the mouth be opened as wide as possible to check for any problem that might involve the jaws. Starting at the very top of the body, the scalp, he will inspect the hair, noting whether your hair has its natural color or if you use hair dyes, and will determine if the hair shafts are fine or coarse, if there are signs of abnormal hair loss, and so on. He also will look for bulges, areas of the scalp that might appear inflamed, and he most likely will apply a bit of mild pressure on the bones of the scalp to see if there are any bony irregularities beneath the scalp—any masses, soft areas, or tender spots. If your complaint is headaches, the doctor might even place his stethoscope on the surface of the head and listen for sounds called bruits, which may indicate an abnormality in the blood circulation in that area. He might carefully pinch one of the muscles of the neck, since disorders involving the head sometimes originate in the neck and many medical mysteries are solved by tracing the source of an illness to another part of the body. The Oriental technique of acupuncture relies on the knowledge of referred pain paths.

Normal Growth of the Skull

The age of a person determines to a great extent what is normal and what's not about the appearance of the head and neck. A baby's head, for example, is relatively large for its body size. A newborn infant's head is about half the size of the head of an average adult, but while the head doubles in size from infancy to adulthood the legs grow to five times their length at birth. The proportions of a human head also change between babyhood

and adulthood, with most of the new growth occurring in the facial area beneath the forehead. If an adult had his facial features arranged in the same manner as those of a baby, his eyes, nose, and mouth would all be crowded into the area normally occupied between the nostrils and the chin, and the rest of the face would be forehead.

Several bones of the head, or more properly the skull, are not completely formed at birth and are separated by soft spots called fontanels. The fontanels are protected by wedges of membrane and usually are closed by growing bone after the first two months of life. However, one fontanel near the front of the skull but well behind the forehead does not close completely until after the first year of the infant's life.

A doctor examining an infant's head may observe pulsations of the heartbeat through the front fontanel, which also may expand or contract when the baby cries. When the fontanels finally are closed by the fusing of separate skull bones, small bony ridges develop along the lines of closure. These bony ridges, known as sutures, sometimes remain long after the skull bones have merged. Such linear bulges on the skull are normal.

Changes in the facial features of a developing human occur as the nasal and sinus cavities of the skull grow and the teeth begin to appear in the child's mouth. The nasal cavity, which is situated almost between the eyes of a newborn child, moves lower as the facial bones develop. By the time a youngster is seven years old, his or her facial proportions are approximately those of an adult. The next change in head size and proportion occurs around the time of puberty, when the features of a boy become those of a man and

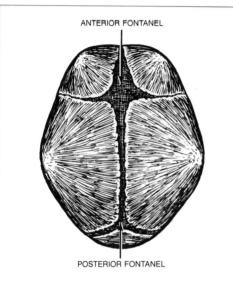

ANTERIOR FONTANEL

POSTERIOR FONTANEL

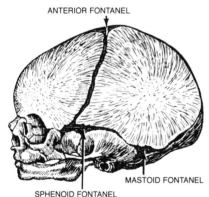

ANTERIOR FONTANEL

MASTOID FONTANEL

SPHENOID FONTANEL

The adult skull bears only a slight resemblance to that of a newborn baby. The baby skull above shows some of the separate bones that later grow together to form a continuous bone surface. The skull bones at birth are separated by fontanels, or "soft spots" where gaps in the cranium are protected only by membranes.

the features of the face of a girl become those of a woman. After adulthood has been reached the skull of the male usually has become larger and heavier than the female skull.

The skull is composed of 22 flat or irregular bones. Eight of the bones form the cranium, which is a Greek word meaning "helmet." Appropriately, the cranium is a helmet-shaped group of bones that protects the brain. The remaining 14 bones of the skull are facial bones that form the cheeks, jaws, and upper bridge of the nose. The lower portion of the nose is composed of cartilage, a material similar to the gristle at the edges of young chicken bones.

There are a number of other bones in the head area not considered parts of the skull. They include a U-shaped bone called the hyoid, which serves as a sort of anchor for muscles that move the tongue, and the auditory ossicles, sets of three tiny bones in each of the ears which translate sound waves into the distinctive vibrations that we identify as music, voices, or irritating noises. The teeth also are excluded from the total bone count of the skull.

The skull and its contents, including three to four pounds of brain tissue, would be a bit more difficult to balance on the top of the spinal column if it were not for the fact that many of the facial bones contain air spaces. The air spaces are known as the sinuses of the head. They are connected to the nasal cavity, which may help explain why respiratory infections lead easily to sinus problems.

Except for the mandible, or lower jawbone which holds the lower teeth, and the vomer bone, which is a part of the nasal septum, the 14 facial bones come in pairs, one for each side of the face. The nasal bone, for example, is composed of two

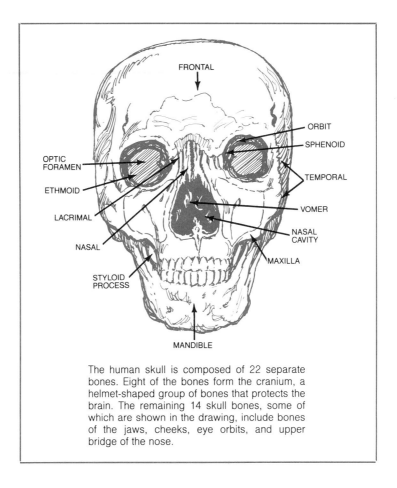

FRONTAL

ORBIT
SPHENOID

OPTIC
FORAMEN

TEMPORAL

ETHMOID

VOMER

LACRIMAL

NASAL
CAVITY

NASAL

MAXILLA

STYLOID
PROCESS

MANDIBLE

The human skull is composed of 22 separate bones. Eight of the bones form the cranium, a helmet-shaped group of bones that protects the brain. The remaining 14 skull bones, some of which are shown in the drawing, include bones of the jaws, cheeks, eye orbits, and upper bridge of the nose.

small oblong bones that are situated side by side on the middle upper surface of the face; the bridge of the nose marks the place where the two separate bones meet. The sizes and shapes of the six pairs of facial bones vary from one individual to the next, and frequently the bones are not quite mirror images of each other.

As a result of this asymmetry we get our distinctive facial features. For most people the facial bones on the right side of the head appear to be somewhat larger, with more prominently molded forehead and cheek features on the right side than on the left. By carefully observing your own face in a mirror, you may find that an eyebrow on one side is a bit different in height or shape than an eyebrow on the opposite side of the face. The same lack of symmetry may be seen in the eyes, mouth, and other facial features. But such variations are more likely to be the normal thing than a sign of abnormality. In fact, if a photograph could be made by combining two left halves or two right halves of a picture of your face, the chances are the person in the photo would not look exactly like you.

The lower jawbone is the largest and strongest of all the facial bones. Although it is a single bone, it develops into its horseshoe-shaped structure from two smaller bones early in life. The lower jawbone goes through several changes during a lifetime. At birth the lower jawbone is like a small shell containing the sockets for several of the baby teeth that will erupt. During childhood the bone becomes longer and thicker, providing space for additional teeth to come and to accommodate the powerful pressure that is exerted by the muscles that must move the jawbone as the child learns to eat solid foods. After adulthood is reached the lower jaw reaches its maximum size and thickness, and even the angle of attachment to the rest of the skull becomes altered somewhat. Thus the angle of the jaw of an adult shows an almost right-angled L shape, with the short side of the L forming the attachment to the skull. In old age the lower jaw gradually returns to the general shape and angle of the infant's lower jaw. As teeth are lost, some of the surrounding bone tissue is absorbed. The length of the jaw may remain approximately the same, but the lower jawbone in old age is considerably reduced in size.

After the lower jawbone, the upper jawbones are the largest bones of the facial structure. The upper jawbones form the roof of the mouth, the bony cavities that house the eyeballs, the nasal bone, and the sockets for the upper row of teeth. Like the lower jaw, the upper jawbones, called maxillae, go through changes in size and strength between infancy and old age, reaching a peak in size during adulthood and contracting in later years when teeth are lost and supporting bone tissue is absorbed.

Next to the large upper jawbones on each side of the skull and bordering the eye sockets are a couple of the body's smallest and most fragile bones. About the size and thickness of a fingernail, the lachrymal bones are a part of the apparatus for releasing the tears that wash the surface of the eye. Each lachrymal bone is attached to an even smaller muscle which has the job of helping to squeeze fluid from the tiny tear sac so it will flow toward the eye.

Muscular Development of the Head and Neck

The upper jawbones are attached to 12 sets of muscles and the lower jawbone to 15 sets of muscles. Although one seldom thinks of the head area as being muscular, the head and neck are literally swathed with layers of muscle tissue. The layers include several rather powerful muscles involved in eating. They include the masseter, a Greek word meaning "chewer," which runs from the cheekbone to the lower jaw, and the temporalis, which connects the lower jawbone with the cranium. Others are small gentle muscles such as one with the jawbreaker name of Orbicularis palpebrarum, which closes the eyelids when you fall asleep. A neighboring muscle of the facial area draws the eyebrow downward and inward when you frown. The muscles around the eyes sometimes contract so firmly that the skin is drawn into folds which produce the wrinkles known as crow's-feet.

A muscle known as Orbicularis oris circles the mouth and is used to purse the lips. A muscle called the external pterygoid contracts to open the mouth after it has been closed by contractions of the masseter and temporalis muscles. There are three sets of muscles that move the outer ear, and six different muscles are needed to move the eyeball, or globe of the eye, upward, downward, inward, outward, or a combination such as downward and outward. A sheet of muscle tissue called the occipito-frontalis runs across the scalp from the area of the nose to the back of the head; it is used to raise the eyebrows as well as to produce the forehead wrinkles that express surprise or fright.

While the names of muscles might seem like complex meaningless words to the average person, the names generally have precise meanings to the doctor. The names generally indicate the shape of the muscle, the body area to which it is attached, or something similar. The name of the temporalis muscle, for example, indicates that it is attached to the temporal bone of the head, the area commonly known as the temple. The occipito-frontalis runs from the occipital bone at the back of the head to the frontal bone at the front or the forehead. The trapezius, a muscle that extends from the back of the trunk to the back of the neck, gets its name from its trapezoid shape, that is, a sort of triangle with one corner cut off.

Because humans seem to have been designed as if to defy the law of gravity, the muscles of the head and neck frequently are subjected to more stress and strain than other muscles of the body. Gravity should pull the lower jaw down so the mouth will remain open when the head is held erect, but powerful face muscles are able to keep the jaw closed almost continuously as long as a person is awake. One explanation for this effect, which sometimes is referred to as muscle tone, is that the individual muscle fibers in the muscle group take turns contracting and relaxing. Thus, half the muscle fibers work to defy gravity while the other half may be resting. In four-footed animals with a similar jaw design there is less demand on the facial muscles to hold the mouth in a closed position.

Muscles along the back of the neck of humans similarly hold the head erect for most of the period the individual is awake, even though the force of gravity tends to pull the head forward and downward. When a person finally is overcome by fatigue, of course, his head may droop into a nodding position and the jaw muscles may relax and allow the mouth to open. It is often the muscles that are required to fight gravity all day that show the first signs of stress and fatigue. The headache that marks the end of a trying day frequently is an ache that originates in the muscles of the neck, such as the trapezius. A person who is under physical or emotional stress may display his discomfort unconsciously by nervous motions of the muscles in his cheeks and jaws.

The bones and muscles of the head and neck are fairly representative of bones and muscles throughout the body. Bone is commonly thought of as lifeless material similar to stone or concrete. Actually, most living bone material is physiologically active tissue like any other organ system of the body. Living cells and blood vessels are found throughout bone tissue; nutrients are being delivered and waste products are being removed constantly. Red blood cells are manufactured in the spongy areas of some bones. Calcium and other minerals are moving into and out of the bone matrix almost continuously.

Living bone is about 20 percent water. Approximately half of bone is mineral and a third is organic matter. The minerals found in bone generally are salts or compounds of calcium, phosphorus, magnesium, and other elements. The organic portion is chiefly collagen, a kind of protein fiber commonly found in connective tissue, tendons, and skin. The organic materials and the minerals are thoroughly mixed together with a natural cement to form a substance that can be as strong as cast iron but much lighter and more flexible. That substance forms the bones of the skull.

The skull bones are different from some other bones of the body in that they are built in layers, like a sandwich with one slice of bread thicker than the other. The outer layer is thicker and tougher than the brittle inner layer. The sandwich filling of the skull bones is a spongy matrix of bony material, which varies in thickness in different parts of the head.

The muscle tissues of the head and neck area are for the most part skeletal, or striated, muscles. Skeletal muscle generally is called that because it is connected, sometimes indirectly through tendons, to parts of the skeleton. Muscle tissues are called striated, or more precisely cross-striated, because the muscle fibers when viewed under a microscope show numerous stripes that run across the width of the fibers.

There are other types of muscles in the body—smooth muscles that do not show the dark and light bands across the widths of their fibers, and cardiac muscle tissue that has some of the characteristics of both striated muscle and smooth muscle. Smooth muscle tissue usually is found in blood vessels, the gastrointestinal tract, and other places where contractions are automatic, as in digestion and response to cold and heat. Contraction of cardiac muscle also is automatic—for example, the heartbeat that continues day and night without instructions from the individual.

Skeletal muscle usually is found in body areas over which we exercise some control, such as making an arm or leg move because we instruct it to move.

Smooth muscle is sometimes identified as involuntary muscle, and skeletal muscle as voluntary muscle, although both obviously are misnomers of a sort. Voluntary muscles frequently move involuntarily, as in reflex actions, and involuntary muscles can be controlled, as has been demonstrated by people who practice transcendental meditation or yoga. In the human body one can find all sorts of exceptions to man-made rules and definitions, and this is just another example.

Human body movements are made possible by a collection of some 600 assorted shapes and sizes of muscles. Some muscles are large enough or sufficiently prominent to be observed in action beneath the skin; these include the biceps of the upper arm and the masseter muscles of the lower jaw. Others are so tiny and fragile that they probably would not be noticed except for the functions they perform, such as the muscles that change the size of the iris in the eye or squeeze the tear sacs to moisten the eyeball.

A single set of muscles can contain millions of individual muscle fibers, each about the thickness of a human hair. The main difference in the sizes of various muscles is the number of fibers bundled together in a muscle. The size also may change when a muscle contracts or relaxes. The biceps, for example, might go unnoticed until you flex the arm and see the biceps bulge outward as it contracts. When a skeletal muscle contracts, the fibers slide together in a sort of telescoping movement. When fully contracted, a skeletal muscle may be only one-half to two-thirds as long as its relaxed dimension.

Muscle fibers can be tremendously strong for their size. Some muscle fibers can support hundreds of times their own weight. A muscle group containing millions of muscle fibers can exert enough force during a contraction to damage a tendon or bone to which it is attached.

There are about six billion muscle fibers scattered throughout the body. Each has a specific action, and in some cases the action is to reverse the action of an opposing muscle fiber, or more precisely the muscle to which it has been assigned by nature. The biceps, for example, has the job of bending the elbow, but it has no way of straightening the elbow joint once it has been bent. For the job of straightening the elbow, there is an opposing muscle called the triceps. The biceps must remain relaxed while the triceps does its job, and vice versa. The same relationship holds true for muscles in other body areas. In the eye, for example, for the action of one muscle there is a counteraction that must be performed by another muscle; one muscle, therefore, dilates the iris of the eye while the opposing muscle is called upon to restrict the size of the iris opening.

In some cases, two sets of muscles that generally are used to produce opposing action can join forces to cause a somewhat different action. The muscles that run from the trunk of the body to the back of the head, the sternomastoid muscles, are used ordinarily to turn the head. These muscles, which are large enough to be felt beneath the skin by pressing them gently, contract to turn the head either to the right or the left; there is a sternomastoid muscle on either side of the body. But when both sternomastoid muscles are contracted at the same time, they pull the head down and forward, as in the action of nodding.

When a muscle fiber contracts, the energy that produces the action is power that came originally from the sun. All animal muscle power depends upon food, usually in the form of carbohydrate molecules called glucose, which is a form of simple sugar. Through a complex series of chemical reactions involving photosynthesis, energy from the sun is utilized by growing plants to combine water and carbon dioxide from the environment into carbohydrate molecules, usually as plant starches or sugars. The plant cells, through some additional chemical magic, can build molecules of fats, proteins, or other substances from the basic sugar molecule. Plants that are eaten by animals may transform those carbohydrate, protein, or fat molecules into still other food substances, such as cholesterol, that are not found in the original plant cells.

Just as carbohydrates can be built into more complex molecules of fats or proteins, the body's chemistry can break down most fats, proteins, and carbohydrate units into simple glucose molecules again. An exception, for humans at least, is cellulose, a giant carbohydrate molecule that can be digested by other animals such as cows but not by the human body alone. The basic glucose molecule becomes the primary fuel for muscle contractions. With the help of other chemical substances in the body cells, the energy that came originally from the sunlight is released to move the muscle fibers. At the same time, like the mythical prince who is returned to life from a frog with the wave of a magic wand, the carbohydrate molecule suddenly becomes once again a bit of water and carbon dioxide.

The preceding explanation, of course, is somewhat simplified. There are other factors involved in producing a muscle contraction. Oxygen, for example, is needed to complete the transformation of the carbohydrate molecule into water and carbon dioxide, just as oxygen is needed to release the energy in gasoline to produce the power required to move an automobile. Anybody who has run a marathon or rushed up a flight of stairs is aware of the sustained need for oxygen in order to pump the muscles for more than a few brief moments.

The oxygen used to release muscle energy came originally into the body cells from air breathed into the lungs. The red blood cells circulating through capillaries in the lining of the lungs capture the oxygen molecules as they are inhaled. Some oxygen molecules may be taken out of the bloodstream and stored in the muscle tissue for emergency use. The substance that makes the red blood cells red, an iron-rich protein called hemoglobin, has a remarkable ability to attract and transport oxygen to the body cells needing it. The muscle tissue containing stored oxygen also has a reddish coloration because of a chemical cousin of hemoglobin, the similar substance known as myoglobin. It is because of the oxygen held by myoglobin that people are able to run races, swim under water, and perform other physical feats which consume oxygen faster than it can be pumped into the bloodstream by the lungs. However, the average human body is able to function without fresh oxygen for only about four minutes, that time period representing the amount of oxygen stored in muscle hemoglobin.

The hemoglobin and myoglobin molecules make it possible for the body to store about 60 times as much oxygen as could be handled by other fluids and tissues. If the body had to depend upon ordinary water to transport oxygen through the circulatory system, for example, one would need about 500 pounds of water in his arteries and veins for just that purpose. When the body's reserve supply of stored oxygen is exhausted, a person feels the same way, suddenly exhausted. After a brisk workout in which oxygen is burned to release energy for the muscles, we usually have to stop for a short period of rapid breathing. This period is sometimes called getting one's "second wind," but it's more accurately a time for replacing the oxygen reserve consumed in the "first wind." If oxygen is not replaced quickly enough the muscles may simply cease contracting on command, or muscle pains may develop because of an accumulation of waste products in the tissues, or both.

Nerves in the Head and Neck

The command for muscles to contract is transmitted from one or more nerve centers along nerve fibers, which actually are long filaments of nerve cells called neurons. A single nerve cell may conduct a command to hundreds of individual muscle fibers. A large bundle of nerve fibers might require connections with hundreds of nerve fibers to insure that all muscle fibers get the same message at the same time. Once a nervous system command reaches a muscle, usually near the center point of the length of the muscle, it spreads toward both ends at a speed of about 10 miles per hour. Although that rate of speed may not seem very swift in terms of today's jet age standards, it is fast enough for a nerve impulse to spread over the longest muscle in the body in roughly 1/10th of a second. For smaller muscles, the travel time of the message is much faster and can be measured in thousandths of a second.

Normally, the muscle contraction message requires that all the muscle fibers go into their act at the same time. There aren't any options; it's either go or no go. However, most skeletal muscles do have a kind of dual control arrangement with the central nervous system. There is an automatic response, such as in reflex action when you move away quickly from a painful or threatening object, whether it be a hot stove or a rock zinging toward your head. In addition to the reflex action, which requires no thinking on your own part about whether to command the muscles to react, there is a free will option that frequently offers a sort of manual override control on muscle actions. By exerting will power, you can hold your hand on the hot stove and endure the pain, or you can refuse to flinch from the rock traveling toward your head.

Command Headquarters: The Brain

Headquarters for the central nervous system is lodged within the cranium in the brain, which is protected by several layers of membranes beneath the sandwich layers of skull bones. The spinal cord extends from the bottom of the brain through an opening in the skull, with branches reaching out at intervals along its length, to the bottom of the vertebral column, or backbone. Other branches of the central nervous system extend from the brain into the sensory organs of the head—the eyes, ears, nose, and mouth—which serve as part of an early warning radar system for the body in its contacts with the outside world.

The human brain contains some 12 billion neurons and weighs about three pounds. Some brains are larger and some smaller than the average. But there is no

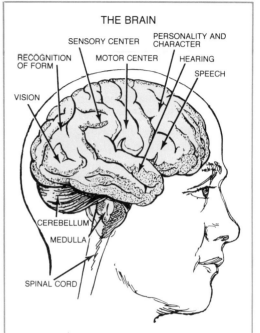

Position of the brain within the skull. Various areas of the brain have been mapped to indicate portions associated with different living functions. Much of the information regarding the location of centers for hearing, speech, and so on, has been obtained from studies of persons who have suffered brain damage in accidents or as a result of strokes.

evidence that a large brain guarantees the possession of talent or intelligence. One of the largest brains ever examined by doctors belonged to a laboring man, while the brains of several of the greatest geniuses of art, literature, and music were found to be of less than average size. One random study of 12 different human brains revealed that the largest brain of the lot, as well as the smallest, belonged to persons who had been examined by psychologists and classified as idiots.

Although the study of the human brain has involved hundreds of scientists for hundreds of years, very little really is known about the exact processes involved at the brain cell level in memory, problem solving, dreaming, and other mental activities. The nerve cells have been counted, nerve pathways have been traced, brain tissue has been examined under the microscope and analyzed in chemical laboratories, but we're still not certain how many simple thought processes occur in the brain tissues.

Studies of the human brain have revealed some indications of how this important organ might have evolved over millions of years. The ancient Greeks were aware that the human brain was divided into several separate structures, or brains, each of which apparently had specific functions. In the area where the spinal cord enters the brain, for example, the cord widens into a structure sometimes identified by the medical term of medulla oblongata, and sometimes called simply the hindbrain. This is the sort of brain found in some very primitive animals that possess a spinal cord of any sort. Located next to the hindbrain in humans and more advanced types of animals with a spinal cord is a bulge of brain tissue known as the cerebellum, or little brain.

The primitive areas of the brain still control certain basic functions in humans, just as they do in simple animals such as worms. The reflex action that occurs when a person touches a hot stove is for practical purposes identical with the reaction of a worm to an environmental threat.

Later in the scale of evolution, the brain acquired the functions necessary for survival as a fish or reptile. Eventually, the brain of mammals evolved with an overgrowth of nervous tissue that became the cerebrum, with its still later developing cerebral cortex that covers the primitive basal brain structures. In some lower animals and in an unborn human child, the cerebral portion of the brain is smooth. But as the brain grows the cerebral cortex becomes folded and convoluted in order to accommodate a greater surface area. The brain surfaces of other "intelligent" animals such as the horse and dolphin have similar convolutions.

The muscles of the head and neck area, like those of other parts of the body, can be thought of as slaves of the central nervous system, which has more than one level of command. The lower level of command, in the old primitive brain area, sends orders along the nervous pathways ordering the muscles to react in a primitive manner to a contact with the environment. The higher command post, in the cerebral cortex, handles muscle activities that depend in part on the will of the mind. Scientists learned in the 19th century that animals with the cerebral cortex removed surgically continued to live but functioned at a primitive level with their basal brains.

The human brain is divided near the top into two, right and left, symmetrical halves. Each of the two halves, in addition to certain individual responsibilities in the area of mental work such as language handling, controls the movement of the body half on the opposite side. That is, the motor cortex, or portion of the cerebral cortex that controls motion, is situated on the left side of the brain and is responsible for muscle action on the right side of the body. And vice versa. Thus, an injury to the motor cortex area on the right side of the brain could result in paralysis or a similar loss of function on the left side of the body.

The relationship actually is much more specific. There are areas on the motor cortex of the brain that correspond to differ-

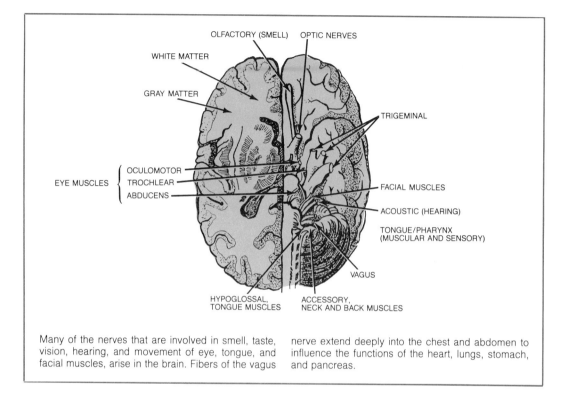

OLFACTORY (SMELL)   OPTIC NERVES

WHITE MATTER

GRAY MATTER

TRIGEMINAL

OCULOMOTOR
EYE MUSCLES   TROCHLEAR
ABDUCENS

FACIAL MUSCLES

ACOUSTIC (HEARING)

TONGUE/PHARYNX
(MUSCULAR AND SENSORY)

VAGUS

HYPOGLOSSAL,
TONGUE MUSCLES

ACCESSORY,
NECK AND BACK MUSCLES

Many of the nerves that are involved in smell, taste, vision, hearing, and movement of eye, tongue, and facial muscles, arise in the brain. Fibers of the vagus nerve extend deeply into the chest and abdomen to influence the functions of the heart, lungs, stomach, and pancreas.

ent body parts. Various motor cortex relationships have been carefully mapped during medical experiments and in work with patients who have suffered brain injuries on the battlefield or perhaps as a result of a stroke. Now doctors can pretty well pinpoint a motor area on the right side of the brain that will cause the muscles on a finger, leg, neck, or another body area on the left side of the body to contract. The relationship can be demonstrated by touching an electrode to one of the motor cortex areas and producing a muscle contraction in one of the mapped target areas of the body.

The nerve pathways, of course, cross from the left side of the brain to the right side of the body, and vice versa, to make this phenomenon possible. This informa-

tion is of more than academic interest to an examining physician because it can help the doctor to diagnose an ailment that may affect muscle function after a stroke or an accident.

Extension of the Brain: The Eye

The brain, in effect, is extended through the nerves that reach to the terminal filaments of nerve cells near the surface of the body, in the skin, and in special sense organs such as the eyes. The eyes, in fact, are probably the most direct extension of brain tissue beyond the cranium. The eyeballs rest in bony cavities in the front of the skull, along with the extraocular muscles that control movements of the eyes, the optic nerve endings, and the lacrimal apparatus which includes the bones, muscles, and glands that produce tears. The "house" of the eye is called the orbit, a cavity formed by several separate skull bones and lined with fat cells and other protective tissues.

The eye itself, sometimes referred to as a globe, is roughly spherical and about one inch in diameter. It has a transparent opening in the front, the cornea, and an optic nerve extending from the back; the rest of the organ is covered with a white tissue called the sclera. The cornea and the sclera are continuous, that is, they are the same membrane, a tough, fibrous tissue layer which is transparent in the area in front of the lens so that light can pass

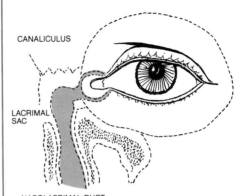

Bones of the skull contain spaces for sinuses and ducts, such as the nasolacrimal duct, which permits tears to drain into the nasal cavity after washing the surface of the eye.

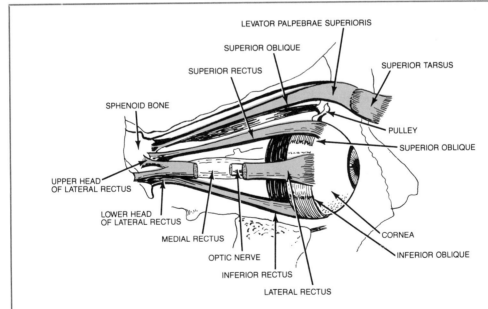

The eyeball is moved by a series of muscles arranged so that by contracting or relaxing their muscle fibers, the eye can be turned to the right or left, upward or downward, without moving the head. When one or more of the muscles fails to function properly, the person may have difficulty in maintaining normal binocular vision. Muscles that force the eyeball outward abnormally create a condition known popularly as walleye; muscles that hold the eyeball pointed inward cause a condition known as crosseye.

through it. This membrane both protects and shapes the eyeball.

A second more or less continuous layer inside the cornea and sclera is known by the medical name of uveal tract. For about 80 percent of the inner surface of the eyeball, this layer contains blood vessels that nourish the other eye tissues. The layer also includes the iris, a membrane that gives the eye its color—brown, blue, green, etc.—and controls the size of the pupil, plus ligaments that change the focus of the lens of the eye.

The retina is the innermost layer of tissue of the eyeball. One surface of the retina is in contact with the blood-rich uveal tract, and the other surface faces the vitreous humor, a transparent, jellylike substance that fills the cavity of the eyeball between the retina and the lens. The retina is composed of light-sensitive, terminal nerve filaments. Some nerve filaments are rod-shaped and are called rods; they are sensitive to light per se and are able to detect faint amounts of light in the environment. If you are trying to find your way in an otherwise dark night, depending only upon moonlight or starlight, the rod-

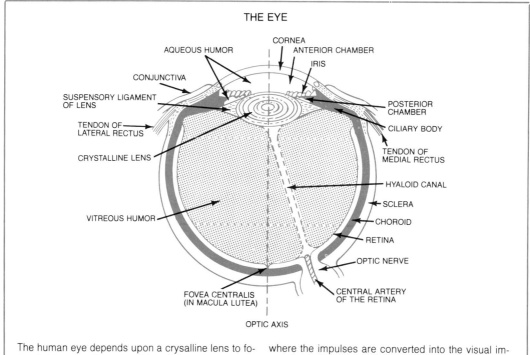

THE EYE

The human eye depends upon a crysalline lens to focus light waves through a thick vitreous humor onto the retina lining most of the interior of the eye. The retina contains nerve cells that translate light waves into impulses carried by the optic nerve to the brain, where the impulses are converted into the visual image "seen" by the individual. Tiny muscles control the shape of the lens and the size of the pupil (iris) to help the eye focus the image clearly before transmitting the impulses to the brain.

shaped nerve endings make it possible to navigate by means of celestial illumination.

The cones, or cone-shaped nerve endings in the retina, are color-sensitive. The cones generally function only when the visible light reaches a certain threshold of brilliance. Colors are difficult to distinguish in faint light. When the light intensity reaches a level that permits the cones to distinguish images in colors, the rods may continue to react to the light impulses, but they probably add little or nothing to the picture in your mind. Animals that sleep during the daylight hours and come out only at night, like owls, have no color-sensitive cones in their retinas.

The nerve fibers of the retina converge at the back of the eyeball to form the optic nerve. A retina usually contains millions of light receptor cells, so the fibers make a rather thick bundle as they extend backward in the optic nerve to centers in the brain that analyze the light messages and form the pictures of the world that we see as vision.

The lens of the eye is a small disk-shaped transparent structure, about 1/3rd of an inch in diameter, at the front of the eyeball but behind the protective cornea. Under a microscope, a section of lens might give the appearance of a slice of onion because it is composed of numerous concentric layers of transparent membrane. The lens is held in a transparent membrane capsule that is somewhat elastic. In the unborn child the lens is almost spherical and has a slight reddish tint. By adulthood the lens has become convex on the back side and is colorless. In old age the lens tends to become flattened on both the front and back surfaces, slightly opaque, and tinted amber.

THE EYELIDS

ORBICULARIS M.

IRIS

MEIBOMIAN GLANDS

CORNEA

EYE LASHES

CONJUNCTIVA

The front surface of the eyeball is protected by the cornea, which is continuous with the scleral layer of the organ, and the eyelids. The meibomian glands secrete an oil. The conjunctival membrane separates the cornea and the eyelids.

A chamber between the lens and the cornea contains a fluid called the aqueous humor. The fluid, which is nearly pure water, flows into the chamber almost constantly and normally flows out again at the same rate. In some individuals the plumbing system for the aqueous humor chamber malfunctions so that the fluid enters the chamber faster than it drains away. The result is a disease called glaucoma.

Earlier, mention was made of the crossover of motor nerves from the left side of the body to the right side of the brain's motor cortex, and from the right side of the body to the left side of the motor cortex. The nerve fibers from the retina are routed to the brain by a similar yet different method. After passing through the opening in the skull bones behind each of the eyes, the optic nerves meet under the front of the brain where there is a redistribution of nerve fibers. The area where the optic nerve fibers meet is called the optic chiasm, and here all the fibers receiving light inputs from the right side of the visual field are routed to the left side of the brain. At the same time, fibers of the retina that receive light stimuli from the left side of the visual field are directed to the right side of the brain. From the optic chiasm, two reorganized trunks of nerve fibers carry the visual stimuli from the retinas toward the area of the brain that is protected by the occipital portion of the skull, at the back of the head. This is where the brain forms the visual images from coded messages it receives in a more or less continuous stream through millions of nerve fibers, which in turn are connected to rods and cones in the retina.

Each eyeball is attached to six extraocular muscles, so called because they are outside the eyeball. Their job is to move the eyeball up, down, across, diagonally, and so on, as required to follow whatever action in the outside world demands attention at the moment. A seventh extraocular muscle in the orbit has the function of raising the eyebrow. The six extraocular muscles that move the eyeball on each side normally are synchronized to go through the contractions and relaxations needed to produce parallel vision in both eyes. However, if the extraocular muscles become unbalanced, one or both eyes may turn in or out, producing the condition commonly called cross-eyes (eyes turned in) or walleyes (eyes turned out). The medical name for the condition is strabismus.

The lens of the eyeball normally focuses light on the retina like a camera lens focuses light on a piece of film. But whereas the camera lens can be moved closer to or further from the object in order to take a sharp picture, the lens of the eye must change its shape in order to produce a sharp image. The ability of the lens to adjust to changes needed in order to produce a clear image is called accommodation; as one gets older, the eye gradually loses its lens accommodation and the image is projected ahead of or behind the retina instead of squarely on the retina. When the image is focused ahead of the retina, the vision problem is called nearsightedness, or myopia; when behind the retina, farsightedness, or hyperopia.

The lens is not always the culprit in problems of accommodation. Occasionally, the lens of the eye is adequate for normal vision, but the eyeball has a shape that causes the image to fall ahead of or behind the retina. That condition is something like having the right lens in the wrong camera. Farsighted individuals may be able to see distant objects clearly without eyeglasses, and nearsighted persons usually can see objects that are close to the face with minimum effort. But most problems of accommodation are easily corrected with a pair of eyeglasses or contact lenses designed to compensate for variations from normal vision.

Color blindness, which affects men more often than women, usually is an inborn condition involving a failure of the cone cells of the retina to develop normally. A person who is born without ability to distinguish colors generally learns to adapt to the color schemes of the world by distinguishing between lighter and darker shades of gray, differences in brightness of lights, or, as in the case of traffic signals, remembering that there is a standard red-yellow-green pattern from top to bottom.

Some color-blind persons cannot distinguish between blue and yellow, but red-green color blindness is the more common form of the condition. There are several simple tests for color blindness, although there is no medical cure for the problem.

Most lenses, whether man-made for cameras or made by nature for the eye, fail to produce a perfect image without some device that will compensate for the fact that the thin outer edges of lenses focus light rays differently from the thicker centers of the lenses. Man-made lenses are corrected by combinations of different kinds or units of glass. In the human eye nature has built in a corrective device in the form of a special shape for the cornea. Normally, the curvature of the transparent cornea compensates for visual errors that would be produced by light entering the eye along the edges of the lens. But even the corneal curvature is not a completely fail-safe device, with the result that many people develop blurred vision because of the cornea. The blurred vision may involve changes in the lens or the shape of the eyeball, but most commonly the cornea surface becomes irregular and the visual difficulty that results is known as astigmatism. Injury or inflammation frequently lead to astigmatism, and a contributing factor may be pressure on the eyelids. Many ophthalmologists believe that frequent rubbing of the closed eyes will eventually distort the normal curvature of the cornea and cause astigmatism.

The Ears

The ears are provided a greater share of protection from the environment than the organs of vision. The eyes are quite literally "out front" and are shielded from injury and infection by the cornea and the eyelids, composed of the thinnest skin layer of the entire body. The organs of hearing, while not invulnerable, are at least recessed in bony caverns of the skull. Even the eardrum, or tympanic membrane, the surface exposed to the outside environment, is located within the skull. The parts of the ear that can be seen outside the skull are the auricle, that portion of skin-covered cartilage which protrudes from the head on either side, and the ear canal, the inch-long tunnel that leads from the external ear to the eardrum.

The human ear sometimes is divided into three sections for purposes of explaining how the sense of hearing works: the external ear, including the ear canal; the middle ear, an air-filled space between the eardrum and the inner ear; and the inner ear, where the sound waves collected by the external ear are finally translated into specific sounds.

The role of the external ear involves the collection of sound waves, which are vibrations of the air at different frequencies. The external ear and ear canal form a sort of funnel which directs the sound waves toward the eardrum or typanic membrane. The sound waves pound on the eardrum's surface, which vibrates at the frequency and intensity of whatever has produced the noise, music, speech, etc.

Humans do not hear the full range of sounds that permeate the environment, and with increasing age the ability to hear even the higher, normally audible frequencies is lost. It is believed that a newborn baby can hear sounds in a range of about 16 cycles per second up to 40,000 cycles per second (CPS). A normal adult usually can perceive frequencies as high as

MIDDLE EAR CAVITY, TYMPANIC MEMBRANE, AND EUSTACHIAN TUBE

TYMPANIC MEMBRANE

MIDDLE EAR CAVITY

EUSTACHIAN TUBE

BONE

CARTILAGE

PHARYNX

Human skull bones provide support and protection for the delicate nerve structures associated with the sense of hearing. This drawing shows the middle ear cavity, surrounded by bone and protected from the outside by the tympanic membrane. The eustachian tube leading from the middle ear to the pharynx, or throat, permits the air pressure in the middle ear to adjust to the air pressure of the outside environment.

20,000 CPS, but in later years hearing is considered normal if sounds of up to 10,000 CPS can be detected. Because most human conversation utilizes frequencies between 250 and 2,000 CPS, the restricted hearing of older persons may be adequate for most purposes.

The intensity of most human conversation is rated at about 60 decibels, which is a technical term for measuring the pressure of sound and simply means loudness. The decibel system of measuring loudness follows a rather complex mathematical procedure that shows that every time the number of decibels of loudness increases by six, the sound pressure actually has doubled. Or more precisely, a sound of 120 decibels is 1,000 times more intense than a 60-decibel sound. As points of reference, a 120-decibel sound is loud enough to cause ear pain but is still less intense than the sound of a jet airplane engine at a distance of 30 feet from the observer.

The middle ear contains three of the smallest bones in the body. They are sometimes identified by their common names of hammer, anvil, and stirrup, and also by their Latin medical names of malleus, incus, and stapes, respectively. Together the three bones are known as the ossicles. They transmit sound from the eardrum to the inner ear and accomplish this task through a unique sort of linkage. The malleus rests against the eardrum and transmits sound wave vibrations by the ear drum membrane to the incus by means of a pounding action which in turn is relayed to the stapes, or stirrup. The stapes acts as a piston that pushes on a tiny window on the side of the inner ear.

Scientists have calculated that nature designed the middle ear so that the ossicles would increase the intensity of sound vibrations between the tympanic membrane, or eardrum, and the oval window of the inner ear by a ratio of 26 decibels. The middle ear, thus, serves as a kind of sound transformer to insure that sound waves trapped in the ear canal are transmitted to the inner ear mechanisms without a significant loss of intensity.

The reason for this kind of mechanical leverage to increase sound intensity is that the inner ear is filled with fluid, which tends to reflect sound waves. If you have ever held your head under water in a swimming pool and tried to understand the conversation of other persons talking in the air above the water, you would have some grasp of nature's need to evolve some mechanism that would allow descendants of marine creatures to understand sounds made by air vibrations.

Mention should be made at this point of

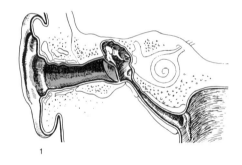

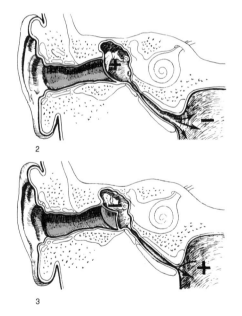

Drawings of the middle ear and surrounding areas show what happens when air pressure within the middle ear becomes out of balance with the air in the environment outside the body. The first picture shows the middle ear under normal conditions; the eustachian tube is open and air pressure inside and outside of the ear is equalized. The second picture shows what happens when a person ascends rapidly in an elevator or airplane: the ear drum bulges outward and air flows down the eustachian tube toward the pharynx. In the third drawing, the ear shows the effects of suddenly descending from a higher altitude: low air pressure within the middle ear causes the ear drum to bulge inward, displacing the tiny bones that transmit sounds, and the eustachian tube closes so that air at ground level pressure cannot enter the middle ear to correct the imbalance. The result is the condition known as barotitis, or middle ear discomfort, which sometimes can be helped by chewing gum, yawning, or sipping a fluid to open the eustachian tube by activating the muscles controlling the airway.

two openings of the middle ear into other areas of the skull. One opening from the middle ear leads to the mastoid air spaces near the ear; the other opening is a connection with the eustachian tube that leads to the back of the throat. The purpose of the eustachian, or auditory, tube is to equalize the air pressure in the middle ear with the atmospheric pressure outside the body. Sometimes during airplane flights, rapid descents in elevators, or as a result of respiratory diseases, the eustachian tube becomes blocked so that air in the middle ear does not become properly equalized with air outside the body. The middle ear connections from the throat to the mastoid areas also offer opportunities for the spread of infections from one part of the head and neck area to another.

A facial nerve trunk passes near the mastoid bone, the middle ear, and the inner ear. The nerve supplies the nerve endings that control the muscles involved in facial expressions. While the position of the nerve may be of no more than aca-

demic interest to the average person, an examining doctor may find the condition of the facial nerve a clue to effects of a disease or injury involving the ear. A health problem affecting the ear could result in partial or complete paralysis of the facial nerve.

The inner ear actually consists of two separate organs. One is the final step in the phenomenon of translating sound waves into nerve impulses, an apparatus called the organ of Corti, or the "true organ of hearing." The other organ is the vestibular apparatus which helps give an individual a sense of equilibrium, or balance.

The organ of Corti is enclosed in a bony structure called the cochlea, a snail-shaped spiral tunnel that coils around about two and a half turns and contains small hair cells. As sound waves from the outside are transmitted through the middle ear to the oval window of the cochlea and translated into fluid vibrations, the fluid movements displace the position of

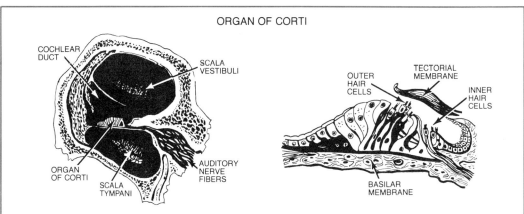

ORGAN OF CORTI

COCHLEAR DUCT
SCALA VESTIBULI
OUTER HAIR CELLS
TECTORIAL MEMBRANE
INNER HAIR CELLS
ORGAN OF CORTI
AUDITORY NERVE FIBERS
SCALA TYMPANI
BASILAR MEMBRANE

The organ of Corti is the true organ of hearing and is located in a section of the inner skull next to the brain. Sound waves translated through the middle ear bones to the inner ear cause vibrations that are sensed by hair cells and transmitted as nerve impulses along the fibers of the auditory nerves.

the hair cells. As the hair cells move in response to variations in frequency and intensity of the fluid vibrations, the movements produce electrical signals that are routed to the brain. The brain receives the myriad signals from the hair cells in the organ of Corti, and translates the bits of data into an audio image that we recognize as some meaningful sound, or in many cases as meaningless noise. An injury or disease affecting any of the steps involved in receiving or translating sound waves, from the eardrum to the ossicles, the fluid in the organ of Corti, or the auditory nerves, can result in partial or total deafness.

The vestibular apparatus extends beyond the cochlea portion of the inner ear, on the other side of the oval window that receives waves of sound pressure from the middle ear. The organ of balance within the vestibular apparatus depends upon fluid movements within three semi-circular canals, or tubes, that are set at right angles to each other. The arrangement is similar to that of three adjacent sides of a cube that come together at one corner. The semicircular canals contain hair cells that are mounted in a gelatinous substance. The hair cells are nerve endings designed by nature to detect movements of the head.

If the head is moved upward, downward, or at some angle, the pull of gravity on the fluid in the semicircular canals is noted by the hair cells as the movement of fluid is "felt" by the nerve receptors. Signals from the vestibular hair cells are carried to the brain by a separate nerve trunk that runs parallel to the nerve that picks up sound messages from the organ of Corti.

In addition to the sense of balance provided by the nerve endings in the semicir-cular canals, two small sacs in the inner ear monitor changes in velocity of the human body when it is in motion. The tiny structures, called the saccule and the utricle, contain small grains of limestone, or calcium carbonate. The grains of limestone rest on a layer of hair cells embedded in a gelatin-like material. Any sudden movement of the head causes the limestone grains to shift position among the hair cells, which are nerve receptors, and this action produces signals to the brain. The sensation you feel when you are in an automobile or jet aircraft that suddenly increases its speed, or comes to a sudden stop, usually is due to the movement of the tiny grains of limestone in your inner ear structures.

The Nose

Two more prominent features of the head are the nose and mouth. The nose has the obvious functions of providing a passageway for air entering and leaving the lungs and of housing the body's organ of smell. The nose contains structures that screen and condition the air entering the lungs, and it offers the head an opening for drainage and for equalizing air pressure in the middle ear and sinuses. Some of these continuing functions are masked by the external nose, the structure of bone, cartilage, and skin that we observe when looking at the noses of other people or at our own nose as it appears in a mirror. The internal nose, the part we seldom if ever see, is where the nasal action is, and it is the area of most interest to a doctor examining the head and neck area.

The internal nose is divided near the midline by a wall of cartilage and bone called the nasal septum. On either side of the septum at the entrance to the nose are

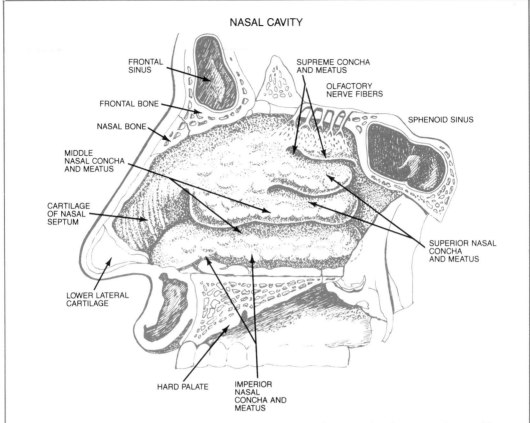

NASAL CAVITY

FRONTAL SINUS

FRONTAL BONE

NASAL BONE

MIDDLE NASAL CONCHA AND MEATUS

CARTILAGE OF NASAL SEPTUM

LOWER LATERAL CARTILAGE

SUPREME CONCHA AND MEATUS

OLFACTORY NERVE FIBERS

SPHENOID SINUS

SUPERIOR NASAL CONCHA AND MEATUS

HARD PALATE

IMPERIOR NASAL CONCHA AND MEATUS

An inside look at a human nasal cavity. Drawing shows two of the sinuses, or air spaces, associated with the respiratory system and the nasal conchae, or convoluted surfaces that help raise the temperature of inhaled air to near-normal body temperature be-fore it continues into the pharynx, trachea, and lungs. At the roof of the nasal cavity are the olfactory nerve fibers which detect odors. The meatus situated in the conchae is an opening into an air cell or other space in the head.

the nostrils, or nares. On the walls of the septum are a series of folds, called turbinates, which have the job of helping to condition the air entering through the nostrils. The folds of turbinate tissue increase the amount of surface exposed to the incoming air so that the temperature of the air can be warmed or cooled a bit before it passes into the throat and lungs.

The internal walls of the nose, including the surfaces of the turbinates, are covered with mucous membrane with cells that secrete mucus. The mucus helps moderate the temperature and humidity of inhaled air. It also traps some of the dust and bacteria entering the body through the nose. In a cold environment the flow of mucus frequently is increased—an effect felt as a "runny nose." If the environment is unusually dry, the mucous membranes may lose moisture too rapidly through mucus secretion and become irritated.

Hairlike filaments called cilia, lining the inner membrane surfaces of the nose, contribute to the business of filtering the incoming air. The cilia wave back and forth rapidly to catch dust and other foreign particles in the air. Another type of hairlike process in the mucous membrane of the internal nose is an olfactory hair, actually a nerve receptor for the sense of smell. The septum is thickly laced with the olfactory hairs, which lead to an olfactory bulb on the floor of the cranium. The olfactory bulb is the front end of the olfactory nerve trunk that extends back into the brain's center for evaluating odors and aromas.

The septum occasionally becomes deviated in its normal location along the midline of the internal nose. A deviated septum can be the result of an injury or a congenital disorder, that is, an abnormal condition existing at birth. The septum can become perforated as a result of a disease such as tuberculosis, from use of cocaine, or by exposure to toxic fumes in an industrial plant. A small perforation of the septum can cause a whistling sound when the individual breathes heavily, a problem that usually can be corrected by surgery. A septum change can alter the sound of one's voice because the individual design of one's nose influences the tone of a person's speech. A network of blood vessels in the septum is vulnerable to injury and is the source of nosebleeds that occur after the nose encounters an immovable object.

The sinuses are irregular air spaces in the bones that border the nasal bone. There are four major sinuses on each side of the nose, and occasionally there may be additional air spaces, depending upon how the facial bones develop in an individual's skull. In some people the frontal sinuses may fail to develop in the forehead area above the eyes; in others the frontal sinus may develop on the right side but not on the left side of the nose. The maxillary sinuses, which are located beneath the eye orbits and alongside the nose on either side, are the first—and largest—sinuses to develop. The sinus cavities usually are lined with the same kind of mucous membrane containing cilia that is found in the two chambers of the nose itself.

The cilia apparently help sweep sinus secretions toward the nasal cavity. Because of the openings to the nasal cavity and the circulation of air from the nose, the sinuses are easily irritated and infected by foreign substances in the inhaled air. Bacteria and viruses may be forced into the sinuses from the nasal cavity when blowing one's nose.

The Mouth

The mouth, like the nose and sinus cavities, helps shape the sound of one's voice by its own shape. The mouth is a source of air when breathing through the nose is difficult, although the mouth lacks the cilia and mucus facilities for conditioning inhaled air. But a primary function of the mouth is mastication, or chewing food, with the sense of taste serving as an auxiliary organ of processing food for the digestive system. The mouth also contains the teeth and tongue, which aid in vocalization as well as in mastication, and the major salivary glands of the body.

The roof of the mouth is called the palate. A hard palate with a bony framework extends over the front two-thirds of the mouth area. The soft palate covering the

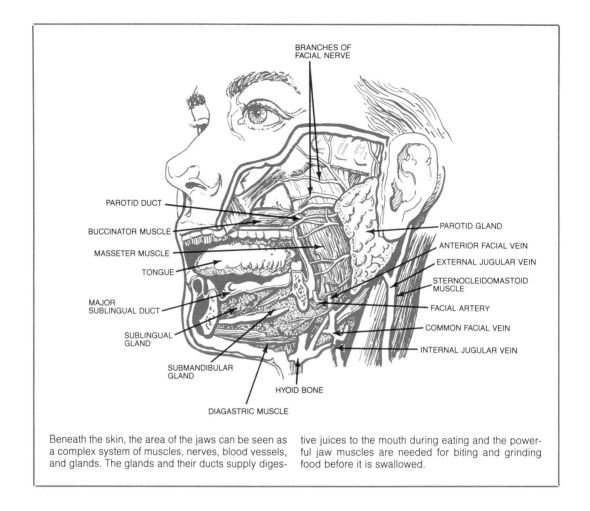

BRANCHES OF
FACIAL NERVE

PAROTID DUCT

BUCCINATOR MUSCLE

MASSETER MUSCLE

TONGUE

MAJOR
SUBLINGUAL DUCT

SUBLINGUAL
GLAND

SUBMANDIBULAR
GLAND

DIAGASTRIC MUSCLE

HYOID BONE

PAROTID GLAND

ANTERIOR FACIAL VEIN

EXTERNAL JUGULAR VEIN

STERNOCLEIDOMASTOID
MUSCLE

FACIAL ARTERY

COMMON FACIAL VEIN

INTERNAL JUGULAR VEIN

Beneath the skin, the area of the jaws can be seen as a complex system of muscles, nerves, blood vessels, and glands. The glands and their ducts supply digestive juices to the mouth during eating and the powerful jaw muscles are needed for biting and grinding food before it is swallowed.

rest of the mouth is composed of muscle and connective tissue. The palate forms a partition between the mouth and the nasal cavity.

The tongue is a bundle of muscle covered with a rough membrane, which contains taste buds. The tongue pretty well fills the mouth, or oral cavity. Being quite flexible and mobile for a muscle, the tongue can change its shape from concave to convex, or vice versa, push against the palate or flat against the floor of the mouth, and can move from side to side. All of these movements are involved in the process of chewing food.

We usually see only the front, or body, of the tongue when we look into a mirror, or examine somebody else's tongue. The root of the tongue, sometimes called the base, has a somewhat different type of surface from the part that is usually visible. The base of the tongue contains dozens of elevations called lingual tonsils, which are associated with the lymphatic system. There also is a blind pouch called the foramen cecum. And along a V-shaped line separating the front of the tongue from the base are about ten large wart-like papillae lined with taste buds.

Other taste buds are scattered over the surface of the tongue as tiny papillae that give the tongue its rough texture. The taste buds are sensitive to four different sensations: sweetness, sourness, salt, and bitterness. Taste buds at the back of the tongue seem to be more sensitive to bitter flavors, while the tip of the tongue appears to be more sensitive to sweet tastes. Taste buds on the sides of the tongue detect sourness and salt. Biologists claim that humans may be less sensitive to food flavors than other mammals; an average human has about 3,000 taste buds scattered about his tongue and mouth, while a cow may have 35,000 taste buds and some wild animals have even more.

Under and behind the tongue, situated between the skull and tissues covering it, are several rather large salivary glands.

The saliva secreted by these glands is a clear, rather viscous fluid that has a number of health functions, including that of maintaining a moist environment for the teeth, tongue, and other surfaces of the oral cavity. Saliva is needed to help humans digest starch, and it contains an enzyme that helps break up large molecules of plant starch so they can be digested. It is not unusual for an average person's salivary glands to produce more than one quart of saliva a day.

The salivary glands may be the source of a variety of health problems. The parotid glands, along the jaws, become swollen and painfully tender during an infection of mumps virus. The parotid and other salivary glands can become swollen as an allergic reaction to certain medicines. The salivary glands also may become swollen as a result of a bacterial infection or blockage of a duct that normally allows a gland to empty into the mouth. The sali-

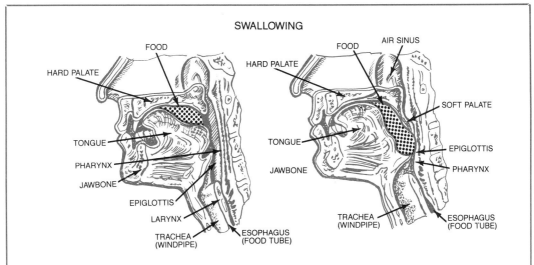

SWALLOWING

The tongue is a powerful mass of muscle that helps in chewing and swallowing food. In swallowing, the tongue presses against the hard palate and pushes chewed food to the back of the mouth where it enters the esophagus while the epiglottis drops over the trachea to keep food out of the windpipe.

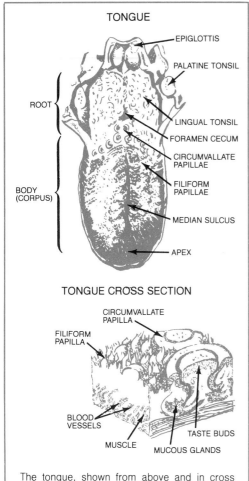

TONGUE

- EPIGLOTTIS
- PALATINE TONSIL
- ROOT
- LINGUAL TONSIL
- FORAMEN CECUM
- CIRCUMVALLATE PAPILLAE
- FILIFORM PAPILLAE
- BODY (CORPUS)
- MEDIAN SULCUS
- APEX

TONGUE CROSS SECTION

- CIRCUMVALLATE PAPILLA
- FILIFORM PAPILLA
- BLOOD VESSELS
- MUSCLE
- TASTE BUDS
- MUCOUS GLANDS

The tongue, shown from above and in cross section, reveals the location and design of the taste buds and tonsils. The taste buds are found in tiny trenches surrounding the centers of the circumvallate papillae. The filiform papillae are covered with hard scalelike cells that may accumulate during digestive upsets to produce the "furry tongue" effect.

vary glands sometimes become the sites for various kinds of tumors.

The Teeth. Humans normally are born with buds for two sets of teeth. The first set, called the deciduous or milk teeth, begin to appear around the age of six months. When a child is about two years old, the complete set of 20 milk teeth usually are in place. The first of the second set of teeth, the permanent teeth, may begin to replace the milk teeth as early in life as the age of five. The last of the set, the wisdom teeth, may not break through the surface of the gums until the age of 25, and in some cases do not appear at all.

The part of the tooth that rests in a socket of the jaw is known as the root. The portion extending above the normal gumline is called the crown. A tooth is not firmly set in the jawbone but instead is held in place by a network of connective tissue which allows for a bit of independent movement by the tooth so it will "give" a little when chewing. The outer surface of the crown of the tooth is covered with a layer of compacted minerals, including calcium, phosphorus, and magnesium. The enamel has no nerves or blood vessels. Beneath the enamel and throughout the root, the tooth is composed mainly of a bony substance called dentine. Within the dentine layer is the pulp cavity, which is filled with nerves and with blood and lymph vessels. The nerves and the blood and lymph vessels are connected through openings in the bottom of the roots, or root canals, with the nervous and circulatory systems of the rest of the body.

The nerve fibers extending into the pulp cavity, beneath the layers of dentine and enamel, are the source of delicate pain when a cavity develops, or when very hot or very cold foods come in contact with the teeth. Tooth enamel is designed by nature to last a lifetime for eating most kinds of meats, vegetables, and fruits, but the enamel is easily penetrated by acids produced by bacteria in the mouth. The bacteria thrive on food particles that remain after a meal, particularly refined sugars, and the acids produced by their bodies are in effect the excrement of the bacteria. If the bacteria can find a small crack or defect leading to the dentine, they can expand the defect all the way into the pulp cavity in a very short period of time.

Our teeth are inherited from prehuman ancestors, so the number and arrangement of the teeth follow a more or less standard pattern. Incisors and canine teeth are located at the front of the jaw for cutting and tearing food into smaller pieces. The molars, at the rear of the jaw, grind and pulverize food. The arrangement of the 32 permanent teeth follows the same general pattern on either side of the upper and lower jaws. Starting from the midline and working toward the back of the jaw, there should be two incisors, one canine, two premolars, and three molars on both sides, upper and lower. If a map were made of the arrangement of your teeth as they should appear when you smile into a mirror, it would look something like this:

MMMPPCII IICPPMMM
MMMPPCII IICPPMMM

with M for molar, P for premolar, C for canine, and I for incisor.

The outside, or third molars, are the wisdom teeth and the last to erupt. Some individuals do not have third molars, which probably are not as important as they once were when humans ate foods that required more grinding and pulverizing before they could be digested. On the other hand, some individuals occasionally

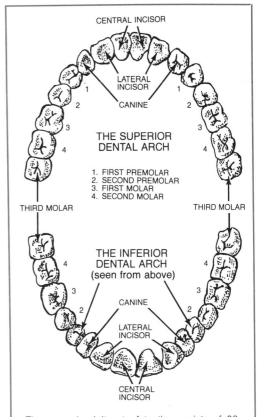

CENTRAL INCISOR

LATERAL INCISOR

CANINE

THE SUPERIOR DENTAL ARCH

1. FIRST PREMOLAR
2. SECOND PREMOLAR
3. FIRST MOLAR
4. SECOND MOLAR

THIRD MOLAR   THIRD MOLAR

THE INFERIOR DENTAL ARCH (seen from above)

CANINE

LATERAL INCISOR

CENTRAL INCISOR

The normal adult set of teeth consists of 32, eight on either side of each jaw. Each group of eight teeth follows a similar pattern, starting with a central incisor at the front of the jaw. Next is a lateral incisor and a canine. The remaining five teeth in each group of eight consists of first and second premolars, and first, second, and third molars.

develop fourth molars, which was standard dental equipment in humans who lived thousands of years ago.

Vital Parts of the Neck

Beyond the teeth and tongue is a mucous membrane-lined muscular funnel that connects the mouth and nose to the passage-

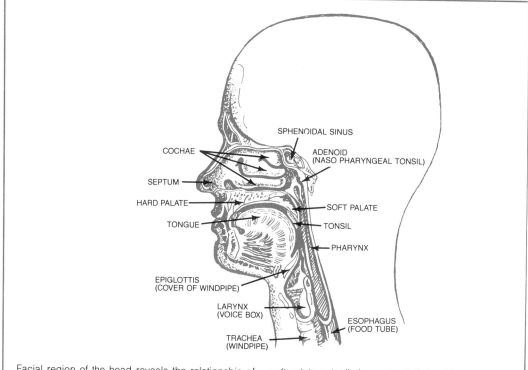

COCHAE

SPHENOIDAL SINUS

ADENOID
(NASO PHARYNGEAL TONSIL)

SEPTUM

HARD PALATE

SOFT PALATE

TONGUE

TONSIL

PHARYNX

EPIGLOTTIS
(COVER OF WINDPIPE)

LARYNX
(VOICE BOX)

ESOPHAGUS
(FOOD TUBE)

TRACHEA
(WINDPIPE)

Facial region of the head reveals the relationship of the pharynx to the nose, mouth, throat, and sinuses. Adenoid tissue in the area of the pharynx above the soft palate actually is a potentially troublesome tonsil that may be infected by organisms entering the body through the nose.

ways inside the neck that lead to the lungs and stomach. The funnel is known as the pharynx. For a part of its length, this tube serves as a common pathway for air, food, and drink. Under normal circumstances the air and food are routed into the proper channels with the help of a flap of tissue called the epiglottis. The epiglottis, at the base of the tongue, drops down over the opening of the trachea when food is swallowed, thereby preventing food or beverage from entering the lungs. Almost everyone has at some time or other experienced a failure of this fail-safe device, an experience marked by mild or possibly severe choking. Much more common and far less serious is the alternative problem of swallowing air, which can be relieved by belching. A piece of food that might be too large to swallow into the esophagus can become lodged over the epiglottis and interfere with normal breathing. The piece of food should be removed as quickly as possible, using approved first aid techniques, because unconsciousness and death can follow within a very few minutes after breathing is interrupted. A person whose breathing is blocked by a piece of food is unable to speak and therefore cannot explain the problem vocally; voice sounds are made by the passage of air over the vocal cords in the larynx, or voice box.

The vocal cords of the larynx are located in the neck between the trachea and the epiglottis. The larynx itself is a funnel-shaped group of cartilages, stacked one above the other, with the trachea opening at the bottom of the stack. The vocal cords are shielded by an incomplete ring of cartilage in the stack that is called the thyroid cartilage by doctors and is commonly known as the Adam's apple. The Adam's apple also participates in the swallowing action; when a person starts to swallow food or beverage, the Adam's apple can be seen moving upward to help seal the closure of the epiglottis.

The vocal cords are two folds of membrane across the open part of the larynx, or voice box. They are held in place by an

FRONT VIEW OF LARYNX

EPIGLOTTIS
HYOID BONE
THYROHYOID MEMBRANE
THYROID CARTILAGE
CRICOTHYROID LIGAMENT
CRICOID CARTILAGE
CARTILAGE RINGS

Front view of the larynx shows the relationship of the cartilage rings and other tissues that form the throat beneath the skin. The larynx extends from the base of the tongue to the top of the trachea, which divides into the bronchial tubes leading to the lungs.

INTERIOR VIEW OF THE LARYNX

BASE OF TONGUE
VOCAL CORD
EPIGLOTTIS
FALSE CORD
ARYTENOID CARTILAGE
GLOTTIS

When the doctor looks into a patient's throat he may see a view like the one in the drawing with the vocal cords separated. During speech, the vocal cords are brought closer together by the arytenoid cartilages. Width of the glottis is a factor in the tone produced by the vocal cords.

attachment to the front of the larynx wall, and at the rear by two pieces of cartilage attached to small muscles. As the muscles contract or relax, tension is increased or decreased on the vocal cords so that they are moved back and forth over the air passageway of the larynx. Ordinarily, the vocal cords are held at the sides of the voice box while air is inhaled and the sounds that become the voice are produced during exhalation. It is the pressure of air being expelled from the lungs that determines the loudness of the voice. The length and tension of the vocal cords determines the pitch of the voice.

The oral cavity, nasal cavity, sinus cavities, pharynx, and other body structures contribute to individual voice qualities by their resonating factors. Longer resonating cavities of the body tend to lower the pitch of the voice, just as changing the size of the resonating cavity of a wind instrument alters the pitch of the music produced. The lips, tongue, and soft palate are coordinated with the vocal cords and resonating cavities to produce words of speech.

While the larynx is rather well known for its role in producing voice sounds, it also has some less well-known functions. For example, the larynx must be closed for an instant before coughing in order to build up enough lung and abdominal pressure to produce an effective cough. Closing the larynx may be necessary to increase internal body pressures for defecation and urination. Even the intra-abdominal pressure utilized in childbirth depends upon an ability to close the larynx, a facility that may be lost in some individuals because of disease or injury.

Medical Problems of the Head and Neck

The head and neck areas probably offer as many varied health conditions as any other section of the human body. Most of the different kinds of medical specialists are involved in treating the head and neck. They include opthalmologists, dentists, plastic surgeons, neurosurgeons, orthopedic surgeons, and so on.

A health problem as ordinary as a headache can involve a wide range of possible causes and effects, including hypertension, contraction of neck muscles, a blocked artery, brain tumor, cerebral hemorrhage, bacterial infection, eye strain, fever, and sinusitis, to name a few of the more common disorders associated with headaches. An examining doctor may have to consider any or all possible ailments of which a headache is a symptom when a patient makes an appointment because of a headache complaint. The small fraction of one's body extending from the top of the scalp to the Adam's apple contains a highly complex combination of networks of blood vessels, nerves, bone structures, skin and connective tissue variations, glands, muscles, special sense organs, and apparatus associated with breathing. In addition, the head and neck areas contain assorted cavities and pathways for infectious organisms to enter the body and spread quickly to other regions.

Besides the disorders that may involve the head and neck areas directly, the diagnosing physician frequently finds clues in examining this region that may help determine or confirm an abnormal health problem involving other parts of the body. A recessed nasal bridge, for example, could be a sign of achondroplasia, a unique sign of a rare hereditary bone disease that may be revealed by careful examination of the head. A soft, raised yellowish plaque on the eyelid may be a sign that the individual may have an abnormally high level of cholesterol in his blood. Swollen bleeding gums may signal a vitamin C deficiency.

The doctor's examination of your head and neck area will include in some detail your hearing, vision, nose, mouth, and pharynx. He probably will inspect the neck, including the skin, and may ask that you tilt your head forward and backward as far as possible, and rotate your head as far to the right and left as possible without moving the shoulders. The doctor may take your head in his hands and gently move the head through the same range of motion tests that you did on your own. If you have complained of pain or injury involving the head and neck areas, however, the doctor may skip the range of motion tests.

The doctor also is likely to palpate the sides of the neck to see if he can find masses under the skin that could be enlarged lymph nodes. These enlargements frequently can be detected by running the fingertips back and forth along the skin below the jaw while the head is tilted backward, and to the opposite side of the area palpated. There are normal structures in the neck that are not lymph nodes, but an experienced doctor usually can tell what's normal and what's not.

Examination of the Eyes

Detailed eye examinations usually are handled by a specialist such as an ophthalmologist. A doctor making a quick check

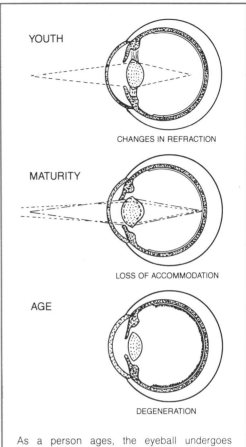

YOUTH

CHANGES IN REFRACTION

MATURITY

LOSS OF ACCOMMODATION

AGE

DEGENERATION

As a person ages, the eyeball undergoes changes that may interfere with normal vision. A common problem is the loss of accommodation due to a loss in the ability of the eye to adjust to far and near images. Changes in refraction also occur during a normal life span and a far-sighted person may gradually become near-sighted. In addition to changes in vision due to altered lenses or corneas, the retina may undergo degeneration, resulting in blindness.

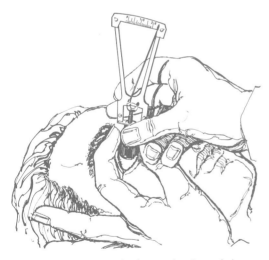

The doctor checks a patient's eyes for signs of glaucoma with an instrument called a tonometer. Eyedrops containing an anesthetic are applied before the tonometer is placed over the surface of the eyeball. The tonometer measures the pressure of fluid within the eyeball. Abnormally high pressure is a cause of glaucoma, which results in blindness if not corrected by medicine or surgery.

of your vision, along with other body functions, may ask you to read a line or two from a newspaper. One eye at a time will be checked, the other eye being covered during the reading test. The test may be repeated for persons who wear eyeglasses—once while wearing the glasses and once without. If one's eyesight is obviously poor, the doctor may try an additional simple test, such as having you count the fingers he will hold a certain distance from the eyes.

The doctor will try to determine if the eyes are steady or if one or both may turn inward or outward, or otherwise lack coordination. This test may be conducted by having the patient follow a lighted flashlight or the doctor's finger through a series of motions. By moving the light or finger from a point near the bridge of the patient's nose straight outward for a distance of several feet, then back again directly toward the nose, the doctor usually can tell whether both eyes track the object together or if one eye turns inward or outward when the moving target is a few inches away from the face.

The doctor may darken the room and sweep a flashlight beam from side to side

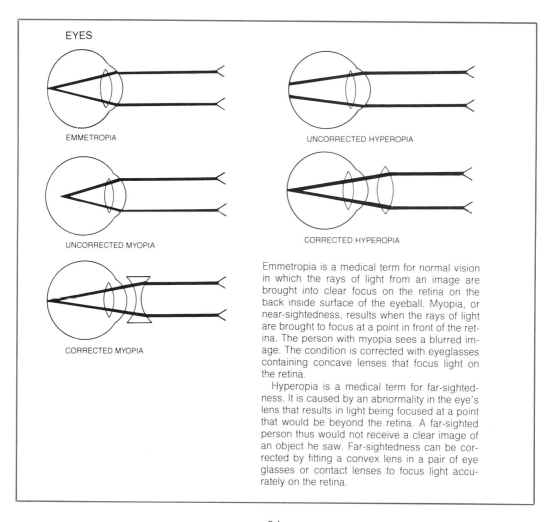

EYES

EMMETROPIA

UNCORRECTED HYPEROPIA

UNCORRECTED MYOPIA

CORRECTED HYPEROPIA

CORRECTED MYOPIA

Emmetropia is a medical term for normal vision in which the rays of light from an image are brought into clear focus on the retina on the back inside surface of the eyeball. Myopia, or near-sightedness, results when the rays of light are brought to focus at a point in front of the retina. The person with myopia sees a blurred image. The condition is corrected with eyeglasses containing concave lenses that focus light on the retina.

Hyperopia is a medical term for far-sightedness. It is caused by an abnormality in the eye's lens that results in light being focused at a point that would be beyond the retina. A far-sighted person thus would not receive a clear image of an object he saw. Far-sightedness can be corrected by fitting a convex lens in a pair of eye glasses or contact lenses to focus light accurately on the retina.

across the face in a slow motion. Normally, the pupil of each eye will contract when the light beam crosses it, after dilating or expanding when the room was darkened. As a substitute for the light in a darkened room, the doctor may place his hands over the patient's eyes so that the pupils will dilate, and then quickly uncover each eye, one at a time, to watch the pupils contract. The pupils should be of the same diameter when dilated or contracted. The pupils of older persons' eyes may react sluggishly to changes from darkness to bright light, or vice versa, and this might be a sign of aging rather than a clue to a health problem. The pupils' failure to constrict from exposure to bright light could be a sign of several kinds of infection, botulism, lead poisoning, or the use of narcotics.

A red reflection from the pupil while testing with a flashlight usually is considered a sign that the lens behind the pupil is normal. A whitish reflection usually is a sign of an opaque cataract in the lens. The pupil should appear black when not reflecting light. The cornea of the eye should be clear and glasslike. A fine, gray, opaque band around the cornea can be a sign of excess lipids, or fatty substances, in the blood of young persons, but they may be considered a normal condition for a person over the age of 60. Scratches, infections such as herpes simplex, and injuries can produce a grayish, lackluster appearance in the normally glistening cornea tissue.

As part of the general eye examination, the doctor usually inspects the eyelids for any signs of crusting pus, xanthelasmas—painless yellow plaques that may indicate a high level of cholesterol in the bloodstream—or reddening that might be a sign of a sinus infection. If there has been injury to the eyelid, producing a "black

CONJUNCTIVITIS

Conjunctivitis is marked by an inflammation of the conjunctiva, the membrane separating the front of the eyeball from the inner lining of the eyelids. See illustration page 76.

eye," or palpebral hematoma, the doctor probably will want to make a further check of the condition of the skull and head tissues. A black eye can appear hours or even days after an injury that does not involve the eyelid directly, and the farther away from the eye the injury was, the greater is the time lapse. A nasal fracture, for example, might result in a black eye within hours after the injury, whereas a fracture of the back of the skull can produce the black eye effect several days later.

Examination of the Ears

Just as a quick examination of the eyes may begin with a simple reading test, a brief check of the ears may start with a basic hearing test. The doctor may hold a watch next to the ear and slowly move it away until it can no longer be heard.

The ear canal is examined with an otoscope, an instrument with a light, a magnifying lens, and a speculum, or funnel-shaped device that gently holds back the tissues along the barrel of the ear canal while it is being inspected with light and lens. Because the external ear canal is slightly curved, the external ear usually has to be pulled a bit backward and upward to straighten the fleshy tunnel. If the ear canal is not blocked by a plug of cerumen, or ear wax, the doctor should be able to inspect the eardrum, or tympanic membrane, while looking into the ear canal with the otoscope. Some doctors use a special kind of otoscope with a rubber bulb attached; the device, a pneumatic otoscope, can move the eardrum a bit with changing air pressure while the doctor observes the effect through a lens.

Since the eustachian tube is associated with the middle ear, the doctor usually will inspect the opening from the throat by inserting a mirror in the mouth. If it appears that the eustachian tube is blocked on either side, the doctor can force a little compressed air through one nostril while holding the other closed to clear the passage. The eustachian tube also can be forced open occasionally by practicing either the Valsalva maneuver or the Toynbee maneuver. The Valsalva maneuver consists of holding the mouth and nose closed while exhaling; the Toynbee maneuver is similar except that one swallows while holding the nose and mouth closed. Under normal circumstances, either swallowing or forcibly exhaling with the mouth closed and the nostrils held shut will open a blocked eustachian tube.

The doctor may give an additional hearing test by holding a vibrating tuning fork an inch or so away from each ear and repeating the test with the tip of the vibrating tuning fork placed over the mastoid bone behind the ear. The results of the test will indicate the relative ability to detect sound as transmitted by air vibrations versus conduction of the same tone by the bone surrounding the ear canal. Then the doctor may place the vibrating tuning fork in the middle of the forehead or on the nasal bone ridge and ask whether the sound can be heard better in the left ear or the right ear. If one has difficulty in hearing, the tuning fork tests can help locate the cause of the problem. A disorder involving the organ of Corti or some other part of the inner ear, including the auditory nerve, will be reflected in better hearing in one ear when the tuning fork is placed midway between the ears, because air conduction will be more effective than bone conduction. If the problem involves the eardrum or the middle ear, hearing will be better when transmitted through the bone than when the tuning fork is held outside the external ear. And sound will be heard in the poorer ear when the tuning fork is touched to the nose or forehead if there is a defect in the eardrum or middle ear bones.

When a patient has a known hearing problem and a simple cause such as excessive ear wax has been ruled out, an examining physician with the proper equipment may want to check the ears in greater detail. One technique is to present tones of various frequencies and intensities through a headphone, starting with the good ear as a relatively normal hearing benchmark. The doctor starts sending tones at a measured loudness, in known decibels, that should be well above the patient's hearing threshold. The tone is repeated for one or two seconds at a time at lower and lower levels of loudness, or intensity, until it can no longer be heard. The intensity usually is raised and lowered a few decibels at a time, above or below the level at which the tone can just barely be heard. After the threshold of hearing for that particular tone has been found, the tests are repeated for various other frequencies. The various tone frequencies and intensities are recorded on a chart called an audiogram, which is used to analyze a person's range of hearing.

If a hearing problem appears to be due to a disease or injury involving the inner ear or the auditory nerve, the same kind of hearing test is conducted. Instead of transmitting the tones through earphones, however, the sounds are sent through a vibrator placed over the mastoid bone behind the ear. Normal hearing levels measured by audiograms are close to zero decibels, although persons whose threshold for certain frequencies may be as high as 15 decibels may be considered to have normal hearing. A variation of more than 15 decibels from the minimum hearing threshold is classified abnormal.

Several ear conditions of varying seriousness may attract special interest by an examining physician. Excessive ear wax, or cerumen, in the ear canal may result in hearing loss, discomfort, and other disorders, including the development of cerumen plaques that may lead to irritation and infection. Infections of the ear canal may be caused by bacteria or fungi. The infections may result when the patient tries to remove ear wax with a hairpin, paper clip, toothpick, or similar object, and gouges a hole in the membrane lining the canal. Fever, pain, and swelling of tissues are common signs of infection of the ear canal. Fungal infections are most likely to develop in warm, humid climates and have similar signs and symptoms.

Irritation of the ear canal, which may be marked by swelling and redness or thick, dry, scaling skin, can be a form of contact dermatitis. The cause may be an allergic reaction to medicines used for treating ear problems. Another common cause of irritation of the external ear canal may be hairsprays, cosmetics, soaps, or perfumes used in abundance about the ears.

When cerumen, or ear wax, blocks the ear canal, the doctor may try flushing out the offending substance by irrigating the tunnel with mild salt water that has been warmed to body temperature. Water that is too cool or too warm will cause a feeling of dizziness or fainting because of its stimulating effect on the neighboring semicircular canals, which are responsible for your sense of balance. The mild, warm salt water usually is squirted into the ear canal with a syringe, but if the cerumen can't be dislodged, the doctor may try to remove it manually. Sometimes the ear wax can be dislodged with an instrument that produces a suction effect in the ear canal.

Young children have a habit of sticking small objects in the external ear canal. The objects may be food, toys, stones, or anything else small enough to enter the ear canal but large enough to become stuck in the tube. Foreign bodies that are not removed immediately can produce complications in the form of pain, infection, and swollen tissues that make removal of the objects even more difficult. When a foreign body cannot be removed from the ear canal without difficulty, a doctor usually will advise that the patient be taken to a hospital or a clinic with facilities for minor surgery; a local or general anesthetic may be required to permit the object to be removed.

The eardrum is easily damaged by infections, injury, or rapidly changing pressures due to underwater swimming or rapid vertical movement during an airplane flight. The membrane may rupture and cause severe pain, bleeding, and loss of hearing in that ear. The pain and bleeding usually will subside after a while, but the membrane must be repaired. Some cases may require readjustment of the middle ear bones before normal hearing resumes. In cases of mild damage the membrane can be healed rather quickly and easily. The doctor may sometimes make a temporary patch with a piece of thin porous paper that has been treated with several chemicals. The membrane generally will mend itself over a period of about three weeks while the paper "bandage" is in place. However, the patient must avoid sneezing or blowing his nose during the period of recovery or the treatment may have to be started over again. Or, as an alternative, a type of surgery called myringoplasty may be required to repair the ruptured ear drum.

The examining physician is unlikely to test the function of the semicircular canals unless there is a complaint that suggests a loss of the sense of balance. A bacterial or viral infection can invade the inner ear, producing symptoms that include tinnitus, or ringing in the ears; hearing loss; and vertigo, a form of dizziness. Two common diseases that sometimes involve such inner ear symptoms are measles and mumps. The symptoms in various individuals may last from a few minutes to a few days, and in some cases the effects may persist for weeks.

One way to test the inner ear function is to introduce either warm or cold water into the external ear canal and watch for signs of vertigo. Vertigo usually is manifested by oscillating eye movements, an effect known as nystagmus. The amount of time that elapses from the instant the cool or warm water is injected into the ear until nystagmus signs appear, and the length of time the nystagmus continues, are the clues that tell the examining physician whether the inner ear's semicircular canals are working normally or abnormally. The full test of the semicircular canals utilizes both cool and warm water in both ears. The examining doctor may have the patient's head tilted in positions that arrange the semicircular canals so that they are either parallel to the ground or vertical. Obviously, such a test requires special knowledge and training.

Examination of the Nose

When the nose is examined, the sinuses usually are checked at the same time because the two areas are so closely related that a health problem affecting one is likely to involve the other as well. A digital examination, using light pressure with the fingers, may be used to detect possible tenderness around the frontal and maxillary sinuses, in the forehead and the cheekbones. In addition, the anterior ethmoid sinuses, located just above the eyes and beneath the eyebrows, may also be tested for tenderness. A digital examination of the nose may be made if the evidence suggests a broken nose. If there is a nasal fracture, the break usually can be located by gently pressing on the bony portion; the bones generally will produce a distinct sensation of rubbing against each other along the fracture line.

The doctor cannot look directly into the sinuses but, using a head mirror and light, he can inspect the interior of the nose as far as the turbinates or bulges within the nasal cavity that help condition inhaled air. The doctor may use a speculum, an instrument to widen the opening of the nostrils, for a better view of the nasal cavity. If necessary, he probably will squirt a medication into the nostrils to shrink swollen membranes that may block his view.

To inspect the back end of the nasal cavity, the doctor will look into the patient's mouth, using a tongue depressor to hold down the tongue while a mirror is held just beyond the back edge of the soft palate. The person being examined usually is asked to breathe through both the mouth and nose during this part of the nose and sinus examination.

There are two commonly used methods of examining the sinus cavities. One is by a technique called transillumination, which means simply that a light is used to illuminate the sinus cavities in a darkened room. This method is most effectively used to check the condition of the maxillary sinuses, situated along the front of the jaw bones on either side of the nose. A light, such as an ordinary flashlight, is held in the mouth while the room lights are darkened, or the patient stands or sits inside a dark closet with a lighted flashlight in his mouth. The light normally will be transmitted through the sinus bones and skin so that any fluid accumulation or large tumors can be observed. The frontal sinuses can be checked by placing a light source near the junction of the nasal bone and the orbital ridge of the eye socket.

The second method of viewing the sinuses is X-ray examination, but this is not likely to be used except when a patient has signs and symptoms of a serious problem, such as a possible tumor in a sinus. When transillumination and X-ray examination cannot be used to locate an apparently serious sinus problem, a third alternative is surgery.

The facial area is richly endowed with blood vessels so that nearly any injury to the nose or face is likely to result in bleeding. Most bleeding from the nose, or epistaxis, occurs from the rupture of a network of small blood vessels near the front of the nose. This type of nosebleed usually can be controlled by pinching the cartilage walls of the nose, which are rather flexible, against the nasal septum. Light packing of the bleeding nostril with gauze also can be helpful. But severe bleeding of any part of the nose should be treated by a physician.

There are many possible causes of epistaxis, including hypertension or high blood pressure, violent exertion, leukemia, injuries, foreign bodies, infections, and tumors.

The Common Cold

An infection caused by the common cold frequently involves more than one part of the overall head structure and can result in inflammation or other disorders of most areas, including the throat, the nasal cavity, sinus cavities, and the middle ear. Common colds usually are caused by one of a large variety of viruses. Unlike certain other diseases caused by viruses, one bout with the common cold does not confer immunity. One reason is that there always seems to be another strain of cold virus to contend with after you have perhaps acquired some immunity to a previous strain. A common cold that spreads into the throat can be expected to produce symptoms of viral pharyngitis.

When a cold virus invades the pharynx, you may or may not develop a fever. But you probably will feel some throat discomfort, and a doctor examining your pharynx will observe small fluid-filled blisters on the lining of the throat. The irritation will be treated with aspirin, fluids, and plenty of rest, unless there is a secondary infection of bacteria.

If bacterial infection occurs in the pharynx, the symptoms can be more dramatic. You might have severe throat pain, a high fever, loss of appetite, difficulty in swallowing, and a general feeling of poor health. There may be small blister-like eruptions on the membrane lining the throat, but instead of being filled with clear fluid they may contain pus. A very serious form of throat infection, diphtheria, may be marked by a white membrane appearing in the throat and by possible bleeding from the tissues beneath. Certain other bacterial infections can produce similar signs and symptoms which require professional medical care, including antibiotics and other medications that must be obtained by a doctor's prescription. Treatment also includes the usual regimen for respiratory infections—plenty of rest and increased intake of fluids.

Because of the location of the tonsils at the base of the tongue and around the top of the pharynx, where they form a sort of ring of lymphatic tissue, infections of the nose, throat, and neighboring regions inevitably involve the tonsils. Ordinarily, the tonsils can cope with a certain amount of bacteria passing through the pharynx, but occasionally the tissue may be overwhelmed by an infection and become the site of a health problem commonly known as tonsillitis. Acute tonsillitis produces similar symptoms to those experienced during a bacterial infection of the pharynx—pain, fever, loss of appetite, etc. The treatment also is similar, including antibiotic therapy. When bouts of tonsillitis recur frequently, the doctor has the option of recommending surgery to remove the tonsils.

GLOSSARY

THE HEAD AND NECK

The following entries define and describe the common and medical names of ailments, anatomical features, and other terms that relate to the head and the neck. Words in italics refer to separate entries in the Glossary that provide further information on the subject.

abscess A collection of pus. An abscess may form in an organ or structure of the head and neck area as a result of an infection. For example, a brain abscess can develop as a complication of an infection of the middle ear. Treatment of an abscess usually requires the administration of antibiotics and, in some cases, surgery.

acoustic neuroma A type of tumor that can interfere with the sense of hearing and also the sense of balance, or equilibrium. Symptoms may include a ringing in the ears and *vertigo*, as well as loss of hearing. Occasionally, an acoustic neuroma will press on nearby nerve trunks to produce other head ailments, such as facial palsy.

acoustic output A term used to describe the total loudness of a sound after being amplified by a *hearing aid*. For example, if a hearing aid picks up a 50 decibel sound and amplifies it an additional 50 decibels, the acoustic output is said to be 100 decibels. Most good hearing aids have a built-in limit of acoustic output which prevents discomfort or further damage to the wearer's hearing if the microphone picks up a very loud noise.

acoustic trauma Injury to the delicate cells in the organ of Corti, the "true organ of hearing," which results in a type of hearing loss. The range of hearing lost generally is in the higher frequencies, above 4,000 cycles per second, but the loss also may be below that point.

Hearing loss may be temporary or permanent and usually is marked by a ringing in the ears, or ear if only one side is involved. The cause of acoustic trauma usually is overexposure to loud noises such as gunfire, jet engine, high decibel music, etc.

acromegaly A chronic condition caused by overactivity of a growth hormone that may be manifested in the head and neck areas by enlarged lower jaw and separated teeth, along with enlarged nose, lips, tongue, and other features. Treatment may be X-ray therapy or surgical removal of a tumor.

actinomycosis A type of fungal infection that may involve the throat with pain and swelling of the pharynx, larynx, and mouth. Treatment usually requires antibiotics and other medications. The disease occasionally invades the salivary glands, in which case the same type of therapy is applied by the doctor.

acute laryngitis Inflammation of the larynx, marked by hoarseness, coughing, general throat discomfort, and redness or swelling of the tissues lining the larynx. The inflammation can be caused by allergy, virus, or bacteria. Treatment may include voice rest, bed rest, aspirin, medications to ease symptoms of cough and/or sore throat, and, where appropriate, antibiotics or removal of the offending causative allergen.

acute rhinitis An acute inflammation of the membrane lining the nose, marked by redness, swelling, sneezing, etc. The ailment can be caused by a virus, such as the *common cold* virus, or a bacterium. Viral infections usually produce symptoms that last from two to ten days, with spontaneous recovery. The only treatment consists of aspirin, increased consumption of fluids, and rest.

Bacterial infections usually are more serious; symptoms include fever, pain, and nasal blockage, and complications involving the tonsils, *sinuses, middle ear,* or pharynx. Treatment may require the administration of antibiotics in addition to fluids, rest, and aspirin.

adenoidectomy Surgical removal of the adenoid tissue, a not uncommon procedure when the tonsil tissue becomes chronically infected and swollen so as to interfere with normal breathing. An adenoid infection is most likely to affect young children, who develop a habit of mouth breathing when the nasal cavity becomes blocked by swollen *adenoids.* The infection tends to spread to the *middle ear,* causing a complication called *otitis media.* An adenoidectomy frequently is performed in conjunction with surgery to remove other tonsil tissue. The procedure may be indicated in medical records as "T & A," an abbreviation for tonsils and adenoids.

adenoids Another name for the tonsil tissue located at the back of the nasal cavity and above the soft palate. A doctor may identify the tissue as the pharyngeal tonsil.

adrenal insufficiency Also known as Addison's disease, a systemic disease with signs that include buccal pigmentation, or dark spots on the inner lining of the cheeks.

aero-otitis A term used to indicate problems of the inner ear caused by changing air pressures. The effect is most likely to occur during an airplane flight, or while an individual rides a rapidly rising or dropping elevator or is diving in deep water. The difference between air pressure in the *middle ear* and that of the environment may cause a feeling of fullness, pain, or partial loss of hearing in one or both ears. The condition usually is relieved by swallowing, chewing gum, drinking a beverage, or yawning. Another name for the problem is *barotrauma.*

allergic rhinitis A common condition of sneezing, runny nose, and general cold symptoms produced by individual allergy to house dust, animal dander, plant pollen, or other irritants. Treatment usually involves the use of antihistamines or similar medications and desensitization therapy. A complication can ensue if the sinuses or middle ear are involved.

anaphylaxis A severe type of allergic reaction that may be life-threatening. Symptoms may include asthma-like breathing caused by muscle spasms of the respiratory system, circulatory failure, and shock. Anaphylaxis can be caused by insect stings, reactions to drugs, or exposure to substances to which an individual may be extremely sensitive. Treatment must be immediate and should be directed by doctors or other health professionals.

angiofibroma A generally harmless tumor that may be associated with a nasal obstruction. The tumor is richly endowed with blood vessels and may be responsible for frequent nosebleeds. An angiofibroma is most likely to develop in a teenage boy and usually regresses, or gradually disappears, by the time the patient has reached adulthood. Some angiofibromas respond to treatment with male sex hormones. Alternative treatments include radiation or surgery, or both.

ankyloglossia A technical name for *tongue-tie.* A tongue-tied person has difficulty in speaking and eating normally because the tongue is literally tied down by a membrane that prevents proper extension of the tip of the tongue. The inborn condition is easily corrected by surgery that permits normal protrusion of the tongue.

anosmia A loss of the sense of smell. The condition usually is caused by damage to the olfactory nerves as a result of an injury to the head, or it may be due to a brain tumor.

antibiotics Medicines such as penicillin which are capable of destroying or controlling the spread of bacteria and some other disease organisms. Certain types of antibiotics are designed to fight specific strains of bacteria or are administered under a particular set of conditions. One type of penicillin, for example, can be absorbed effectively with meals, while another type is intended for use between meals. Antibiotics generally are not effective for treating viral disease such as a common cold infection.

antihistamines Medicines designed to reduce the effects of histamine, a substance released by body tissues in cases of allergy, hay fever, and asthma. Histamines may be associated with certain kinds of headaches.

antrum A term sometimes used to identify a sinus cavity, particularly the *maxillary sinus.*

aphasia A loss of ability to use language or speech effectively, usually due to a brain injury which might be caused by a blow to the head, a brain tumor, an infectious disease, a stroke, or similar insult to the brain tissue. Aphasia can appear in many different forms, including inability to understand written words, or an inability to understand spoken language, or, in some cases, a compulsion to repeat words spoken by other persons without understanding the meaning of the words. An aphasic person often can speak or write but has difficulty in naming common objects such as a piece of furniture or an item of silverware. Mild cases of aphasia may be treated by speech therapy.

aphthous ulcer A medical term for *canker sore,* which appears on the tongue, usually as a small lesion with a white base and yellow margins. It may be caused by a virus infection, a food allergy, or in some cases by emotional stress.

arched palate A palate with an abnormally high arch that may be a sign of several hereditary disorders.

arcus senilis A band of gray opaqueness on the *corneas* of the eyes. The band eventually develops into a grayish circle and is considered a sign of aging.

arteritis A disorder marked by a throbbing, pulsating headache and prominent appearance of the arteries involved. The disorder commonly occurs in the area of the temples, in which case it may be identified as temporal arteritis. The exact cause is unknown but the problem seems to be triggered by an inflammation of the arteries. Women of menopausal age are most likely to be afflicted with arteritis. Untreated, the condition can lead to blindness.

atrophic rhinitis A condition marked by loss of supporting soft tissues beneath the mucosal membrane lining the inside of the nose. The membrane surfaces tend to become dry, crusted, and infected. Therapy usually includes frequent irrigation of the nasal membranes and increased humidity of the patient's surroundings in order to reduce the drying effects of the environment.

audiogram A record, usually in the form of a chart, in which results of hearing tests for an individual are kept.

audiometer An electrical device for producing sounds of controlled pitch and loudness to test a person's hearing ability.

auditory canal The tubular structure that runs from the external ear to the eardrum and helps direct sound waves toward the eardrum.

aura Generally a warning sign or premonition of a convulsion or epileptic fit. An aura also is associated with migraine headaches. The migraine aura may vary somewhat with different patients but can be characterized by visual disturbances, a weakness or numbness in the face, arms, or legs, and dizziness or brief loss of consciousness. The type of aura experienced by a migraine headache patient tends to repeat its pattern with each attack; that is, a patient who experiences visual disturbances usually has the same kind of visual aura each time.

auricle The portion of the ear that extends beyond the head; also called the external ear.

auricular hematoma Hemorrhage under the skin of the external ear, or *auricle,* usually as a result of injury. For cosmetic reasons, an auricular hematoma should be drained carefully by a doctor. If not properly treated the external ear may acquire the *cauliflower ear* deformity associated with professional boxers.

bacterial conjunctivitis A bacterial inflammation of the *conjunctiva*, a delicate membrane that separates the eyeball from the inside surface of the eyelid. The disease is manifested by a discharge from the eye that can result in crusting of the eyelids and cause them to stick together at times. The disorder sometimes is called "red eye" or "pink eye" because the inflammation produces a reddish appearance about the eyes. An examining physician usually will try to identify the species of bacteria involved and prescribe an antibiotic ointment or drops that can be applied to the affected area.

bacterial myringitis A bacterial infection of the eardrum, usually accompanied by pain, swelling of the tissues, pus formation, and hearing loss. Antibiotics usually are administered to control the spread of the infection. Drainage of the pus through the external ear canal is required in most cases. If not treated, the infection can progress to rupture of the eardrum.

Barany rotation test A medical test of a patient's equilibrium, or sense of balance, by seating the subject in a chair that is whirled about rapidly for about 20 seconds, then suddenly stopped. The duration of the period of dizziness after the chair has stopped is used as an indication of the individual's sense of equilibrium.

barotitis media One of several terms used to identify the feeling caused when rapidly changing air pressure outside the body affects the middle ear space. It may occur as the result of flying in an airplane, diving in deep water, or riding in a fast-rising or -dropping elevator in a tall building.

barotrauma Another name for *aero-otitis*, the effects of changing air pressure on the middle ear; also called barotitis.

Bekesy The name of a type of audiometry equipment used in diagnosing hearing disorders that may involve the *middle ear*, the *inner ear*, the auditory nerve, or other causes. The device automatically produces a record of one's hearing that is called a Bekesy *audiogram.*

Bell's palsy A disorder involving a facial nerve in which some control over the nerve's normal function is lost. The disorder may be marked by pain, a weakness of the facial muscles, and loss of ability to blink the involved eyelid. The problem may begin with pain and swelling along the facial nerve, sometimes after exposure to extreme cold. Most patients recover within one to three months, although there may be some nerve degeneration in certain cases.

benign Descriptive term for a growth that is not malignant or cancerous.

binaural A term used to indicate hearing in both ears, or on both sides of the head. The term for hearing on just one side, or with one ear, is monaural.

biopsy A medical procedure in which a sample of tissue is removed from a patient for microscopic or other detailed examination. For example, a tumor in the mouth might be sampled in this manner in order to determine whether it is benign, or relatively harmless, or whether it is malignant and therefore cancerous tissue.

black tongue A fungal infection of the tongue that results in an appearance of black hairlike growths on the surface that are threads of the fungus. The patient experiences no symptoms with the infection, which may be treated by the use of antibiotic medicines to inhibit the growth of the normal bacteria that would destroy the fungus.

blepharitis A condition, also known as granulated eyelids, marked by scales, crusts, and general inflammation of the margin of the eyelid. The condition can be caused by a bacterial infection or a form of seborrhea similar to the sebaceous gland activity associated with dandruff of the scalp. Treatment may include a cream containing cortisone, with antibiotics used to control a bacterial infection and dandruff-control shampoo used to control the seborrhea form of blepharitis.

blink reflex A stimulus response of infants to a sound used in testing the child's hearing. An examining doctor may create sound by clapping his hands or producing an *audiometer* tone of known loudness and frequency near the ear of an infant. If the child blinks, the response is considered a proof that the hearing is normal.

bone conduction hearing This refers to the ability of bone tissue to conduct sound. Bone conduction through the mastoid bone to the inner ear makes it possible for persons to hear part of the normal range of sounds when the air conduction leg of their hearing apparatus is not functioning. Bone conduction of sound usually eliminates some frequencies at the high and low end of the scale received by people with normal hearing.

branchial cyst A type of tumor that appears on the neck just below the mandible, or lower jawbone. The cyst may be soft and resilient, or hard and inflamed. It usually is filled with a fluid that is oily and contains cholesterol.

branchial fistula A blind tube that develops on the neck muscle below the lower jawbone, opening to the outside but extending as far as the tissues surrounding the pharynx. The fistula can be a complication of a previous *branchial cyst* that was drained. Medical attention usually is needed to repair the opening and to prevent infection.

buccal cyst A cyst that occurs on the membrane lining the inner surface of the cheeks. A buccal cyst commonly is caused by an obstruction in a mucous gland. The cyst usually is translucent and has a bluish dome.

buccal ulcer An ulcer that develops on the inner surface of the cheek.

bullous myringitis A medical term for inflammation of the eardrum. The complaint usually is marked by a pain in one or both ears but without loss of hearing. The cause is a viral infection that produces blisters on the eardrum, or *tympanic membrane*. Treatment usually is limited to relief of the symptoms and may include applying heat to the ear and inserting warmed drops of analgesic medications. If the condition lasts more than two or three days, you should have a doctor check for complications involving a possible bacterial infection.

caloric test A test for the body's function of determining its orientation in space or equilibrium by introducing warm or cool water into the external ear canal. The test material also could be warm or cool air. The principle of the test involves the fact that the temperature difference of the test material produces a feeling of *vertigo* or dizziness in the subject. The effect can be measured by eye movements of the person being tested after the dizzy sensation begins. Doctors determine what's normal and what's not about the person's equilibrium by the amount of time it takes for the eye movements, called *nystagmus*, to begin and by the length of time required for the person to recover from the sensation.

canal Usually refers to the external *auditory canal* that extends from the outer ear to the eardrum.

canker sore A type of ulcer that appears on the tongue, usually as a result of a food allergy, emotional stress, or a herpes virus infection.

cannulation A procedure for treating sinus infection or inflammation by inserting a tubular instrument, a cannula, into the sinus and irrigating the sinus cavity.

carcinoma A type of malignant, or cancerous, tumor. The ear, lip, nose, and tongue are among sites where carcinomas of the head may be found.

carotid arteritis A condition associated with pain in the neck that occurs when swallowing. It may be a throbbing pain that extends from the ear or lower jaw and usually develops in association with a viral infection of the pharynx.

The carotid artery, which passes through the area, may be quite tender, and pressing on the artery can cause the pain to spread along the route of the blood vessel. The complaint may involve just one side of the neck or both.

cartilage An elastic semihard tissue, commonly known as gristle, that forms parts of the features of the head, such as the ears, the nose, and the pharynx.

cataract A progressive clouding of the normally transparent lens of the eye. The clouding eventually can result in blindness by blocking the passage of light to the *retina* of the eye. Most cataracts are associated with degenerative processes of aging, but the condition may be congenital or caused by an accident, drugs, disease, or exposure to radiation. The only symptom may be a gradual dimming of vision in one or both eyes.

Since nearly all adults experience a certain amount of opaqueness in the lens, a doctor usually makes a study of the amount of vision lost before recommending treatment. The condition can be corrected by surgically removing the natural lens and replacing it with an implant of a plastic lens. The alternative is the use of contact lenses or thick eyeglass lenses designed to focus light on the individual's retinas so that normal vision is restored.

CAT scanner A type of X-ray equipment that directs pencil-thin beams in a semicircle around a portion of the body being examined, with the picture projected onto a television screen rather than on a piece of film. By making a series of consecutive scans at slightly different positions, the device can produce a series of "slices" of a body part or organ, thereby enabling a doctor to "see" inside tissues that may be injured or diseased. A CAT scanner may be used to look inside a patient's skull, for example, to inspect the *optic nerve,* or to look for a possible brain tumor. The abbreviation CAT stands for Computerized Axial Tomography.

cauliflower ear A common name for a deformity of the outer ear resulting from hemor-

rhages inflicted by blows received in fighting or by similar injuries.

cellulitis A type of bacterial infection of the subcutaneous tissues that can involve the external ear, the ear canal, the mastoid area, and the face. The disease can spread rapidly through tissues beneath the skin, producing red, swollen, painfully tender effects; the infection may be accompanied by fever. Prompt medical care is needed to control the spread of the infection, and treatment usually includes antibiotics, bed rest, and application of warm, moist packs to the affected areas.

cerebellar system test A test of neurological function that may be conducted by an examining doctor. One common form of the test is to ask the patient to close his eyes and place the index finger of each hand on the tip of the nose. Another variation requires that the patient, with eyes open, touch the finger of one hand to the finger of the examining doctor, then move the finger to the patient's nose and back to the doctor's finger, which finger will have moved to a different position. The patient's cerebellar brain function is considered normal if he can perform such tasks quickly and accurately with both hands.

cerebellopontine angle tumor A long medical term used by some doctors to identify a group of tumors that may involve the cellebellum portion of the brain and/or several cranial nerves of the head. Most tumors of this kind, sometimes simply called angle tumors, involve nerve fibers in the inner ear. Symptoms usually include ringing in the ears with some hearing loss plus dizzy spells and headaches. If not treated in early stages, the tumor begins to produce facial paralysis and loss of the normal eye-blinking reflex when the cornea is touched. Surgical treatment is required to correct the condition.

cerebral hemorrhage Severe bleeding, usually from a ruptured blood vessel, in the brain tissue. Symptoms frequently include a sudden, severe, generalized headache that can be associated with vomiting, and loss of some muscle or other body functions controlled by the area of the brain involved. The effects of cerebral hemorrhage usually are determined by the precise site of the bleeding and the extent of brain damage. Some victims who slip into a coma may recover with only symptoms of mental confusion that may persist for several weeks; others quickly lose consciousness and die after the first signs and symptoms appear.

cerumen A medical term for ear wax. Cerumen is produced by a specialized type of sweat gland located in the ear canal. Excessive cerumen production is not an abnormal condition, but if the substance is allowed to become hard and impacted, complications ranging from hearing loss to infections can result. However, caution must be exercised in removing cerumen because of the hazards of damaging the eardrum at the end of the canal, or tearing the membrane lining the canal. Cerumen frequently can be removed by irrigating the ear canal with a mild saltwater solution warmed to body temperature.

chalazion A round swelling or lump under the skin of the eyelid caused by an enlarged eyelid gland. The lump usually causes no pain unless it becomes infected, but it may be drained by a doctor if it causes a cosmetic problem. In most cases, a chalazion will gradually regress without treatment.

chancre An ulcer-like lesion that may develop on the lip or tongue as a result of a syphilis infection. A syphilis lesion in the area of the mouth is relatively rare, but it may begin as a small pustule that soon ruptures and develops into a rather distinctive lesion with a button-like plaque imbedded in the tissue at the bottom of the ulceration. The chancre generally is not painful and there is little or no pain associated with the swelling of nearby lymph nodes. Blood tests for syphilis may indicate an absence of the disease during the stage at which the chancre appears.

cheilitis An inflammation of the skin around the corners of the mouth. The disorder sometimes is related to a vitamin B complex deficiency and is treated with large doses of B vitamins and application of a steroid hormone ointment.

chemosis Another name for edema of the *conjunctiva*, characterized by a transparent, swollen appearance of the conjunctival membrane that lines the eyelids and extends to the surface of the eyeballs. Chemosis can be a sign of a systemic disease involving the thyroid gland.

chemotherapy The use of chemicals to treat a disease. The chemicals generally are of a type, such as antibiotics, that destroy the source of the disease organism without causing serious harm to normal body tissues.

choanal atresia A condition caused by development of a membrane at the rear of the nasal cavity that interferes with normal breathing through the nose. The problem may result from injury or an infectious disease, although the condition can be congenital, or present at birth. If an infant is born with the disorder, immediate steps usually are necessary to provide breathing by mouth; otherwise, the child may be unable to breathe and could die within a few minutes. Emergency treatment may involve inserting a sharp, curved instrument to puncture the membrane so that air can pass between the nose and the trachea, or windpipe.

cholesteatoma A tumor that can develop from the skin lining the ear canal, damaging the eardrum and eventually eroding the surrounding bone structures, particularly the mastoid bones which border on the internal ear structures. The tumor gets its name from the term cholesterol because the growth contains the substance in large amounts. A cholesteatoma frequently is the cause of chronic *otitis media*, or inflammation of the middle ear.

chondrodermatitis A medical term for a nodule that may occur on the external ear surface. The growth can be painful and usually must be removed by surgery.

choroid One of three basic tissue layers of the eyeball. The choroid layer contains blood vessels that supply nourishment to eye tissues, as well as a pigment that helps exclude light rays that might otherwise enter the eye through tissues beyond the lens.

cigarette paper patch A term sometimes used to describe a type of dressing used to repair a perforated eardrum. A small circle of thin porous paper, similar to cigarette paper, is treated with medical chemicals and placed over the eardrum while the membrane goes through its natural healing process.

cleft lip Another term for *harelip*, a deformity of the upper lip. The defect may be associated with other abnormalities of the body such as *cleft palate.* The cleft in the lip is usually corrected by plastic surgery shortly after a baby is born.

cleft nose A congenital defect marked by a small vertical depression at the tip of the nose. It is caused by a failure of nasal cartilage to fuse normally before birth. The condition can be corrected with plastic surgery.

cleft palate An opening along the midline of the hard palate, the front portion of the roof of the mouth. It is a congenital defect caused by a failure of those parts of the fetal maxillary bones to fuse while the infant skull is being formed. A cleft palate frequently is accompanied by a *cleft lip*, or *harelip*.

cobblestone tongue The common name given to the tongue when the *papillae* on the surface become red and swollen, usually as a result of a vitamin B deficient diet.

cochlea A spiral structure of the inner ear that contains the organ of Corti, the sensory unit that transmits sound to the brain.

color vision test A test used by doctors during eye examinations to determine the ability of a patient to discriminate between colors.

One common test consists of 15 colored pictures composed of dots of different sizes. A sample picture may show the number 12 in red ink on a blue background that a red-green color-blind person might not be able to decipher properly. The patient usually is allowed two seconds to view each of the colored pictures and describe what image could be observed in the dot pattern. An additional test may consist of samples of yarn in various colors such as pale green and bright red, along with the so-called confusion colors—beige, olive, and brown—that color-blind persons find difficult to identify.

Comberg technique A special type of X-ray examination that may be used to locate a foreign object in the body when the object is made of a substance that doesn't show up on ordinary X-ray film. Dental X-ray film that is "bone free" or permits a view of the interior of a bone structure may be used in the procedure. The Comberg technique might be employed to find a foreign body inside the globe of the eye.

common cold A term commonly used to refer to *acute rhinitis*, or an inflammation of the nasal mucous membrane. The common cold type of inflammation usually is caused by a viral infection, but similar symptoms can be produced by several types of bacteria as well as tobacco smoke and chemical fumes. More than one variety of virus may be responsible for acute rhinitis. The onset of an infection can be aided by exposure to cold weather, low humidity, fatigue, and other factors that lower a person's resistance to disease in general.

Symptoms of the common cold include an incubation period of from one to three days, during which a dry, irritated sensation is felt in the throat or nasal cavity. The nasal mucosa generally becomes red and swollen, and the patient feels congestion, a mild general illness, with sneezing and a runny nose. The infection generally is self-limiting and the symptoms subside in about a week.

Treatment includes plenty of rest, increased fluid intake, increasing the humidity of the environment if needed, and the use of aspirin, nasal decongestants, and other appropriate medications. Antibiotics and antihistamines are not recommended for a viral infection except to control complications such as a bacterial secondary infection or allergy. One of the most effective methods of preventing the common cold is to avoid people who have the cold.

congenital anomaly A deformity or defect present at birth. The condition may be hereditary, that is, transmitted by the genetic material of one or both of the parents, or caused by a factor that interferes with normal embryonic or fetal development, such as a German measles virus.

conjunctiva A delicate mucous membrane that lines the insides of the eyelids and the front of the eyeball.

conjunctivitis An inflammation of the conjunctiva. See illustration page 95.

contact ulcers Lesions of the vocal cords associated with improper control of the voice.

contusion A bruise, usually the result of bleeding beneath the outer layer of the skin after an injury. Cold compresses applied to the area of the contusion generally will relieve some pain and swelling, but professional medical care should be requested for a contusion that involves a fragile or vital area such as the eyes.

coriolis illusion A serious loss of orientation, often accompanied by dizziness, that can result when the body's sense of equilibrium is subjected to two different conflicting forces. An example is the effect produced on the semicircular canals when a person in an airplane bends his head forward while the aircraft is going through a turning maneuver.

cornea The transparent but firm outer coat of the eyeball. The cornea is a part of the sclera, or outer white covering of the eyeball, but it normally is clear to permit light to enter the lens of the eye, directly behind the cornea.

corneal abrasion Scratches on the cornea produced by foreign bodies and attempts to remove them, or by children scratching their eyes. Superficial corneal abrasions usually can be healed within a few days by professional medical treatment. In some cases of deep corneal damage, a doctor may prescribe the use of antibiotic eye drops during the healing process.

corticosteroid A chemical that is similar to or mimics the effect of a steroid hormone produced naturally by the cortex of the adrenal gland. Corticosteroids may be prescribed by a doctor for treating a variety of disorders in the head and neck area, including severe *allergic rhinitis*, edema of the larynx, or eczema of the external auditory canal.

coryza Another word for *rhinitis*, or inflammation of the mucosal lining of the nose.

craniotabes A softening of the skull bone associated with a variety of disorders ranging from rickets and syphilis to hypervitaminosis A, a condition resulting from adding too much vitamin A to one's diet.

craniotomy Surgery performed on the cranium, the part of the skull that encloses the brain.

cricoarytenoid arthritis A form of rheumatoid arthritis that affects the cartilage rings supporting the trachea. Symptoms may include hoarseness and shortness of breath.

cricoid A cartilage ring of the pharynx, below the larynx, or voice box. The trachea is situated immediately beneath the cricoid cartilage. When a *tracheostomy* is performed to provide emergency breathing for a patient, the opening into the trachea usually is made at the level of the cricoid.

CROS hearing CROS is an acronym, or combination of letters, standing for Contralateral Routing Of Signals. This fancy phrase means simply that sound is received by a microphone or hearing aid device placed near a deaf ear and is transmitted all the way around the head to an earphone placed near the good ear. The system provides a kind of stereo sound pickup for people who normally can hear on only one side of the head. The CROS hearing device usually is concealed in the framework of a pair of eyeglasses.

croup An inflammatory disease that invades the soft tissues of the trachea below the vocal cords. The symptoms include a distinctive croupy cough and swelling of the tracheal tissues to the point where breathing may be obstructed. Treatment usually requires increased humidity of the environment, antibiotics, and steroid hormone medications. Serious cases generally require hospitalization and surgery to open the trachea if necessary.

culture A sample of body substance, such as a discharge from the nose, taken for laboratory or microscopic examination. The sample, or specimen, is used to start a colony of the infectious organism in an artificial medium under controlled conditions. The laboratory personnel can then examine the colony, which is the actual culture, to identify the strain of germ involved, the number of microorganisms per milliliter, and other data that is needed to help determine what antibiotic or other medication should be used to fight the infection.

cycloplegic A term used by doctors to identify drugs used in certain kinds of eye examination in which it is necessary to cause temporary paralysis of the ciliary muscles, which control the size of the pupils. An example of a cycloplegic drug is atropine, the substance contained in eye drops used to dilate the pupils. A cycloplegic eye examination also may be referred to as a static eye examination.

dacryocystitis A long medical term for obstruction of the tear duct. The area of the lacrimal, or tear, gland and duct, between the eye and nose, becomes inflamed, tender, and swollen. The condition frequently results from a bacterial infection. It can be aggravated by exposure to smoke and dust. Pus from the infection can spread to the conjunctival lining of the lower eyelid.

deafness The loss of ability to hear sounds. Conductive deafness results from disease or injury involving the portions of the ear that transmit sounds from the external ear to the oval window of the inner ear. The parts include the ear canal, the eardrum, the eustachian tube, and the ossicle bones of the middle ear. Neurosensory deafness, also called nerve deafness, involves loss of hearing because of a disorder of the inner ear, which contains the organ of Corti, or the nerves that transmit impulses from the organ of Corti to the hearing centers of the brain. A mixed hearing loss or mixed deafness would be one that was partly conductive and partly nerve deafness.

decibels A system of measuring the relative loudness of different sounds. Decibels generally represent a ratio between pressures of various sounds and have no absolute value. As a general rule, doubling the sound pressure increases the loudness or intensity by six decibels.

decongestant A medicine that reduces congestion or swelling.

deglutition A technical term for the act of swallowing, which is partly voluntary and partly involuntary. Moving food to the back of the mouth toward the opening of the esophagus, utilizing the muscle power of the tongue and cheeks, is a voluntary action. Once the food reaches the end of the oral cavity, the act of swallowing becomes involuntary, or automatic.

delayed feedback test A test for hearing loss that depends upon the fact that a person normally is unable to read material into a microphone if his voice is delayed slightly and fed back to him through earphones. The delayed feedback test is used sometimes when doctors are unable to find any physical, or organic, disorder to account for a person's hearing loss. An example of nonorganic deafness would be psychogenic hearing loss.

Delphian nodes Lymph nodes that grow near the thyroid gland in the neck. They usually are of interest to an examining doctor because the nodes can become enlarged as a sign of a disease involving the thyroid gland.

dental ulcer An ulcer that develops along the sides or under the tongue where the tongue rubs against a protruding tooth or poorly fitted dentures. The dental ulcer sometimes has a trough-like appearance rather than a rounded area. The ulcer usually heals within a few weeks after the cause of the irritation has been removed. If not treated at an early stage, the ulcer could develop into a cancer.

depth perception The ability of the eyes to perceive the environment in three dimensions, an ability that may be lacking in persons with good vision in only one eye. Generally, the vision in both eyes must be coordinated in order to produce a three-dimensional image in the brain. However, many individuals who lack binocular vision are able to accommodate to the real, three-dimensional world without difficulty.

A commonly used test of depth perception requires that a patient view a series of black stripes on a white background, with two of the stripes in one plane and the third either in front of or behind the other two in a different plane of vision. The third stripe may be narrower or wider than the other two in order to trick the patient who may lack true depth perception but has learned that objects farther away should appear smaller.

dermoid cyst A whitish opaque cyst that may occur under the tip of the tongue or on the floor of the mouth.

detached retina A disorder of the eye in which a portion of the retina containing the rod and cone cells necessary for seeing colors and shades of brightness separates from the part of the eyeball lining that contains the eye's nutrient supply. The rod and cone nerve endings cease to function, and there is a danger that the entire retina eventually will separate. If that happens, all vision in the eye will be lost.

The cause of a detached retina usually is the seepage of fluid between the rod and cone cells and the nutrient layer. A detached retina is re-paired by draining and stopping the seepage of fluid and by causing the retina to fall back into its normal position. The retina cannot be stitched together but it can in effect be glued to the layer behind it through the use of cryosurgery, intense light beams, or other surgical techniques which produce a scar tissue that creates a sort of adhesive effect.

dewlap A fatty tumor that may develop near the base of the neck, just above the breastbone. The fatty mass of tissue gets its name from its resemblance to the fold of skin that grows under the throats of dogs, cows, and other animals.

diphtheria A serious bacterial infection that generally invades the pharynx and tonsils. A gray membrane spreads over the pharynx and tonsils, and occasionally to other areas of the throat lining; removing the membrane causes bleeding. The patient has symptoms of sore throat, headache, fever, swollen neck, and occasional breathing problems. Diphtheria can be prevented by immunization. Once the disease is contracted, treatment includes injections of diphtheria antitoxin and antibiotics, bed rest, and intravenous fluids.

diplacusis A technique for diagnosing an inner ear problem by placing a vibrating tuning fork at an equal distance from the ear canal on each side of the head. If the cochlea of the inner ear and its contents are normal, the tone should sound the same on either side. Distorted sound received at a higher pitch and less smoothly on one side indicates the presence of a lesion of the inner ear.

diplopia The medical term for double vision, caused by the inability to focus both eyes together.

dizziness The common word that means about the same as *vertigo*, a term the doctor may prefer. There are many possible reasons for dizziness, which may involve a sensation of light-headedness rather than the whirling sensation of true vertigo. Causes of dizziness might include fluid in the middle ear, *glaucoma* and other eye disorders, effects of alcohol or nicotine, and ear wax or a foreign body pressing against the eardrum.

Doefler-Stewart test A test for functional, or nonorganic, deafness or hearing loss in which the patient must judge the loudness of speech that is transmitted at levels above the minimum level of loudness the patient claims he can hear distinctly.

dyslalia Abnormal speech sounds due to loss of hearing or structural defects of the body parts involved in producing voice sounds.

dyslexia A condition marked by the inability to read printed words correctly. The cause is believed to be the result of abnormal development of the left hemisphere of the brain, the area that controls sequential reasoning, or a lesion in that brain area. Because of confusion about proper sequence of letters, particularly those with similar shapes, patients tend to see words as if some of the letters are transposed or reversed. Treatment of the disorder may involve the use of programmed learning techniques that start with simple combinations of letters and progress toward more complex word arrangements.

dysphonia A type of hoarseness that occurs when the false vocal cords close over the true vocal cords of the larynx. The effect can be the result of a tumor that blocks the movement of the true vocal cords, arthritis of the tracheal cartilages that immobilizes the true vocal cords, or abuse of the larynx.

dyspnea The term means simply shortness of breath, which can be caused by a number of different factors, including obstruction of the larynx. Laryngeal dyspnea is marked by ease of exhaling but difficulty in inhaling because the incoming air forces the vocal cords to close over the trachea. The harder the patient tries to inhale, the more difficult the breathing becomes. The problem usually is resolved by resorting to quiet breathing while the laryngeal disease responsible for the original obstruction is cured.

edema The presence of abnormally large amounts of fluid in the tissue spaces of the body, usually as a result of an injury or disease.

emmetropia A medical term that means refraction of the eye is normal. *Myopia*, for nearsightedness, and *hyperopia*, for farsightedness, are abnormal alternatives.

encephalitis An inflammation of the brain tissues. One form of encephalitis is caused by a virus carried by mites or mosquitoes. Signs and symptoms include tremor of the lips, tongue, and hands; severe headache; stiff neck; sudden high fever; and nausea. Treatment involves bed rest and use of medications to relieve the symptoms. Encephalitis also can be a complication of infections by *herpes simplex*, measles, and chicken pox viruses.

endolymph The name given the fluid in the *inner ear.*

entropion A disorder of the lower eyelid in which the lid turns inward. It may be the result of an inflammation of the eye or because of the contracture of scar tissue. When the lower lid turns outward abnormally the condition is called ectropion.

episcleritis A type of conjunctivitis that involves the sclera, or white covering, of the eyeball. It is a painful ailment that usually requires analgesics to relieve the discomfort and cortisone drops for the affected eye.

epistaxis The medical word for a bloody nose, or nosebleed.

epulis A type of fibrous tumor that grows out of the gums and may emerge between the teeth. The tumor is benign and may develop in association with an infection of the roots of a tooth. It is simply cut away by an oral surgeon.

erysipelas A bacterial infection of the skin that frequently affects the ears, nose, and other facial features. Symptoms include sudden chills and fever plus a sensation that the skin has tightened. The skin acquires large reddish areas with sharply defined and elevated borders. Treatment requires the administration of antibiotics and medications to relieve the symptoms of the infection.

erythema A medical term used to describe the redness of the skin caused by a congestion of blood vessels at the site of an injury or infection.

erythema multiforme A disease characterized by eruptions on the lips and lining of the mouth. The eruptions usually begin as small blisters that turn into raised, reddish lesions which bleed and form crusts. The eruptions usually affect only children and young adults, and may be associated with one of several infectious diseases. Treatment consists of steroid hormones and medications that relieve the discomfort of the symptoms, including lozenges that have an anesthetic effect.

esophageal speech A method of producing voice sounds after the larynx has been removed because of cancer or a similar reason. Persons who have undergone a laryngectomy are left without the ability to produce normal speech and must breathe through an artificial opening in the neck. These patients are taught to communicate by esophageal speech, which involves swallowing air into the esophagus or stomach and belching the air back up the esophagus. By controlling the air burp, the walls of the pharnyx can be made to vibrate and produce sounds. The lips, tongue, and palate can be trained to convert those sounds into speech that is understandable, although not normal.

Esophageal speech consists of gutteral sounds and sentences that are interrupted after short word sequences while more air is swallowed in order to produce additional words. A laryngectomized patient can learn to function in society with esophageal speech.

esophageal strictures A narrowing of the opening of the esophagus that can result from inflammation or ulceration of the membrane lining the food tube, and from a number of different diseases. If the stricture is not associated with a malignant tumor, a doctor will expand the opening with specially designed instruments or devices that can be swallowed by the patient and retrieved for a repeat performance of the procedure.

esophageal varices A condition somewhat like having varicose veins in the wall of the esophagus. The dilated veins are caused by abnormally high pressure in the blood vessels. The varices may make their presence known through internal bleeding or by appearing as a string of beads on an X-ray film following a barium meal. The condition can be treated by surgery or injection of a chemical solution.

esophagitis Any inflammation of the lining of the esophagus. The causes range from highly seasoned or hot foods and beverages to vomiting or *hiatus hernia* that permits a backwash of stomach acid into the esophagus.

esophagoscopy Examination of the esophagus, usually conducted with instruments that can be inserted through the mouth and down the food tube.

ethmoid sinus A sinus cavity in the bone that forms the roof of the nasal cavity. A sinus infection involving the ethmoid sinuses may cause pain across the bridge of the nose as well as in the eyes.

eustachian tube A thin tube that extends from the back of the throat to the middle ear to help equalize the air pressure of the middle ear with that of the atmosphere outside the body.

exophthalmos A medical term used to indicate eyeballs that seem to bulge from their sockets. The condition may develop as a result of an overactive thyroid gland.

extraocular movements A reference to the half-dozen separate muscles that control the directions in which the eyeballs can be turned.

exudate The waste products of an inflammation deposited on or in the surface of a body tissue. An exudate may contain fluid, tissue cells, or the remains of dead cells, or a combination of different kinds of organic debris.

eye muscles There are six muscles attached to each eyeball that move the eye in the various directions normally used for vision. If one or more of the muscles does not function properly, the patient may have one or both eyes that turn inward or outward, as in cases of crossed eyes or wall eyes. In addition to the external muscles, there are tiny muscles within each eyeball that open and constrict the pupil and help the lens to focus on images. See also *strabismus.*

eyestrain A condition that may occur when the muscles that move the eyeballs have been held in sustained contraction for a prolonged period. The effect frequently is a localized headache that follows the path of nerves radiating from the area of the eye toward the back of the head.

facial paralysis An occasional complication of *otitis media,* an inflammation of the middle ear. Because the facial nerve passes through a natural opening in that area of the skull, an infection of the middle ear can eventually involve the facial nerve. The nerve may become swollen, or pressure from the diseased middle ear tissues can press on the nerve and produce the paralysis. If the problem arises during an early stage of otitis media, simply controlling the middle ear infection with antibiotics usually will restore normal functions of the nerve. At a later stage of otitis media, when the disease may have spread to the surrounding bone, treatment generally requires surgery to relieve pressure on the facial nerve.

field of vision The area around your body in which you can perceive an object while the eyes are focused on a certain spot. The area includes the fringes of vision in which you may be able to detect the location of a fixed or moving object even though you may not be able to see the object distinctly. People suffering from glaucoma have a smaller "fringe area" of vision than people whose eyes permit a normal field of vision.

finger identification A test of vision for people whose eyesight is so poor that they can't read an eye chart. The examining doctor may hold up one finger or more and ask the patient to count them. The patient's vision in such cases is not recorded as 20/20 or 20/100, but rather as V.O.D. = 2 F (for fingers) at 3 feet, or whatever distance was used. V.O.D. are the initials for vision oculus decter.

foramen A natural opening or passage into or through a bone. The skull contains a number of foramens through which nerves and blood vessels pass.

Fordyce spots Painless and harmless sebaceous cysts that appear on the mucous membranes of the lips, cheeks, and tongue as tiny white or yellowish spots.

forehead wrinkles Of some interest to an examining physician because the patterns can suggest certain systemic or congenital disorders. Persons suffering from a thyroid disorder, for example, may not produce the usual furrowing of forehead skin when raising their eyebrows.

fortification spectrum Part of the image associated with the aura of migraine attacks. The patient sees zigzag, colored patterns which resemble the outline of an ancient fortress. The pattern may be so vivid that the patient can trace the pattern by looking at a piece of paper and drawing a pencil line along the zigzag pattern.

fovea A slight depression in the retina at the rear of the eyeball. A line drawn through the eye so that it would pass through the center of the lens would also pass through the fovea. There are no rod cells in this portion of the retina, only cones. The area also is known as the fovea centralis, since it lies along the optic axis of the eye.

frenulum A fold of tissue along the midline of the undersurface of the tongue, attaching the bottom of the tongue to the floor of the mouth. In some persons the frenulum is abnormally short, a condition that produces *tongue-*

tie. The remedy is to have the frenulum cut so the tip of the tongue can be moved about normally.

Frenzel glasses Special eyeglasses placed over the eyes of patients during tests of inner ear function. The lenses in the Frenzel glasses are so powerful the patient can't focus on anything in the room. However, the lenses permit the doctor to study the iris and cornea of the patient's eye, or eyes, while the tests of equilibrium—as measured by *nystagmus*, or involuntary eye movements—are being conducted.

frequency The number of vibrations per unit of time. In the case of hearing, sound usually is measured in cycles per second or Hertz. The terms usually are abbreviated in medical records; for example, 500 CPS or 500 Hz. Most human speech sounds range from a frequency of 500 CPS to about 2,000 CPS.

frontal sinus The sinus cavities of the lower forehead, above the nose and between the eyes. Infection of the frontal sinuses usually results in pain and tenderness just above the eyes.

functional hearing loss A type of deafness that may be considered psychological because examining doctors find no damage to the ear structures to account for the hearing loss.

furry tongue The same as hairy tongue or *black tongue*, a condition marked by the appearance of dark hairy growths on the surface of the tongue. The effect actually is produced by a fungal infection.

furuncle A painful skin nodule caused by a bacterial infection. A furuncle usually is associated with a hair follicle, which offers the bacteria a passageway to the lower skin layers.

gag reflex An automatic gagging reaction occurs when the pharynx is touched. The reflex may be tested by an examining physician doing neurological checkups. The gag reflex is controlled in the medulla portion of the brain.

gaze A term used sometimes in examining a patient for normal or abnormal vision. A person with abnormal gaze may turn his head to the right or left in order to focus on an object in front of him. Or he may tilt his head upward in order to move the eyes above the horizontal, if he suffers from failure of normal vertical gaze.

Gelle test A type of hearing test used to analyze the condition of the ossicles of the middle ear. A vibrating tuning fork is held against the skull while air pressure is raised in the external ear canal and against the eardrum. If the individual's hearing is normal, the tuning fork's sound will diminish as the pressure on the eardrum is increased. If there is a problem in the middle ear that immobilizes the ossicles, or tiny bones, in that part of the skull, the person tested will not notice the pressure effect on the sound level.

geographic tongue A relatively harmless condition marked by the appearance on the tongue of bright red areas with light yellow fringes. The pattern may change within several days so that yellow-fringed red areas appear on a different part of the tongue surface, while the originally affected region returns to a normal appearance.

gingivitis An inflammation of the gums, which doctors and dentists may refer to as the gingiva. Gingivitis may take a variety of forms and be characterized by redness, swelling, ulceration, easy bleeding, etc. Some kinds of gingivitis are marked by color changes or pigmentation. The appearance of a gray line along the gum margin, for example, could be a sign of lead poisoning.

glaucoma A visual disorder caused by abnormally high fluid pressure within the eyeball. There are several forms of glaucoma, but all generally result from an obstruction to the normal drainage of fluid from the anterior, or front, chamber of the eyeball, the region between the lens and the cornea. Fluid called aqueous humor flows into the chamber continuously and normally flows out at the same rate, but when the fluid does not drain properly it accumulates, and the pressure can cause a wide assortment of visual problems. In chronic cases of glaucoma the increased pressure may be painless, and damage to the eye can be so gradual that the patient is not aware that he is becoming blind until he notices specific signs such as halos that appear around lights, or the "tunnel vision" effect of a narrowing field of vision. Acute attacks of glaucoma, on the other hand, are marked by severe pain in the eyes, nausea and vomiting, and loss of vision.

Glaucoma can be detected easily during a physical examination by the use of a tonometer, a device that measures the fluid pressure within the eyeballs. Treatment may be with drops of medicine that stimulate the drainage of fluid from the anterior chamber, or surgery to provide passageways for the outflow of fluid, or both.

glomus jugulare A generally harmless tumor that can develop in the area of the middle ear. Although this tissue growth seldom becomes cancerous, it can produce a variety of problems such as hearing loss, a pulsating ringing in the ears, pressure on nerves that pass through the middle ear region of the skull, and bleeding from the ear. The tumor must be removed surgically.

glossitis An inflammation of the tongue; commonly called red tongue. Glossitis can be caused by a wide variety of health problems, from an infection of the pharynx that involves the tongue to scarlet fever. The tongue can become not only red but swollen and tender; it may have a burning sensation, especially when spicy foods are eaten. Treatment generally depends upon controlling the cause of the symptoms.

glue ear A common name for a hearing problem involving the middle ear. Fluid that has accumulated in the middle ear may develop a jelly-like consistency and result in moderate to severe hearing loss when the ossicles are unable to move freely. The disorder sometimes is due to blockage of the eustachian tube.

goiter An enlargement of the thyroid gland. The normal thyroid gland is firm but not hard, with a lobe on either side of the throat just beneath the larynx. In a case of goiter the gland may grow very large so that it protrudes on either side of the front of the neck, or in some cases on both sides. An examining doctor usually will palpate the thyroid gland to check its condition, including the presence of firm, rounded masses of nodules which usually are a sign of thyroid gland tumors. The normal size of a goiter can vary somewhat according to several factors such as age, sex, and the region of the country in which one lives. Female thyroid glands may be affected by pregnancy and menstrual periods.

granuloma A type of tumor, usually malignant, that may develop in the upper respiratory tract, with lesions involving the larynx, pharynx, soft palate, or nasal cavity. Treatment usually requires radiation, chemotherapy, steroid hormones, and, when necessary to control secondary infections, antibiotics.

gustatory Refers to the sense of taste. Taste buds that are sensitive to the basic taste sensations are generally located on the inner walls of gustatory pores on the surface of the tongue, and occasionally on the soft palate and epiglottis.

halitosis A term referring to bad breath that may be caused by poor oral hygiene, including irregular brushing of teeth after meals, tobacco smoking, and eating aromatic foods such as garlic, or by sinus infections involving post-nasal drip, acute infections of the mouth, nose, and throat, or tumors in the same areas. Treatment in most cases involves simply removing the cause and practicing good oral hygiene. A medical term for bad breath, seldom used even by doctors, is fetor ex ore.

Hand-Schuller-Christian disease A type of tumorous bone disease sometimes associated with diabetes and involving the middle ear.

harelip Another name for *cleft lip*, the term harelip is derived from the resemblance between the human lip deformity and the lip of a hare, or rabbit.

Harvard word list A list of about 200 phonetically balanced words, that is, words selected to contain one-syllable speech sounds used in normal conversation. The list is used to test the quality of speech a person with hearing loss can understand. The patient is asked to repeat the words he hears after they have been pronounced by an examiner. A similar word list contains a series of two-syllable test words.

hay fever A common name for a type of *allergic rhinitis*, or inflammation of the nasal cavity, caused by sensitivity to a plant pollen.

headaches A common term used to describe the symptoms of a disorder that might be caused by a very wide variety of health problems, ranging from allergy to injury. Doctors who are asked to treat a headache usually need to ask quite a few questions about the frequency of the headaches, their exact location, the intensity of the pain, how long a period of headaches may last, whether there is any warning before the pain begins, whether there are any other symptoms associated with the headache attacks such as nausea or vomiting, runny nose, etc. The doctor also will want to know if the headaches occur during periods of anxiety or stress, if the headache symptoms began after an injury or other triggering factor, and so on.

Some doctors classify headaches according to problems that are considered "extracranial," that is, outside the head, such as headaches caused by contractions of muscles in the neck and shoulders; and those that may be "intracranial," or due to involvement of arteries and nerves in the head. However, the task of determining whether the headache is caused by intracranial or extracranial factors can be difficult for a doctor. Headaches frequently occur without any physical signs such as a tumor, lesion, inflammation, or a similar warning flag that will show up on X-ray film, by palpation or visual examination, or in laboratory tests.

Among the common causes of headaches are nose or sinus infections, migraine, neuralgia, injury, allergy, high blood pressure, eye disease, dental problems, anxiety or tension, muscle contractions, dilated arteries, fever, and histamines.

hearing aid A compact electronic device designed to amplify sounds for persons with hearing loss. A hearing aid contains four basic parts: a microphone, a power supply, an amplifier, and an earphone or receiver. The microphone receives sound waves directed toward the user; the power supply, consisting of a small battery, helps the amplifier increase the sound that has been converted to electrical impulses by the microphone; and the earphone or receiver translates the electrical signals back into sound waves at a level that can be heard by the person using a hearing aid. A hearing aid may be designed to conduct sound through the external ear canal by air conduction, or to transmit the sound through the mastoid area by bone conduction, if the cause of hearing loss involves the tympanic membrane of the *middle ear*.

hemangioma A noncancerous blood vessel tumor that may develop on the tongue or in the nasal cavity, or other areas of the head. A form of hemangioma occurs occasionally in the larynx of infants, producing signs of hoarseness, breathing difficulty, and a croupy cough. Treatment of a hemangioma in the larynx usually requires radiation of the tumor, and surgery if radiation is inadequate.

hematoma A medical term for bruise. Hematomas are caused by bleeding under the surface of the skin.

hemotympanum A medical term for an unusual condition also known by the common name of blue eardrum. The eardrum has a blue or blackish coloration and usually is associated with a loss of hearing. The cause in many cases is a chronic case of *otitis media*, or inflammation of the middle ear.

herpangina The name of a virus that sometimes is associated with acute infection of the pharynx. The infection usually is characterized by sore throat, a feeling of dryness, and in some cases, fever. Tobacco, alcohol, and other substances may aggravate the symptoms of the infection, which is treated with bed rest, aspirin, increased fluid intake, and antiseptic lozenges or throat spray.

herpes simplex The name of a virus responsible for cold sores, which may involve the lips, nose, and other features of the face. A herpes infection usually begins as an area of irritation, soon followed by small blisters that contain a watery fluid. The infection generally is self-limiting; symptoms subside within ten days to two weeks. Therapy is directed mainly toward soothing the affected skin or mucous membrane areas with cold-sore lotions or salves. The discharge from the sores should not be allowed to contact the eyes because the virus can produce permanent damage to eye tissues.

herpes stomatitis Another name for the herpes simplex viral infection of the lips and mouth. See *herpes simplex.*

herpes zoster oticus A type of viral infection that may be marked by pain around the ear and the appearance of blisters resembling cold sores about the external ear canal. The infection can be more serious than some herpes diseases because the virus can cause paralysis of the facial nerve, along with some loss of taste and the ability to salivate or produce tears on the affected side of the head. Additional complications can include partial hearing loss, vertigo, and nausea and vomiting when neighboring nerve trunks become involved in the disease.

hertz A term used in hearing tests to indicate cycles per second, or the *frequency* of the sound as measured in hertz—for example, a tone of 2,000 Hz.

hiatus hernia A physical condition associated with the symptom of heartburn. There are several variations of hiatus hernia, but all involve a protrusion of the upper end of the stomach through a hernia, or opening, in the diaphragm, the muscular wall that separates the chest from the abdomen. The condition permits a reflux of gastric acid into the esophagus from the stomach.

hippus A condition in which the pupils of the eyes fluctuate in size. The problem may be associated with the tone of the muscles controlling the dilation and contraction of the pupils.

histamine cephalgia A medical term for histamine headache, also commonly known as a cluster headache because the attacks occur in clusters. The patient experiences brief, severe headaches several times a day or week, followed by a relatively long period without headaches. The headaches apparently are caused by dilation of the artery supplying blood to the side of the head, where the pain usually is felt. The ailment is sometimes identified as a histamine headache because it can be triggered by an injection of histamine, although there is little or no evidence that histamines occurring naturally in the body are a cause. Treatment usually involves the prescription of ergot-type medications.

histoplasmosis of the larynx A fungus infection that involves the larynx, usually in association with histoplasmosis of the lungs. The fungus may produce deep ulcers in the ears, the tongue, the lips, and the pharynx. Symptoms of the disease may include weight loss and diarrhea with abdominal cramps.

hoarseness A sign of a disorder involving the larynx, or voice box. The possible causes are myriad and commonly include overuse, as from shouting; infection involving a disease such as diphtheria, which invades the throat; burns from hot liquids; irritation from tobacco smoke; tumors or ulcers on the vocal cords; compression of the larynx by an enlarged thyroid gland; alcoholism; gout; and so on.

hordeolum A medical term for a stye in the eye caused by infections of glands in the eyelids. A stye can develop into a painful lump in the skin of the eyelid, with an *abscess* that can break through the skin and drain pus. A stye usually is treated by applying hot, moist packs. A doctor may recommend draining the abscess and applying antibiotic ointment to prevent possible spread of the infection to the brain or other areas of the head. Analgesics usually are taken to relieve pain symptoms.

hot cross bun skull A common name given to a congenital skull deformity characterized by two deep troughs, or fissures, that cross the cranium at right angles, producing four bulging bones separated by a thin depression shaped like a cross. The deformity usually is due to a syphilis infection of the mother.

hydrocephalus A rare condition that may be congenital or acquired later in life in which an obstruction in the body prevents the normal circulation of cerebrospinal fluid. The patient may experience headaches, nausea, weakness, and lack of coordination in the arms and legs. The most obvious signs are enlargement of the head and thinning of the bones of the cranium.

hydrops A term sometimes used to describe the effects of a disorder involving the vestibular apparatus of the inner ear that is responsible for the sense of balance. The person feels a fullness in the ear, occasional severe attacks of vertigo accompanied by sweating and nausea, and a ringing in the ears. The disorder sometimes is identified with *Meniere's disease* and is treated with antivertigo medicines and diet. The patient should observe general rules for good health such as abstinence from smoking, and getting plenty of rest and exercise.

hyperopia A medical term for farsightedness. A farsighted, or hyperopic person usually sees objects in the distance better than objects nearby. Eyeglasses that correct for the error in natural light focusing are needed to enable the person to have normal vision.

hypertensive headaches Headaches sometimes associated with periods of blood pressure changes. The source of the pain may be in muscle contractions or in dilated arteries supplying blood to the head. The pain frequently is centered at the back of the head, but may involve other areas. Despite the suggestive name of the disorder, some patients experience hypertensive headaches when their blood pressure is lower than usual, rather than higher.

A doctor may diagnose a hypertensive headache by palpating the carotid arteries, which run alongside the neck just below the chin; when the arteries are depressed the headache usually disappears. However, the digital technique is not recommended as a way of treating hypertensive headaches because the two carotid arteries are a vital source of blood to regions of the head, and depressing them for more than an instant can have damaging effects.

hypertrophic An enlarged or overgrown organ due to an increase in the size of the cells of the tissues forming the organ.

hypoglossal paralysis A loss of function of a nerve that controls the movements of tongue muscles. As a result of an injury, tumor, or infection involving the nervous system, the hypoglossal nerve will lose its ability to control motor functions, and the tongue will tend to move to one side. The affected side of the tongue, meanwhile, will gradually degenerate, impairing the patient's ability to eat and speak normally.

hypopyon An accumulation of pus in the anterior chamber of the eye, behind the cornea. The cause could be an infection of scratches on the cornea or the spread of *conjunctivitis* from the outside surface of the eyeball.

hyposmia A decreased sense of smell. The partial loss of the sensation of smell can occur naturally in older persons as part of the aging process. It also can be a sign of diabetes or the result of taking certain drugs.

inner ear A small complex organ encased in bones of the skull and containing two separate organs, one related to hearing and the other involved in the sense of balance. One is the organ of Corti, sometimes called the "true organ of hearing," which translates sound vibrations received from the *middle ear* into electrical impulses or signals that are carried by the auditory or acoustic nerve to the brain cells, which interpret the signals as speech, music, noise, etc. The organ for the sense of balance, sometimes called the vestibular apparatus, consists of three semicircular canals set at right angles to each other, like the edges of a box coming together at a corner. Fluid in the canals moves whenever the head moves, and the fluid signals the nerve endings in the canal regarding the position of the body.

intensity A physical measure of sound wave pressure that helps determine what people interpret as the loudness of sound.

intranasal Referring to the inside of the nose. A doctor usually wears a head mirror that allows him to focus light into the nose while making an intranasal examination.

intraocular A medical term meaning inside the eyeball. The term generally is used in connection with intraocular pressure measurements during eye examinations. Abnormally high intraocular pressure, caused by fluid flowing into the anterior of the eye faster than it drains out, is a sign of the disease known as *glaucoma*.

iris A thin, colored membrane, circular in shape, that gives the eye its normal coloration, that is, blue, brown, etc. The iris controls the amount of light entering the lens behind it as the opening in the center of the iris forms the pupil. The fine muscles of the iris expand or contract to change the size of the pupil.

iritis An inflammation of the iris. An infection involving the iris may be marked by a pus col-

lection in the bottom of the anterior chamber. Another complication of iritis can be an adhesion of the iris to the lens of the eye.

Jaeger test A test of vision in which the person is asked to read blocks of sentences printed in different sizes of printer's types on a card. The Jaeger test usually is employed to determine how well a person can read small type at a close distance. It is commonly used by opticians or optometrists during the fitting of eyeglasses.

keratitis An inflammation of the *cornea* of the eye. The inflammation can be associated with a viral or bacterial infection, a fungus, or an allergy. A viral infection of the cornea can result in scarring. A bacterial infection can produce ulcers that rapidly perforate or erode the cornea. Fungal and allergic forms of keratitis also can produce scarring that will reduce the vision of the patient. Treatment depends upon the cause of the keratitis, such as the strain of bacteria involved; in the case of a viral infection, the organism usually is the cold-sore virus, *herpes simplex*. If the cornea is severely damaged by an attack of keratitis, a corneal transplant may be needed.

Kobrak test A variation of the caloric method of testing one's vestibular apparatus, or sense of balance, with an injection of water against the eardrum. The water used in the Kobrak test usually is a few degrees lower than body temperature. A diagnosis of the condition of one's vestibular apparatus is based on the amount of time that passes before the effect of the water on the eardrum begins and the amount of time required for the patient to recover.

Kocher's test A test for the effect of a *goiter* on the trachea. A goiter, the result of an enlarged thyroid gland, sometimes compresses or displaces the path of the trachea. A harsh vibrating sound may develop in one's breathing during a Kocher's test if a doctor applies a bit of pressure to the side of the thyroid gland when it has displaced the normal path of the trachea.

Koplik spots Small white spots that appear on the inner surface of the mouth, most commonly near the molars, as a diagnostic sign of measles. Each white spot is surrounded by a narrow band of red. The traditional measles rash usually appears a day or two following the Koplik spots.

k.p. A doctor's notation that has nothing to do with military duty in the kitchen. The abbreviation stands for keratic precipitates, cellular debris found on the cornea during an attack of *keratitis*.

labyrinthine function The term refers to one's ability to orient himself in space and means the ability to resist feelings of vertigo or dizziness when moving rapidly in a vertical, horizontal, or rotary direction—for example, in a chair that is whirled around or in an airplane going through acrobatic maneuvers. Some people are slower than others to experience vertigo, and some recover more rapidly than others under such conditions. What is normal and what's not in this category depends pretty much on some arbitrary standards that have been developed from *caloric tests*, the *Barany rotation test*, or *vestibular function tests*.

labyrinthitis A term used to designate inflammation of the inner ear. The cause may be a bacterial or viral infection, or a nonspecific factor associated with an infection in another area of the body. The symptoms may include ringing in the ears and *vertigo*, plus some degree of hearing loss, in viral and nonspecific cases. Bacterial labyrinthitis can be a very serious disease resulting in meningitis and death if immediate medical treatment is not provided.

laceration A wound that results from a tearing of the skin and subcutaneous tissues. Lacerations about the head and face frequently are self-inflicted, as in trying to remove ear wax with a paper clip or hair pin. Such lacerations generally are mild injuries, but they can

lead to infections. A severe laceration with bleeding should be treated by a doctor.

lacrimal apparatus A term used to describe a collection of structures near the eye—a gland, a sac, and several ducts—that enables one to cry. The lacrimal gland that produces tears, known technically as lacrimal fluid, is a small almond-shaped organ in the skull. The tears pass through ducts to the conjunctival surface of the eye, and drain through another duct to a sac that collects the used tears and passes them along into the nose.

LaForte fracture A type of facial fracture in which the maxillary portion, the upper jawbone, becomes separated from other bones of the face. The fracture line may extend upward to include the nasal bone. It is a serious type of fracture that usually requires wiring the pieces together and prolonged therapy.

laryngeal cartilages The several rings of cartilage that shield the vocal cords and shape the general structure of the larynx, or voice box. The laryngeal cartilages form a shape that is seen in the skin of the neck as the Adam's apple.

laryngeal paralysis Paralysis of the nerve that controls the voice box. The symptoms may be loss of voice intensity and some voice fatigue. Another form of the disorder can be more serious because the vocal cords, which lie across the middle of the trachea, can interfere with normal breathing if they do not move naturally when the person inhales. If only one vocal cord is involved, somewhat normal breathing will continue. A person with both vocal cords "frozen" by paralysis of the laryngeal nerves usually cannot get enough oxygen for doing anything more active than resting in bed. A *tracheostomy* generally is required to restore normal breathing.

laryngeal polyps Mucous membrane tumors, usually noncancerous, that form on the vocal cords. The polyps may be the result of vocal abuse, an allergy, or irritation. The treatment is surgical removal of the growths.

laryngeal stenosis A disorder of the larynx caused by scar formation, the result of injury or disease. The scar tissue may interfere with normal breathing and speaking. In severe cases, surgery is needed to treat the condition.

laryngocele A diverticulum, or air sac, in the wall of the membrane around the larynx. The pocket may extend outward from the wall of the larynx or inward. An internal laryngocele may cause hoarseness or breathing difficulties, while an external diverticulum might only appear as a swelling on the neck. The air sac might be found on the throat of a person whose work requires increased pressure in the trachea, such as glass blowers or musicians who play wind instruments. If a laryngocele becomes a health or cosmetic hazard it can be repaired surgically.

laryngomalacia A congenital deformity in which the cartilages of the larynx fail to develop properly. The cartilages are soft and flexible and may tend to be sucked inward when the child inhales. The resulting sign is a rasping sound that occurs with breathing. The deformity gradually corrects itself during the first six months of life, and in most cases no further treatment is required.

laryngoscopy Direct examination of the larynx and surrounding areas with special instruments that can be inserted into the region of the voice box. The examination is done while the patient is under a general or local anesthetic, depending in part upon how apprehensive the patient might be about having a doctor poking about his larynx while he is fully conscious.

leiomyoma A type of noncancerous tumor that may develop in the lining of the lower half of the esophagus. Symptoms may relate to a possible problem in eating or swallowing, including discomfort that is associated more with solid than with liquid foods. An examination, including a barium X-ray, usually will confirm the presence of the growth. An esophageal tumor usually is removed by surgery or by instruments inserted into the food tube, depending upon the type and size of the tumor. Radiation treatment might be used in some cases.

lens A small, disk-shaped transparent structure about one-third of an inch in diameter, which focuses images on the retina of the eye. The lens of the eye is suspended by ligaments that help change the shape of the lens in focusing on near or distant objects.

leprosy A chronic infectious disease marked by nasal discharge, loss of appetite, hoarseness, and loss of feeling in some skin areas. The disease also is characterized by the appearance of nodules and other lesions on the forehead, cheeks, and ears.

leukoplakia A white plaque that forms in the membranes lining the mouth, frequently in association with heavy drinking and smoking. The plaques frequently regress if the person cuts down considerably on his smoking and drinking and practices proper oral hygiene. Otherwise, the leukoplakia plaques may develop progressively into cancers. Small areas of leukoplakia may be removed surgically as a preventive measure against cancer of the mouth.

lichen planus A disease of the mucous membrane lining the mouth. It usually appears as a white, lacey pattern of lesions on the tongue, palate, and other surfaces. The disease causes no physical discomfort, although the person plagued with the disorder may be concerned, particularly if he is hypochondriacal. The membrane lesions may suddenly disappear without treatment, or they may persist for months or years despite all kinds of treatment. Therapies that have appeared to be helpful range from administration of steroid hormones to applications of vitamin A in large doses on the lesions.

A variation of the oral cavity type of lichen planus may occur as intensely itching eruptions on the arms, legs, lower back, genitals, and other skin areas. When lichen planus appears in the mouth, the doctor usually looks for signs and symptoms of the disease elsewhere on the body.

linea alba A horizontal white line that appears on the membrane of the inner surface of the mouth, at the level where the teeth meet. The effect is related to rubbing of the inner surface of the cheek on the molars and generally is no cause for alarm.

lingual thyroid A small mass of thyroid tissue that occasionally appears at the base of the tongue. The wild growth of thyroid tissue occurs at that spot as a mild deformity that developed during embryonic life. It may be removed surgically but the doctor usually will order tests before taking such action to make certain there is adequate thyroid tissue where nature intended, around the Adam's apple.

lingual tonsils A mass of tonsil tissue at the root of the tongue. The tonsils are composed of lymphatic tissue and appear as several dozen, to as many as 100, elevations on the surface of the rear third of the tongue.

Lombard test A test for bilateral functional hearing loss, or deafness in both ears that cannot be associated with organic damage. Earphones are placed over both ears of the person being tested and he is asked to read aloud. While the person is reading, a noise is played into the earphones and the intensity of the noise is increased and then decreased gradually. If the patient's voice changes or fluctuates as the noise level changes, the doctor assumes that the person can hear the background noise on the earphones. A person with a true loss of hearing presumably would not be aware of the background noise.

lop ears A common name for protruding external ears. The ears that protrude abnormally are usually inherited, and the offspring of persons plagued by lop ears also may have the same problem. The condition is harmless, but for cosmetic effect the protruding ears can be made to appear normal by plastic surgery. A few less obvious errors of ear design by nature can be concealed by long hair.

loudness A psychological measure of the intensity of sound. Technically, sound is produced by the vibration of air or other molecules, and the vibrations travel in waves. The greater the pressure of the wave, the greater is the intensity of the sound, and the greater is the loudness received and translated by our hearing organs. The range of the human ear is so great that conventional sound pressure measurements are inadequate to cope with the variations. For that reason, human hearing of loudness usually is measured in *decibels*, a mathematical ratio between sound intensities; a scientist, on the other hand, might measure sound intensities in dynes per square centimeter.

lumpy jaw The common name for a fungal infection that may develop in the mouth. The infection leads to the formation of multiple lumps in the soft tissues. The lumps contain pus that drains through the sinus tracts leading to the skin. A prolonged bout of antibiotic therapy is one form of treatment; the alternative is surgery.

lupus erythematosus A systemic disease characterized by fever, symptoms of rheumatoid arthritis, and pain in the chest and/or abdominal area. The persons afflicted by this disease, of unknown origin, frequently develop reddish skin on both sides of the nose in a pattern that vaguely resembles a butterfly.

lupus vulgaris A tuberculous lesion of the skin of the nose, apparently caused by invasion of tuberculosis germs through a break in the skin. Reddish brown lesions appear on the nose and gradually progress through a stage of soft nodules to ulcers that heal with scar tissue. A person who develops this sign of tuberculosis probably will be examined closely by a doctor for other signs and symptoms of tuberculosis, and he will be treated with drugs designed to control that disease.

lymphatic tissue A part of the system that carries lymph, a watery fluid closely resembling blood plasma, throughout the body. Lymph vessels collect blood plasma that has seeped from blood capillaries into tissue spaces where it has nourished body cells and returns it to the veins. The lymph vessels pass through lymph glands or nodes, which tend to become enlarged when a disease organism enters the system.

macroglossia A congenital deformity in which the tongue is enlarged to the point of interfering with normal functions of the mouth. In certain cases the tongue may be reshaped surgically and excess tissue removed.

macula The point of clearest vision on the retina of the eye. It sometimes is called the macula lutea because of its yellowish coloration, although it actually may appear as a small, dark red spot to a doctor examining the interior of the eye. It is located along the optic axis at the opposite end from the lens of the eye. Variations in the appearance of the macula can provide clues to diseases, such as diabetes, which may show a sign of tiny red spots. A person afflicted with Tay-Sachs disease may have a white macula with a bright red spot in the center.

malleus One of the three bones of the *middle ear.* It sometimes is identified by its common name of hammer, an appropriate designation since its job is to hammer on the next bone in the chain, the incus, or anvil, with vibrations it receives from the eardrum. The malleus is firmly fixed to the membrane of the eardrum for normal hearing function. In some cases of hearing loss, the malleus and other middle ear bones must be removed and repositioned as part of the treatment.

malocclusion The failure of the teeth of the upper and lower jaws to mesh properly. In severe cases the faulty alignment of the upper and lower rows of teeth can interfere with proper mastication. The cause of malocclusion can be a result of a child inheriting the upper jaw of one parent and the lower jaw features of the other parent. Most cases of malocclusion can be corrected by an orthodontist, a dentist who specializes in realigning teeth.

masking A term used to describe a technique used in hearing tests when doctors want to shield a good ear from sounds directed toward an ear with hearing loss. Because sound vibrations can be transmitted around the head by bone conduction, it becomes necessary to feed a masking noise into the good ear to eliminate the crossover effect of bone conduction.

masseter One set of muscles that works the jaw when a person chews food.

mastication A term referring to the chewing of food. The process of chewing requires the action of four different sets of muscles that move the jaws, plus the motion of the tongue muscles in pushing the food between the rows of teeth in the upper and lower jaws.

mastoid A region of spongy bone around the middle ear and the opening of the eustachian tube into the middle ear. Because the mastoid is a close neighbor of the eustachian tube and middle ear, it is subject to involvement with infections that invade those organs. Some infections of the mastoid such as mastoiditis can be very serious, requiring hospitalization and surgery.

mastoidectomy A type of surgery performed to remove diseased mastoid bone.

maxillary sinus The cavity in the maxillary bone, which forms the facial bone surface of the upper jaw on either side of the nose. The maxillary sinuses are the largest in the skull, and they also are the first sinuses to develop in the newborn child.

median rhomboid glossitis A fancy medical mouthful used to describe a raised slick area on the tongue. The smooth bump may be of interest to an examining doctor looking into the mouth of a person who has a median rhomboid glossitis feature, because it occasionally is mistaken for a tumor. However, the firm, elevated bit of tissue is a harmless congenital defect for which there is no real reason for concern.

Meniere's disease A collection of signs and symptoms associated with degeneration of the inner ear; also known as *hydrops*. The patient may experience *vertigo*, nerve deafness, headaches, ringing in the ears, and nausea and vomiting. The disease may be triggered or aggravated by emotional upsets. The cause of Meniere's disease is unknown.

middle ear An air-filled space between the eardrum and the *inner ear*, or true organ of hearing. The middle ear is not sealed against the outside world but is connected to the nasal cavity by way of the eustachian tube, which makes it possible for the pressure in the middle ear to adjust to the air pressure of the surrounding environment. The middle ear contains nerves that communicate between the brain and the face and tongue, and the ossicles, or tiny bones that transmit sound vibrations from the eardrum to the inner ear. Because the facial nerve passes through the middle ear, a disease or injury involving the ear can result in facial paralysis.

migraine A rather common type of headache, particularly for younger women. The pain is caused by a dilation of arteries supplying the head. The attacks sometimes are associated with food allergies, menstrual cycles, or personality patterns. Migraine headaches tend to occur in families. The attacks of migraine frequently are preceded by an aura, or warning sign, that may include flashing lights, blind spots in vision, or other phenomena. There also may be symptoms of nausea, dizziness, and tenderness on the side of the head affected; the attacks frequently involve only one side at a time although both will be affected alternately during a series of migraine attacks.

Treatment is by administration of medicines containing ergot. The medications also may contain caffeine, which has the effect of constricting the dilated arteries that produce the pain symptoms. For migraine patients who are unable to take the drugs orally because of nausea and vomiting, the medications also are given in suppository form so they can be administered through the other end of the digestive tract.

mirror examination A term sometimes used by doctors to mean that they wear a head mirror to direct light into the mouth, throat, or nasal cavity while checking for tumors, ulcerations, infections, or congenital defects—which frequently are clues to the presence of possible problems elsewhere in the body.

monaural loudness balance test A hearing test in which the patient tries to balance the loudness of two different tones directed to the same ear. The test usually is conducted when there is some hearing loss in both ears and the examining doctor wants to find which frequencies of sound are within the hearing range of the patient. The patient is presented with two tones of different frequencies that are sounded alternately; he signals the examiner when he feels the two tones are of the same loudness.

mucocele A cyst that can form on the inner surface membranes of the lips or cheeks. The cyst can be quite soft or about as hard as a rubber ball. It generally grows in size until the cyst has to be removed surgically.

myopia Nearsightedness, or clear visual perception of objects close at hand and blurred vision for objects at a distance. The problem, which may be a hereditary defect in some cases, is caused by images being focused by the lens of the eye on a point ahead of the retina instead of on the retina. Myopia is relatively easy to correct with eyeglasses that bend the rays of light entering the eye so that they focus on the retina. The eyeglass lens usually is concave on both sides to compensate for the error in the eye structure that results in nearsightedness.

myringitis A medical term for inflammation of the eardrum. The condition may be nonspecific in that the cause is not immediately known, or it may be due to a specific bacterial or viral infection. A nonspecific case of myringitis typically is marked by a red and swollen tympanic membrane, and the patient may complain of a dull aching pain in the region of the ear, with some hearing loss. Treatment usually is limited to application of soothing ointments or ear drops to help relieve the symptoms.

A case of bacterial myringitis has similar signs and symptoms but with the added factor in some cases of pus formation. Treatment for bacterial myringitis generally is more rigorous because of the possibility that the disease organism might perforate the eardrum and spread into the mastoid and *middle ear*. Any pus accumulation is drained carefully and regularly, and antibiotic medications are applied.

myringoplasty A name for plastic surgery of the tympanic membrane. The procedure generally is limited to temporary repair of perforated eardrums. Small perforations usually are self-healing over a period of time, and the myringoplasty technique involves simply placing a porous paper patch or piece of skin over the eardrum to hold the membrane in normal position while the healing action is under way.

myringotomy An incision made through the eardrum.

nasal polyps Small gray masses that hang from the roof of the nasal cavity near the turbinates, the cone-shaped structures that help condition inhaled air. Since the polyps are not easily visible, even by looking into the nose, the doctor checking into possible causes of mucus drainage, blocked breathing, or sinusitis, may spray a decongestant into the nasal cavity to shrink the surrounding membranes and bring the polyps into the open—if they are present. Treatment is surgical removal under a local anesthetic.

nasal septum A wall that divides the two chambers of the nose. The front half is made of cartilage and the back half is of bone. The septum is easily injured at almost any time in life, and any disease or injury can result in breathing difficulties. A deviated septum, for example, can narrow the flow of inhaled air through this passageway, forcing the individual to depend upon mouth breathing. Most septal problems can be corrected by surgery. The septum also is the site of a complex of blood vessels and is the source of nosebleeds when the nose is injured.

nasopharynx The part of the pharynx that extends beyond the back of the mouth, up into the rear end of the nasal cavity. The soft palate is at the bottom of the nasopharynx, the adenoid tonsils are on the roof, and the openings into the eustachian tubes are on the rear wall of the cavity.

neurinoma A tumor that arises on a nerve. Acoustic neurinoma, for example, is a tumor involving the nerve that is associated with the inner ear. Symptoms include a ringing in the ears followed by gradual loss of hearing, beginning with difficulty in hearing higher tone frequencies. Other symptoms might include vertigo and headaches.

night vision test As the name suggests, this is a test for persons whose night vision may be deficient. The test is conducted in a darkened room in which the person to be tested must adapt to total or near total darkness for about 30 minutes before the test begins. The adaptation may be helped by having the subject wear dark goggles for a half hour preceding the test. After the person has adapted to the darkness, he is asked to identify characters or other images printed in radioactive ink or paint that glows in the dark. A diagnosis is made on the basis of how many items the person can identify in the dark and the distance required for seeing the characters distinctly. The closer to the images that the viewer must be, the lower is the score.

nystagmus Any involuntary rapid movement of the eyeball. The effect is commonly produced during periods of vertigo, or dizzy spells. See also *positional nystagmus.*

ocular A term referring to the eye, such as an ocular injury for an eye injury. The term usually is further extended to tell medical personnel whether a word refers to the inside of the eyeball or the outside. An extraocular muscle, for example, is attached to the outside of the eye. An intraocular muscle is one that performs a function within the eye, such as the intraocular muscles that adjust the size of the pupils. An eye injury also may be designated as extraocular, as in the case of a cut involving the eyelid, or intraocular, such as a foreign object inside the globe, or eyeball.

odontoma Medical term for a dental problem in which a tooth fails to erupt because of a tumor at that point in the gumline.

olfactory function The sense of smell. The human sense of smell is directed from an olfactory organ at the top of the nasal cavity. It is a long bulb of tissue with nerve endings that extend through tiny holes in a bony ledge that supports the organ. The nerve fibers terminate as a layer of hair cells in the mucous membrane of the nasal lining. The olfactory receptor cells are sensitive enough to detect certain substances that have been diluted to as much as one part in 30 billion. Before any substance can be detected as an odor, however, a few molecules of the substance must be dissolved in the mucus secreted by the nasal membrane.

Humans are less effective as smellers than other animals which depend more upon odors and aromas. The average dog, for example, has an olfactory membrane area that is about 40 times the size of the human olfactory function area.

ophthalmoscope An instrument used to examine the interior of the eyeball. The doctor using an ophthalmoscope can inspect the cornea, the lens, the aqueous humor in the chamber between the lens and the cornea, the vitreous humor in the eyeball behind the lens, and the retina with its arteries, veins, and disk, or head of the optic nerve.

ophthalmometer An instrument used to measure images reflected from the cornea of the eye. It is used by an examining eye doctor to determine the degree of astigmatism in the cornea.

optic atrophy A type of deformity of the retina in which the optic disk, at the point where the optic nerve leaves the back of the eyeball, appears white rather than a normal reddish color when examined with an ophthalmoscope. The pale coloration of the disk frequently is a sign of pressure in or around the brain tissue, such as a brain tumor.

optic nerve The nerve trunk, on either side of the head, that transmits visual images from the retina to the brain. The optic nerve begins at the back of the eyeball as a sort of cable formed from nerve fibers extending from the retina.

orbit The bony cavities of the skull that house the eyeballs, and associated structures such as the muscles that move the eyes, the glands that secrete tears, etc.

oropharynx The back part of the mouth, between the soft palate and the epiglottis.

ossicular chain The three little bones of the middle ear, also known as the ossicles, which transmit sound vibrations from the eardrum to the inner ear. The bones are the malleus, incus, and stapes, also called by their more common names of hammer, anvil, and stirrup, respectively.

osteitis deformans A medical term for *Paget's disease*, which is marked by changes in the bone tissue of the afflicted person. The skull becomes abnormally enlarged with thickened bones at the top, in contrast with normal-sized skull bones. The disease is characterized by other signs and symptoms, such as pain in the bones and bowed legs, but the changes in head shape are among the first and most obvious effects. Some victims of Paget's disease, in fact, become aware of the onset of the disorder when they discover that their hats no longer fit properly.

osteogenesis imperfecta A medical term used to identify an inherited disorder in which the bones are abnormally brittle and are easily broken. The disease sometimes is characterized by such signs as otosclerotic deafness, involving the middle ear bones, or by a bluish coloration of the normally white area of the eyeball surface.

osteomyelitis An inflammation or infection of the bone tissue. The onset of a bone infection is usually sudden and involves severe pain and high fever. Acute osteomyelitis is treated promptly with antibiotics.

otalgia A medical term meaning simply an earache. An earache can be an early warning signal of damage to the upper part of the spine, a forerunner of facial paralysis, or a symptom that occurs just before the onset of *Bell's palsy*. Earache also may be associated with disease or injury involving the teeth, tonsils, sinuses, or larynx, as well as with health conditions affecting a half-dozen different nerve trunks of the head and neck.

otitis externa An inflammation or infection involving the *auricle*, or external ear.

otitis media A general term used to indicate an inflammation or infection of the middle ear. The disorder may be identified further as acute or chronic, and serous or purulent. Serous otitis media is characterized by the appearance of a generally clear fluid in the middle ear; purulent otitis media is marked by the formation of pus in the middle ear. The purulent form is associated with a bacterial infection and may be accompanied by severe pain and hearing loss in the affected ear.

otolaryngologist A physician who specializes in the treatment of disorders of the ear, nose, and throat.

otomycosis If you see this term on a medical record, it means that fungus was detected in the external ear.

otorrhea A discharge of a substance, such as pus, from the ear.

otosclerosis A disease that involves the formation of an abnormal bone structure that inactivates the stapes bone of the *ossicular chain*. When this occurs, the stapes is no longer able to transmit sound vibrations into the inner ear, and the result is a loss of hearing. The problem tends to become progressively worse unless treated by surgery.

otoscope A medical instrument used to examine the ear.

ototoxicity A term usually applied to drug reactions that affect the sense of hearing. Aspirin and quinine, for example, can cause a temporary hearing loss when used in large doses. Antibiotics of certain kinds can cause permanent damage to inner ear mechanisms. The treatment for ototoxicity is to stop using the medications that cause the problem.

oxycephaly The medical term for a pointed head. This is a true skull malformation that can occur because of the premature union of the sutures separating the bones of the cranium. A common name for the deformity is steeple skull.

ozena A term sometimes applied to a crust that forms on the mucous membrane due to an infection. Ozena may be noted by a doctor examining the nose or throat for signs of infection.

pachydermia Although the term suggests circus elephants, it actually translates into something like "thick skin" and is used to identify a disorder of the larynx that is marked by an overgrowth of the membrane tissues around the vocal cords. The symptoms, including hoarseness, are similar to those of chronic laryngitis. The treatment usually requires excision of the excess tissue, and the patient must avoid abuse of the vocal cords, and abstain from the consumption of alcoholic beverages and tobacco products, until the problem is resolved.

Paget's disease The common term for *osteitis deformans*, a crippling deformity involving abnormal growth of bone tissue.

palate perforation A hole in the hard palate, which may be the result of a disease such as syphilis, or due to radiation therapy. A perforated palate could be related to a *cleft palate* problem.

pansinusitis A medical term used sometimes to note that more than one sinus is inflamed or infected. The term suggests only that two or more sinus cavities are involved, without identifying which sinus cavities.

papillae Tiny nipple-shaped protuberances on the surface of the tongue. Some papillae are of the filliform type, which means that they resemble the fine hairs of a velvet fabric, and others are of the fungiform type, so called because they look like fungi. At the back of the tongue a V-shaped row of eight to 12 larger papillae, called vallate papillae, are lined with taste buds.

papilledema Another term for choked disk, a form of disk edema similar to *papillitis* but different in that the optic nerve function is not impaired and vision remains essentially normal. However, some of the same causes of papillitis can be responsible, such as infectious diseases or reactions to toxic substances.

papillitis A disease caused by inflammation of a portion of the optic nerve that results in a swelling of the optic disk, at the point where the optic nerve leaves the eyeball. There usually is loss of vision as the disorder progresses. The inflammation may be the result of metabolic disorder, a wide variety of diseases ranging from multiple sclerosis to mumps, or reactions to toxic substances such as methyl (wood) alcohol.

papilloma A wart-like growth, usually noncancerous at the beginning but capable of undergoing changes to become malignant. A papilloma may develop from the skin of the vestibule in the nose. The tumor is quite distinctive in that it bleeds easily, and bleeding can be started simply by touching the growth.

paranasal sinuses The name for bony cavities in the skull that have connections with the nasal cavity.

parasomia A term meaning a distorted sense of smell. The condition can be caused by inflammation of the olfactory organ tissues in the nasal cavity or by certain hormonal imbalances. A distorted sense of smell also can be the result of emotional problems.

parotid gland One of the pair of salivary glands located just in front of and below the ears.

parotitis Inflammation of a *parotid gland*. A classic example of parotitis is the effect of the mumps virus on the parotid glands, causing tremendous and painful swelling to the extent that the patient sometimes finds it difficult even to open his mouth.

patching A common technique for helping a child overcome a condition of amblyopia, sometimes called lazy eye. Even though the child's eyes seem perfectly normal, the child may depend upon the use of just one eye so much that visual acuity in the other eye is gradually lost, along with normal binocular vision which depends upon the two eyes working together. By having the youngster wear an eye patch over the good eye, the so-called lazy eye is forced to focus on objects in the child's environment and, in theory at least, to become trained to work as well as the good eye. In some cases patching is effective in correcting a lazy eye problem, but in others it fails to work out as well as expected. Surgery frequently is used instead of, or in addition to, patching in order to correct the lack of binocular vision that is marked by crossed eyes or squint.

pediatric audiometry The name given to a group of tests and procedures used to determine whether an infant has a normal sense of hearing. Since a small child is unable to communicate with examiners conducting tests of hearing loss, the diagnosis of an infant's ear functions must be done indirectly. The precise techniques vary with the age of the child. For example, if the child is old enough to respond to the sound made by a squeeze toy or to his own name, that particular sound or word can be directed toward the child to see whether he responds by turning his head. A child less than three months of age might be checked with a jerk or blink reflex action when a sound of known intensity and frequency is directed at his ear from a distance of a few inches.

pemphigus A form of rare skin disease characterized by large blister-like lesions or eruptions on the inside of the mouth and throat. Unless controlled by special medications such as steroid drugs, the disease tends to spread and become increasingly debilitating. The cause of the disorder is unknown.

periodontosis Another word for *pyorrhea*. A related term, periodontist, is the name given to the dental specialist who corrects periodontosis, or pyorrhea.

peritonsillar abscess Another name for the condition sometimes called *quinsy*. The disorder is characterized by severe pain around the soft plate and walls of the pharynx; the discomfort may be felt in the neck as well. The person afflicted may find it difficult to open his mouth. The cause of the disorder is the spread of a bacterial infection from the tonsils. The treatment will include antibiotics to control the infection, incisions to drain the pus from the abscess, saltwater throat irrigations, and plenty of bed rest.

pharyngitis Inflammation of the pharynx, usually marked by throat pain or discomfort, difficult swallowing, loss of appetite, and fever. The inflammation usually is caused by an infection such as the common cold virus, although the infection could be the result of an uncommon bacteria like diphtheria. A case of pharyngitis in which a white membrane appears in the pharynx, with bleeding when the

white membrane is stripped, should receive immediate attention by a doctor.

phonation The production of speech sounds.

pink eye A common name for *conjunctivitis*, or inflammation of the conjunctiva of the eye.

plate set A term used sometimes to identify the series of plates, or printed pictures, for testing color vision; or more specifically, pseudoisochromatic plate set. A standard plate set contains 14 different colored pictures with images that are not easily detected by persons with red-green color blindness. The set also includes a 15th plate that is used to demonstrate how the test is conducted. The person being tested is given about two seconds to find the image hidden in the color pattern of each plate.

politzerization A long word meaning a technique for opening the eustachian tube by pumping air into it. The way it works is this: one nostril is pinched shut and a device called a politzer bag is used to pump air into the other nostril, forcing air into the eustachian tube and the middle ear space.

polypectomy The surgical removal of polyps from the nasal cavity. The procedure is done while the patient is under a local or general anesthetic. In some cases, the surgery is performed at a hospital.

positional nystagmus Also called positional vertigo, this condition is an unusual health problem in which *nystagmus* or *vertigo* is experienced only when the head is held in a certain position. There is no nausea or hearing loss associated with the nystagmus the person feels when the head is moved in a particular direction. The disorder is related to the type of loss of balance or vertigo experienced when seated in a chair that is whirled around rapidly.

A doctor examining a patient for possible positional nystagmus usually will place the patient on an examining table in a sitting position, then rapidly move the person to a supine position, that is, flat on the back. Next the head is moved quickly to the right and to the left. Finally, the person is raised rapidly back into a sitting position. At some point in the test a person afflicted with positional nystagmus will exhibit the rapid eye movement sometimes accompanying a dizzy spell within a few seconds after a quick change of head positions. Generally, a case of positional nystagmus will be self-limiting, that is, it will clear up within a few weeks or a few months. If the condition continues beyond three months, a more detailed examination will be recommended because of the possibility of disease or injury to the central nervous system.

postnasal drip A common complaint associated with inflammation of the nasal cavity and pharynx. Postnasal drip can be a sign or symptom of the basic problem, which can be either an infection or an allergic reaction. Doctors, who usually develop some expertise in sorting out postnasal drip characteristics through years of practice, will note that a watery postnasal drip associated with watery eyes and sneezing probably is due to an allergy. If the postnasal drip is thick and contains pus, the doctor usually will determine that the cause is an infection. An infectious postnasal drip frequently is associated with a sinus problem, with the drip coming from the sinus infection. If the cause is an allergy, the doctor usually will try to determine the substance causing the irritation so that the patient can avoid the allergen in the future.

presbyopia A vision problem that is associated with growing older. The crystalline lens that focuses an image on the retina of the eyeball loses its elasticity and therefore its ability to change shape and accommodate distinct viewing of images at different distances. The problem is corrected by the use of reading glasses designed to permit clear vision at whatever distance is appropriate for the person's usual job performance.

prosthesis An artificial body part. In the head and neck area, a prosthesis could be an artificial replacement part for a damaged ossicle in the middle ear. The incus and stapes occasionally are rebuilt from plastic and/or metal, as in a *stapedectomy.*

pterygium A triangle-shaped tumor that may grow near the nasal edge of the cornea of the eye. The fleshy growth is not a malignant, or cancerous, tumor, but it can cause local irritation and eventually interfere with normal vision. In that case a pterygium can be easily removed by surgery.

ptosis A drooping of the upper eyelid. There can be a variety of causes, such as myasthenia gravis, a neurological disease; an injury to the muscle that controls movement of the eyelid; or an injury that resulted in scarring of the lid. If the disorder is a sign of a disease or injury involving the lid or nearby tissues, the treatment usually is directed toward correcting the original problem. However, in some cases ptosis can be relieved by eyelid surgery.

ptyalism A fancy term for increased saliva secretion, a condition that can be caused by teething in a child, a rabies infection, smoking tobacco, reactions to certain foods or medications, diseases of the mouth and throat, or emotional stress.

pyorrhea A term referring to the loss of supporting tissues around the teeth, usually as a result of infection and poor dental hygiene. The condition tends to spread from one tooth to the next until the entire set becomes involved, unless professional dental care is started to control the disorder. If the pyorrhea damage becomes extensive, the restoration of the teeth becomes extensive and expensive.

quinsy A commonly used term for *peritonsillar abscess,* an infection that spreads from the tonsils to the neighboring areas of the nose and throat.

radiation injury An area of skin or other tissue that has been overexposed to X-ray or similar radiation therapy may appear like a sunburn, that is, reddened, perhaps swollen, and oozing a thin, clear fluid.

radium plaque A device used in tests for night vision. It may contain a display of images, geometric patterns or characters, printed with a radioactive material which allows the images to be seen in total darkness by a person with normal night vision.

ranula The name of a bluish-reddish cyst that may develop under the tongue. Although a ranula is not cancerous, it must be removed surgically.

raspberry tongue A peculiar reddish color that appears on the tongue as the result of certain diseases, such as scarlet fever. The color is caused by toxins that produce an inflammation of the papillae on the surface of the tongue.

recruitment An unusual sensitivity to loud sounds by a person whose hearing otherwise is impaired. A person with signs of recruitment frequently can hear loud sounds better than a person with normal hearing.

reflex An involuntary response to a stimulus. Reflex tests are used to determine if a child too young to speak may be suffering from a form of deafness. A sudden burst of sound in the form of a controlled tone at a specific intensity, for example, should cause an infant with normal hearing to blink or jerk its limbs in a reflex action.

refraction The ability of substances to bend rays of light. In the eye the cornea, the aqueous humor in the chamber between the cornea and lens, the lens itself, and the vitreous humor behind the lens all have a bending effect on light entering the eye. When all parts of the eye bend the rays of light so that the image of an object you are looking at is focused sharply on the retina of your eye, your refraction is rated as normal. The medical term for normal refraction is emmetropia. If the cornea, lens, or other parts of the eyeball—including the general shape of the eyeball itself—fail to produce normal refraction, eyeglass lenses are prescribed to compensate for the natural errors of vision. Concave lenses generally compensate for nearsighted errors of refraction, and con-

vex lenses usually are prescribed for farsighted errors of refraction.

retina A thin layer of light-sensitive nerve receptors lining the inside of the eyeball. The receptors are attached to nerve fibers that extend from the back of the eyeball to form the optic nerve.

retinal atherosclerosis A sign of disease in the blood vessels as observed by a doctor examining the interior of the eyeball. The artery walls normally are transparent when seen in the retina of the eye. As atherosclerosis develops, however, the blood vessel walls become thicker and the fatty deposits may give the vessels a milky white appearance. At a point of moderate accumulation of fatty deposits, the vessels may have the coloration of burnished copper. The condition of the arteries in the retina generally indicates the extent of the disease elsewhere in the body. The retinal arteries might not represent the state of atherosclerosis in other areas, but they are one of the best clues to the condition that a doctor can find without actually examining arteries directly, as in surgery.

retinitis An inflammation of the retina which usually results in visual disturbances. Blood, urine, and other laboratory tests usually must be conducted to determine the cause of the inflammation so that the proper kind of treatment can be prescribed.

retinopathy A term used by doctors to indicate certain distinctive signs that appear in the retina in association with a disease. In the case of hypertension, for example, the blood vessels in the retina may appear during examination of the eye to be abnormally narrowed or constricted.

rhagades A name for white scars that may appear at the corners of the mouth, radiating outward in thin lines, caused by a disease such as syphilis.

rhinitis An inflammation of the lining of the nose. The cause can be a viral infection, like the common cold, or irritation from tobacco smoke or chemical fumes, or an infection involving bacteria. See also *acute rhinitis; allergic rhinitis; atrophic rhinitis; vasomotor rhinitis.*

rhinolalia A term sometimes used to identify nasal speech sounds produced by a person suffering from paralysis of the pharynx and/or palate.

rhinophyma A medical term for the overgrowth of skin and sebaceous glands on the tip of the nose. The condition is usually associated with acne rosacea, or "whiskey nose."

rhinoscopy Examination of the nasal passages.

Rinne test A tuning fork test of hearing used by an examining doctor to tell whether the hearing problem is in the middle or external ear, or in the inner ear. The vibrating tuning fork is held about one inch away from the external ear, then placed against the mastoid bone. If the tuning fork is heard more easily when the tip is placed against the mastoid, it indicates a hearing loss in the air-conduction system extending from the eardrum through the middle ear bones. If the sound is heard more easily when the tuning fork is held near the ear, it is a sign of damage to the inner ear.

Ritter unit A piece of equipment that uses compressed air to open a blocked eustachian tube. The patient is instructed to swallow or to pronounce the letter "K" several times while compressed air is forced into one nostril, the other nostril being held closed at the time.

saddle nose The common name sometimes used to identify a sunken bridge of the nose. The cause usually is an injury that damages the nasal septum, an abscess of the septum, or a disease that produces a similar effect.

salivary duct calculus A disorder that has nothing to do with higher mathematics but is due to the formation of a stone in a salivary duct or gland. A calculus most often develops in the maxillary gland and causes some pain and swelling while the person is eating. The symptoms subside after a short period of time. An examining doctor often can detect the location of a salivary gland stone by palpation, or feeling the gland through the skin.

salivary gland tumors The salivary glands can be targets for either cancerous or noncancerous tumors. The parotid gland is the most common tumor site for abnormal growths in the salivary glands. The tumors can develop in a person at any age. Treatment generally is by surgical removal of the growth.

salpingitis An inflammation of a tube of body tissue. An inflammation of the eustachian tube might be recorded by a doctor as eustachian salpingitis.

scintillating scotoma A mouthful of medical terminology that identifies a type of visual disturbance sometimes associated with migraine headaches. The person afflicted may see wavy lines that resemble the "heat waves" rising from the pavement on a hot day.

scleritis A type of inflammation of the sclera, or white outer coat of the eyeball. The disease can be a painful spinoff of conjunctivitis or an allergic response to a disorder involving other areas of the body. The disorder frequently is associated with rheumatoid arthritis. Some forms of scleritis are marked by the appearance of nodules or ulcers on the sclera.

sense of smell The *olfactory function* of the nose.

septoplasty An operation performed to straighten a deviated nasal septum.

sialadenitis An inflammation of a salivary gland by a viral, bacterial, or fungal disease. Bacterial infections of salivary glands are not uncommon and may be characterized by severe pain, swelling, and tenderness. Before antibiotics were available, bacterial infections of the parotid gland could be life threatening. Treatment today is generally quick and effective when the disease organism has been identified so that the proper medication can be used.

Mumps is a good example of a viral infection of the salivary gland. Although the painful swelling of the jaws associated with mumps usually occurs in children, it also can affect adults who have not been immunized.

Allergic sialadenitis usually is caused by a reaction to medicines being taken for some other disorder. The allergic swelling usually subsides as soon as the offending substance has been identified and discontinued.

sinus An irregular air space in the bones that surround the nose. There are roughly a dozen sinuses on each side of the nose, but the exact number may vary. Some people, for example, have a frontal sinus on each side of the nose, others have a frontal sinus on just one side, and still others have no frontal sinuses at all.

Snellen test A vision test for persons who can read letters of the alphabet. It is the standard eye chart test, which has just one large letter, such as a capital E, at the top and successive rows of letters below, each row or line of letters being somewhat smaller in size than those above. Under ideal test conditions, a person with normal distance vision can read from a distance of 20 feet a line of letters that most people with good visual acuity can read. Such a person is said to have 20/20 vision. If the person tested can see well enough to read only the line which an individual with normal vision can read at a distance of 40 feet, his vision is recorded as 20/40. The lines of type generally are printed in rows that are readable by a person with normal vision from distances of 200, 100, 70, 50, 40, 30, 20, 15, and 10 feet.

In order for the person being tested to give an accurate response, he should be exactly 20 feet from the eye chart. When examining rooms aren't large enough to permit eye chart reading from a distance of 20 feet, equivalent methods may be used. For example, smaller sets of letters are projected on a screen, or the patient reads the chart by looking in a mirror 10 feet away from a 20-foot distance chart. Patients with poor vision who can't see even the largest letters on the chart from a distance of

20 feet may have to try from perhaps 8 feet—in which case their visual acuity is recorded as 8/200.

speculum An instrument used by doctors to view a passage or cavity in a body. For examining the head and neck area, there are special speculums designed to look into the ears and nose.

sphenoiditis An inflammation of the sphenoid sinus, which lies in the center of the head. An infection of this region can be marked by severe deep-seated headaches, fever, loss of appetite, and a general feeling of illness. While not a common ailment, sphenoiditis can be very dangerous because the infection can spread into the brain with fatal results. Treatment usually involves the administration of antibiotics and decongestants, plus drainage and irrigation of the sinus.

stapedectomy An operation to correct a defect in the ossicles, or bones of the middle ear, by removing the stapes, or stirrup. The stapes and its footplate are replaced during the operation with a prosthesis, or artificial stapes, built of materials such as wire and plastic. The operation usually is performed when bone growth invades the stapes footplate and immobilizes it so that sound vibrations cannot be transmitted to the inner ear.

stereo orthopter A device used by eye doctors to check the way in which the human eyes coordinate. It also may be used to strengthen eye muscles and to correct eyes that do not work together properly.

stomatitis An inflammation of the mucous membrane lining the mouth.

strabismus A medical term meaning that the two eyes do not work together properly, usually because of a muscle imbalance. The effect of the two eyes failing to coordinate is known commonly as cross-eye or walleye, depending upon which way one or both eyes may deviate from the normal. If the eye deviates inward, or toward the other eye, the condition sometimes is called esotropia; if the eye wanders outward, it is known as exotropia; and if the eye wanders upward, the condition is called hypertropia.

Strabismus may be marked by a gross deviation of one or both eyes at all times. In other cases, an eye will wander only when the individual is ill or fatigued. The condition frequently is corrected by surgery that alters the muscles of the wandering eye; other corrective measures can include *patching*, eye exercises, or an eyeglass prescription designed to reduce muscle imbalance. A child born with strabismus may be given all of the corrective procedures because failure to correct the muscle imbalance problem can result in amblyopia, or a loss of normal vision in the eye not used properly.

stridor A wheezing or rasping noise made when a person inhales or exhales. The cause generally is an obstruction in the air passages between the nose and the lungs; most often stridor is caused by a problem in the larynx.

submucous resection An operation to correct a deviated septum in the nose.

symblepharon Adhesion of the eyelid to the eyeball, a situation that sometimes occurs after an acid or alkali is accidentally splashed into the eyes. The doctor treating a chemical burn of the eyes will apply an ointment to the conjunctiva in order to keep the surfaces lubricated and less likely to stick together.

syncope A medical term for fainting. Fainting sometimes is caused by decreased circulation of blood to the brain. This problem can be the result of hardening of the arteries, an injury that causes a loss of blood, or heart disease, among other factors. The lightheadedness that many people experience when they suddenly rise to a standing position after lying on the back is a syncope symptom. Persons who are syncope sensitive usually learn to move slowly from a resting to a standing position; otherwise they may "pass out" and fall to the floor.

systemic disease A disease that affects the body as a whole. A systemic disease often produces signs and symptoms that may appear at first to be only an inflammation or infection of a small area of the body. For example, a disease known as scurvy affects the entire body, but it may be discovered because of tender or bleeding gums, which are among the signs and symptoms of the vitamin C deficiency disease.

T & A Commonly used abbreviation for tonsillectomy and adenoidectomy, or tonsils and adenoids. A doctor may recommend surgical excision of the tonsils if a person, usually a young child, has repeated attacks of tonsillitis, or infections of the tonsils. Other reasons for a tonsillectomy may include tonsillitis complicated by other diseases such as rheumatic fever, or diphtheria when doctors find an antibiotic-resistant form of the bacteria that seems to settle in the tonsil tissue. Tonsils usually become less of a problem after the age of 12 years, and thus there is less likelihood of surgical excision in an older youngster.

An adenoidectomy commonly is performed at the same time as a tonsillectomy, although the problems associated with adenoid disorders, such as nasal obstruction or middle ear infection, do not appear to be directly related to pharyngitis. However, adenoids are tonsil tissue located high in the nasopharynx, and an organism that invades one tonsil is likely to spread to the others as well. Adenoids atrophy when a child approaches puberty and, with a few exceptions, adenoidectomies usually are not performed on youngsters after they become teenagers.

taste The sensations of sweet, sour, bitter, and salt as perceived through taste buds located in the tongue, the palate, the lining of the cheeks, and in some cases, on the walls of the pharynx and epiglottis. The taste buds are nerve receptors which relay their information through two different nerve trunks to the brain.

threshold The point at which a stimulus just barely produces a sensation. The normal human ear is most sensitive to sounds with a frequency of about 1,000 cycles per second. Sounds of lower or higher frequencies generally must be louder to reach the just barely heard stage.

thrush A common name for moniliasis, a fungal infection of the mouth and pharynx. It is characterized by a white plaque that may cover any area of the inside of the mouth but most often appears on the pharynx and soft palate. Symptoms can include a feeling of discomfort and dryness of the mouth. The person who is afflicted with thrush frequently is one who has been treated with antibiotics for another disease; the antibiotics not only destroy the disease bacteria but the "good" bacteria of the body that normally keep the fungi of the mouth under control.

tic douloureux Another name for trigeminal neuralgia, a severe type of nerve pain that affects the middle of the face. The area affected can range all the way from the eye to the lower jaw but most often involves the upper jaw. The attacks are easily triggered by seemingly insignificant stimuli such as touching the face, exposure to cold, or brushing the teeth. Tic douloureux attacks are rare in young people and are most likely to affect persons who have reached middle age. The attacks of pain usually do not last long, but they can become increasingly severe as they are repeated.

Treatment of various kinds may be tested in the search for one that provides continuing relief for a victim of the nerve disease. The therapies usually include the administration of sedatives, tranquilizers, narcotics, and other medications; inhalation of trichloroethylene, an anesthetic; injections of vitamin B 12, alcohol, or boiling water; and, finally, surgery to cut the sensory nerve involved in the disorder.

tinnitus The medical term for a ringing in the ears. There are several variations of tinnitus as experienced by different people. Some describe the sensation as high pitched, others as low

pitched; the ringing also can be steady, intermittent, or pulsating. Tinnitus may be caused by exposure to loud noises, a blocked eustachian tube, or a middle ear infection. The effect also can be a sign of a brain tumor, a tumor of a cranial nerve, or a disease of the inner ear.

TMJ An abbreviation for temporomandibular joint, the "hinge" of the skull where the lower jaw is attached to the upper jaw. The mandible is the lower jaw, the part that moves when the mouth is opened or closed. The action is controlled by several groups of muscles that can move the lower jaw up, down, or sideways.

TMJ problems are many and can be either of an organic or functional nature. Organic disorders may include a fusion of the joint, usually as a result of an injury, or destruction of the temporomandibular joint by arthritis. Functional disorders can include a variety of facial pain complaints, including a type of ear pain that radiates to the temple or neck, usually on one side of the head, and is aggravated by chewing motions. TMJ complaints sometimes can be traced to dental disorders; a missing tooth or an improper filling may cause the affected patient to favor one side of the jaw so that coordinated action of TMJ's on both sides of the skull becomes unbalanced. Stress and tension effects, such as grinding of the upper and lower sets of teeth together or clenching of the jaw, can lead to muscle fatigue or spasm, which in turn may become a functional complaint.

Most functional TMJ problems can be relieved by simple measures such as eating soft foods, applying heat to the affected area, and taking medicines that relax muscles and relieve pain.

tongue-tie A congenital disorder in which a person is born with an abnormally short piece of tissue holding the tongue to the floor of the mouth; the medical name is *ankyloglossia*. In some severe cases a tongue-tied patient cannot move the tip of his tongue far enough to touch the roof of his mouth. Because of the immobilized tongue, speaking and eating may be difficult. However, the problem is rather easily solved by surgery.

tonometer An instrument used to measure the intraocular pressure of the eyeball. One type commonly used is the Schiotz tonometer. It is placed over the *cornea* of the eye after the eye has been anesthetized. The instrument has a small weight attached and works as a sort of balance in measuring the pressure exerted against it by the fluid between the lens and the cornea. Other tonometers work by electronically measuring the intraocular pressure or by blowing a puff of air against the cornea to measure resistance.

torus palatinus Another fancy medical term for a minor medical problem. The problem is a cartilage or bone protuberance that may appear in the midline of the hard palate. A torus palatinus is a harmless growth that ordinarily requires no treatment, unless it interferes with the fitting of dental plates.

tracheostomy The name for an operation in which a hole is made in the trachea by surgery so that a tube can be inserted to improve the flow of air to the lungs. A tracheostomy is usually performed when there is an obstruction to breathing in the upper part of the pharynx. The procedure also may be used occasionally for other purposes such as to suction foreign matter from the bronchial area between the trachea and the deep lung tissue.

transconioscopy A technique for examining the larynx by inserting a small telescope into the throat.

trench mouth A common name for *Vincent's angina*, an infection of the pharynx that is marked by sore throat, a mild fever, and a bad taste in the mouth. The tonsils, gums, and other mucous membranes of the mouth and throat may be covered with grayish patches. Treatment requires antibiotics as well as other medications.

trismus Difficulty in opening the mouth due to pain, muscle spasms, or a problem involving nerves that control the muscles of the mouth.

tuning fork tests A variety of tuning fork tests are used by doctors to check problems of hearing loss. The most common tests involve placing the tip of a vibrating tuning fork on the mastoid area of the head to check bone conduction of sound as compared with air conduction through the external ear, or placing the tip of the vibrating tuning fork at the midline of the forehead to determine whether the sound is heard better in one ear or the other. Tuning forks also are used to test functional hearing loss, as in cases of persons who claim they are deaf although doctors can find no evidence of disease or injury to account for the reported hearing loss.

tympanic membrane The eardrum. If the eardrum is perforated as a result of disease or injury, doctors sometimes help the healing process by patching the perforation with pieces of porous paper that have been soaked in medicinal chemicals. An alternative procedure, called *myringoplasty*, involves repair by surgery, using a skin graft from the patient.

tympanoplasty A term meaning surgical reconstruction of the ossicles, or bones that transmit sound vibrations through the middle ear. The tympanic membrane usually is involved in the reconstruction and is rebuilt with a skin graft or transplant of other tissue from the region of the ear. The ossicles may be rebuilt or replaced with wire or plastic parts, and repositioned so they will transmit sound vibrations in a normal manner to the oval window of the inner ear.

uveitis An inflammation involving the choroid layer of the eyeball, or the *iris* and ciliary body of the eye, the three structures which comprise the uveal tract. The condition sometimes is marked by the appearance of deposits of white or yellow flecks on the inner surface of the cornea.

uvulitis An inflammation or infection of the uvula, the flap of tissue that dangles from the end of the soft palate at the back of the roof of the mouth.

vasomotor rhinitis A general term used by doctors to identify any inflammation, irritation, or infection involving the nose or nasal cavity when the exact cause is unknown.

vertical gaze failure A lack of ability of a person to gaze upward, usually because of a disorder of the nervous system. Since the eyes cannot be moved upward without moving the head, the affected person must tilt his head backward to see objects above a line that would be on the same plane as his eyes.

vertigo Technically, a failure of the body to orient itself in space. Actually, the person with vertigo feels dizzy or has the sensation of falling or spinning around. The causes of vertigo can be disorders of the middle ear or inner ear, or lesions of the brain or nerve trunk that connects the ear to the brain.

vestibular function tests Vestibular, or labyrinthine, tests are used to check on the normal or abnormal condition of the semicircular canals of the inner ear, which control one's sense of balance. Most tests involve either whirling a person about in a chair or injecting water that is slightly warmer or cooler than normal body temperature against the eardrum. Either test method can produce a feeling of vertigo or dizziness that causes a rapid movement of the eyeballs. The eye movements, or *nystagmus*, are supposed to begin a certain number of seconds after the stimulus and stop within a fixed period of time if the semicircular canals are in normal condition.

vestibular neuronitis The medical term for a disorder involving the nerve cells of the inner ear that are associated with the sense of balance. The illness is characterized by severe attacks of *vertigo* with nausea and vomiting. The person afflicted requires bed rest with a minimum of body movement, since any change of position can trigger an attack. After the first week the symptoms subside, but an additional two to three weeks of bed rest may be needed for complete recovery. Treatment during the illness usually is limited to antivertigo medicines, which may have to be given by injection

or suppository during the early stages marked by severe nausea.

Vincent's angina Medical term for *trench mouth*, an ulcerating disease that can affect almost any part of the oral cavity from the gums to the throat.

vocal nodules Sometimes known as singer's nodes, the growths are inflammatory reactions to abuse of the vocal cords. The condition is marked by hoarseness and a voice that cracks when speaking or singing. The nodules are removed by laryngoscopy. The patient is advised to give the voice a long rest and take lessons to properly control the voice in speaking or singing.

voice tests A term that is something of a misnomer because the voice tests used by doctors actually are tests of the patient's ability to hear rather than to speak. Voice tests usually are conducted with the subject facing away from the examiner while words are spoken at a whisper or at a normal speaking level from a fixed distance. If the person being tested can hear a spoken or whispered voice at a distance of 15 feet, the response is recorded as 15/15. If the patient needs to be 10 feet from the examiner in order to hear as well as a person with normal hearing from a distance of 15 feet, the hearing acuity would be listed as 10/15.

Voice tests for hearing ability generally have been replaced by electronic audiometry equipment that can generate tones of controlled frequencies and intensities. These are more accurate than voice tests, which require a bit of guesswork on the part of the examiner.

watch test A hearing test in which a patient is asked to listen for the ticking sound of a watch from a fixed distance. Like the so-called voice tests, it is not very accurate.

water provocative test One of the tests used in diagnosing *glaucoma* in a patient who shows a high intraocular pressure when examined with a *tonometer*. The subject is weighed and then asked to drink a measured amount of water, depending upon the weight of the person being tested. The amount of water consumed usually ranges from the equivalent of three drinking glasses of fluid for a 100-pound individual to about six glasses of water for a person weighing 200 pounds or more. If the patient has glaucoma, the intraocular pressure should rise with the intake of fluid. The intraocular pressure in water provocative tests may be measured by electronic tonometry, using equipment that produces a tracing on a chart showing the amount of pressure change following water intake.

Weber test A hearing test in which a vibrating tuning fork is placed at the middle of a patient's forehead to determine whether the hearing is better in one ear or the other.

Wharton's duct The name given salivary gland ducts. They are of more than academic interest when blocked by salivary gland stones, or calculi, causing pain, tenderness, and swelling. In some cases the salivary stones must be removed by surgery.

wick The term sometimes used to identify strips of gauze soaked in medicine and inserted into the external ear canal to treat an infection or chemical irritation.

xanthelasma Soft yellowish plaque that may appear on the eyelids. It usually is a sign of hypercholesterolemia, or an abnormally high level of cholesterol lipids in the blood.

xanthoma A relatively large plaque that may vary in color from yellow to red or brown, associated with a disorder of fat metabolism by the body's tissues. Like xanthelasma, a xanthoma usually is a sign of hypercholesterolemia. The xanthomas may appear on the face and scalp, among other body sites for the plaques.

A somewhat different form of xanthoma may appear on the face and scalp as small reddish-brown plaques that are closely packed together. These tiny plaques, too, are associated with an abnormally high level of cholesterol in the blood.

xerostomia The condition of dry mouth. This medical term refers to a dry mouth that results from decreased activity of the salivary glands. A dry mouth can be caused by a number of factors, including X-ray therapy for treatment of tumors in the area of the mouth, emotional stress, diseases such as diabetes, physical exercise, decreased fluid intake, and an assortment of drugs such as tranquillizers and antihistamines.

QUESTIONS AND ANSWERS

THE HEAD AND NECK

Q: *What kind of antibiotics can I take for a head cold?*
A: If the head cold is caused by the common cold virus it is unlikely that any antibiotic would be helpful, except to control a secondary infection caused by bacteria. Antibiotics are weapons against bacteria but are generally useless in fighting a virus infection.

Q: *Is it possible to have a migraine-type aura without a headache?*
A: Yes, it is possible. But usually as an aura subsides, a head pain develops on the side opposite the eye in which the aura was experienced. In cases of an aura without a headache, such as the zigzag, colored lines that may appear in the vision, there may be an annoying stimulus such as a bright light shining in one's eyes.

Q: *My husband is color-blind. Does this mean our children also will be color-blind?*
A: There are several kinds of color blindness, and female offspring are seldom affected directly. However, the daughters can become carriers of the gene for a form of color blindness, and about half their sons in turn may become color-blind. The patterns of color-blind inheritance are somewhat like those of inherited balding patterns, with the effect appearing in every other generation. If your own sons turn out to be color-blind, it would suggest that your own father was color-blind, with you, the mother, as a carrier of the gene.

Q: *Is a color-blind person really blind to all colors?*
A: It's a bit difficult to tell exactly what colors a color-blind individual may see. However, recent research seems to discount the old idea that color-blind persons see everything in shades of gray. It seems more likely that color-

blind people simply confuse gray with other colors, such as green, blue, or red. They may also confuse brown and black with red, or greenish-blue with purple, and so on. The confusion increases with pale colors rather than deeper hues.

Q: *What is the best home treatment for a black eye?*
A: Emergency treatment for a black eye should be limited to the application of a cold pack, which can be made by wrapping small pieces of ice in a clean towel or cloth. However, any injury severe enough to cause bleeding in the tissues around the eyeball—which is the source of the dark discoloration—may result in fractures of the bony walls around the eye, damage to the optic nerve, or other complications, such as infection. Therefore, a black eye injury should be checked by a doctor as soon as possible.

Q: *Is there a cure for dandruff?*
A: There probably is some confusion about the cause and cure for dandruff because what most people think of as dandruff is not the same condition that a doctor considers to be dandruff. Real dandruff, in the medical sense of the term, involves a serious inflammation of the scalp with irritation and itching, and perhaps some activity of the sebaceous glands. For real dandruff, the doctor treats the disease rather than the effect. The white flecks that most people see in their hair from time to time are merely dead skin cells that have been sloughed off; they are the same kind of epidermal scales, or cells, that are rubbed off or washed off the rest of the body each day in countless numbers. The use of regular shampoos, perhaps twice a week or so, will help rid the hair of the dead skin cells almost as fast as they accumulate. Washing too often, on the

other hand, may dry out the scalp and accelerate the flaking off of skin cells. The use of oily ointments may simply trap the dead skin cells in the hair and make the condition appear worse than it actually is.

Q: *Is there any protection against diphtheria?*
A: Immunization against diphtheria is so common these days that the disease itself is uncommon. The immunization shots for diphtheria usually are given to children routinely, but older persons may not have had the opportunity to get diphtheria shots. If the disease attacks a person not already immunized, a doctor usually administers a diphtheria antitoxin instead of the shots that offer immunity. Diphtheria can be a very deadly disease, causing the formation of a whitish membrane over the back of the throat that can result in suffocation. The disease organism also can damage the heart.

Q: *When I have a toothache, I crush an aspirin tablet and pack it into the cavity. Somebody told me this is not a good way to handle a toothache. What do you think?*
A: I think if you have a tooth cavity large enough to hold a crushed aspirin tablet you should run, not walk, to your nearest dentist. Although many people have packed crushed aspirin into an aching tooth for many years, it is not a good idea for at least two reasons. One is that aspirin works best when it is consumed with a glass of water and allowed to kill pain by circulating through the bloodstream by way of the digestive tract. Secondly, the aspirin might irritate exposed tissues in the tooth pulp, including the nerve that causes the pain.

Q: *Why are tonsils a problem with young children?*
A: Tonsils usually do not become a problem unless they are overwhelmed by an invasion of disease bacteria. The function of tonsils is to help guard against germs that might enter the body through the nose and mouth. They contain lymphatic tissue with white blood cells whose job is to destroy germs. However, the tonsil tissue does not win all the battles and, in fact, there may be occasions when the germs win and make the tonsils a breeding ground for more germs. When tonsils are no longer effective in preventing disease, a doctor may recommend that they be removed. On the other hand, most kids eventually outgrow their need for tonsils, and the tonsil tissue gradually atrophies so it is no longer a potential problem.

Q: *What causes a stye and what can be done about it?*
A: A stye is caused by an inflammation of a tiny gland, and sometimes of several glands, along the edge of the eyelid. A bacterial infection usually is involved, with the result that pus forms and the glands become swollen and painful. The stye eventually ruptures and the pus is discharged. The stye should be treated carefully because of the possibility that the bacteria causing the problem can spread to other tissues surrounding the eye, and the consequences can be additional sties, or worse.

Q: *What causes a person to cough or sneeze?*
A: A cough and a sneeze actually are quite similar, although the noise produced by the violent expulsion of air from the lungs by the two actions may be quite dissimilar. Both are protective reflex actions, methods that nature has for protecting the respiratory system. A sneeze is triggered by an irritation of the mucous membrane of the nose; a cough is triggered by an irritation of the mucous membrane beyond the nose. The irritation can be produced by a variety of stimuli ranging from a blast of cold air to a bit of dust or dirt in the air. The irritant results in the person taking a deep breath, after which the vocal cords close briefly, then open after the explosive outward blast of air begins. To illustrate the power of a cough or sneeze, it has been calculated that the blast of expired air from the lungs travels at about the speed of sound.

Q: *Is 20/20 vision perfect?*
A: Vision that is rated at 20/20 by a Snellen chart test is normal, but a visual acuity of 20/15 is also normal, although one would be

able to see farther with a 20/15 rating than with 20/20. Your question in effect raises another question: just what is normal? A person can have 20/20 vision but at the same time have other visual problems, such as glaucoma, so it would be difficult to argue that normal visual acuity is the same as perfect vision. In fact, it would seem that one could have eyesight that is normal for one set of values, but for other factors the same eyes could be abnormal. The idea that 20/20 should represent normal human vision needs almost an entire book chapter in itself to explain, but briefly, it is based on the assumption that a person looking at two stars in the night sky, separated by only one minute of arc, would see two stars, while a person with less than 20/20 vision would see just one star. Normal, therefore, may not mean perfect, but it also means your eyesight is O.K.—so don't worry.

Q: *Does astigmatism develop only in nearsighted people?*
A: Astigmatism generally involves a visual aberration caused by a cornea that is not evenly curved. It can occur in addition to either farsighted or nearsighted visual defects, or it might be the only problem in otherwise normal eyes. The image seen by a person with uncorrected astigmatism has been compared to the reflection one sees in an amusement park mirror that distorts sizes and shapes.

Q: *Is nearsightedness caused by too much reading?*
A: No. This is a common misconception probably based on the fact that the problem usually is discovered in children who spend a lot of time trying to read with schoolbooks close to their faces. The notion that reading causes nearsightedness is as erroneous as the belief that wearing eyeglasses causes a loss of visual accommodation in middle age; presbyopia, or loss of accommodation, occurs naturally beginning in middle age, whether one wears glasses or not.

Q: *Does hay fever occur only in the summer or can you get the symptoms at other seasons of the year?*

A: Hay fever actually is a form of allergic rhinitis, meaning an irritation of the nasal cavity. There are certain plant pollens, usually from trees, that can produce hay fever effects in the spring. Fungus spores and grass pollens usually account for hay fever symptoms during the summer months. The well-publicized ragweed pollens cause hay fever effects in the late summer and early autumn. Hay fever that seems to occur at any time of the year may be due not to plant pollens but to food, household dust, animal dander, or fumes from chemicals at work or around the house.

Q: *I have trouble with bleeding gums. Could this be a sign of a vitamin deficiency?*
A: Bleeding gums could be a sign of a vitamin deficiency. But there can be other causes, also, and a close examination of the teeth and gums is necessary to diagnose the actual cause. One type of vitamin deficiency, lack of vitamin C, can result in gums that are inflamed and bleeding, but in a rather distinctive manner—the gums are enlarged with little sacs of blood and the teeth generally are loosened, along with other signs and symptoms. In cases of pellagra, caused by a lack of a B vitamin called niacin, the gums become inflamed and bleed easily, and the lips usually are red and cracked, the tongue turns a bright red, and the mouth feels "burned" and develops ulcers. But inflamed gums also can be associated with leukemia, diabetes, pregnancy, reactions to chemicals and drugs, and pyorrhea.

Q: *I develop a sore tongue after using one of the popular brands of mouth wash. Could I be allergic to something in the mouth wash?*
A: Yes. It is not unusual for a person to become sensitized by a substance in a mouth wash. Change brands and see if the problem goes away. If changing mouth wash does not correct the situation, try changing your toothpaste. Some people have been known to develop allergic reactions to substances in toothpastes.

Q: *My friend has little lines that radiate from the corners of his mouth. Does this mean he might have had a venereal disease?*

A: While syphilis sometimes is a cause of the lines that can occur at the corners of the mouth, it is only one of many possible factors. The cracking or fissuring of the skin around the edges of the lips also can be due to a lack of B vitamins in the diet, a habit of licking the lips, or an infection of a nonvenereal disease such as cold sores.

Q: *A man working at my company seems to be spitting all day, like he has quarts of saliva in his mouth. Is it normal for a person to produce so much saliva?*
A: What's normal saliva secretion is about two to three pints a day. What's not normal is up to 10 quarts a day, but hypersecretion of saliva in tremendous amounts does occur in some people. There can be a number of possible reasons for hypersecretion of saliva. They include several kinds of disorders of the nervous system, irritation of the mouth from poorly fitted dentures, excessive use of tobacco, and reflex stimulation from the stomach or liver. Some cases of sialorrhea are caused by reactions to medications taken for other health problems.

Q: *My son developed a hematoma of the nasal septum after a football injury. Our doctor recommended that the hematoma be drained. Is it always necessary to have the blood drained from a hematoma?*
A: A hematoma is caused by bleeding under the skin or surface membrane, and the pooled blood forms what is sometimes called a blood blister. In many kinds of hematoma, it isn't necessary to make an incision to drain the blood, for the blood eventually is absorbed by the surrounding tissues. However, it's usually wise to have a septal hematoma drained because the injury at this site is easily infected. An infection of the nasal septum can become an abscess that spreads quickly to the brain and causes death. A septal abscess can be painful along with other symptoms and would have to be drained in most cases anyway.

Q: *What is the best way to apply nose drops? I have trouble getting my head tilted back far enough to get the drops into the nasal cavity.*

A: You probably are trying to instill nose drops while your body is in an upright position. To instill nose drops most effectively, you should lie on your back on a bed or sofa, with your head extended over the edge and your nose pointed upward.

Q: *My doctor said I have hyperkeratosis of the larynx from smoking too much. Is there really such a disease that can be caused by smoking?*
A: Yes, there is a condition called hyperkeratosis of the larynx that can be caused by smoking as well as by an infection or abusing the voice. The discomfort and hoarseness that usually go along with the condition result from an increased thickness of the membrane surface of the larynx, and that in turn is due to whatever produces the irritation. Your doctor probably wants you to stop the irritating process by giving up your tobacco habit. The condition can become quite serious if not corrected because hyperkeratosis can lead to leukoplakia, a premalignant disease. In other words, hyperkeratosis is nature's way of telling you to quit irritating your throat.

Q: *My wife hasn't been able to speak above a whisper since I went on a vacation without her. Our doctor claims there is nothing wrong with her throat. Could her loss of voice be psychological?*
A: Without examining your wife, it would not be possible to make a diagnosis. However, there is a condition called dysphonia plicae ventricularis in which a person seems unable to use the vocal cords to produce normal speech sounds. The false cord area folds over the glottis, or opening of the larynx, to prevent speaking except in a whisper. Before determining that the problem is psychological a specialist should be consulted to make sure there is no evidence of laryngeal paralysis or a similar reason for vocal cord failure. Speech therapy sometimes will help a patient to regain normal use of the larynx.

Q: *I have difficulty in getting my children to use a vaporizer or inhaler when they have a cold. They complain that the medicine that's* mixed with the steam hurts their eyes. Is there some way to avoid the eye irritation that goes with vaporizing?

A: Yes. And it's quite simple. Just make a funnel-shaped shield out of a towel, a piece of thin cardboard or a paper sack, and fit it to the child's head so that the vapors reach the mouth and nose but do not bathe the areas beyond.

Q: *Can anything be done about an eye that waters for no apparent reason?*

A: You didn't mention the age of the individual with the watery eye. In infants the problem frequently is a congenital defect in the nasolacrimal duct that generally regresses, or fades away, during the first year. In middle age a watery eye usually is caused by a similar situation involving the nasolacrimal duct that fails to drain properly. In most cases a doctor can drain or flush out the duct, ending the condition. Otherwise, if the condition is one that interferes with employment, a new drainage route can be constructed by a surgeon so that the tears flow directly into the nasal cavity.

Q: *How does bleeding under the skin of the ear (hematoma) result in a cauliflower ear?*

A: One hematoma is not likely to produce a cauliflower ear. But repeated bruising of the external ear, which can happen to professional or amateur boxers, interferes with the normal blood circulation to the cartilage that gives the ear its original natural shape. (And it is the bleeding under the skin that causes the abnormal skin coloration we call a bruise.) If the cartilage fails to get its normal blood supply on a regular basis, it atrophies. It is the atrophied cartilage that gives the cauliflower ear its deformed shape.

Q: *I have just recovered from a bout with red eye (acute conjunctivitis) and would like to know how one can avoid it in the future.*

A: Acute conjunctivitis can be caused by quite an assortment of viruses and bacteria, which frequently are the same types that cause infections in other parts of the body. The disease is transmitted in the same general manner as most other infections, such as direct contact with a person suffering from the disease, using a face towel or other item that has been used by an infected person, touching the area around the eye with your own unwashed hands, swimming in water containing the disease organism, or getting a bit of infected dirt or fluid in your eye. This answer may not be very comforting since it doesn't leave many options for avoiding infections of the conjunctiva. On the other hand, most bookies would give you good odds against getting conjunctivitis again in the near future.

Q: *Is the human ear more sensitive to certain tones or frequencies of sound than others?*

A: Some experts contend the human ear was designed to receive sounds in the area of a few thousand cycles per second. Indeed, the threshold of hearing for humans is the lowest, or most sensitive, at about 1,000 CPS. The threshold of painful noise also is lowest at around 3,000 to 4,000 CPS, by more than 10 decibels. Human conversation ranges from around 125 CPS to more than 12,000 CPS, and orchestral music covers an even greater span of tone. But, again, we are most sensitive to sounds at frequencies that are in the 1,000 to about 4,000 CPS range.

Q: *When a surgeon removes the adenoids, which are above the soft palate, does he cut through the nasal cavity or the mouth?*

A: Although the adenoids aren't easily visible by looking through the mouth, they are accessible to a surgeon who uses an instrument with a cutting blade that is at right angle to the handle. By making a sort of backhand movement after inserting the instrument, called a curette, into the back of the mouth, he can easily trim off the adenoid tonsil tissue. It's partly a matter of knowing human anatomy that makes this possible; the oral cavity, which includes the mouth, and the nasal cavity, which includes the nose, are actually more or less one cavity divided for most of the space by the palate. The easy access from the mouth to the nose, and vice versa, also may explain how disease organisms can quickly move from one to the other.

Q: *At what age should a child with a cleft palate undergo an operation to repair the defect?*
A: Many surgeons recommend that cleft palate repair surgery be done when the baby is about 12 months of age, or before he begins to talk. Until plastic surgery is done to correct the defect, the child will have trouble eating and breathing. Normal suction can be very difficult for the infant, so breast or bottle feeding may have to be handled with extreme care. In some cases, feeding may be done by tube or with a specially designed spoon. As in surgery for correcting a harelip, the baby may have to be restrained with padded splints during the recovery period to prevent it from poking its fingers into the freshly repaired tissues.

Q: *What is a rodent ulcer and what does it have to do with rodents?*
A: A rodent ulcer has nothing to do with rodents and it's not really an ulcer. It is a common name for a type of cancer that may develop, among other places, on the eyelid, starting as a saucer-like bulge in the skin. A suggested cause is overexposure to sunlight and a recommended cure is surgery.

Q: *What causes drooping eyelids in some children and adults?*
A: Drooping eyelids, called ptosis by doctors, can be a congenital defect in some children; the condition also can be the result of disease or injury. It is one of the first signs of a disease known as myasthenia gravis, which affects the nerves and muscles. If the ptosis is a sign of myasthenia gravis, the disease should be treated immediately, before other areas of the body become involved. If the drooping eyelid is congenital, it should be corrected by plastic surgery so it will not interfere with normal vision. A doctor can determine rather quickly whether a drooping eyelid is a sign of myasthenia gravis by administering a drug that will cause the eyelid to open if the disease is the causative factor.

Q: *When my son got a bit of sand in his eye at the beach, the doctor in town put eye patches over both eyes even though only one eye was injured. Is this standard operating procedure?*
A: In emergency treatment of eye injuries, it's always best to patch both eyes, even when only one eye is involved. The double eye patch helps relieve discomfort by keeping out light and restricting movement of the eyes. When the injured person can't use either eye, he is less likely to move the injured eyeball and aggravate the injury. The eye patch should be applied without any pressure since even a slight force on the eye could increase the risk of permanent injury.

Q: *What is "tunnel vision" that seems to affect people with glaucoma?*
A: The term, "tunnel vision," refers to the restricted peripheral visual field that is one of the effects of glaucoma, especially in cases where proper treatment has been neglected. The fluid pressure in the eyeball causes gradual destruction of the optic nerve endings, with the result that vision for objects in the fringe areas of the visual field are lost. As the disease progresses, the glaucoma victim can see less and less of objects at either side of the head, or above or below what is straight ahead. Eventually, he literally sees the world as if looking at it through a tunnel. Glaucoma, incidentally, is one of the more common causes of blindness.

Q: *I have been told that a person can have atrophic rhinitis without being aware of the problem. True?*
A: True, unless his best friends avoid the person as a hint that the disease usually is accompanied by an objectionable odor. Ironically, however, the disorder also damages the mucous membrane of the nasal cavity, so the person may lose his own sense of smell and won't detect the odor.

Q: *How can you tell if a headache may be caused by a brain tumor?*

A: A physician usually can learn whether a headache might be caused by a brain tumor by making a careful diagnosis based on a number of bits of information. One bit of information is whether the headache is a deep, aching pain that usually is steady and occurs every day. Another bit of information is whether changing the body position affects the intensity of the pain. Many bits of information are needed before a diagnostician can be certain of the cause of a headache.

Medical textbooks contain many pages of signs and symptoms associated with various types of headaches. Even the textbooks do not agree on all points. Some authors claim, for example, that the tendency for migraine headaches is inherited, like eye color or hair color. Others contend that migraine headaches are psychosomatic and occur only in persons who are meticulous, ambitious achievers. The patient with a headache usually could care less about the arguments of experts and would prefer a quick simple remedy. But first we must find the cause.

4
THE CHEST

A standard part of nearly any general physical examination is the doctor's probing, listening, X-ray filming, and general viewing of the chest area of the body in a search for health clues. You may have a stethoscope pressed against the flesh, be asked to breathe deeply, and feel the doctor tap the chest wall a few times.

The doctor also may inspect the breasts when that part of the chest examination is appropriate; and he may look at the spinal column and ribs. It's all an important part of the general checkup; everything the doctor does in examining the chest, or thorax, as he may call it, is for a good reason.

Chest pains may rank second only to headaches as a common complaint that will induce a person to visit a doctor. Frequently the chest pain is compounded by concern that the cause of discomfort might be heart trouble or lung cancer, diseases that have been well publicized as silent assassins that attack through the chest organs.

The heart and lungs are the major organs of the chest, so when they are injured or diseased, the entire body may be in big trouble. Other tissues in the chest include bones that ring the chest cavity from top to bottom, in front and along the back and sides. The ribs are attached to muscles, and a large muscle sheet, the diaphragm, forms a sort of floor for the chest cavity. There are important organs and blood vessels in the chest as well, including the end of the windpipe, or trachea, and the food tube, or esophagus, which extends all the way through the chest to the stomach, which is just beneath the diaphragm. In fact, there are so many things in the chest that one might wonder how this part of the anatomy every acquired the apparent misnomer of chest cavity.

It is partly because of the maze of organs and other tissues in the chest that a doctor frequently has to do some careful checking of the patient's chest anatomy in order to locate a source of chest pain. The examining doctor may ask whether the pain is felt near the surface of the chest or deep within the chest. A pain near the surface could be an inflammation, an injury, or a tumor. There might be bruises, cuts, ulcerations, masses or growths under the skin, and so on, which could be good clues to the nature of a chest pain. In some

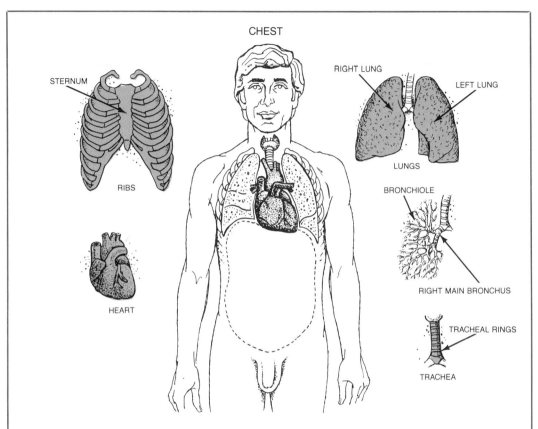

CHEST

STERNUM

RIBS

HEART

RIGHT LUNG

LEFT LUNG

LUNGS

BRONCHIOLE

RIGHT MAIN BRONCHUS

TRACHEAL RINGS

TRACHEA

The chest is protected by a bony cage composed of 12 pairs of ribs, extending from the top of the shoulders to the roof of the abdomen. The top ten pairs of ribs are attached by strips of cartilage to the sternum, a dagger-shaped breast bone at the front. At the back, the ribs are attached to the spinal column. The bottom ribs, the 11th and 12th pairs, are attached only at the back and are called floating ribs.

The heart is a fist-size bundle of muscle that contracts and relaxes alternately about 72 times a minute, or 40 million times a year for a lifetime. By contracting and dilating, the heart squeezes blood returning from the veins into the lungs on either side for fresh oxygen and then back again into the arteries leading to tissues throughout the body. It pumps more than 4,000 gallons of blood daily.

The lungs on either side of the heart are composed of hundreds of millions of tiny air sacs which give these organs a sponge-like appearance. Air is forced in and out of the lungs by the contraction and relax-

ation of the diaphragm, a dome-shaped muscle just beneath the lungs, and muscles of the chest wall. Together, these muscles pump the lungs like a set of bellows, as we inhale and exhale air.

Air enters and leaves the lungs through a tree of tubes called bronchioles. The bronchioles lead to the bronchi, which are branches of the trachea. At the other end of each bronchiole is a cluster of alveoli, or tiny air sacs; blood capillaries running through the walls of each alveolus release carbon dioxide and water vapor to the exhaled while absorbing fresh oxygen which has been inhaled into the lungs.

The trachea, or windpipe, continues below the larynx and well into the chest area where it subdivides into bronchi leading to the lobes of the lungs. A series of cartilage rings, called tracheal rings, hold the windpipe open. The bronchi, which divide from the trachea near the level of the heart, also are held open by cartilage rings. The smaller air tubes have muscle tissue in their walls.

cases the problem might involve the tissues of the breasts.

Since the chest is a rather flexible structure, despite the usually sturdy construction of ribs connected to the backbone and breastbone, or sternum, a movement of the chest can increase the intensity of a pain caused by an injury or inflammation. The old saying goes, "It only hurts when I laugh," but in such cases it also can hurt when one coughs, sneezes, or takes a deep breath.

Pain that increases when part of the chest is moved can be caused by a disorder of the ribs, cartilage, muscles, nerves, or pleura. The pleura is a sac-like membrane that separates the lungs from the inner chest wall. When the pleura is inflamed, as during an infection, the condition sometimes is called pleurisy. Pleurisy is easily aggravated by such simple actions of the chest as coughing or deep breathing.

Muscular Movements in the Chest

There is quite an assortment of muscles available for moving the chest in breathing, laughing, coughing, or sneezing. First, there are 12 pairs of ribs attached to the spinal column, the stack of vertebrae extending from the base of the skull to the pelvis. The top 10 pairs of ribs, starting below the clavicle, or collarbone, are attached to the breastbone in the front. The dagger-shaped breastbone, or sternum, is not directly attached to the ribs, but is connected by strips of flexible cartilage. The rib connections to the spinal column also are through cartilage strips.

This flexibility is an important factor in normal breathing as well as in forced breathing. It permits the various parts of the rib cage to move somewhat independently. In forced breathing, for example,

the intercostal muscles which connect one rib to the ribs above and below it help increase the capacity of the chest by relaxing, thereby extending the space between ribs or pairs of ribs. When you take a deep breath, notice how the muscles pull upward and outward, starting with the top level of ribs and continuing with a ripple effect to the bottom ribs. In forcibly exhaling as much air as possible from the lungs, the muscles contract to make the chest capacity smaller.

The lower two pairs of ribs, incidentally, are attached to the spinal column at the back but have no front attachment to the sternum. For that reason they sometimes are referred to as "floating ribs."

The intercostal muscles between the ribs can be the source of chest pains. Neuralgia, or nerve spasms, involving the intercostal muscles often trigger fear of a "heart attack." More than half of all adults experience intercostal neuralgia at one time or another, and a goodly percentage of older persons seek medical help because of chest pains caused by nerves in the intercostal muscles. The symptoms generally are harmless, but any chest pain is worth a visit to the doctor's office, even if the cause is nothing more serious than intercostal neuralgia.

Sources of Pain in the Chest

A pain in the chest that is centered in a particular area and is aggravated by breathing or other movements of the chest wall can suggest several clues to the doctor examining a patient. If the painful area is particularly sensitive and the pain is quite sharp, the doctor may check for evidence of a rib fracture. The doctor might palpate the area carefully with his fingers, trying to detect vibrations made by the broken ends of bones rubbing together.

However, a rib fracture may not always be the cause of such symptoms. A dislocated cartilage might produce similar effects by rubbing against an adjacent rib. A recent injury such as a blow to the chest could be a cause of a rib fracture; a dislocated fracture might be due to an old injury that did not heal properly. In either case, the pain might be more severe under conditions such as heavy breathing.

Muscular strain or muscular irritation might trigger pain in the chest, and the problem might not be easily apparent on X-ray film. Lifting a heavy bag of groceries or a baby, as well as physical labor, can lead to chest pains related to muscle strain. The chain-reaction effect of rib motions can aggravate an inflamed intercostal muscle on the lower chest wall when the shoulder muscles are moved. Thus, even the repeated lifting of the arms may produce mysterious chest pains under certain conditions.

Another cause of chest pains that might be unexpected by a patient is a herpes infection that involves the nerves of the intercostal muscles. Herpes zoster, a close relative of the virus that causes fever blisters or cold sores, is responsible for a type of nerve inflammation commonly known as shingles. Shingles usually is marked by a reddening of the skin along the path of a nerve in the chest wall, or more specifically in the muscles that connect the ribs. The reddened skin may be preceded by the appearance of small blisters, or vesicles, that resemble the cold sores occasionally seen around the lips and nose. The vesicles eventually break and then slowly heal, but a burning pain in the chest muscles can persist for days, weeks, or even

months. A doctor examining the chest for causes of painful discomfort probably would recognize the red marks or sores that follow the route of a nerve in the chest wall, but a person not previously troubled by shingles might miss that clue.

Function of the Diaphragm

The major muscle mass involved in normal breathing is the diaphragm, the layer of muscle fibers that separates the chest cavity from the abdominal cavity. The diaphragm is attached to the sternum in front, the spinal column at the back, and to the lower ribs along the side of the body.

When you inhale, or breathe air into the lungs—a more or less continuous process that occurs unconsciously—the chest cavity expands because the muscle fibers of the diaphragm contract. This action draws the dome-shaped diaphragm roof down toward the abdomen and creates a partial vacuum within the chest walls. Air rushes into the lungs through the nose and/or mouth to fill the vacuum. When you exhale, or breathe out, the diaphragm simply relaxes and pushes upward against the lungs, squeezing the air out of the myriad tiny air sacs in the lung tissue.

The diaphragm can be the source of certain types of chest pains. For example, there is a disorder known as diaphragmatic pleurisy that is marked by sharp shooting pains in the chest wall when a person afflicted with the ailment laughs, coughs, or merely takes a deep breath. Another effect of an inflamed diaphragm can be a pain in the neck, literally. This situation can result because the nerves that serve the muscle fibers of the diaphragm also run to the neck and shoulders. Similar symptoms can be produced as a result of irritation of the diaphragm by the esophagus, which passes through a tight opening in the diaphragm on its way from the mouth to the stomach. The opening in the diaphragm, called a hiatus, sometimes is widened by pressure from the stomach pushing upward; the condition is called a hiatus hernia. A reflux of stomach acid back up into the esophagus may be responsible for a type of chest pain occasionally called "heartburn."

Chest Pains Caused by Heart Disease

Despite some of the easily available clues, it is not always simple for a doctor to determine immediately if a chest pain is due to a heart disorder, a broken rib, a dislocated cartilage, shingles, intercostal neuralgia, or one of many other possible alternatives. A pain that is felt as a "deep" chest pain, behind the sternum, might involve the stomach, gallbladder, esophagus, the duodenum (the first segment of the intestine leading from the stomach), or a major vein or artery near the heart, as well as the heart itself.

Angina pectoris, one form of heart disease, may be felt as a burning, stinging, aching pain accompanied by pressure in the chest that begins after a period of exertion. The pain may be steady and last from one to ten minutes, then subside after a period of rest or the use of a prescribed medication such as nitroglycerine. However, the pain of angina pectoris, caused when the heart muscle does not receive enough freshly oxygenated blood, can occur anywhere from the neck to the lower part of the chest. The intensity of the pain can range from mild to severe. In addition to exertion, angina pains can be

produced in some people by exposure to cold, by intense excitement or emotion, after a period of heart flutter or rapid heartbeat, or after eating a large meal.

Among clues the doctor may check are lag times preceding the onset of pain after a period of exertion and the start of relief from pain after a period of rest. The lag time factor is a common clue to angina pains, which may typically begin after a certain amount of exertion and subside after a fairly predictable amount of rest. An even better clue can be the effect of a dose of nitroglycerine on a patient suspected of suffering from angina pectoris. If the pain is relieved with a dose of nitroglycerine that is strong enough to cause a headache and flushing, there is a better than average chance the chest pain is a symptom of angina. Most of the other possible causes, including myocardial infarction, the critically severe type of heart attack caused by an interruption of normal blood flow to the heart muscle, would not be relieved by a dose of nitroglycerine.

Myocardial infarction pains are quite similar to those of angina pectoris. The deep, steady pain is accompanied by a feeling of constriction or pressure in the chest, and it may be felt anywhere from the top of the abdomen to the neck and arms. In addition, the intensity of pain can be quite severe, and be accompanied by sweating, nausea, and vomiting. Myocardial infarction pains are not always triggered by exertion, and they are not relieved by either a period of rest or the administration of nitroglycerine. Also, while angina pains usually do not continue beyond ten minutes or so, myocardial pains can continue for hours.

A serious chest pain should not be allowed to continue any longer than necessary. An acute myocardial infarction is an extremely serious condition that requires immediate professional medical care. Time is very important in saving the life of a myocardial infarction patient. His blood pressure can fall rapidly to such low levels that shock will follow. With the heart muscle deprived of its blood supply, heart failure and death can occur quite suddenly. The best hope for saving a heart attack victim is to get him to a doctor's office or the emergency room of a hospital as quickly as possible. Laboratory and other tests at the hospital will be used to determine the extent of damage to a heart muscle and the outlook for quick recovery.

Besides angina pectoris and myocardial infarction, there are heart disorders that overlap the two types of cardiac problems just mentioned. For example, a condition called pre-infarctional angina can be an intermediate disorder between angina pectoris and myocardial infarction, or it could be an angina attack that is progressing into myocardial infarction. There also are angina pectoris-like symptoms that may be experienced by persons recovering from myocardial infarction. The many variations in chest and heart signs and symptoms do not make it easy for a doctor to find quick answers to a patient's concern about thoracic discomfort.

Normal Functions of the Heart

To help put heart problems in a somewhat simple perspective, you might think of the heart as a fist-size bundle of muscle tissue nestled between the right and left lungs, and connected to the lungs by several large arteries and veins. The heart can be thought of as a double pump with two separate blood circulation routes, although the two routes actually form a continuous pathway for the blood.

The blood carries oxygen and nutrients to the trillions of body cells between the soles of the feet and the scalp of the head. The blood also removes the waste products that result from the feeding and watering of the myriad cells on a continuous lifetime basis. A normal heart contracts and dilates about 100,000 times a day from embryonic life until death—and in some cases even after the legal death which is determined by brain activity.

Some medical experts have calculated that the work done by the heart muscle is comparable to the energy expended by the muscles of both legs while running a foot race. And though the leg muscles eventually are allowed to rest, the heart is allowed to rest for only a fraction of a second at a time—the time between heartbeats. Obviously, that leaves little opportunity for the heart muscle to take a break in its daily routine. If the heart does skip a beat once in a while, you probably will be more aware of that brief change of pace than you are likely to notice the months or years of work performed by the heart without missing a beat.

The contractions of the heart muscle literally squeeze the blood through the many miles of blood vessels that form a meshwork touching every area of living body cells. The squeezing action normally occurs at a rate of about 72 times a minute, and the rate is considerably faster during periods of exertion. Each time the heart contracts to squeeze blood into the major arteries, the action is called a systole. When the heart muscle relaxes to allow another batch of blood to return to its chambers, the action is a diastole. It is from these two words that the terms used

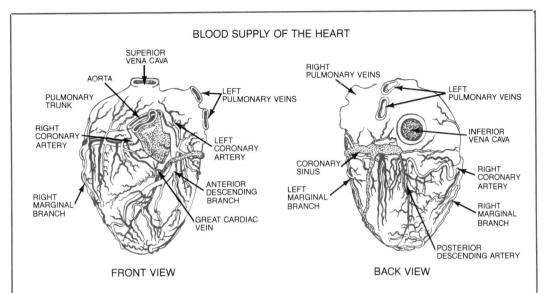

BLOOD SUPPLY OF THE HEART

FRONT VIEW

BACK VIEW

The heart, which pumps blood to all living cells of the body, is itself a major consumer of blood because the heart uses about ten percent of all the oxygen received by the lungs. And since it works continuously, contracting 100,000 times a day with no rest period, its nutrient needs are about twice those of the leg muscles of a runner competing in a marathon. The heart is richly endowed with arteries and veins in order to insure optimum blood circulation, as shown in the illustration. Blood from other areas of the body enters the heart through the vena cava and leaves from the aorta to arteries that supply body tissue. Pulmonary vessels carry blood between the lungs and the heart.

in measuring blood pressure—systolic and diastolic—are derived.

The human heart has four chambers or compartments; some lower animals have two or three compartments. The human heart's chambers are arranged in two pairs, with two at the top and two at the bottom. The top heart chambers are called atria, or atrium if referring to just one of the top chambers. Those at the bottom of the heart are called ventricles. Because of the double pump system of the human heart, the left atrium and left ventricle work as one team, while the right atrium and right ventricle work as a sec-ond pump. A wall of muscle separates the right and left pumps on the inside of the heart, and valves separate the atria from the ventricles to prevent a backflow of blood when the heart contracts.

Circulation of the Blood

The reason for the double pump function of the heart is that each drop of blood must move through the heart two times after it has been returned through the veins following a trip around the tissue cell circuits of the body. The "used" blood, which sometimes is described as blue blood because of the bluish coloration it gives the veins, has given up its oxygen to the tissues that require oxygen in order to function normally. If you have accidentally cut a blood vein, you may have noticed that the "blue" blood suddenly turned red when it was exposed to the oxygen of the air. This used or blue blood is routed into the right atrium of the heart. From the right atrium it is allowed to enter the right ventricle which, on the next contraction, squeezes the used blood into arteries that extend into the lung tissue.

In the lungs the blood is routed into the microscopically thin walls of tiny air sacs where the blood cells give up their load of carbon dioxide and water vapor collected on the trip around the body cells. At the same time, the red blood cells take on a fresh load of oxygen molecules, making the blood red again.

Each batch of blood squeezed through the lungs pushes the previous batch ahead through the fine network of capillaries in the lung tissue and back towards the heart again. On the second trip through the heart, however, the freshly oxygenated blood is routed into the left atrium. From the left atrium, the fresh blood goes into the left ventricle, and on the next squeeze it goes back out into the general circulation network of the arteries, which branch into smaller and smaller blood vessels extending to the tips of the fingers and toes, and reach the deep organs of the body as well as the surface areas.

The heart is almost pure muscle tissue. It is composed of layers of muscles. Some of its muscle fibers run in circles and some run in spirals, but the pattern always is part of a design that allows the heart to work most efficiently and effectively in squeezing blood through the various valves and vessels each time the muscles

contract. Since the ventricles have the biggest work load in moving blood, the walls of the ventricles are thicker than the walls of the atria, which serve mainly as reservoirs or holding chambers for blood waiting to move into the next stage of circulation.

The function of the valves is to control the direction of blood flow during the systolic phase of heart action. The tricuspid valve—so called because it is made up of three flaps, or cusps, of tissue—is pulled closed by a set of tiny muscles when the right ventricle begins to contract. The stoppage prevents the used blood from being pushed back up into the right atrium during the muscle squeezing. Instead, the dark blood is directed into the pulmonary arteries that run into the right and left sides of the lungs.

When the blood returns from the lungs into the left atrium, it waits an instant before being dropped into the left ventricle through the opening of the bicuspid, or mitral valve. Then the mitral valve flaps are pulled closed by tiny muscles to prevent backflow when the ventricle contracts the next time.

There are other valves throughout the human circulatory system, including so-called semilunar valves located in the major arteries leaving the heart, and small valves in some of the veins.

The valves in the internal veins of the lower extremities, the legs, have the responsibility of helping the circulatory system overcome the pull of gravity. Just as gravity pulls water downhill, it also tugs on the body's blood supply, pulling it towards the feet when a person is standing. If a person spends a lot of time standing or sitting, the blood in the veins tend to accumulate in the veins of the lower legs, while the valves in the veins try to prevent the blood from pooling by holding it back. People who are on their feet a good deal of time but who do a lot of walking or running are more likely to overcome the pull of gravity on the blood in the legs, because some leg muscles help pump the blood upward through the veins by squeezing the veins each time the muscles contract. A person who is seated can get a similar benefit by performing simple exercises that contract the lower leg muscles, thereby squeezing blood that needs fresh oxygen back toward the heart and lungs.

When valves in the veins start to fail, the condition is called varicosities, or varicose veins. Valves in the heart also are subject to stresses and occasional failures. But for most individuals the valves last a lifetime with a minimum amount of wear and tear. They do a remarkably smooth job of maintaining a precise amount of blood in each of the heart's chambers. The amount of blood in the right ventricle, for example, must equal the amount of blood in the left ventricle, at least under normal conditions. This is because the amount of blood entering the lungs through the pulmonary arteries should equal the amount of blood returning via the pulmonary veins. In certain disorders of the circulatory system, however, there is a problem of one pump getting out of step with the other.

Blood vessels that carry blood away from the heart always are identified as arteries. Vessels that carry blood to the heart always are called veins, regardless of whether they carry fresh red blood or used dark blood. Thus, when a doctor speaks of a pulmonary vein, he is thinking of blood that is freshly oxygenated; and when he speaks of a pulmonary artery, he is referring to a vessel carrying used blood to the lungs. For the rest of the body, arteries carry the red blood and veins carry the dark blood. But between the heart and the lungs, names of certain blood vessels seemingly contradict the general scheme of circulation.

At some point in the capillary beds of the body, the smallest arterial branches become the smallest veins when the blood starts its return journey to the heart. At this point the blood vessels are so tiny that red blood cells, which measure less than 1/30,000th of an inch in size, must pass in single file. In order to reach all of the trillions of body cells needing oxygen and nutrients, the circulatory system needs literally thousands of miles of capillaries. In fact, the capillary network of an average human body is so vast that it could swallow the entire blood supply if something went wrong with the arterial distribution system. What prevents such an accident is a complex arrangement of valve-like muscles which feed blood into different capillary beds in a sort of round-robin pattern.

The Heart's Appearance and Location

Pumping blood through thousands of miles of plumbing obviously is a tough job for any fist-size bundle of muscle that must work continuously for scores of years. The left ventricle, which does most of the work, needs more of the muscle power of the heart. For that reason the left ventricle appears much larger on the outside of the heart than the right ventricle, even though the interior chambers of the ventricles are of the same capacity.

The heart's left ventricle bulge gives the organ an appearance that only faintly resembles the heart used as a design for Valentine's Day cards. Also, it is not usually located as far on the left side of the chest as one might be led to believe by watching where people place their hand over their heart when the flag is passing by. Actually, for most people the heart is located just to the left of center of the chest, with the atria situated mainly behind the breastbone, or sternum, and the ventricles extending to the left side. The tip of the ventricles usually does not point downward, as in children's drawings, because the heart rather rests on its side.

This description of the heart is not intended to disillusion people who like to think of the human heart as a bright red, cone-shaped object with a pointed tip that is aimed toward the ground. Rather, it is intended to help explain why your doctor may check for normal or abnormal heart sounds and signs in areas of the chest where you usually do not place your hand during patriotic ceremonies.

The Doctor's Examination of the Heart

Your doctor may look to the left of your sternum, or breastbone, when checking your heart because that is where the heartbeat usually can be seen or felt, or both. There is a point on the wall of the chest for many, if not most, individuals where the heartbeat is visible as a brief push against the intercostal muscle separating the fifth and sixth ribs, counting downward from the collarbone. That point can be located in most individuals along an imaginary line that runs straight down the left side of the chest from about the middle of the collarbone.

For a man the point is slightly below the left nipple and toward the breastbone. For a woman the point might be concealed beneath a breast, and the doctor would have to move the breast to find the point in some individuals. For some people the visible heartbeat is apparent while they are in a sitting or standing position. For others it may be necessary to lean forward in order to make the heartbeat visible.

Why make the heartbeat visible? The doctor obviously does not have to see the heart beating to determine whether it is still working. But the trained physician can tell quite a bit about the quality of the heartbeat by simply observing how it appears on the chest wall. Significant characteristics of the heartbeat might be whether the beat comes like a gentle tap against the skin from inside the chest or if the push is more diffuse, whether the push of the heartbeats covers a small area or a large area of the chest wall, and so on. If the pericardial sac, a membrane bag that covers the heart, should become filled with fluid, for example, the doctor probably would not be able to see the effect of the heartbeat on the chest wall, and that would be a clue to the health of the patient.

If the heartbeat is not visible at that point on the chest, which would mark the maximum point of impulse from the normal action of the heart, the doctor probably will palpate the area—that is, he will feel for the heartbeat with his fingers. In a severe case of fluid accumulation around the heart, palpation might fail to locate the point where the thrust of the heart pumping action should be felt. In that case the doctor usually can solve the problem by using his stethoscope and shifting the position of the patient. When the patient changes body positions, the fluid should shift away from the area in which it seems to interfere with the clear transmission of heart sounds that can be detected with the stethoscope.

Enlargement of the Heart When the heartbeat is observed or felt farther to the left than is usual, it can be a clue that the heart is enlarged, so that the end of the ventricle is beyond the normal point of maximum pulsation. If the heart is enlarged, the cause may be a continued overloading of work for the left ventricle that may be the result of hypertension. Chronic hypertension can reduce the bore of the blood arteries, so that the ventricle has to work harder in order to pump blood through the smaller opening. A weaker than normal heartbeat that appears over a larger area of the chest wall could suggest an enlarged heart caused by ventricular dilation.

Percussion Technique If the doctor suspects an enlarged heart on the basis of his early examination evidence, he frequently can determine which of the four heart chambers may be involved by a technique called percussion. Percussion is a way of producing vibrations in the chest wall by tapping with the finger. The technique is somewhat like the method used by carpenters who try to locate studs, or 2 by 4's, in the wall of a house by tapping on the wall and listening to the hollow or solid sounds returning from beneath the layer of plaster.

The examining physician does not tap on a patient's chest directly with his finger; instead, he taps one finger of the right hand upon a finger of the left hand while holding the left hand against the patient's chest. Of course, if the doctor is left-handed, he taps with his left-hand finger on a finger of the right hand. Because of his experience and training, the doctor usually can tell from the pitch of the percussion vibrations—their length, dullness,

PERCUSSION

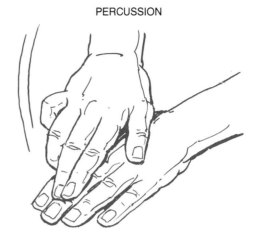

During a medical examination of the chest, the doctor often uses the technique of percussion to check the condition of the heart and lungs. By tapping the fingers of one hand on the fingers of the opposite hand placed at a strategic point on the chest wall, the doctor can tell by resonant sounds produced by the tapping the precise location and size of a patient's heart.

strength, and so on—what's normal and what's not about tissues inside the chest.

By having a patient inhale and exhale during percussion, a doctor frequently can picture the borders of the lungs, how far the diaphragm moves within the chest, the location of the upper border of the liver, and the general size and shape of the heart.

Heart Sounds Most people are familiar with the heart sounds as heard through a stethoscope. They are used occasionally in radio and television programs involving doctors and hospitals. The sounds sometimes are spelled out as lubb-*dup*, with the lubb sound being longer and having a lower pitch than the *dup* part. The lubb sound is made by the closing of the tricuspid and bicuspid valves that separate the atria and the ventricles on each side of the heart during contraction of the ventricles. The *dup* sound represents the closing of the valves of the aorta, the major artery carrying blood to tissues throughout the body, and of the pulmonary arteries when blood is squeezed into the general circulation system and the lungs. During the brief pause between the end of one *dup* sound and the next lubb, the atria release more blood from their reservoirs into the ventricles.

The lubb-*dup* sounds of heart action are what might be regarded as normal heart sounds. What's not normal might be a sound something like pul-lubb-*dup*. That kind of sound might be a clue to a doctor checking with his stethoscope that something could be amiss with a ventricle.

To pinpoint a heartbeat problem more specifically, the doctor moves his stethoscope around the chest to sort out various possible sources of off-beat heart sounds. If an abnormal sound is heard near the aorta, which usually is located in the region of the chest where the second rib joins the sternum, the cause could be a disorder involving the left ventricle. Heard more distinctly on another part of the chest wall, a pul-lubb-*dup* sound might indicate a disorder of the right ventricle. But these are only clues that are small pieces of the picture of a patient's health. One strange heart sound doesn't necessarily explain a pain in the chest or imply a possible disorder of the circulatory system.

Other sounds produced by the heart may have other meanings in a doctor's diagnostic picture. Instead of a lubb-*dup* or a pul-lubb-*dup* sound, a heartbeat may be heard as a lubb-*dup*-puh sound. A doctor might also hear clicking sounds or heartbeats that appear to be slurred and mushy. A heart murmur might be felt by a doctor palpating the chest as a vibration quite similar to the purring of a happy cat. Such rapid vibrations also may be referred to as thrills and are frequently associated with defects in the valves; the valves may fail to close tightly, or they may not open quickly enough or far enough to let the blood flow evenly from one chamber to the next. Heart murmurs can occur somewhat like eddies in a river when the liquid flow, or in this situation the blood flow, is uneven because of countercurrents produced by obstacles to the main stream of the channel.

Some heart murmurs are normal and some are not. In many instances a heart murmur may be a caution signal but not a cause for great alarm. An eddy type of heart murmur, for example, may be a functional disorder that can develop in a heart which has valves that are in very good condition. Sometimes a murmur is heard when air moves into the lungs during a heartbeat, which also can be a "normal" type of heart murmur.

A murmur caused by a defect in the septum, the wall that separates the right and left heart pumps, generally is a sign of serious trouble. Since the left ventricle is more powerful than the right ventricle, each contraction of the ventricles can result in a backflow of blood from the left side to the right side of the heart.

Some abnormal heartbeats are more serious than others. A rapid heartbeat, which a doctor may describe by its medical name of tachycardia, might be the result of using tobacco, alcohol, or caffeine beverages such as coffee. Even among heartbeats that are normal, the rate may be as slow as 40 per minute or as rapid as 100 per minute. The average is around 70 per minute.

What frequently makes an abnormal rapid or slow heartbeat is how the source of the unusual rate disturbs the normal rhythm of the heart. The atria and ventricles may get out of phase with each other, for example. The ventricles might respond to every second, third, or fourth impulse of the atria if some factor causes the upper heart chambers to develop a rapid rate of contraction. Or the ventricles may contract at an abnormally rapid rate while the atria continue to function at their usual pace. Or the ventricles may contract prematurely, that is, out of step with the rest of the heart.

In a condition known as ventricular fibrillation the ventricles may contract wildly at a rate of as much as 300 beats per minute, but at the same time the ventricles may not actually pump any blood. When ventricular fibrillation occurs, emergency treatment is needed in order to restore an orderly heart rhythm. Otherwise, with no blood being pumped through the body's vital organs, the patient will lose consciousness quickly and death will follow.

Still another strange sound that may occur within the chest because of the action of the heart's pumping role is the result of blood flow turbulence. At a point just above the heart, for example, blood pumped by the right ventricle toward the lungs must move either into the right lung or the left lung, because the right and left pulmonary arteries branch out from the main pulmonary artery there. As might occur in any rapid flow of fluid in a stream bed or plumbing system, blood smashing against the point of artery bifurcation produces a turbulence that may be detected as the sound of a heart murmur. However, the blood turbulence in the pulmonary arteries is another normal happening which may be repeated on a smaller scale at points where other arterial branchings occur.

See also Chapter 17: *Heart Disease.*

Electrocardiogram Many questions about heart condition today are resolved with the use of electrocardiograph equipment. An electrocardiogram has become a part of the standard physical examination record of many patients, even those in good general health, since the written record of a patient's heart condition can be used as a benchmark for measuring possible future changes in the health of the heart. The basic electrocardiogram, recorded during a period of normal health, serves somewhat like a record of your normal or average temperature, blood pressure, and so on. Thus, in future examinations or periods of illness, the doctor can tell whether changes in your physical condition are major or minor variations from the normal or typical readings for your own body.

An electrocardiogram is a record of the performance of the heart's muscles that is based on tiny electrical impulses generated by contractions of the atria and ventricles. The electrical impulses are detected through electrodes that are attached to the chest and limbs of a patient. The electrical changes produced by the muscle contractions and detected by the electrodes are relayed through a galvanometer, a common device used to measure small amounts of electricity. The electrical impulses received by the galvanometer are translated into a written record by tracing pens on a sheet of moving graph paper.

The electrocardiogram electrodes are placed on the body in certain patterns that not only detect the impulses but the direction in which the electric current generated by the muscles moves. A current moving toward the galvanometer, for example, causes the tracing pen to swing upward, while a current moving away makes the pen deflect downward on the graph paper. The resulting picture on the graph paper appears as waves, with one wave representing the contraction of the atria and the others showing the contraction and relaxation phases of the ventricles. The relaxation phase of the atria generally does not produce enough electric current to make a tracing on a standard electrocardiogram.

The various wave forms on an electrocardiogram (frequently abbreviated as ECG or EKG) are identified by letters of the alphabet. A "P" wave, for example, represents the contraction of the atria; a "T" wave records the relaxation of the ventricles. Other actions of the heart muscle produce waves that are designated as "Q," "R," and "S."

There are several variations in the way in which electrodes can be aligned on the chest and the arms or legs, as well as the number of electrodes used. Depending upon the equipment and the specific information needed about the heart, an ECG may be made with one electrode on the chest and one on each arm, or, in some cases, by using six different electrodes on the chest. Regardless of the number and positions of the electrodes employed, an ECG can yield a considerable amount of data about one's heart condition, such as any abnormality in the rate and rhythm of the heartbeat, any injury to the heart muscle, an abnormality in the size of a ventricle, and so on. In a case of a myocardial infarction, an electrocardiogram might pinpoint the site on the heart muscle where the infarction, caused by a block-

age in the flow of blood from the coronary artery, has occurred.

What's Normal and What Isn't About the Lungs

Because of the close proximity of the heart and lungs, it is not too surprising that the health of one organ might affect the normal functioning of its neighbor. As we already have noted, certain suspicious sounds detected in the chest when listening through a stethoscope may be due to the interdependence of the heart and lungs as a team, working well or working poorly together.

The lungs fill the rib cage from a point slightly above the collarbone to the bottom of the diaphragm, which is tied by ligaments to the bottom of the rib cage. The right lung is divided into three lobes—an upper, middle, and lower lobe. The left lung has only two lobes, an upper and a lower. However, there is a portion of the left lobe that corresponds to the middle lobe of the right lung; it sometimes is identified as the lingula.

Each lobe is divided into smaller units, called lobules. Each lung lobule has a bronchial tube, nerves, blood vessels, lymph vessels, and a bunch of tiny air sacs called alveoli. The bronchial tubes eventually branch into smaller tubes, or bronchioles, with a cluster of alveoli at the end, resembling a bunch of grapes on a stem.

The pulmonary arteries spread throughout the lung tissue like the branches of a large oak or maple tree. The larger branches support increasingly smaller branches, finally ending as tiny twigs at the tips of the smallest branches. At the ultimate end of the pulmonary arteries are capillaries so small that the red blood cells passing through them are separated from the air in the lungs by only one layer of cells in the tissue-thin membranes of the alveoli. At this point the blood is so close to the air from outside the body that small differences in pressure between the circulatory system and the atmosphere allow carbon dioxide molecules to pass from the red blood cells into the air spaces in the alveoli, and permit fresh oxygen molecules to be pulled through the layer of alveoli cells to become attached to the red blood cells.

The arrangement of alveoli clusters on the bronchioles is one of nature's tricks for cramming as much membrane surface as possible into a limited amount of tissue space. About 100 quarts, or 95 liters, of air are pumped into and out of the lungs every minute during the normal breathing of an adult. During periods of peak physical activity, the amount of air passing through the lungs, which means into and out of the microscopically tiny air sacs, may amount to 500 quarts per minute. During that same period a tremendous amount of blood must flow through the thin walls of the alveoli to expel carbon dioxide and water vapor, and to pick up fresh oxygen molecules.

Fluid or other substances in the air, or in the walls of the alveoli, can interfere with the normal exchange of oxygen and carbon dioxide. Fluid in the alveoli, for example, can cause a disorder known as pulmonary edema, which results in a fluid barrier to the flow of oxygen from the air to the red blood cells. Carbon monoxide, a toxic gas produced by combustion of fossil fuels, is more strongly attracted to the red blood cells than oxygen. As a result, carbon monoxide in the atmosphere from automobile exhaust or other sources can fill up all the spaces reserved for oxygen molecules in the red blood cells and render

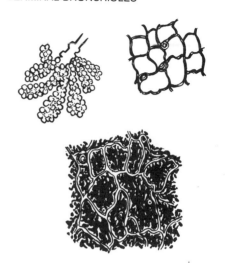

TERMINAL BRONCHIOLES

Drawings show what happens inside the alveolar sacs of the lungs when an infection such as lobar pneumonia invades the breathing apparatus. The object in the upper left, resembling bunches of grapes on a stem, is a cluster of alveoli, or tiny air sacs, at the end of a bronchiole; bronchioles carry oxygen to the alveoli and provide an exit passageway for carbon dioxide and water vapor when a person exhales. The sketch at the upper right represents a more highly magnified view of a group of alveoli, with tiny blood vessels running through the membrane walls. During normal breathing, the sacs contain the air being inhaled or exhaled. The illustration at the bottom indicates the condition of the alveoli when they become filled with pus and/or fluid during a lung infection. Since oxygen cannot enter the alveoli, the tiny air sacs have no way of getting rid of the carbon dioxide and water vapor waste products delivered to the lungs by the circulatory system. The result is a feeling of suffocation by the person with the lung infection.

the blood cells useless. Thus, oxygen needed for the life support systems of tissue cells in the brain, heart, and other organs simply doesn't get through.

Toxic gases also can cause pulmonary

edema by damaging the walls of the alveoli. A feeling of shortness of breath, sometimes called dyspnea by the doctor, is just one symptom of pulmonary edema. Asthma-like attacks, coughing, and difficulty in breathing can interrupt normal sleep patterns. In mild attacks the patient may find that getting up at night and walking about seems to reduce the symptoms so that sleep can be resumed. In more severe cases, such as those involving failure of the heart to pump blood out of the lungs as fast as it enters the capillaries of the alveoli, the fluid portion of the blood may become trapped in the alveolar walls and complicate the condition. The attacks of breathlessness and coughing spells then become more serious, and the patient may spit up blood-tinged sputum.

Nitrogen Gas One of the major gases in the atmosphere we breathe is of no particular use to the human body, but it poses no serious problems except for persons who go too high in the sky or too deep in the ocean, or enter similar environments where atmospheric pressure is significantly different from the one in which humans have learned to live normally for the past several million years. The gas is nitrogen. It makes up nearly 80 percent of the air we breathe, which also contains in addition to oxygen small amounts of carbon dioxide, water vapor, and other substances. Nearly one quart of nitrogen is carried in the blood of an average adult; it becomes dissolved in the fluid portion of the blood as a result of breathing a nitrogen-rich atmosphere. During normal breathing some nitrogen is expelled into the alveoli, but at the same time it is replaced by nitrogen absorbed from the alveoli.

Most people are not aware of the nitrogen in the bloodstream until they encounter a situation where the atmospheric pressure is changed, such as in a pressurized aircraft or a pressure chamber deep below the surface of the earth, or while using equipment for deep-water diving. Even then the nitrogen causes no problems as long as the pressure changes gradually and nothing goes wrong with the equipment. But if a diver rises to the surface too rapidly, the dissolved nitrogen, or other gas, may form bubbles in the blood vessels. The bubbles can produce severe pains, especially around the body joints. The pain sometimes is called "the bends," and the condition is referred to as decompression sickness or caisson disease.

Oxygen Reserves In addition to the quart of nitrogen, most people carry at all times in their bodies about two quarts of oxygen. Some of the oxygen is in the blood, some in the alveoli, and some in the body tissues. In an emergency, such as a blocked windpipe caused by choking on food, the reserve supply of oxygen should be enough to keep most of the body functioning normally for around four minutes.

The reserve supply of oxygen also helps an athlete during peak periods of performance. During a footrace, for example, the body may consume more oxygen than the lungs can supply for a short period of time. The oxygen reserve in the muscles, lungs, and blood is thrown into the fray. When the reserve supply is exhausted, the muscles usually quit working and become painful because of an accumulation of waste products that can't be carried away fast enough by the blood.

Then there also is the matter of the "second wind" during which a person breathes deeply, heavily, and rapidly for several minutes while he repays the oxygen debt acquired by borrowing from the body's reserve supply of the vital gas. The heavy breathing associated with repaying one's oxygen debt also requires an extra effort by the heart. It has to work harder to keep the blood circulating in order to deliver fresh oxygen to the depleted tissue stores and to help unload the accumulated waste products of tissue metabolism.

The business of making the heart and lungs work hard enough to develop a "second wind" is part of the theory behind the "aerobics" type of exercise program. Most aerobic exercises are designed to produce some huffing and puffing, especially for people who are not in top physical condition.

Blood Clots Besides providing a means for blood cells to have close access to the atmosphere, the lungs have a little-known function of helping the circulatory system to get rid of blood clots. The lung tissues do this with enzymes that help dissolve the blood clots. It is not unusual for tiny clots to form in the veins and be carried to the lungs. The clots are called emboli, or an embolus if there is only one. A small embolus normally will be trapped by the filtering apparatus of the lungs and dissolved before it can do any harm such as blocking an artery.

A large embolus, however, can overwhelm the filtering system of the lungs and become lodged in one of the pulmonary artery branches. If a branch of a pulmonary artery becomes blocked by an embolus, circulation to the tissues beyond that point will be interrupted. The disorder is called a pulmonary embolism, the seriousness of which depends upon the amount of lung tissue deprived of blood circulation.

The pulmonary embolism can produce what is known as a pulmonary infarction. The lung tissue deprived of blood circulation will die, and a form of pleurisy probably will follow. In a mild case the patient may appear relatively normal, and the chest pain associated with the pleurisy usually will not appear until some time later. Or there may be mild to severe chest pain, depending upon the size of the embolus and the area affected; if it is a relatively large pulmonary embolism, the signs and symptoms can be quite similar to those of a myocardial infarction. If a major part of the pulmonary circulation is blocked, the effect may be similar to that of heart failure, with a general circulation interruption and rapid death.

Most pulmonary emboli begin in the legs and frequently signal their development with pains, swelling, and tenderness, sometimes accompanied by discoloration of the skin in the area of the blood clot. The blood clots usually can be dissolved at an early stage of development by the use of anticoagulent drugs.

A blood clot in the leg may be called a thrombus. One thrombus frequently heralds the development of other blood clots, with small clots being followed by the development of larger clots. In many cases early and careful preventive treatment of blood clots in the legs can help prevent the threat of an embolus traveling to the lungs.

Persons with sluggish blood circulation, perhaps because of a heart disorder, lung congestion, surgery, or illness, are likely to be threatened by the development of blood clots in the veins. Thus, people who are bedfast or who spend very little time in a standing or walking position should exercise their legs for several minutes every waking hour in whatever way is feasible for them.

Pulmonary Disorders Another disorder involving a link between the heart and lungs, and one that often is associated with bronchitis or emphysema, is pulmonary arterial hypertension. The disease may be aggravated by cigarette smoking, air pollution, or exposure to cold weather. Pulmonary arterial hypertension is similar to the kind of hypertension commonly associated with high blood pressure, the difference being that the hypertension involves blood circulation through the lungs rather than in the rest of the circulatory system. In some cases, pulmonary arterial hypertension can be a result of emboli that disrupt the normal circulation of blood through the lungs. The symptoms may include chest pains, fatigue, and shortness of breath.

One form of pulmonary arterial hypertension is pulmonary heart disease, sometimes called cor pulmonale. It is characterized by the rupture of some walls of the alveoli, so that several of the tiny air sacs become one larger air sac. This situation reduces the amount of alveolar surface available for the exchange of the main respiratory gases, oxygen and carbon dioxide. As a result, the right side of the heart has to work harder in order to get the same amount of blood oxygenated with less alveolar surface exposed to the oxygen in the lungs. Eventually, the right ventricle becomes enlarged and susceptible to failure.

Another complication of pulmonary heart disease is that the body's efforts to compensate for a loss of alveolar surface can be an overproduction of red blood cells. Since the red cells can be sticky, blood that contains an excess of red cells usually does not flow smoothly. The excessive red cell condition, called polycythemia, theoretically should permit a smaller amount of blood to carry a normal amount of oxygen, but it actually places an increased burden on the left ventricle, which must push the thick, sticky type of blood through many miles of tiny blood vessels.

The patient with pulmonary heart disease will experience some wheezing and other breathing difficulties if untreated. He also may suffer from such effects as trembling hands and mental confusion because of poor blood oxygenation. He may become barrel chested and develop clubbing of the fingers. Eventually, he may need a readily available supply of oxygen and an oxygen mask, plus diuretics, heart drugs, and antibiotics to control respiratory infections. Pulmonary heart disease patients can have reasonably comfortable lives, but they must avoid smoking, air pollution, exposure to cold and damp environments, and they must receive prompt medical attention for respiratory infections.

See also Chapter 18: *Strokes and High Blood Pressure.*

Forced Breathing As a further example of the close relationship between the heart and lungs, the lungs get their cue for breathing from the amount of carbon dioxide circulating in the bloodstream. The blood flows through a respiratory center in the brain that measures the level of carbon dioxide and calls for deeper and more rapid breathing when the carbon dioxide level increases. Another respiratory center in the central nervous system measures the level of oxygen in the bloodstream, and when the percentage of oxygen drops below a certain level, it stimulates increased respiration.

Forced breathing can deplete the carbon dioxide level of the blood so that breathing ceases temporarily; a chemical signal to the brain suggests that the body has enough oxygen for a while. The reaction can be followed quickly by dizziness and loss of consciousness. Ordinarily, the victim recovers from a forced breathing "blackout" within a few minutes after the carbon dioxide accumulation returns to a level that triggers normal breathing. However, forced breathing before diving into a swimming pool could be dangerous since the depletion of carbon dioxide might result in a loss of consciousness while the person is beneath the surface of the water.

Some individuals who suffer severe emotional stress may "pass out" as a result of forced breathing and carbon dioxide depletion. Too much carbon dioxide, on the other hand, also can result in a loss of consciousness. The amount of carbon dioxide needed to maintain normal breathing is rather critical. The alveoli normally contain about five percent carbon dioxide; but if the level is increased to more than ten percent carbon dioxide, loss of consciousness will occur.

Breathing Measurements The amount of air passing into and out of the lungs during normal quiet breathing is called tidal air. The amount of air that can be inhaled and expelled from the lungs during forced breathing is called vital capacity. Both the amount of tidal air and vital capacity may be measured during certain kinds of physical examinations, such as checkups involving the respiratory system. The vital capacity for an average young adult man is around five quarts, but that amount usually declines with age.

The vital capacity of women generally is less because of their smaller average body sizes. The capacity of the lungs of trained athletes, as might be expected, is greater than average.

In addition to the amount of air that may be measured in terms of vital capacity or tidal volume, the human lungs usually hold about one and a half quarts of residual air. This air remains in the lungs even after forced breathing to measure vital capacity. Residual air is a normal factor in studies of respiration since it represents air trapped in the bronchioles and alveoli because of pressure of respiratory muscles which close some air passages during forced breathing.

The tidal air of a person may be measured with a machine called a spirometer. A peak flow meter frequently is used to measure vital capacity.

Bronchoscopy A doctor may examine the upper part of the respiratory tract by ordering a bronchogram, a special kind of X-ray that shows the condition of the main air tubes leading from the end of the trachea to the lobes of the lungs. The doctor also can examine the main bronchi by administering a local anesthetic to the interior of the throat and trachea so that the air tubes can be inspected with instruments equipped with lights, mirrors, and lenses that magnify the tissues. Such an examination is called a bronchoscopy. It allows the doctor to see inside the respiratory system to about the level of the second pair of ribs, where the main bronchi branch away from the trachea.

GLOSSARY
THE CHEST

The following list of medical terms relates to the anatomy and disorders of the chest; words in italics refer to other entries in this Glossary.

abdominal breathing A term used to describe breathing in which the diaphragm muscle plays a major role. Abdominal breathing sometimes is differentiated from thoracic breathing, in which the intercostal muscles between the ribs are more actively involved in expanding and compressing the lungs. Women are more likely to depend upon thoracic breathing than men.

achalasia A neurological disorder of the esophagus. It may be marked by chest pain and the regurgitation of food, particularly while lying down. Complications can result from inhaling regurgitated food, resulting in pneumonia or other respiratory problems. Treatment of serious cases may require surgery.

acute coronary insufficiency A condition that may be described as somewhere between *angina pectoris* and *myocardial infarction.* The pain may be that of angina, but more severe and beginning suddenly with little or no exertion. It may begin during a period of rest. Treatment usually is designed so as to prevent or lessen effects of the onset of myocardial infarction; immediate rest and medications are prescribed to reduce the risk of blood clots forming in the coronary arteries.

adiposis dolorosa A medical term sometimes used to identify a form of obesity that is marked by painfully tender fat lobules that develop about the thorax and limbs.

adrenalin A drug, also known as epinephrine, which may be used in emergencies to stimulate the heart and increase blood pressure. Adrenalin also is used to relax bronchial wall spasms during attacks of asthma. However, its value generally is limited to situations in which a quick response is needed because the effects last for only a short period of time.

adventitious sounds Noises a doctor may detect while examining one's chest with a stethoscope. The sounds may be produced by the movement of fluid in the lungs, the rubbing of broken rib bones, or other sounds not produced by ordinary breathing or the voice apparatus.

air As generally used, the term refers to the mixture of gases in the atmosphere we breathe—about 80 percent nitrogen and 20 percent oxygen, with small amounts of carbon dioxide, water vapor, and other gases. In an individual medical case, however, the composition of the air may be somewhat different. A person with chronic bronchitis, for example, might be administered "bottled" air containing from 25 to 30 percent oxygen. Other patients under special circumstances might require humidified pure or nearly pure oxygen. Air in the alveoli normally contains around five or six percent carbon dioxide, or many times the less than one percent level of the air outside the body. Generally, the human body can tolerate for short periods air that contains at least 13 percent oxygen and no more than 10 percent carbon dioxide. Too little oxygen or too much carbon dioxide can result in loss of consciousness and death.

air hunger A common term used to identify deep breathing sounds that resemble repeated sighs. The deep sighing sounds sometimes accompany the breathing of patients suffering from pneumonia and other respiratory diseases.

alveolar cell carcinoma A rare type of malignant tumor that grows in the walls of the *alveoli.*

alveoli The tiny air sacs that give the lungs an appearance resembling a sponge. The alveoli (plural for alveolus) occur in clusters like a bunch of grapes at the end of a terminal bronchiole, the final tube of a series of branches and sub-branches extending from the trachea. Air that is inhaled through the nose, or mouth, passes down the trachea to the bronchi, and from the bronchi to the bronchioles, until it reaches the alveolar pouches. The walls of the alveoli are very thin and contain blood vessels. Oxygen molecules from the inhaled air pass through the alveolar walls and are "captured" by red blood cells in the tiny capillaries within the membranes. At the same time, carbon dioxide and water vapor molecules are released from the blood through the alveolar walls to be expelled during the next phase of respiration when air is exhaled from the lungs. See illustration page 161.

aminophylline A drug commonly used in the treatment of asthma because it relaxes the spasms of the bronchial walls and provides relief from the wheezing and coughing attacks associated with the disease. The medicine, which also may be identified as theophylline ethylenediamine, can be administered by mouth, by injection, or in a suppository.

amphoric breathing Respiratory sounds that are similar to the noises produced by blowing over the mouth of a bottle or jug. Amphoric breathing sounds can be clues to a possible abnormality in the lungs or bronchial tubes.

aneurysm A stretching or ballooning of a major blood vessel, such as the *aorta*. If the aneurysm is not controlled, it may rupture and cause sudden death. An aneurysm may be felt by the patient as a severe pain in the chest accompanied by a sensation of internal tissues being torn apart. The pain may be felt both in the front and back, and as far down as the abdomen, depending upon the area of artery damage. The patient usually is pale but sweating, and has a rapid pulse rate. Emergency treatment is directed toward lowering blood pressure and relieving pain. The damaged artery can be repaired later by sewing the blood vessel or replacing a section with a *Dacron graft.*

Some aneurysms produce no symptoms of pain but are detected during X-ray examinations for other complaints which may or may not involve the aneurysm. In some cases the ballooning blood vessel may press against a neighboring organ such as the lungs, esophagus, or larynx, with the result that breathing or swallowing difficulties, or hoarseness, become clues to the presence of the aneurysm.

angina pectoris A disorder characterized by severe pains in the chest, accompanied by a steady feeling of pressure or squeezing. The condition is caused by a reduced flow of blood through coronary arteries of the heart because of a partial obstruction of the blood vessels. The pain and pressure may be induced by physical work, emotional upset, or another factor such as eating a large meal.

The pain may radiate to the left shoulder and arm, or to the jaw, and last from one to 20 minutes. The patient may experience feelings of fear or apprehension. Nausea and perspiration may accompany the pain. The symptoms usually are relieved by the use of nitroglycerine medication or a period of rest. The condition is diagnosed with the help of *electrocardiograms*, examination of the heart region of the chest, and the administration of nitroglycerin to determine its effects on the symptoms.

angiography A technique for examining blood vessels by X-ray. An opaque dye, one that will be easily visible on X-ray film, is injected into an artery that is to be examined and an X-ray picture is made. Any constriction or narrowing of the blood vessel can be located on the X-ray film. The technique may be used to study the coronary arteries, in which case it is referred to as coronary angiography.

aorta The major blood artery which feeds blood from the left ventricle of the heart to organs and tissues throughout the body. The aorta divides shortly after leaving the left side of the heart into a system of arteries which further divide into *arterioles*. The arterioles finally subdivide into capillaries, the smallest of the blood vessels carrying blood away from the heart.

arrhythmias A medical term meaning irregular or abnormal heartbeats. An example of arrythmia is an abnormally rapid heartbeat, which doctors called *tachycardia*. Another kind of arrythmia might be a disorder called premature ventricular contractions, caused by the heart ventricles contracting before their turn in the heart pumping cycle.

arterioles Small arteries which have a narrow bore but thick, muscular walls; they are a link between the regular arteries and the thin-walled capillaries, which are the ultimate end of the fresh blood distribution system that trickles down from the *aorta*.

asbestosis A lung disease that can result from prolonged exposure to asbestos, or magnesium silicate dust. The microscopic fibers of the mineral can be inhaled deeply into the *alveoli*, where they interfere with the exchange of gases, stiffen the membrane walls, and in general reduce the volume of air that can be handled by the lungs. Asbestosis also is associated with various types of lung tumors and the greater risk of lung cancer among cigarette smokers. While persons who work with asbestos, such as insulation installers, are more likely to develop asbestosis, there is some evidence that people who live near asbestos plants or who live with asbestos workers also may develop the disease.

Treatment of asbestosis generally is limited to relief of the symptoms, which may include pain and breathing difficulties. Certain forms of tumors associated with asbestosis can be removed by surgery, but one of the more common types, mesothelioma, seldom can be treated surgically.

aspergillosis A type of fungus infection that can affect the lungs. The infection can produce symptoms of asthma, but it may produce no serious effects. In lungs previously damaged by another disease, such as tuberculosis, aspergillosis may result in a condition known as mycetoma, or a ball of fungus in a lung cavity. A mycetoma may remain untreated if it causes no serious effects, or it may have to be removed surgically.

asphyxia A term used to describe a lack of oxygen in the body tissues. While commonly used to indicate a lack of oxygen available to the lungs, asphyxia technically includes conditions in which oxygen is present in the atmosphere or lungs but cannot reach tissue cells in the body organs. Carbon monoxide poisoning, for example, can prevent oxygen molecules from being transported from the alveoli to the various tissue cells of the body by combining with the hemoglobin of the red blood cells.

asthma A respiratory disease marked by attacks in which the patient has difficulty in exhaling normally. The disease is due to spasms of the bronchial muscles and *edema*, or fluid in the mucosa lining the bronchial tubes. Unlike *bronchitis* or *emphysema*, in which the breathing obstruction problem is more or less continuous, asthma generally occurs sporadically with periods of normal breathing between attacks. The asthma attacks are characterized by bouts of wheezing which occur almost entirely while breathing out, the expiration phase of breathing.

A typical asthma attack may last an hour or two and be accompanied by sensations of pressure in the chest and of suffocation. It may be necessary to hold the body in an upright position in order to breathe in a somewhat normal manner, and breathing may become increasingly rapid. The lungs tend to become distended with air, which enters the lungs faster than it can be expelled because of the bronchial obstruction. In severe cases the patient may temporarily lose his normal coloring because blood flowing through the lungs fails to obtain enough fresh oxygen to maintain a normal red color. At the end of an attack, the patient may cough up a large amount of thick sputum.

Asthma that seems to be due to external agents, such as house dust or cat hairs, sometimes is identified as extrinsic asthma; asthma attacks that are not related to external allergens are classified as a sign of intrinsic asthma. When acute attacks of asthma continue for several days or more, the condition is called status athmaticus. Another variation of asthma, in which the patient suffers a mild chronic form of the disease for a number of days, may occur during a period when a seasonal allergen is present—for instance, during the hay fever season.

asystole A medical term used to describe faulty contractions of the heart's *ventricles*.

atelectasis Collapse of a lobe of the lung or a portion of a lobe. The condition can be an effect of bronchopneumonia.

atrial fibrillation A type of arrythmia in which there are rapid, irregular contractions of the atria that are independent of contractions of the ventricles.

atrial flutter A condition similar to atrial fibrillation but with very rapid, regular contractions occurring at a rate of as many as 300 per minute. The ventricles try to maintain a regular rhythm but manage to respond to every second, third, or fourth contraction of the atria.

atrial septal defect A failure in the wall that separates the right atrium from the left atrium, the two top chambers of the heart. The defect can result in the two atria acting as a single reservoir chamber and in an increased flow of blood through the pulmonary artery, which gets its blood supply from the right side of the heart; since the left side of the heart is more powerful, the pressure difference forces blood from the left to the right side. Small defects may not produce any symptoms until after middle age, when the defects can contrib-

ute to development of arrythmias or congestive heart failure.

atrioventricular block A term used by doctors to describe a failure of the normal nerve impulse that controls heart contractions passing from the atria to the ventricles. Failure of the nerve message to reach the ventricles results in a missed heartbeat. The missing heartbeat sometimes is called a dropped beat.

auscultation A method of checking the condition of the heart by listening to and analyzing sounds made by the heart while its four chambers, the two atria and two ventricles, are contracting and relaxing, and while the various heart valves are opening and closing. The doctor frequently uses a stethoscope to listen to heart sounds, applying a bell-shaped device on the end of the stethoscope to detect low-pitched sounds, and using a shallow, wide device to analyze high-pitched sounds. By listening at four different points on the patient's chest, the doctor can hear the sounds of four different heart valves.

bagpipe sign A sign of a defective respiratory system that is marked by the sound of air continuing to be exhaled from a person's lungs after the actual effort at breathing out has been completed. The sound usually indicates a partial obstruction in the bronchial tubes.

benzocaine A drug occasionally used as a local anesthetic to reduce pain or discomfort during exploration or treatment of the trachea and bronchi of a patient suffering from a respiratory disorder. The benzocaine can be administered in several different ways. It may be taken orally in the form of a lozenge, or the doctor might spray the anesthetic into the patient's throat, and in some cases a patient might receive a benzocaine spray after taking a benzocaine lozenge.

beta-blocking drugs Certain nerve receptors in the heart and bronchial muscles are stimulated by hormones such as adrenaline; doctors refer to these sites as beta receptors. When a drug such as propanolol is administered to a patient, the molecules of the medicine are attracted to the beta receptor sites and prevent or minimize the stimulating hormones from using the nerve receptors. As heart medications the beta-blocking drugs slow the heartbeat and reduce the work load of a cardiac patient's heart by blocking the beta receptors.

black lung disease The common name for a type of pneumoconiosis that occurs in coal miners and causes the lungs to become black. It is caused by an inflammation of the lungs resulting from prolonged inhalation of coal dust.

blebs A name applied to dilated air sacs in the lungs. The sacs occasionally burst and cause a condition known as a *pneumothorax*.

blood gases Levels of oxygen and carbon dioxide in the blood are measured during laboratory testing. The exact procedure is rather complicated, but the information produced by analysis of the gas molecules in the blood sample often can help diagnose a wide variety of disorders, ranging from lung diseases to central nervous system problems.

blood pressure The pressure produced in the bloodstream by the pumping action of the heart. Blood pressure can be measured directly in a laboratory by inserting a tube into an artery and allowing the pressure of the blood flow to force a column of mercury to rise in a glass straw at the other end of the tube. A doctor measures blood pressure in an indirect fashion by fastening an inflatable cuff around the patient's arm. As the cuff is inflated by pumping a rubber bulb attached to it, the cuff squeezes on an artery in the arm, and the blood pressure in the artery pushes back and forces a column of mercury upward in a glass tube. The higher the mercury rises in the glass straw, or tube, the higher is the measure of blood pressure. In actually measuring one's blood pressure, the doctor pumps air into the cuff until the pulse below the cuff can no longer be detected, indicating that the inflated cuff has exerted enough pressure to stop the flow of blood, much as a tourniquet tied around the arm would stop blood flow in the artery. Then the doctor gradually releases air from the cuff until the pulse can just be detected again. This is the high mark of the blood pressure, indicating the force of the thrust of the blood squeezed from the heart. The doctor records this as the systolic blood pressure. Next, the cuff is further deflated until the sound of the pulse, as heard through a stethoscope, becomes muffled and disappears. The level of the mercury in the glass column at the point where it is last heard is recorded as the diastolic blood pressure.

The blood pressure information generally is written as something like 130/80. The numbers stand for the level of the mercury in the tube as measured in millimeters when the systolic (130) and diastolic (80) levels were observed. Blood pressure figures generally are lower for young people, starting with perhaps 80/60 for a baby, and increase to 140/90—a level sometimes regarded as the upper limit of normal blood pressure—in later adult years. Blood pressure readings higher than 140/90 usually are a cause for concern for persons of any age, since they suggest a tendency towards hypertension, or high blood pressure disease.

bone crepitus A sound heard through a stethoscope held against the chest when the two edges of a fractured bone rub against each other. The sound, which is a grating noise, frequently is a clue that a fractured rib is the cause of a pain in the chest.

breastbone A common name for the sternum, a dagger-shaped bone at the front of the rib cage. The heart is partly concealed behind the breast bone.

breast masses A doctor examining the breast usually checks for abnormal masses of tissue by looking for dimpling, bulges, flattened contours, and other clues. The examination involves palpation by pressing the hand against the chest, compressing tissue between the thumb and forefinger, and transilluminating the breast by holding a small flashlight under it. Each type of mass may provide its own clues during a breast examination. A fluid-filled cyst, for example, may appear as a somewhat transparent area in the breast during transillumination.

breast quadrants A term used by doctors to locate sites of possible abnormal tissue in the breast. If imaginary lines are drawn across a female breast so that a horizontal line and a vertical line intersect at the nipple, the "geography" of the breast would be divided into four quadrants. The two upper quadrants may be identified as the upper medial (toward the sternum) and upper lateral (toward the outside). The lower quadrants can be called the lower medial and lower lateral. A protrusion of breast tissue that extends toward the armpit from the upper lateral quadrant sometimes is called the axillary tail.

bronchial lavage A surgical technique that may be used to treat certain types of respiratory diseases in order to clear the bronchial tubes. Thick mucus blocking the bronchial tubes is carefully washed out so that normal breathing can be resumed.

bronchiectasis A condition in which the smaller branches of the bronchi become dilated, usually as a result of an infection such as bronchopneumonia or whooping cough. The disorder is accompanied by the secretion of large amounts of pus. The patient coughs up a sputum that separates into several layers. Treatment includes placing the patient in a postural position that aids drainage of the pus and administration of antibiotics to control the infection responsible for the condition.

bronchitis A medical term for inflammation of the trachea, or *windpipe*, and of the bronchial tubes extending from it into the lungs. Bronchitis can be acute or chronic and is caused by either infectious agents such as bacteria or by physical or chemical agents, including tobacco smoke.

Acute bronchitis frequently is a complication of a common cold or a similar virus infection of the nose and throat, and it may be associated with a bacterial infection of tissues originally inflamed by a virus. While coughing generally is identified with bronchitis, a cough may be a signal that acute bronchitis is just beginning. The disease also can include such symptoms as chills, fever that reaches above 100 degrees Fahrenheit and continues for several days in severe cases, sore throat, and muscle pains. There also may be difficulty in breathing, and wheezing after a siege of coughing. Treatment usually consists of bed rest, increased fluid intake, and the use of medications that relieve pain and inflammation symptoms. A steam vaporizer can help speed recovery, which usually occurs within three weeks. Bronchopneumonia can be a complication of acute bronchitis.

Chronic bronchitis is a term sometimes used to describe a form of the disorder that is associated with prolonged exposure to irritants of the bronchial tree. It may be accompanied by a set of signs and symptoms that include persistent coughing and production of large amounts of mucus from the throat, along with structural damage to the bronchial tubes. See also *mucopurulent chronic bronchitis; tracheobronchitis.*

bronchodilator A drug administered to relax the smooth muscles of the breathing passageways. There are a number of different bronchodilators, usually administered as an aerosal spray, with varying potencies, lengths of action, and other factors such as side effects.

broncholiths Tiny particles of calcium or other minerals that are coughed up in the sputum of patients suffering from respiratory diseases such as *silicosis* and histoplasmosis. The rocklike particles usually are formed from deposits of minerals in the lymph nodes of the bronchial tree. Broncholiths sometimes are associated with bloody sputum.

bronchus One of the two bronchi, or air tubes, which branch from the bottom of the trachea, or windpipe. One bronchus extends into the left lung and one into the right lung. Each bronchus subdivides into smaller tubes, called bronchioles, in a pattern somewhat like limbs and branches of a tree. The larger bronchial branches are protected and supported by rings of cartilage, which help hold them open for the passage of air during breathing.

bundle branch block A term used by heart specialists and other doctors to identify a certain type of failure of nerve impulse to complete a circuit as required for normal heart contractions. A result of bundle branch block is that the two ventricles are out of step with each other in heartbeat rhythm, one contracting slightly ahead of the other.

byssinosis An occupational disease that affects people who work with textiles. Dust and other foreign particles, such as molds and fungi, from cotton, flax, and other fabric materials produce a wheezing and feeling of tightness in the chest. The ailment sometimes is called by its common name of brown lung disease.

capillary The nearly microscopically small blood vessels that carry blood with oxygen and other nutrients to the individual body cells and carry away the waste products of the cells' metabolic activity, thus linking the arteries and veins of the circulatory system. The human body may contain literally thousands of miles of capillaries, most of them so thin that red blood cells must pass through them in single file.

cardiac arrest This means simply that the heart has stopped. Signs of cardiac arrest are an absence of a pulse in the carotid or femoral arteries, a sudden loss of consciousness, dilation of the pupils of the eyes (although this is not a sure sign), an ashen or grayish-blue complexion, and gasping for breath or cessation of breathing.

When cardiac arrest occurs, emergency measures such as external cardiac massage or mouth-to-mouth resuscitation must be started immediately. If a second person is available, he or she should summon professional medical help by the quickest means possible. Irreversible brain damage can occur if heart action and blood circulation are not restored within four minutes, but efforts to restore normal breathing and heart action should be continued be-

yond that time unless a doctor advises that further emergency aid is useless.

cardiac catheterization A technique for studying the activity of the heart by inserting fine catheters into the chambers of the heart. The patient is given a sedative and perhaps an anesthetic before a catheter is inserted into a blood vessel in an arm or leg; the exact blood vessel selected as the starting point depends upon which chamber of the heart is to be studied for blood pressure or other data. The catheters used are radio-opaque, meaning that they can be seen with X-ray equipment and guided as they are threaded through an artery to the heart. The heart chambers and all major blood vessels attached to the heart can be examined by cardiac catheterization.

cardiac heave A term used to describe the effect of the heart action which in some individuals can be so powerful that it causes the sternum or ribs to move with each beat. Some doctors use the term "cardiac lift" for the same effect.

carina The angle where the bronchi branch away from the bottom or lower end of the trachea.

carotid sinus A structure in the carotid artery, which carries blood from the heart to the head. The carotid sinus contains nerve receptors that can measure the levels of oxygen and carbon dioxide in the blood passing through the artery. Signals from the carotid sinus receptors to the brain help control one's rate of breathing, according to the need for more oxygen or to expel more carbon dioxide from the lungs.

CCU An abbreviation sometimes used to identify a Coronary Care Unit, an area of a hospital that may be specially equipped with modern life-saving devices and staffed by personnel who have had special training in caring for patients suffering from heart diseases.

central tendon A sheet of flat fibrous tissue attached to the muscles of the diaphragm. When muscles of the diaphragm contract, their action pulls the central tendon down toward the abdomen. This in turn creates a partial vacuum in the lungs so that air rushes into the alveoli, resulting in inhalation.

cervical rib syndrome An extra rib that develops in some people above the usual first rib. The cervical rib may press on nerve tissue that passes from the neck to the arm, causing pain and numbness in the arm. Treatments include postural exercises and surgery.

chemotherapy drugs Chemicals designed to kill or control the growth of cancer cells. The drugs frequently are used to ease the discomfort of lung cancer patients.

chest aspiration A technique for draining fluid from a lung. A hypodermic syringe and needle, with a length of rubber tubing and a small valve attached, is inserted into the chest wall. As the plunger of the syringe is pulled back and the valve is turned on, fluid in the lung is siphoned into a container.

Cheyne-Stokes breathing A pattern of respiration in which the breathing becomes deeper and deeper until a maximum is reached and the respirations diminish until respiration ceases briefly. Then the pattern, which may last two or three minutes, begins again. This type of breathing is associated with a failure of the respiratory control center to make an accurate measurement of the carbon dioxide level in the patient's blood. Cheyne-Stokes breathing is a sign of a disorder involving the left side of the heart.

chronic obstructive lung disease A term used to describe any of several diseases, such as bronchitis, asthma, or emphysema, in which breathing is difficult because of such factors as a general narrowing of the bronchial tubes or loss of normal function of lung tissue.

cilia Small hair-like projections lining the trachea. The cilia are covered with mucus, produced by bronchial glands, which helps them to trap dirt and other foreign particles that may be inhaled. The cilia help move foreign materi-

als upward toward the throat and away from the lungs.

clavicle The medical name for the collarbone, a slightly curved, slender bone that extends on either side of the base of the neck from the sternum, or breastbone, to the shoulder joint.

closed chest cardiac massage Sometimes called external cardiac massage, this is a method of restarting heart action after cardiac arrest. The hands are placed, one atop the other, with the heel of the lower hand on the lower end of the breastbone. The breastbone, or sternum, is then depressed forcefully and repeatedly at a rate of about 70 times per minute, slightly faster than one push every second. The procedure is continued until signs of heart action, such as a pulse in the carotid artery, are observed, or until a physician advises that further effort is useless.

Closed chest cardiac massage can be quite tiring for the person applying the technique, so it is helpful if other persons are available to take turns. The rescue technique must be done carefully since too much pressure can damage other organs, such as the liver, particularly when cardiac massage is applied to children. For very small youngsters, closed chest cardiac massage frequently can be applied with only the thumbs, one atop the other, at a rate of about two compressions per second, or 120 per minute.

closed heart surgery Certain operations involving the heart and blood vessels and valves near the heart are performed while the heart continues to pump blood. Closed heart surgery may be used to increase or reduce the blood flow in a pulmonary artery carrying blood from the heart to the lungs, or to remove an obstruction in a major artery. This type of surgery differs from open heart surgery in that the heart and lungs are temporarily replaced by an artificial pump and oxygenator while open heart surgery is performed.

clubbing A condition in which the soft tissues at the ends of the fingers become swollen and the skin becomes shiny; the fingernails may become more curved at the same time. The clubbing effect occurs as a sign of a variety of different heart and lung disorders, such as emphysema and congenital heart disease.

coarctation of the aorta A defect in the aorta, usually a congenital condition, in which the artery is narrowed at a point just beyond the heart so that normal blood flow is restricted. The disorder frequently is accompanied by a defective valve in the aorta. The condition may not produce any serious signs or symptoms in early life and frequently is not detected until the adult patient is examined by a doctor for hypertension or another circulatory problem.

coccidioidomycosis A fungus disease involving the lungs. It is caused by inhaling spores of a type of mold that grows in hot, dry areas such as the southwest desert of the U.S. and some regions of Latin America. The symptoms of the disease may resemble those of the common cold or influenza. Treatment involves bed rest and the administration of antibiotics to prevent or control secondary infections of bacteria.

congestive heart disease A disorder marked by difficulty in breathing and retention of salt and water by the body. Treatment includes diet, rest to reduce demands on the heart, administration of drugs such as digitalis to strengthen heart muscle action, and diuretics to help eliminate edema, or the accumulation of fluids in the body.

costa fluctuans A Latin term sometimes used by medical personnel to identify a "floating rib," one of four ribs that aren't attached to the sternum, or breastbone.

costal A term that refers to a rib; for example, a costal cartilage is a piece of cartilage connecting a rib to the sternum.

costochondritis An inflammation of the joints formed by the ribs and their cartilage connections. The upper ribs of the chest generally are involved, and the symptoms include chest pains and tenderness in the area of inflammation.

cough fracture A fracture of the ribs, usually near the lower end of the chest, as a result of coughing. The patient may notice chest pains associated with breathing or tenderness in the area of the fractured rib, which may not be revealed by X-ray pictures of the chest.

cyanosis A bluish complexion that results from lack of oxygen in the blood.

cystic fibrosis An inherited disease that is marked by the accumulation of abnormally thick mucus and abnormal secretion of sweat and saliva. In the lungs the mucus can block the small bronchial tubes and interfere with normal breathing. Inhaled air may become trapped in the alveoli, and the walls of the tiny air sacs may collapse. Since the mucus is too thick to flow easily, it tends to collect bacteria rather than help to rid the body of disease organisms; the mucus thus tends to trap infectious diseases in the respiratory system. Cystic fibrosis is inherited as a recessive trait, meaning that both parents must be carriers of the gene that causes it.

Dacron graft A short length of Dacron plastic tubing that can be substituted for a diseased or injured portion of a major blood vessel. A Dacron graft for example, may be used to replace a section of the aorta that has been damaged by an aneurysm.

defibrillator An electrical device that is used to apply an electric shock to the heart to stop abnormally rapid rhythms, or fibrillations. The machine produces a large jolt of direct current (electricity) which is applied to the chest of the patient through insulated "paddles" held by the operator. In some cases the shock is planned to be applied at a particular stage of the normal heart action cycle to help adjust the rhythm to a normal beat and pattern again. But in a real emergency, when every second is important in saving the patient's life, the rescue team does not have time to synchronize the shock with the heart rhythm.

dermatophagoides A long word for a tiny insect, or mite, sometimes found in house dust, which may be responsible for asthma attacks in persons who are allergic to house dust.

Devil's grip Common name given the symptoms of sharp pains in the chest and abdomen resulting from a viral infection. The pain apparently is caused by the friction of pleural membrane layers that rub against each other.

dextrocardia A heart that is positioned backward in the chest so that the bottom of the ventricles extends beyond the sternum on the right side rather than on the left side. In some cases other body organs also are reversed. The condition may or may not be associated with organic defects of the heart.

diaphragm A sheet of muscle tissue that forms the floor of the rib cage and supplies the muscle power for the act of breathing. Contraction of the diaphragm muscles pulls the dome-shaped sheet of tissue down toward the abdomen, creating a partial pressure difference in the lungs so that air rushes into the alveoli. When the muscles relax, the diaphragm pushes upward against the lungs again, squeezing air out of the alveoli.

diaphragmatic hernia A hernia of the diaphragm in which a part of the stomach pushes up through the opening in the diaphragm intended for the esophagus to pass through from the throat to the abdomen. See *hiatus hernia.*

diastole The relaxation phase of heart action after each *systole.* It is during this period of the heart pumping cycle that blood flows from the *atria* into the *ventricles;* at the end of the diastole, the atria contract to force more blood into the ventricles.

digitalis intoxication A condition marked by nausea, diarrhea, muscle weakness, loss of appetite, and visual disturbances, all of which are adverse side effects associated with the use of digitalis, a drug commonly used to strengthen heart action in the treatment of heart failure.

digoxin A form of digitalis prescribed by some doctors for the treatment of heart failure.

dropsy A somewhat obsolete word sometimes used to identify the condition of *edema,* or fluid accumulation in the body, that can result in certain cases of heart failure. The amount of fluid that may accumulate can be remarkably large, amounting to well over a gallon before it becomes noticeable. One of the more common effects of dropsy is a swelling of the feet and ankles when the patient is standing or walking.

dry pleurisy A painful disorder caused by inflammation or irritation of the pleura, the two-layer membrane which covers the lungs and lines the inner wall of the chest. The pain results from the rubbing together of the membrane layers when the patient breathes. Dry pleurisy can result from a variety of conditions ranging from injury to the chest wall to pneumonia or tuberculosis. The patient usually rests propped up in bed and is given mild analgesics to relieve the pain, along with a heating pad applied as needed to the more sensitive areas of the chest.

ductus arteriosus A blood vessel that joins the aorta, or main artery, to the pulmonary artery, which circulates blood to the lungs. In the fetus, or unborn child, the ductus arteriosus is a part of the normal blood circulatory system because the lungs are not used before birth. After birth, the vessel normally is closed; otherwise, higher pressure in the aorta can divert blood to the lungs and cause serious heart and circulatory problems in an infant. The abnormal condition, called patent ductus arteriosus, can be corrected surgically.

dynamic lung volume The measurement of the forced vital capacity of the lungs during breathing tests over a fixed period of time. For example, the test might measure the amount of air that a person can expel from his lungs during the first second of blowing into a spirometer, an instrument used to measure lung capacity; or it might measure the volume of air the person's lungs can handle per minute.

dysphagia Difficulty in swallowing. The complaint might be a symptom of a lung cancer that causes pressure on the esophagus.

dyspnea A medical term meaning shortness of breath (pronounced dis-nee-uh or disp-nee-uh). The condition may be characterized by symptoms of coughing or wheezing, especially after arising in the morning, or the need to get a "second wind" while walking up a hill or hurrying along a level path.

dysrhythmia A medical term meaning a disturbance in the normal rhythm of the heartbeat or brain waves.

Ebstein's disease A disorder, usually congenital, caused by a failure of the tricuspid valve, the three-flap valve that separates the right atrium from the right ventricle. The faulty valve permits blood in the ventricle to be regurgitated into the atrium during ventricular contractions. Treatment is by surgery.

ECG Abbreviation for *electrocardiogram.*

echogram A recording of ultrasound waves made to assist the diagnosis of tumors in the chest area. The ultrasound pattern can help identify the type of tumor—for example, whether it is a fluid-filled cyst or a solid tumor.

ectopic beats Heartbeats that start at some point other than the sino-atrial node, a point where the *vena cava*, the major vein returning blood from the body organs, empties into the right atrium of the heart. Ectopic beats also may be identified as premature beats or contractions, which occur on occasion in persons with normal hearts; however, these dysrhythmias are more likely to be found in individuals who have experienced a myocardial infarction.

edema Abnormal accumulation of fluid in the spaces between the body tissues. It frequently is a sign of congestive heart disease or heart failure. An examining physician sometimes can estimate the amount of edema in a patient's body by pressing his thumb against the skin above a lower leg bone, then removing the thumb. The indentation in the skin made by the thumb will remain for a short period of time, and the depth of the impression can be used to estimate the extent of fluid accumulation.

EKG Another abbreviation for *electrocardiogram.*

electrocardiogram A record made of the normal or abnormal activity of a patient's heart as it goes through its repeated cycles of contractions and relaxations. The electrocardiogram records the tiny electrical charges made when the nerve impulse that triggers the heart's systole and diastole phases spreads from the sino-atrial node, or natural pacemaker, of the heart to the ventricles. The sino-atrial node is located near the junction of the *vena cava*, the major blood vein into which all the smaller veins eventually empty, and the right atrium of the heart.

The electrical changes caused by the spread of the signal and the contractions of the muscle fibers of the heart are detected by a sensitive galvanometer, which translates the electrical activity into pen tracings on a continuously moving sheet of squared graph paper. The electrical activity is fed into the galvanometer from electrodes placed in strategic locations on the body. The electrodes usually are arranged in pairs, which helps the galvanometer determine the direction of the electrical flow in the heart. Each pair of electrodes is a lead (pronounced "leed") and each lead makes a separate trace on the electrocardiogram. The number of leads used and the location of the electrodes on the chest and limbs is determined in part by what sort of information about a patient's heart is needed.

The trace lines made on the electrocardiogram appear as a series of waves, each wiggle of which indicates a specific action of a heart muscle. One part of the pattern, called a P wave, for example, represents the contraction of the atria; other wiggles, called Q, R, and S waves, represent contraction of the ventricles. And a T wave on an electrocardiogram shows the relaxation phase of the ventricles.

An EKG can provide the doctor with a great deal of information about the heart rate and rhythm, as well as the paths taken by the electrical impulses involved in heart activity. Some doctors advise that electrocardiograms be made during routine physical examinations, so that a record of a patient's heart activity while he is young and healthy can be used as a baseline for comparing later EKG data, or for detecting subtle changes in the heart as the person grows older.

embolism The blocking of an artery by a blood clot or a piece of foreign matter circulating in the bloodstream. In addition to a blood clot, an embolism can be produced by an air bubble accidentally introduced into a vein, by a drop of fat entering the bloodstream after the fracture of a bone, or by bacteria and its toxic material that has drifted away from the site of an infection. See also *thromboembolism*.

emphysema Enlargement, usually accompanied by destruction, of the alveoli, or air sacs, at the ends of the bronchioles in the lungs. Some stretching of the lung tissue and loss of elastic recoil ability occurs normally with age, as in senile emphysema. However, the condition can be accelerated and aggravated by diseases such as asthma and bronchitis, as well as by cigarette smoking. The destruction of the alveoli can involve the formation of cysts, the rupture of membrane walls so that several small air sacs become one larger alveolus, or the appearance of fluid-filled blisters on the walls of the membranes. Any loss of alveolar membrane surface reduces the ability of the lungs to absorb oxygen from inhaled air, and to expel carbon dioxide and water vapor that have accumulated in the body's trillions of tissue cells. See also *familial pulmonary emphysema*.

empyema An accumulation of pus in a body cavity, such as the lungs, because of a bacterial infection.

endocarditis An inflammation of the endocardium, the membrane lining the heart and covering the heart valves. The inflammation can be caused by a bacterial infection, a fungal infection, or by another category of disease such as rheumatic heart disease. The heart valves are often involved in endocarditis. The infection can be quickly overwhelming in acute cases, requiring immediate treatment with antibiotics. In cases of less serious infections of the endocardium, the disease may produce no symptoms, although the effects, such as damaged heart valves, may appear later.

endocardium A single layer of cells that forms a lining for the chambers of the heart and also covers the heart valves.

ephredrine A medication given to asthma and bronchitis patients to help alleviate the wheezing effect of their breathing problem.

extrinsic asthma A form of the respiratory disease that is associated with allergic reactions to substances in the environment, such as dog hairs, house dust, pollens, molds, shellfish, chocolate, etc.

Fallot's tetralogy A congenital heart defect that involves four different problems: an opening in the wall, or septum, dividing the two ventricles; an enlarged right ventricle; and abnormalities of the aorta and the pulmonary artery valve. Because blood is shunted from the right side to the left side of the heart, the patient, usually an infant, acquires a cyanotic, or bluish, complexion due to the lack of oxygenated blood in the lung capillaries. The problem frequently is not apparent in a newborn child with Fallot's tetralogy, but as the youngster grows older and larger, the right ventricle may become enlarged and more blood is diverted from the right side to the left side of the heart, resulting in the cyanotic effect.

There are several variations in Fallot's tetralogy and many degrees of severity. In most cases, the defects can be corrected by surgical reconstruction of the affected heart areas, although the procedure may be carried out in stages, beginning with correction of the aorta and pulmonary artery abnormalities.

familial pulmonary emphysema A form of emphysema that appears to be hereditary and associated with the deficiency of a blood serum substance bearing the unmemorable name of alpha-1-antitrypsin. The symptoms of *emphysema* appear when the patient is in the 20's or 30's, and this disorder is more likely to afflict women than is other forms of emphysema. The familial form requires the same general pattern of treatment as that required for other victims of emphysema, including early control of respiratory infections, use of bronchodilator medications, and avoidance of cigarette smoking or other kinds of air pollution.

farmer's lung A respiratory disease that occurs among persons who work with hay, grains, or livestock. The disorder is associated with the inhalation of spores of fungi from the grain, hay, or livestock feed. It is characterized by breathing difficulty, fever, headaches, and a feeling of "tightness" in the chest. The disease is seldom fatal but it can be severely disabling for a person afflicted with an attack. Treatment consists primarily of having the patient avoid exposure to moldy hay or grain, and the administration of medications to control mold growth and relieve symptoms.

fibrosis A disease caused by the formation of fibrous tissue in organs that normally do not contain fibrous tissue. Fibrosis of the lining of the heart, for example, can spread into the heart muscle and cause heart failure. Fibrosis of the walls of the air sacs of the lungs can interfere with breathing and cause death by suffocation. See also *cystic fibrosis*.

flow-volume A test used by doctors when diagnosing certain types of respiratory diseases. The test measures the amount of air that can be handled by a patient's lungs during a fixed period of time, measured in seconds. The patient may be asked to breathe in as much air as possible and then exhale as much as possible while a spirometer, a device used to measure air flow, is held to the mouth. The data produced by the flow-volume test can help the examining physician to determine how severe the case of respiratory disease might be, provide information about obstructions in the upper or lower portions of the respiratory system, and test the effectiveness of bronchodilators used by the patient.

foramen ovale An opening between the right atrium and left atrium of the heart of a fetus. The opening allows blood to flow from the right to the left side of the heart as part of the normal fetal circulation, when the lungs are not needed to oxygenate the unborn infant's blood. The opening normally becomes closed after birth, removing the umbilical circulation pattern. In some babies, however, the foramen ovale does not close properly, and the disorder in circulation results in cyanosis, a bluish complexion, in the infant. The child is commonly identified as a "blue baby." However, the defect can be corrected by surgery so that the child's development will eventually be normal.

fremitus A term sometimes used to identify the sounds or other signs of *friction rub*, a vibration effect produced by two tissue surfaces rubbing against each other.

friction rub A term used by doctors to describe the chest sound made by the two layers of the chest's pleural lining rubbing against each other during breathing; the abnormal effect is a sign of *dry pleurisy*. The patient may feel the friction rub as symptoms of chest pain and shortness of breath. The condition can be the result of an inflammatory lung disease such as pneumonia, an infection of the pleural membrane, or a heart disorder. The treatment for the condition is related to therapy for the disease causing the friction rub, but generally it involves bed rest, relief of pain, and in some cases strapping the chest with adhesive tape or covering the chest with an elastic bandage.

FVC (forced vital capacity) A test of respiratory function in which the patient inhales as deeply as he can and then exhales as rapidly as he can. The volume of expelled air in a normal person is greatest during the first second of exhaling and usually amounts to more than three-fourths of the total amount of air that can be expelled from the lungs.

gallop rhythm Sometimes when the doctor is listening to heart sounds in the chest, he may hear three sounds that occur in a pattern resembling that of a galloping horse. The gallop pattern may or may not be serious, depending upon the location on the chest wall where the triple sound pattern is heard and the order in which the three heart sounds occur.

galvanometer An instrument that can measure electric current such as the tiny electrical impulses generated by muscle contractions. Galvanometers are used in electrocardiograph equipment to translate heart contractions and relaxations into the wave graphs of electrocardiograms.

gas exchange A technical term referring to the exchange of oxygen for carbon dioxide and water vapor through the membranes of the alveoli. The efficiency of the alveolar membrane in releasing carbon dioxide and water vapor in the "used" blood from the pulmonary artery and allowing fresh oxygen to pass through the thin cell walls to the red blood cells in the capillaries of the alveolar walls can be an important factor in the prognosis of many diseases. Several kinds of tests can be used by doctors to determine the gas exchange efficiency of a patient's lung tissue.

Geiger counter An electronic device for detecting radioactivity used occasionally in laboratory tests that analyze the distribution of air in a patient's lungs and bronchial tubes. After the patient inhales a radioactive gas such as xenon, the Geiger counter can follow the gas molecules throughout the respiratory system. The test might be used to locate an obstruction or to determine how deeply into the alveoli an individual's inhaled air normally travels.

giant cell pneumonitis A type of inflammation of the lung tissue marked by the appearance of giant cells in the alveoli. The giant cells actually may be a "merged" group of several cells with a number of separate nuclei, but without definite walls or membranes separating the individual cells.

glucose A simple sugar molecule present in the blood and body tissues. Contractions of muscles, including the heart muscles, are possible because of the energy released by the glucose molecules when they combine with oxygen in the blood. The glucose and oxygen form new molecules of water and carbon dioxide when the energy for muscle action is released.

Goodpasture's syndrome A disorder involving the lungs, marked by severe bleeding in the alveoli. The patient usually becomes aware of the problem by coughing up blood, and he also suffers from breathing difficulty as the disease progresses. The cause is unknown and there is no effective cure.

gynecomastia A tongue-twister sometimes used by doctors to identify an enlarged breast on the chest of a man. While it is uncommon for a man to have breasts like a female, or even one enlarged breast, the condition does occur. Gynecomastia generally is a noninflammatory condition resulting from a hormone imbalance, although the cause is unknown. It can be associated with a wide variety of diseases, including cirrhosis of the liver, leprosy, leukemia, and lung cancer. Gynecomastia may result from the use of drugs used to treat prostate cancer, heart disease, and psychiatric problems.

head bobbing In infants and small children, the head may bob or flex with each breath inhaled. This can be a sign of labored breathing or respiratory distress. The sign is most easily observed when the youngster's body is positioned so that the head and trunk are elevated; gravity tends to overcome the head bobbing effect when the child is lying flat in bed.

hematemesis The medical term for vomiting of blood. Under some conditions it may be difficult to determine whether a patient has vomited or coughed blood. However, vomited blood usually is darker, is acidic because of gastric acid in the stomach, and may be mixed with food particles. In contrast, blood coughed up from the lungs generally is pink or bright red and frothy, and also may be mixed with sputum. *Hemoptysis* is the medical term for coughing blood, which may be a sign of lung cancer, tuberculosis, pneumonia, pulmonary embolism, or left-sided heart failure. However, hemoptysis may be only a sign of violent coughing rather than a serious heart or lung disease.

hemoglobin A complex chemical molecule composed of protein material and an iron-rich pigment with a tremendous affinity for oxygen. Hemoglobin is the substance that gives red blood cells their coloring, particularly when the cells are carrying their full complement of oxygen molecules. Blood theoretically can carry about 20 percent of its volume in oxygen, although it seldom contains the maximum possible amount even after exposure to oxygen in the air. Without hemoglobin, a person would need about 60 times as much blood fluid in his arteries in order to transport the same amount of oxygen to all the tissue cells in the body.

hemoptysis The medical term for coughing blood, which may or may not be the sign of a serious disorder. It is distinct from the vomiting of blood, or *hematemesis*.

hemorrhage The escape of blood from a broken or cut artery, vein, or capillary. The bleeding can be from an external wound that breaks the skin, an internal injury beneath the surface of the skin, or a body cavity as a result of injury or disease involving a deep organ. Bleeding from a capillary usually oozes from the injured site, bleeding from an artery is marked by spurts of bright red blood, and bleeding from a vein generally is characterized by the appearance of dark blood that flows in a rather steady stream.

hemothorax This medical term refers to the presence of blood in the pleural cavity separating the lungs from the inner chest wall. The blood does not clot, but because of movement of the lungs during respiration the fibrin in the blood, which normally forms clots, forms a coating on the pleural membrane. The usual procedure for treating hemothorax is to have the patient lie flat in bed while the blood is removed by aspiration, or siphoned out of the pleural cavity. Antibiotics are administered to prevent the development of a bacterial infection in the blood. When the bleeding, which may be due to a chest injury or surgery to repair a chest problem, continues and aspiration seems inadequate, doctors may advise opening the chest wall to control the source of bleeding.

heparin A drug administered by injection that helps prevent blood clots. Heparin has no effect on clots already formed, but it prevents coagulation of blood in the vessels and thus helps to avoid the formation of new clots.

heterograft A term sometimes used to describe a heart valve transplant when the valve is taken from a nonhuman source such as a pig. A homograft is a heart valve transplant from another human, a deceased person who has agreed to donate his body organs after death.

hiatus hernia A hole in the diaphragm that permits an abdominal organ, the stomach, to protrude above the diaphragm into the chest cavity. The hernia occurs at the opening in the diaphragm through which the esophagus passes on its way from the throat to the abdomen. In serious cases of hiatus hernia, a portion of the intestine may push through the sheet of muscle and fibrous tissue making up the diaphragm. Hiatus hernia frequently produces the symptom commonly called heartburn, a dull steady pain that may resemble a symptom of angina pectoris.

hiccups Also spelled as hiccoughs, and known by the medical term of singultus, this condition is caused by sudden contractions of the muscles of the diaphragm. A number of possible stimuli can trigger hiccups, including heart disease, an obstruction of the respiratory system, an intestinal obstruction, damage or disease affecting a part of the nervous system, and emotional problems. More frequently, the problem of hiccups results from something recently ingested, such a food or beverage, that irritates the stomach or the esophagus. There are many home remedies for hiccups, some of which may work—for example, holding one's breath and sipping water—and some of which won't—for example, increasing the carbon dioxide content of the lungs by rebreathing one's own expelled air. Hiccups that interfere with sleep, eating, or work may require medications or surgery to control.

His bundle More commonly referred to as the bundle of His, a band of muscle fibers connecting the atria with the ventricles of the heart and serving as a conduit for the transmission of the electric nerve impulse that triggers contractions of the heart chambers. The bundle of His is located on the septum that divides the ventricles and has branches that spread to the left and right sides of the lower heart chambers.

humidifier Respiratory disorders sometimes are aided by adding water vapor to the atmosphere breathed by the patient. The water vapor, which may or may not have soothing medications added to it, helps to prevent secretions of mucus from drying in the tracheobronchial tree, the breathing passages that extend from the throat to the alveoli. There are many different types of humidifiers available in drug stores and other merchandise outlets.

hyaline membrane disease A disorder that affects newborn infants, most often premature babies or those of low birth weight, by the formation of a membrane that blocks the terminal passageways of the bronchial tubes. Because air cannot reach the alveoli through the obstructive membrane, the lungs may collapse. Treatment involves supplying the lungs with oxygen under pressure and feeding the baby through a stomach tube until the condition clears up, which usually is a matter of a few days if the therapy is successful. Antibiotics may be administered to prevent lung infections.

hypertension Another term for high *blood pressure*. Blood pressure may be considered mildly severe if it is in the range of 140/90 to 160/95, compared to a normal adult level of around 130/80. Blood pressure consistently measuring over 160/95 sometimes is classified as moderate to severe hypertension. About nine out of ten cases of hypertension are associated with such factors as heredity, overweight, smoking, use of table salt with meals, and/or an aggressive personality. Most of the remaining cases are linked with another disorder, such as a disease of the artery supplying the kidneys with blood. When hypertension is associated with another disease, it may be called secondary hypertension. If the exact cause cannot be determined, such as in a case associated with overuse of table salt, the disorder is called primary, or essential, hypertension.

Hypertension frequently is controlled by the use of drugs, diet, and weight control. Drugs prescribed for hypertensive patients generally are designed to prevent salt and water reabsorption by the kidneys, and to dilate the smooth muscle walls of the blood vessels so that less pressure is required to push the blood through the circulatory system.

hyperventilation A condition marked by a feeling of faintness and partial loss of consciousness resulting from a period of deep breathing that may have depleted the normal amount of carbon dioxide in the blood. The problem most commonly is due to anxiety or emotional upset, although hyperventilation also can be caused as an adverse side effect of certain medications. Immediate treatment may require only that the person breathe into a paper bag so he will inhale some of his own carbon dioxide, thereby building up normal blood levels of the gas. If the problem occurs often, the cause of the anxiety or emotional tension should be treated.

hypotension Abnormally low *blood pressure*. The effect may occur briefly in an otherwise normal person who experiences a sudden drop in blood pressure when changing body position, particularly while using certain types of medications. If the individual sits up in bed or stands suddenly after spending some time in a sitting or lying position, he may feel dizzy or lose consciousness because of an inadequate flow of blood to the brain while the body is adjusting to the changed postural position. The effect sometimes, in fact, is called postural hypotension.

hypoxemia A condition that can occur when a person is exposed to high mountain altitudes or similar conditions in which the atmosphere contains less than an optimum amount of oxygen; also called altitude sickness. The condition is marked by insufficient oxygen in the blood, and it may be associated with diseases such as pneumonia and chicken pox, or with congenital heart diseases that result in a lack of oxygen in the circulating bloodstream.

infarction An area of dead tissue caused by an artery obstruction that cuts off the supply of fresh blood to the tissue. A *myocardial infarction* involves damage to the heart muscle because of interruption of the blood supply to a portion of the heart. A pulmonary infarction involves an obstruction of the blood supply to a portion of the lung, resulting in death of the lung tissue deprived of fresh blood.

influenza A commonly used medical term derived from the Italian word for "influence," as in the "influence of the cold." The disease, also known as grippe, is an acute infection of one of several closely related types of viruses. The symptoms include chills and fever, a dry, sore throat, muscle pains, coughing, a runny nose, and headache. The disease may cause complete exhaustion. There is danger of secondary infections, particularly of the respiratory system, but exposure to one of the viruses generally offers immunity against another attack. The catch is that one of the viruses responsible for influenza may mutate, or undergo a genetic change, so it may cause another epidemic in a slightly different form. Persons who are likely to be seriously affected by an influenza infection can be immunized against one or more of the prevalent viruses. After the disease has attacked, treatment is directed towards relieving the symptoms.

infundibulum The end of one of the terminal bronchioles in the lungs. It branches into a group of alveoli, looking somewhat like a tiny bunch of grapes at the end of a twig.

inspiration A term frequently used to describe the act of breathing in or inhaling air.

intercostal muscles Muscles that are connected to the ribs along their inner and outer borders for the length of the rib cage. These muscles are involved in breathing since they can expand or contract the lung space within the rib cage. Intercostal nerves and blood vessels supply the intercostal muscles. The intercostal nerves frequently are a cause of chest pains which mimic heart disease and other disorders.

intermittent claudication A painful circulatory disorder affecting the legs and sometimes the arms, particularly in older men. The disorder is similar to the condition that causes angina pectoris, in that insufficient blood flow and fresh oxygen to the muscle tissue results in a painful cramp. The problem may be relieved by resting the legs when the pain is caused by walking; special exercises and medicines also may help relieve the symptoms.

interventricular septum A muscular wall that separates the left *ventricle* of the heart from the right ventricle. See also *ventricular septal defect.*

intrinsic asthma A form of asthma that develops in some persons in late adult life. It is not associated with allergic reactions as is *extrinsic asthma.*

IRDS (infant respiratory distress syndrome) An assortment of breathing problems that may be observed in newborn infants, usually within the first few hours after labor. The child may flare its nostrils, grunt, retract the chest wall during inhalation, or show other signs of breathing difficulty. The causes may be *hyaline membrane disease*, underdeveloped muscles of the chest wall, or abnormally small alveoli. Premature infants are most likely to be victims of IRDS. Treatment may include administering oxygen under pressure to the child until it has adapted to normal breathing.

Korotkoff sounds The sounds of blood pulsing through an artery when a stethoscope bell is pressed against the skin above the artery. When a doctor checks a patient's *blood pressure*, he listens for the Korotkoff sounds of an artery to determine the systolic and diastolic blood pressure levels.

Kussmaul breathing The name given to a type of respiration associated with air hunger. It is characterized by deep, regular sighs. Kussmaul breathing is a sign of several types of disorder, including diabetic acidosis, *hemorrhage*, pneumonia, and peritonitis.

Kveim test A skin test sometimes used in the diagnosis of sarcoidosis, a disease characterized by the development of fleshy lesions in the lungs and other organs. The lesions are similar to those that occur in tuberculosis. The test also may be called the Nickerson-Kveim test, after the doctors who developed the technique.

kyphosis An abnormal curvature of the chest in which the spine is bent forward. The defect can result in an internal chest size and shape that might affect heart and lung function, especially in later life.

laryngeal swab A piece of cotton on the end of a wire that may be placed over the larynx, at the base of the tongue, to catch bits of sputum during a patient's coughing spell. The sputum can be examined in a laboratory to determine what sort of disease organism has invaded the lungs and bronchial tubes.

lipid pneumonia A type of lung tissue inflammation caused by the accidental inhalation of oily substances. The situation may result, for example, from careless use of nose drops containing oil. The oil can form patchy lesions that resemble lung cancer signs, and the patient usually coughs up a sputum that contains oil droplets.

lobar pneumonia A term sometimes used to indicate an inflammation of one or more lobes of the lungs because of an infection of *pneumococcus*, or pneumonia-causing, bacteria. The disorder may have a rather sudden onset; the patient can feel well in the morning, yet be overwhelmed by noon with fever, chills, coughing, and a sharp pain in the chest. Fibrin and blood cells from the blood may flow into the alveoli during the early stages of the disease. Treatment includes complete bed rest, a liquid diet, antibiotics, and medicines to help rid the body of the accumulation of sputum, which in serious cases may have to be aspirated, or siphoned, from the lungs. Pain-killing drugs also may be required.

lobectomy Surgical removal of one of the lobes of the lungs. The procedure sometimes is performed to prevent the spread of cancer from one lobe to another. The human body normally has five lung lobes, three on the right side and two on the left. Removing one lobe reduces the patient's breathing capacity but not as seriously as removing an entire lung, which is called a *pneumonectomy*.

lung scan A technique sometimes used in diagnosing conditions such as pulmonary infarction when the normal blood supply to a portion of the lung tissue has been interrupted. A radioactive substance is injected into arteries carrying blood into the lungs. Radiation detection devices are placed over the chest to locate areas in which the blood flows normally and areas that apparently are deprived of normal blood flow. An X-ray picture of the blood circulation in the lungs also can be made by injecting into the arteries a radio-opaque dye that will make the blood vessels that are still functional stand out in contrast to areas in which blood flow is obstructed.

maltworker's lung A disease of the respiratory system, marked by wheezing and other breathing difficulties, due to an allergic reaction to fungus spores. It is similar to *farmer's lung* and mushroom worker's lung, which are caused by spores of a different type of fungus found in agricultural products.

mammography A type of X-ray technique used to detect breast cancer in women. Proponents of the use of mammography claim that when women are able to detect the presence of a breast tumor by self-examination, the growth usually is about one inch in diameter, whereas mammography is able to find the tumors when they are approximately half that size. Studies of the use of mammography also show that the detection rate of breast cancer with X-rays is about six times that of physical examination alone. Some doctors recommend a combination of regular examination by a physician plus mammography to insure early detection of breast cancers. Recent research has led to development of mammography equipment that provides better X-ray pictures with smaller doses of radiation and shorter patient exposure times than was possible with earlier types of equipment.

Mantoux test A test for signs of exposure to *tuberculosis* by injecting a small amount of fluid prepared from tuberculosis organisms under the skin of a person's arm. The size and firmness of the welt, showing the patient's reaction to the injection, when examined two or three days later, will indicate a positive or negative response.

manubrium The top part of the sternum, or *breastbone*.

Marfan's syndrome A hereditary disease involving bones, muscles, and other parts of the body, including the major blood vessels. The aortic valve of the heart may become defective, and there may be aneurysms of the aorta in Marfan's syndrome victims.

mediastinoscopy An examination of the *mediastinum* by direct viewing of the structures between the sternum and the spinal column with a special scope that is inserted through an incision made above the sternum, or *breast-*

bone. The examination usually is performed while the patient is under a general anesthetic. The procedure may be performed in connection with installation of a heart pacemaker, as well as to check for signs of cancer, tuberculosis, or other diseases among organs and tissues of the chest.

mediastinum A term used to describe the contents of the chest outside the pleural membranes that enclose the lungs. The mass of tissues and organs includes the trachea, esophagus, the heart and its large vessels, the lymph nodes, and the thymus—but not the lungs. The mediastinal areas of the chest can be the sites of tumors or other disorders that may show up on a chest X-ray but do not involve lung tissue directly. Nearly one-fourth of mediastinal tumors, for example, involve tissues of the thyroid and thymus glands; more than half of all cases of Hodgkin's lymphoma have enlarged lymph nodes in the mediastinum.

miliary tuberculosis Now a rather uncommon form of *tuberculosis* characterized by the spread of tuberculosis germs through the bloodstream to organs of the body other than the lungs. The germs form tubercules the size of millet seeds in the brain, kidneys, lungs, and other tissues.

mitral stenosis A disorder, either congenital or the result of a disease such as rheumatic fever, involving the function of the heart's mitral valve between the left atrium and left ventricle. In a case of rheumatic heart disease, the cusps, or flaps, of the valve become inflamed and stick together. *Fibrosis* develops along the edges of the cusps so that the opening becomes smaller and less blood can be moved from the atrium to the left ventricle.

mucopurulent chronic bronchitis A chronic recurrent form of bronchitis that is characterized by the presence of sputum containing mucus and pus. The attacks may be marked by long periods of coughing, expectoration, and a soreness behind the breast bone. Treatment can involve administration of antibiotics and drugs that help reduce the urge to cough, as well as medications that help eliminate purulent sputum.

mucoviscidosis A medical term for *cystic fibrosis.*

mycoplasmal infections Diseases caused by tiny organisms that cause a respiratory disorder known as mycoplasma pneumonia, or atypical pneumonia. Symptoms include fever, sore throat, coughing, and nasal congestion. Headaches occur in some cases that appear more like the common cold or influenza infections. Mycoplasmal organisms are resistant to penicillin but can be treated with other antibiotics such as tetracyclines.

mycotic aorta disease A disease condition in which an embolus, or bit of infected material, resulting from a case of endocarditis may break away from the heart and become attached to the inner wall of the aorta.

myocarditis An inflammation of the heart muscle. Diphtheria and rheumatic fever are among more than a half-dozen infectious diseases that can cause myocarditis.

myocardial infarction See *infarction.*

myocardium Another name for heart muscle. The myocardium has some characteristics of both skeletal muscle, the kind that works the arms and legs, and smooth muscle, the kind that is found in the digestive tract. The heart muscle is somewhat unique in that its fibers run in several different directions in order to squeeze blood into the pulmonary arteries of the lungs and into other arteries running throughout the body, whereas skeletal muscle fibers generally run in a single direction for moving a bone or flexing a joint.

nasal flaring An occasional sign of respiratory distress. It is particularly significant as a clue to breathing difficulty among infants and small children.

neurogenic tumor One of the most common

tumors of the *mediastinum*, the region of the chest outside the lungs. Symptoms may include bone pain or feelings of pressure from the growth of the tumor.

nitrogen One of the gases in the atmosphere we breathe. *Air* is roughly 80 percent nitrogen and 20 percent oxygen. The air reaching the alveoli, where oxygen is absorbed into the bloodstream, contains nearly the same proportions of nitrogen and oxygen. Nitrogen is an inert gas that is of no particular value to the bloodstream or to the cells that receive the materials carried in the blood. Some nitrogen is absorbed by the blood passing through the alveoli; a similar amount is released by the lungs with each respiration.

Divers and others who breathe air under greater than normal atmospheric pressure acquire increased amounts of oxygen and nitrogen. While the oxygen can be consumed, the nitrogen can accumulate in the blood and body tissues, forming bubbles when the individual inhaling pressurized air returns to a near sea-level atmosphere. The nitrogen bubbles in the blood and tissues can produce severe pain, tenderness, or inflammation in the joints. The symptoms, sometimes called the bends, can be avoided by limiting the depth and time spent with pressurized breathing apparatus while diving, and by returning gradually to a normal atmosphere.

node A small collection of tissue mass, sometimes providing a special bodily function. The sino-atrial node, for example, is a collection of muscle fibers near the top of the heart which originates the heart rhythm. The atrio-ventricular node, farther along the organ, sometimes serves as the pacemaker for heart contractions when the sino-atrial node has failed to function properly.

nosocomial A fancy medical term meaning a disease acquired by being in a hospital. While hospitals make every effort to prevent nosocomial infections, such as pneumonia, from developing, infections can be transmitted occasionally by microorganisms that are concealed in bed linens, draperies, the hands of hospital personnel, or in the air circulating through rooms and corridors.

oat cell tumor One of the common types of tumors responsible for lung cancer. Oat cell tumors are small, grow quickly, and spread to other body organs early in the disease. Cancers of the oat cell type are harder to control than slow-growing tumors.

open heart surgery An operation performed on the heart or adjacent tissues in which the heart and lungs are removed temporarily from their normal functions and are replaced by a mechanical pump and artificial oxygenator. Open heart surgery is used to repair a number of heart defects, including damage from rheumatic heart disease and aneurysm of the aorta.

orthopnea A breathing difficulty sign associated with aortic stenosis. In addition to dizziness or loss of consciousness as a result of exertion and becoming easily fatigued, the patient has periods of breathlessness even while lying down to rest.

oscilloscope An electronic device similar to a television set except that the picture tube shows the kind of information about a patient's heart that would be recorded on an *electrocardiogram.*

Osler's nodes Small tender swellings in the fingers and toes of persons suffering from certain types of heart disease. The nodes are due to emboli, or blood clots, in the small vessels.

oxygen The gas which constitutes only 20 percent of the natural atmosphere but is one of the most important elements in sustaining life. Oxygen is required for most of the vital functions of all living body cells; it combines with glucose in the cells to provide the energy needed for muscle contractions and body heat. The normal human body carries enough dissolved oxygen to keep the body functioning for about four minutes. If the body is deprived of oxygen for a longer period, the various vital organs can suffer irreversible damage, beginning with brain damage, and death can follow quickly.

A person who is physically active requires much more oxygen than a resting individual; a trained athlete requires from 40 to 50 times as much oxygen per minute while running a footrace as he does while sleeping. Oxygen, in fact, is the limiting factor in many athletic events; the person competing in an event frequently reaches a point where he cannot breathe enough oxygen into his tissues to keep his muscles performing efficiently.

oxygenator A machine that artificially puts fresh oxygen into the blood of a patient while he is undergoing an operation, such as open heart surgery. There are several different types of oxygenators. One kind bubbles oxygen through the blood; another type has a membrane that separates the oxygen from direct contact with the patient's blood in a manner similar to the way in which oxygen and blood are separated by the membrane of an alveolus in the lung.

oxymeter A device sometimes used to measure the amount of oxygen in the blood. The oxymeter resembles a bulky earring that clips onto the lobe of the ear. It has a light that shines through the flesh of the ear lobe and an electronic counter on the other side. The amount of light passing through the ear lobe is translated by the oxymeter into the amount of oxygen moving in the capillaries while attached to red blood cells.

Paget's disease of the breast A cancerous disease marked by the appearance of a tumor that begins in the nipple of the breast and slowly grows into an oozing ulcer, while the nipple enlarges and becomes fissured.

Pancoast's syndrome A disease that begins with a tumor at the top of a lung or in the upper *mediastinum,* or top of the chest cavity. Symptoms may include pain and weakness in the shoulder and arm, with atrophy of the muscles on the side affected by the tumor.

paroxysmal dyspnea You can call it acute shortness of breath, because on a medical record it means just that. If it occurs at night, the condition is called paroxysmal nocturnal-dyspnea.

PEEP (positive end expiratory pressure) A method used to prevent the collapse of alveoli by maintaining a preset breathing pressure that is higher than the atmospheric pressure surrounding the patient. Without PEEP, some bronchopneumonia patients would experience collapse of a lung or a portion of a lung.

PEF (peak expiratory flow) A term sometimes used in testing the respiratory system for a possible obstruction. The patient breathes out as hard as possible into a peak flow meter which records the amount of air in liters.

percussion Part of a technique used by an examining physician to diagnose a chest ailment. The doctor lays one finger of one hand on the skin of the chest and hits it with the middle finger of the other hand. The sounds or vibrations made by the percussion help the doctor to determine, for example, the density of a lung area, whether a portion of the chest contains air or fluid.

pericarditis An inflammation of the pericardium, the fibrous sac that surrounds the heart and adjacent vessels. The inflammation can be caused by a wide variety of infectious diseases including rheumatic fever and pneumonia; causes also can include injury or a heart attack. The symptoms may be breathing difficulty and a sharp or dull pain radiating to the neck and/or arm, and as far as the abdomen.

pertussis A medical name for *whooping cough*, a respiratory disease caused by a germ called Hemophilus pertussis.

phonocardiogram A graph that records heart sounds and murmurs, somewhat like an electrocardiogram records a wavelike pattern of heart activity. A phonocardiogram and an electrocardiogram can be used together to diagnose a patient's heart condition.

phrenic nerves The nerves that make the diaphragm contract in breathing. The phrenic nerves run from the spinal cord in the area of the neck and pass along the inner side of each lung to reach the diaphragm.

pleura A continuous double membrane that encloses each of the lungs. One surface of the membrane, called the *visceral pleura*, covers the outer surface of lung tissue and passes between the lobes so that each lobe is separately enclosed. The second membrane, the parietal pleura, covers the inside of the chest wall. Between the two layers of membrane is an airspace known as the pleural space. Certain diseases cause the pleural membrane layers to become dry and rub against each other, causing painful *friction rub*.

pleurisy An irritation or inflammation of the pleural membrane. Pneumonia, tuberculosis, or pulmonary infarction can produce a condition known as *dry pleurisy*, which is characterized by painful breathing because the inner and outer layers of the pleural membrane rub together. Pleurisy with effusion, also known as *wet pleurisy*, results from an inflammation associated with fluid in the pleural space. Wet pleurisy is treated by draining the fluid. Dry pleurisy is treated by strapping the chest to restrict movement and giving the patient analgesics to relieve pain.

pneumococcus The name of a bacteria responsible for a common variety of lung infections. One such disease is pneumonia, although pneumonia actually can be associated with any substance or organism causing an inflammation of the lung tissues. See also *lobar pneumonia*.

pneumonectomy Surgical removal of an entire lung when necessary to solve a severe respiratory problem such as lung cancer.

pneumothorax A term used to describe air that may enter the space between the parietal and visceral layers of the pleural membrane. Air in the pleural space is not a normal thing and can result from a wound or a rupture of a pleural membrane during violent exercise. The patient may feel pain and shortness of breath. If the lung collapses, treatment will be directed toward reinflating it so that normal breathing can be resumed. Any foreign air in the pleural space must be aspirated, or pumped out, slowly and carefully.

psittacosis A severe form of lung inflammation caused by an organism transmitted by birds of many kinds, including pigeons, chickens, and turkeys, as well as parakeets, parrots, and canaries; commonly called parrot fever. Symptoms and signs of the disease are fever, coughing, and enlargement of the spleen. Prompt treatment by antibiotics is required.

pulmonary embolism An obstruction of a pulmonary artery by an embolus, such as a blood clot. With circulation to the lung tissue blocked, the affected portion of a lung lobe is effectively destroyed.

pulmonary fibrosis A condition in which the pliable lung tissue gradually is replaced by inelastic fibrous material that makes normal breathing difficult. Pulmonary fibrosis sometimes results from infiltration of the lung tissue by inflammatory lesions of *sarcoidosis*, a disease similar to tuberculosis.

pulmonary infarction The result of a pulmonary embolism, that is, local death of lung tissue where normal blood supply has been blocked. See *infarction*.

pulse The pulsation of the heart contractions as felt through the walls of an artery. The pulse usually is observed in the radial artery where it passes through the wrist. It also can be found in the carotid artery along the neck, at the side of the hip bone, at the temple, and at several other points along the exterior anatomy.

pursed lip breathing A way of slowly exhaling through the mouth with the lips partially closed. It is observed occasionally in patients with breathing difficulties.

pyopneumothorax A disease involving the formation of pus in the pleural space between the lungs and chest wall. The infection can re-

sult from a tubercular growth that has forced a tear or rupture in the pleural membrane.

radiography A method of viewing the inside of the body or a portion of the body by *X-ray* or similar techniques. The exact form of radiograph used will depend in part on what the doctor is trying to learn about a problem inside the body without exploring the area or organs involved by surgery.

Positional X-ray can obtain several different views by taking repeated X-ray pictures while the patient's body is turned to several positions. Fluoroscopy allows the doctor to view the body organs while they are functioning normally; the picture is projected on a television-type screen.

Tomography is similar to positional X-ray except that the patient remains in one position while the X-ray equipment moves in a pattern relative to the film so that the picture reveals a "slice" of the body or the organ being studied. By making a series of pictures of these "slices," a detailed examination of the inside of the body or an organ can be completed without so much as making a single nick in the patient's skin.

Still another form of radiography is the radioactive scan, in which a radioactive chemical is injected into an organ or area of the body and a picture is made of the distribution of the substance. It may show, for example, a blocked artery or a tumor that absorbs a huge amount of blood. The picture is made by allowing the radioactive particles to expose a piece of film placed near the skin, or by placing a radiation detector over the organ or area to be scanned.

radiotherapy The use of radiation, such as *X-rays* or emissions from radioactive chemicals, to treat tumors or other disorders. Radiotherapy may be used, for example, to control the growth of a tumor that presses on a blood vessel or organ.

rales Crackling sounds or vibrations that can be detected by a doctor examining a patient's chest by *auscultation* if the patient has an inflammatory lung disease. The crackling or bubbling sound may vary with different types of respiratory diseases, thereby offering clues as to the part of the lung affected.

residual air The air that remains in the lungs after as much air as possible has been expelled by forced breathing. The alveoli generally hold about one and a half quarts of residual air. The bronchioles, the tubes at the end of the respiratory tree, are forced closed by the muscle pressure of exhalation; the residual air therefore is trapped in the alveoli and cannot be expelled by natural breathing.

respirometer A device that measures the amount of air inhaled by a patient. In some severe cases of bronchitis the bronchioles are blocked with thick mucus so that inspired, or inhaled, air is unable to reach the alveoli. The respirometer indicates this and doctors armed with the data shown on the instrument can decide how to go about opening the passageways to the alveoli.

rheumatic heart disease A form of the bacterial infection, rheumatic fever, that results in damage to the heart valves and other permanent heart defects. In addition to fever, sore throat, loss of appetite, and painful swollen joints associated with a rheumatic fever attack, there may be chest pains, friction rub of the pericardial membrane, heart murmurs, and abnormal tracings on an electrocardiogram—signs and symptoms which indicate cardiac involvement of the infection.

Rheumatic heart disease, while less common than in previous generations, still accounts for about half the reasons for rejecting men from military service for heart disorders. Also, it probably is the most common cause of heart abnormalities among young children. In many cases damage to the heart is not detected at the time of the rheumatic fever attack, but the abnormalities appear in later life.

rheumatoid lung disease Many persons afflicted with rheumatoid arthritis also show signs or symptoms of respiratory disorders. The signs frequently include inflammation and *fibrosis* of lung tissue, involvement of the pleural membrane, and infrequently the appearance of nodules which are revealed by X-ray pictures of the chest. Rheumatoid arthritis also may be associated with circulatory disorders such as aortic regurgitation and *pericarditis*.

rhonchus A term used by doctors to indicate a musical whistling or wheezing sound heard in the chest of a patient with a respiratory disorder.

sarcoidosis A somewhat mysterious disease that is marked by the appearance of tubercle-like growths or lesions in various organs, the lungs being a common target of the disorder. The exact cause of sarcoidosis is unknown, although it has a higher than average rate of incidence in persons who have been infected by tuberculosis. In many cases the patient experiences no serious symptoms and is unaware of the disease until it begins to affect one of the vital organs.

When sarcoidosis involves the lungs, the patient may experience coughing and breathlessness, and a doctor examining the chest may detect the bubbling or crackling sounds called *rales* when listening with a stethoscope. An X-ray picture will reveal the lung lesions associated with sarcoidosis. Treatment usually depends upon the organs involved and the seriousness of the infection, but generally it may include the use of steroid hormone medications.

scalene node One of the lymph nodes in the neck. During diagnosis of certain diseases, such as *sarcoidosis*, a doctor may remove a scalene lymph node for biopsy, or study of the tissue under a microscope.

scoliosis A lateral bending of the human spine. Often there are two curves in the spine, the original bend that was congenital and an acquired curve that developed through the unconscious effort of the afflicted person to compensate for the original curvature. Scoliosis sometimes can alter the internal dimensions of the chest so as to interfere with normal heart and lung functions.

shortness of breath The common name for the type of breathing difficulty doctors may refer to as *dyspnea.*

silicosis An inflammation of the lungs caused by the inhalation of dust from sandstone, granite, coal, or other mined products.

sino-atrial block A failure of the *sino-atrial node* to begin the heartbeat. When this occurs it can truthfully be said that the heart skips a beat.

sino-atrial node A group of tissue cells near the junction of the heart's right atrium and the superior vena cava, the major blood vein entering the heart from the upper part of the body. The sino-atrial node normally is the site of the origin of the electrical nerve impulse that triggers each heartbeat. The impulse spreads over the heart to the ventricles in the rhythmic pattern that makes the atria and ventricles contract and relax in a double-pump action.

sphygmomanometer The instrument used by a doctor to measure your *blood pressure.* The measurement is made in terms of millimeters of mercury, which is the vertical distance in millimeters that blood pressure will raise a column of mercury enclosed in a glass tube. An aneroid sphygmomanometer, which usually has a round dial with numbers around the edge, also is calibrated to show blood pressure in terms of millimeters of mercury even though the instrument does not have a mercury column.

The first number recorded when blood pressure is measured with a sphygmomanometer is the systolic pressure; the second number is the diastolic blood pressure. The figures usually are written, for example, as 135/80, and are read as "135 over 80."

spine The chain of vertebrae, or backbone units, stacked at the back of the body, including the back side of the chest wall; also called

the spinal column. The spinal cord runs through openings in the vertebrae and sends out nerve trunks through the openings between the vertebrae.

Starr-Edwards valve A plastic artificial heart valve that consists of a small ball in a cage. The valve is designed so that the ball sinks to allow blood to pass, then rises in its seating to prevent a backflow. Starr-Edwards valves are installed in the hearts of certain patients to replace the mitral or aortic valves as an alternative to surgical repair of the natural heart valves.

status asthmaticus A condition experienced by some asthma patients in which asthma symptoms persist for days despite treatment, and the patient becomes exhausted and debilitated. If recovery is delayed, intensive care is ordered to prevent respiratory failure.

Stokes-Adams syndrome A form of heart disease in which the victim experiences epilepsy-like attacks. He may suddenly feel dizzy or become unconscious or have a convulsion. He may have no pulse and develop a cyanotic complexion, indicating lack of oxygen in the blood, then just as suddenly regain consciousness when heart action and blood flow resume. The cause may be a briefly temporary failure of the heart to contract or the onset of ventricular fibrillation, the rapid, irregular contractions of the ventricles. Emergency treatment, as in a case of cardiac arrest, is recommended. Although the patient may recover without treatment, he may just as easily die if there is no effort to resuscitate him.

stridor A breathing sound observed in some patients with breathing problems. The wheezing sound occurs during inhalation and is caused by an obstruction or narrowing of the opening in the trachea.

stroke volume A technical term for measuring the amount of blood pumped with each heartbeat. For a resting adult, the stroke volume over a period of one minute totals about five quarts of blood. For each heartbeat, the volume amounts to a little less than three fluid ounces.

suberosis A type of lung inflammation caused by exposure to a mold allergen in cork.

surfactant A thin film secreted by cells of the alveoli to help maintain the elastic properties of lung tissues. A deficiency of surfactant can alter the ability of the air sacs in the lungs to withstand the air pressure changes involved in breathing, a condition that can result in lung collapse. A surfactant deficiency is believed to be one of the causes of breathing difficulties among premature babies.

sympathectomy An operation in which sympathetic nerve fibers are removed to provide relief from the symptoms of a disorder such as Raynaud's disease, a circulatory problem marked by cold, painful spasms of the small blood vessels in the fingers, toes, or other body areas. The surgery has some temporary benefits in improving the blood flow to the affected areas.

syphilis A venereal disease that can affect the circulatory system if not properly treated in the early stages of an infection. The disease can produce inflammation of the blood supply to the aorta wall, causing it to weaken and stretch, and in some cases to develop an *aneurysm*, or rupture of the wall of the aorta.

systemic lupus erythematosis (SLE) A type of arthritis that can involve many parts of the body, including the lungs. Signs and symptoms include blood-tinged sputum, *pleurisy*, and *pulmonary infarction*. Many SLE patients complain of respiratory difficulties despite X-ray examination of the chest which may show no abnormalities. SLE's effects on the respiratory system sometimes are referred to as "lupus lung."

systole A term used to describe the part of the heartbeat in which the cardiac muscle is contracted. Usually systole, or systolic, refers to contraction of the ventricles of the heart, an action that squeezes blood into the aorta and pulmonary artery. When reference is made to contractions of the atria, an action that precedes ventricular systoles, the activity is identified as atrial systole.

tachycardia A term used to indicate an abnormally rapid heartbeat. What may be considered normal is a heartbeat of less than 100 beats per minute. Ventricular tachycardia may be characterized by a rate of 150 or more beats per minute, and accompanied by other aberrant factors such as dissociation with the atrial rhythm. A tachycardia involving the atria may be marked by a rate of 160 or more beats per minute. As the rate increases a point is reached at which the heart beats wildly but does not pump blood, causing the circulatory system to fail.

tachypnea An abnormal respiration pattern characterized by rapid shallow breathing.

thoracentesis A technique sometimes used to aspirate, or drain, fluid from the chest cavity by inserting a needle through the muscle layers between a pair of ribs.

thoracic breathing A type of respiration that utilizes the intercostal muscles (between the ribs) to expand and contract the chest.

thoracic cage The bony framework of the chest, consisting of the sternum, or breastbone, at the front, 12 pairs of ribs connected in the front to the breastbone (except for the two lower pairs of "false" or "floating" ribs) and to the 12 thoracic vertebrae of the spinal column at the back of the chest. The ribs are connected to the vertebrae and breastbone through cartilage joints which allow a certain amount of flexibility to the various tissues of the thoracic cage.

thoracoplasty A surgical technique once used in the treatment of certain lung diseases, such as tuberculosis, by removing portions of the ribs on one side and deliberately collapsing a damaged lung or lobe. The treatment is no longer used but some persons with respiratory problems may have undergone the surgery in past years.

thoracoscopy A method of examining the surface of the lungs by inserting an instrument through an opening in the wall of the chest. The technique may be performed with only a local anesthetic, and the doctor might manage some minor treatment of the lung or pleural membrane during the procedure.

thrills Vibrations or sounds produced in the chest near the tip of the *ventricles*. The vibrations have been compared to the purring of a cat. Thrills in the chest often are a sign of a heart murmur.

thromboembolism Obstruction of a blood vessel by a blood clot, or thrombus, or by other material transported in the bloodstream from the point where it formed. A thrombus can block the blood vessel entirely or become attached to the inner wall of the blood vessel. A thromboembolism problem can be treated either by medications that dissolve blood clots, or by surgery or other techniques such as the use of elastic stockings. Before treatment, the doctor tries to learn as much as possible about the size of the blocked blood vessel, location of the blood clot, and other factors that can determine the therapy to be employed.

thymoma A tumor of tissues of the thymus gland. More than ten percent of the tumors of the *mediastinum* are thymomas, and the abnormal growths often are associated with myasthenia gravis or other diseases.

thymus A gland located in the *mediastinum*, the part of the chest cavity outside the lungs, and behind the upper portion of the sternum, or breastbone. It is involved in immunity and hormone functions, and it apparently has a more important role in human life functions during the fetal and early childhood stages of life. Changes in the size and activity of the thymus in later life are associated with a variety of health problems, including rheumatoid arthritis, Hodgkin's disease, myasthenia gravis, and lowered resistance to infections.

tidal volume The amount of air that passes through the lungs in a single respiration during normal, quiet breathing. Tidal volume usually is measured by having a patient breathe through a device called a *respirometer*. Tidal volume also can be measured by attaching chest electrodes, such as those used in making an electrocardiogram, to a machine that monitors changes in air volume as the chest expands and contracts during respiration.

Tietze's syndrome A disorder marked by pains in the chest near the junction of the sternum and the ribs. There may be inflammation and swelling of tissues around the cartilage joints between the ribs and sternum.

tracheobronchitis A rather common type of respiratory infection which is most likely to occur during the winter months in cool, damp climates among persons who smoke cigarettes or are exposed to industrial fumes. A viral infection usually is the cause of the disease, although sometimes bacteria may be involved.

The person has a fever, a feeling of rawness in the throat as far down as the breastbone, and a cough. The infection frequently is self-limiting and the symptoms subside within one or two weeks if treatment is provided. Without treatment, however, the infection may spread into the bronchioles and other deep lung tissues. Bed rest and relief of the symptoms with cough syrup, aspirin, large amounts of hot drinks, and steam inhalation form the basis for treatment, along with antibiotics which may be needed to control secondary infections.

tracheostomy An operation performed to open a passage to the alveoli, or air sacs, of the lungs when the normal route for air exchange is obstructed. A hole is cut into the trachea, below the larynx, bypassing the nose, pharynx, and larynx. The tracheostomy may be performed to clear the obstruction if it is an accumulation of mucus in the bronchial tubes, or to permit the insertion of a tube to pump oxygen deep into the lungs.

Tracheostomy patients sometimes have difficulty in swallowing, and food or beverages ingested by mouth may enter the trachea by mistake. To test the possibility that food can be aspirated into the lungs, a patient can be given water containing a harmless dye. If fluid colored by the dye can be suctioned from the opening in the trachea, normal oral feeding is delayed until the leakage can be corrected.

tropical eosinophilia A fancy medical term for a type of asthma that some people develop in warm, humid climates. The disease is associated with hypersensitivity to tropical insects or other organisms that thrive in such climates.

tuberculosis An infectious disease of the lungs caused by a germ that thrives in damp, poorly ventilated places. While the disease is rare in North America, it still is a rather common disease in some tropical countries where it is estimated that millions of people still carry the disease organism. Infection is spread by persons inhaling or ingesting the bacterium. The severity of the infection can depend upon the degree of exposure and the individual's ability to resist the infection.

When the disease organism has entered the body tissues, it may become encased in a protective lesion, called a tubercle, which gives the disease its name. The tubercle eventually becomes covered with fibrous calcified tissue. Sometime later, and in some cases many years later, the fibrous capsules may break down and release the tuberculosis bacilli into the bloodstream. The bacteria can then spread through the lungs or other nearby organs. The sputum of the infected person contains the tuberculosis germs which can be spread to other persons when the infected person coughs or spits. One does not have to be in the direct line of fire of the coughing or spitting to become infected; the germs can survive for days in house dust or on cooking and eating utensils.

Tuberculosis can be difficult to diagnose since its signs and symptoms resemble those of many other diseases. The clues to a tuberculosis infection can include shortness of breath, unexplained weight loss, coughing up blood, fever and sweating at night, fatigue, pneumo-

nia-like symptoms that fail to respond to antibiotic treatment, and pleurisy. Children may develop tuberculosis without signs of respiratory problems. The tuberculosis organism may invade other tissues and organ systems, including the bones and joints, kidneys, nervous system, glands, and skin.

Treatment of tuberculosis includes hospitalization and bed rest, plus administration of antibiotics and other medications until the infection is under control and the disease organism does not appear in sputum samples. The patient eventually is allowed to return to his home and work, but treatment may be continued on an outpatient basis for a year and a half or more. The longer the treatment is continued, the less likelihood there is of a relapse.

ultrasound A diagnostic technique used in the study of certain types of chest disorders, such as pulmonary embolism and lung cancer. A device that generates ultrasonic waves, at frequencies higher than 20,000 cycles per second, is placed over the intercostal spaces of the rib cage, and the high-pitched sound is directed toward the lungs. The reflected sound waves provide a "picture" of the size and location of any abnormal tissue areas. The procedure is relatively harmless and free of discomfort to the patient.

vagus nerve A nerve from the brain that is involved in controlling respiration. It transmits impulses or messages between the bronchi and the respiratory center in the brain. The vagus nerve endings can become irritated by foreign substances inhaled into the air passages, triggering the response of sneezing or coughing.

Valsalva maneuver A breathing procedure that involves closing the glottis, the opening in the larynx, while forcefully exhaling. The effect is similar to that produced while forcing a bowel movement by holding one's breath at the same time that abdominal and diaphragm muscles are coordinated to fill the lungs and put pressure on the abdomen. A patient may be asked to perform the Valsalva maneuver during certain diagnostic tests such as chest X-rays, because the effect on air passages and blood vessels can make the X-rays more distinct.

valvotomy As the name suggests, a term meaning a "valve job" on the heart. The mitral valve in the left ventricle, for example, may undergo correction of cusps that have fused and thereby reduced the flow of blood on the left side of the heart. The operation may be performed as a closed-heart procedure, meaning that surgery is done while the heart is pumping blood.

VC (vital capacity) The amount of air one can expel from the lungs after taking a deep breath.

veins Blood vessels that carry blood towards the heart, as contrasted with arteries, which carry blood away from the heart.

vena cava The major vein of the body which drains "used" or "blue" blood from all parts of the body into the heart's right atrium, so that it can be pumped into the lungs to receive fresh oxygen molecules. The superior vena cava collects blood from veins above the heart; the inferior vena cava collects blood from veins below heart level.

ventilation A term sometimes used by doctors to describe the exchange of air between the lungs and the outside atmosphere.

ventilator A mechanical device to aid breathing in a patient with respiratory difficulty. Most ventilators fall into one of two categories: negative-pressure ventilators and positive-pressure ventilators. Negative-pressure ventilators include apparatus such as the "iron lung" which aids breathing by creating a vacuum over the chest of the patient; the vacuum causes the chest to expand so that outside air will rush into the lungs. The positive-pressure equipment forces air into the lungs by direct pressure. Ventilators work automatically at a rhythm that is comparable to the normal breathing cycle of the patient.

ventricle The lower chamber of the heart.

The normal human heart has two ventricles, one on the left side and one on the right. The right ventricle receives blood from the right atrium and pushes it into the pulmonary arteries leading into the lungs. The left ventricle receives via the left atrium blood that has passed through vessels in the lung and must be pumped to the tissues throughout the body. The left ventricle is larger than the right ventricle because it has a bigger work load—that is, squeezing blood through thousands of miles of arteries, arterioles, and capillaries—whereas the right ventricle must move blood only through the pulmonary circulation of the lungs.

ventricular fibrillation Rapid contractions of the ventricles of the heart without coordination with the heart's normal functions. If the irregular contractions are not corrected, as with an electric defibrillator, cardiac arrest and death can follow quickly.

ventricular septal defect A defect in the heart's muscular wall that normally separates blood in the left ventricle from that of the right ventricle. The result is that blood is circulated without the benefit of fresh oxygen since the "used" blood from the veins can be pumped back into the general body circulation without going through the lungs.

venturi A name sometimes used to identify the jet of an oxygen mask. The jet of oxygen enters the mask through openings near the venturi and dilutes the pure oxygen to the proportion prescribed for the care of the patient requiring an oxygen mask. The mask sometimes is called a venturi mask because of the way in which it is designed to draw in precise amounts of outside air to mix with the oxygen supply.

venules Blood vessels that drain blood from capillaries into the veins after the blood has given up its oxygen and other nutrients to the cells of the body and has collected waste products of cell metabolism such as carbon dioxide and water.

vertebral foramen A medical term for the spinal cord hole in a vertebra.

vestibular breathing A type of shallow breathing marked by a long inspiratory phase, or period of inhalation, followed by a short expiratory, or exhalation, phase. When the doctor listens to the breathing sound through the chest with his stethoscope, he may hear a peculiar wheezing or whistling noise that accompanies the inhalation phase.

visceral pleura The inner pleural membrane layer that covers the lungs; the outer pleural membrane layer, the parietal pleura, faces the inside of the chest wall.

weaning A bit of medical jargon relating to the care of respiratory disease patients—but not to nursing infants. The term is used to describe the procedures for training a person who has been breathing with the help of a mechanical ventilator to function normally, or nearly normally, without the need for artificial breathing equipment.

wedge A term sometimes used to describe a balloon that can be inserted into an artery, such as the pulmonary artery, to help control the blood flow and pressure. When the balloon is inflated, which can be done remotely through a catheter, it becomes a wedge in the artery.

wet pleurisy Sometimes called pleurisy with effusion, this is a condition marked by the appearance of a clear fluid in the space between the pleural membrane layers of the chest. A sample of the fluid usually is taken by a needle tap through the chest wall so it can be analyzed in the laboratory. If signs of infection are found, antibiotics can be injected through the needle tap into the pleural space. The cause of wet pleurisy can be due to cancer, a chest wound, pneumonia, tuberculosis, kidney disease, heart disease, or an abscess.

wheezing An abnormal breathing sound produced by the rapid flow of air through a narrowed passageway. Wheezing can be a sign of asthma, bronchitis, emphysema, pulmonary edema, a pulmonary embolism, or a tumor or foreign body in the respiratory airways. Wheezing also may be associated with colds or exposure to smoke, dust, or allergens.

whooping cough A highly infectious respiratory disease that is characterized by coughing attacks that end with a whooping or crowing inhalation sound. The victims, who number in the hundreds of thousands each year, are usually young children. The disease is marked at the onset by a runny nose and fever along with a slight cough. These symptoms last about two weeks and are followed by chills, nausea, and coughing attacks that deplete the air in the lungs. The patient may become cyanotic because of air hunger before the series of coughs ceases. The long whooping or crowing sound occurs when the patient finally stops coughing and takes a deep breath.

Pneumonia, emphysema, and other lung disorders can become complications of whooping cough. The disease is self-limiting and runs its course in about six weeks. However, the symptoms may return with subsequent respiratory infections. The disease is preventable with a pertussis vaccine that can be given in an immunization series, beginning at two months of age and including a booster shot given before the child begins school.

windpipe A common name for the trachea, the tube connecting the nose, mouth, and pharynx with the bronchi.

xiphoid process The bottom part of the sternum, or breastbone. The main part of the sternum is called the body; the top of the three sections is called the manubrium.

X-rays Sometimes called roentgen rays, they are electromagnetic rays used for both diagnostic and therapeutic purposes by medical personnel. Because X-rays penetrate some tissues of the body better than others, they can produce images of bones, organs, foreign objects, and other items on a piece of photographic film placed on the other side of the body.

QUESTIONS AND ANSWERS

THE CHEST

Q: *Is it possible to have tuberculosis without having symptoms?*
A: Yes. Many cases of tuberculosis are discovered through routine skin tests, such as those administered to school children, and through chest X-rays which reveal symptomless lesions.

Q: *I have heard that older people can develop tuberculosis after taking certain kinds of medicines. Can this be true?*
A: What actually happens is that a latent case of tuberculosis is reactivated by medications such as steroids. In other words, the older person already has the infection, acquired perhaps as a youngster, but the disease remains dormant until stimulated to resume activity many years later. The medicine is not really the cause of the disease.

Q: *Is a pulmonary embolism always fatal?*
A: Studies show that between 80 and 90 percent of the half-million cases of acute pulmonary embolism recorded each year in the United States have a favorable outcome. More victims of pulmonary embolism probably could be saved with early treatment and preventive therapy to control the development of thrombi in deep leg veins, where most emboli begin.

Most deaths associated with pulmonary embolism occur before doctors can diagnose the problem and begin treatment. Persons at greatest risk are those who are overweight and physically inactive, although unfortunately many patients are inactive because of a serious medical problem such as stroke, heart disease, broken leg, etc. However, when a thrombus develops in a leg vein the threat of pulmonary embolism generally can be controlled by the use of anticoagulants and other medications.

Q: *Can a person have angina pectoris without severe chest pain?*
A: Yes. Many patients, in fact, describe the symptoms of angina pectoris in terms of heavy chest discomfort or distress, sometimes extending as far as the jaw or elbow, but they do not include pain among their symptoms.

Q: *My doctor has suggested that exercise programs could help my angina problem. Isn't it a bit late to start exercising after angina has developed?*
A: Not at all. While we don't know all of the necessary details of your own case, it is true that modern medicines generally will help control the symptoms of angina so that you can tolerate increased physical activity. The exercise training, in turn, can improve the tone and efficiency of your muscles and circulatory system so that you are less likely to be bothered by angina symptoms.

Q: *I feel heart palpitations once in a while, even while resting. Is this a sign of heart disease?*
A: The palpitations you feel probably are what doctors call ventricular premature beats. Whether they might be associated with any form of heart disease would depend upon other factors requiring a careful physical examination, as well as your age and lifestyle. Ventricular premature beats are more common in older persons and perhaps pose a greater risk for a person 65 years of age than for the same individual of 35. Anxiety, stress, and use of caffeine, alcohol, and tobacco can cause heart

palpitations in some people. Also, overwork can result in the premature beats. Some individuals seem to experience heart palpitations for no apparent reason. But in your case, only your doctor can help you know for sure.

Q: *A doctor has diagnosed my coughing spells as hypersensitivity pneumonitis and said I probably am allergic to parakeets. This doesn't make any sense to me. Could he be correct?*

A: Hypersensitivity pneumonitis is a fancy medical term which is equivalent to another just as fancy medical term, extrinsic allergic alveolitis, which means simply that you may indeed be allergic to a substance associated with your parakeet. Yours is not an unusual situation since many people develop allergies to birds and other pets.

Breathlessness, coughing, fever, and more serious respiratory disorders can result because of sensitivity of the bronchioles or alveoli to mold spores, dust, or dander in the atmosphere of the home or workplace. If there is a way in which you can enjoy the presence of the parakeet without inhaling whatever irritant is produced by the bird, your problem may be solved. Otherwise, you may have to decide whether to get rid of the pet or face the possibility of progressive lung inflammation and eventual respiratory failure.

Q: *Both my wife and I have asthma and take theophylline for it, but the doctor has prescribed different doses of the medicine. Is this because one of us is more sensitive to the drug?*

A: Doctors adjust drug dosages for different patients for a number of good reasons. For example, theophylline doses are based on body weight of the patient; bigger people, in other words, get bigger doses. Children usually get larger doses because they metabolize the drug faster. People who have liver disorders may get smaller doses because they metabolize the drug more slowly. The fact that prescription drug doses are likely to be tailored for a partic-

ular patient is another good reason why it's not wise to use a medicine that was prescribed for another person.

Q: *How can the bronchial tubes become blocked with mucus when a person has asthma or a similar disease?*

A: Most people who do not have a respiratory disorder are not aware of the amount of mucus normally produced in the bronchi; it amounts to nearly four fluid ounces each day and is gradually pushed up the trachea by cilia lining the respiratory tract and into the pharynx where it is swallowed into the stomach.

Individuals who suffer from asthma and similar diseases are more familiar with the mucus, which sometimes is thick and is not easily moved by the hairlike cilia that have the job of cleaning out the air passageways. The smallest bronchi have a diameter about the size of a straw; the bore of a bronchiole is about half that diameter. If the mucus is allowed to accumulate it forms "plugs" which must be coughed up in order to open the airways between the alveoli and the outside air. Irritants like tobacco smoke aggravate the situation by increasing mucus production and preventing the cilia from functioning properly.

Q: *A newspaper story reported recently that you can get a lung disease by breathing the air blowing over ocean water. Could this be true?*

A: Yes. Strange as it seems, a bacterium that causes lung infections lives in sea water and has been found to be carried inland in water droplets by sea breezes. People living along the Florida gulf and east coasts have shown high levels of sensitivity to the disease organism.

Q: *If you have tuberculosis, do you have to go to a special hospital for treatment?*

A: In recent years the trend has been toward treating tuberculosis in general hospitals near the patient's home and releasing the patient as early as possible. In general hospitals the tuberculosis patient may be located in an isolation ward or a chest-disease ward for two to three weeks while chemotherapy is administered to control the infection. When the patient is well enough to leave the hospital, treatment is continued on an outpatient basis; the patient reports to a clinic for regular checkups until the infection is no longer a serious threat to the individual and his community.

Q: *While getting a checkup at a neighborhood medical clinic, I noticed the letters COPD on my records. What does it mean?*
A: COPD is an abbreviation for Chronic Obstructive Pulmonary Disease, which can include asthma, bronchitis, emphysema, and dilation of one or more bronchi. The term sometimes is used when a patient has two or more of the conditions, a situation that is most likely to occur in men over the age of 50.

Q: *I had a bad case of influenza and I am over it now. But food doesn't have the same taste that it did before. Can a disease like flu destroy the taste buds?*
A: Some food flavors are detected through their aromas rather than by the taste buds, and it's quite possible that the respiratory infection had a temporarily adverse effect on your ability to evaluate aromas. The nerve receptors for the sense of smell are at the top of the nasal cavity, and that area of mucous membranes may not have recovered as yet from the inflammation. This is not an uncommon occurrence, and if you can tell the differences between sweet, sour, and salty flavors of food, this would indicate that the olfactory receptors in your nose rather than the taste buds were affected by the infection. The olfactory sensations should return to normal within a few days.

Q: *The doctor told me my heart is enlarged. Will it return to normal size eventually?*
A: The answer depends upon what caused the heart enlargement. Some hearts become larger than normal because of the heavier work load they must adjust to, as in the hearts of athletes and people who do heavy physical labor. The heart is composed of muscle and grows to meet the demand, just as arm or leg muscles are larger for individuals whose arms and legs get a good physical workout. Such an enlargement generally would not be a health threat. And it probably would not get much smaller. A heart enlarged because of a circulatory disorder, however, could be dilated as a result of an overloading of effort and weakened muscle. A dilated heart might eventually become reduced in size through rest and medical care for the cause of the abnormal enlargement.

Q: *During a physical examination my doctor held a lighted match near my mouth and asked me to blow it out without pursing my lips. Could you explain what the test proves?*
A: That was the so-called match test for respiratory function. The test was started a generation ago as part of a diagnostic procedure for emphysema cases. A lighted match from an ordinary paper matchbook is held about six inches from the patient's mouth while he takes a deep breath and tries to blow out the match with his mouth wide open. If the patient is unable to extinguish the match, it indicates he probably has a vital capacity of less than one and a half quarts of air per second, or about half the normal breathing capacity of a healthy young person.

Q: *Why is blood pressure measured on arteries rather than veins, which usually are easier to find?*
A: One good reason is that you can't find a palpable pulse on a large vein. Although the heart maintains pressure in the veins as well as the arteries, artery pressures are about 16 times as great as blood pressures in the veins. For the same reason blood spurts from a cut artery but flows slowly from a cut vein.

Q: *Our doctor recommended that my wife use a steam vaporizer to help loosen the mucus in her bronchial tubes when she has breathing problems with a head cold. But the steam vaporizer seems to make her coughing attacks worse. Is it possible that some people have an adverse reaction to steam inhalation?*

A: You did not explain what sort of steam vaporizer you use or what medications, if any, you add to the water to be vaporized. However, it is possible that your wife is allergic to something that is produced by the vaporizer other than the water. There are instances of vaporizers that are not properly cleaned before using, with the result that bacteria, molds, or other organisms are dispensed along with the steam by the vaporizers.

5

THE ABDOMEN

Perhaps you call it the belly. Some people refer to that part of the anatomy as the gut. Chances are your doctor and his colleagues use the term abdomen when describing the region that fills the space between the diaphragm and the floor of the pelvis.

The abdomen does contain the gut, or the bulk of the digestive system. However, it also is "home" to an assortment of other organs and structures of the body, including the liver, spleen, kidneys, and bladder, and, in the female body, the uterus, ovaries, and Fallopian tubes. The last named structures, of course, are absent from the lower portion of the male abdomen; his sex-related bits of internal anatomy consist mainly of the prostate and its accompanying ducts and vesicles.

The abdomen frequently presents a unique challenge to the examining physician because of the assortment of organs and systems located there, each of which might be the site of a disease or disorder causing discomfort to a patient. Also, the techniques used in examining the skin, head, and chest may be of little help in diagnosing a problem deep in the abdomen.

A disease of the skin, eye, nose, or throat frequently can be observed directly. A chest problem can be identified by examinations using X-rays, stethoscopes, and some knowledge of normal heart and lung function. But a bellyache could be due to a myriad of possible causes that might elude stethoscope and X-ray.

Locating the Abdominal Organs

The doctor might begin an abdominal examination by visualizing the geography of the abdomen in four sections, called quadrants. The imaginary division lines run vertically from the tip of the xiphoid process, the pointy bottom of the dagger-shaped breastbone, through the umbilicus, or belly button, and horizontally at right angles to the first line so that the two lines intersect at the umbilicus. The four quadrants of the abdomen divided in this manner are identified as upper right, upper left, lower right, and lower left. The quadrants are not equal in area; the upper quadrants, in fact, extend into the lower part of the rib cage, because the liver, spleen, kidneys, adrenal glands, and pancreas are partially protected by the lower five or six ribs.

When you are in the supine position, which means lying flat on your back, the abdomen takes the shape of a shallow, oval basin. The spinal column and back muscles form the bottom of the basin. The sides of the basin are formed by the front of the pelvic bones and ribs and by the muscles that extend from the chest to the hips along the sides. The front of the abdomen, or top of the basin, is composed of flat bands of muscle and connective tissue covered with skin.

In the upper right quadrant of the abdomen are most of the liver, the gallbladder, the right kidney and adrenal gland, and part of the pancreas. The stomach, spleen, left kidney and adrenal gland, most of the pancreas, and part of the liver are located in the upper left quadrant. The urinary bladder is at the bottom of the abdominal cavity, along a vertical line from the sternum through the belly button. The female reproductive organs are in the lower two quadrants, as are the male prostate and its associated structures, which lie very close to the urinary bladder.

The intestines, from the duodenum to the colon, are distributed through all four quadrants, although the large intestine normally begins in the lower right quadrant, where the appendix is attached, and loops up and across the upper quadrants, and back down on the left side to the rectum, which is behind the bladder, looking from front to rear.

Some doctors go beyond the four quadrants in laying out the geography of the belly and further subdivide the region into nine sections, like the plan for a game of tic-tac-toe. In the nine-section layout, the abdomen has one center square around the belly button that is identified as the umbilicus. The area directly above the umbilicus is called the epigastrium, and the portion below is known as the hypogastrium, or suprapubic region. The left and right sides of this abdominal checkerboard are labeled, from top to bottom, hypochondrium, flank or lumbar, and iliac—each term being preceded by left or right, as may be appropriate.

Exploring the Abdomen

Most patients with a bellyache probably could not care less what sort of geography game is played by the examining physician as long as he ends their discomfort as quickly and inexpensively as possible. The reason for explaining all of this belly patterning here is to help the reader understand why the doctor goes about his examination procedure as he is likely to do. If he pokes gently into the upper right quadrant (or right hypochondrium), for example, he may be probing for the edge of your liver. If you are very careful, you might be able to locate your own liver by pressing your fingers gently along the lower right edge of your rib cage.

When the doctor checks your liver, he usually asks you to take a deep breath. That is because filling the lungs tends to push the liver downward so it is palpable below the rib cage. Also, the doctor usually holds his hand gently over the upper right quadrant, near the edge of the ribs, and waits for the liver to descend during a deep inspiration. Because of his experience in palpating livers, the examining physician frequently can gain a good bit of information about the shape, size, and consistency of the liver. He also can tell something about the tenderness of the area by your reaction as the liver is palpated. If the doctor looks into your face in-

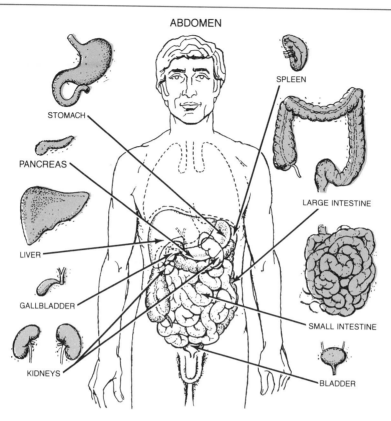

ABDOMEN

SPLEEN

STOMACH

PANCREAS

LARGE INTESTINE

LIVER

GALLBLADDER

SMALL INTESTINE

KIDNEYS

BLADDER

The abdomen contains the organs of digestion, such as the stomach which has glands that secrete pepsin, hydrochloric acid, and other digestive juices. The stomach walls are composed of three separate layers of muscles so the organ can contract and relax in three different directions while churning food particles in the digestive juices.

The pancreas, situated just beyond the stomach, secretes additional substances involved in the digestion of food, including insulin which is necessary for the conversion of sugar to glycogen which can be stored by the body, and enzymes needed to further digest carbohydrates, proteins, and fats.

The liver is a virtual chemical factory involved in numerous digestive activities, including the tearing down and rebuilding of amino acid units for protein molecules, converting sugar to glycogen, converting or storing vitamins A, B, and D, producing bile, urea, and a number of blood components, and removing poisonous substances from the bloodstream.

The gallbladder is a small pouch that stores bile produced by the liver, releasing it as needed to help digest fatty substances in a meal. Bile from the gallbladder enters the small intestine through a common duct that also carries digestive substances from the pancreas.

The kidneys are two bean-shaped organs at the back of the abdomen which have the job of filtering excess water and waste products, such as urea, from the bloodstream. Normal kidneys automatically adjust their filtering activity so that essential fluids and substances are restored to the blood.

The spleen is the only major organ in the abdomen that is not primarily associated with digestion or excretion. In the unborn child, the spleen produces red blood cells, a function taken over by the bone marrow after birth. During periods of stress, however, when red blood cell resources of the body are taxed, the spleen contracts to release its stores of the cells. It also functions somewhat like the kidneys and liver in removing unwanted substances from the bloodstream.

The large intestine forms a loop about five feet long from the point where it collects material from the small intestine, in the lower right corner of the abdomen; it travels upward along the right side of the abdomen and across the front, just below the stomach, and descends downward along the left side of the abdomen to a point where it makes a jog in its path to form the sigmoid-rectal segments of the colon.

The small intestine, which actually is four times as long as the large intestine although smaller in diameter, is lined with millions of tiny fingerlike villi which absorb the nutrients from digested food. The final stages of digestion, including the breakdown of pro-

teins, fats, and carbohydrates, takes place in the small intestine.

The urinary bladder is a hollow muscular organ that stores urine until it is convenient to excrete the waste product collected from the kidneys. Long tubes with muscular walls, the ureters, carry urine from the kidneys to the bladder. A single tube, the urethra, carries the urine to the outside. Circular sphincter muscles control the flow of urine by relaxing to permit emptying of the bladder during the process of urination.

stead of at your abdomen while checking your liver, he probably is watching for a sign that he has found a tender spot, assuming you are not ticklish there.

By imagining the location of various organs in the abdomen's four quadrants or nine tic-tac-toe squares, and by using his experience and knowledge of anatomy and physiology, the doctor can indeed learn quite a bit about a patient's abdominal organs by carefully palpating the area with his palms and fingers. He may be able to tell whether the patient has a distended urinary bladder, feces in the colon, or atherosclerosis in the aorta. Tumors or other tissue masses can be detected by the doctor, who frequently can determine whether the mass is a part of an organ or is attached to the abdominal wall if it moves as the patient breathes. Some tissues move a bit during respiration and others do not. The doctor's knowledge of anatomy provides other clues since some organs, such as the liver and pancreas, are solid, while the stomach and intestines are normally hollow.

In some patients, particularly those with thin abdominal walls, the doctor may be able to observe contractions of the stomach and peristalsis of the intestines.

Peristalsis is the name given the undulating contractions of the intestinal tract as the contents are moved along from the stomach to the descending colon, where feces begin to accumulate. Sometimes the doctor will tap the abdominal wall with his fingers to trigger a wave of digestive tract contractions. The doctor looks for contractions of the stomach or intestine in order to tell from the wave action whether the digestive activity appears to be normal, or if there is a possible obstruction in the large or small intestine or at the pylorus. This is the muscular valve through which stomach contents empty into the duodenum, the first segment of the small intestine beyond the stomach.

When the aorta can be observed, the doctor frequently can estimate the size of the bore, or opening, within this important artery. Often the doctor can detect the presence of an aneurysm, or ballooning or rupture of the aorta wall, or of a circulatory murmur.

The external examination of the abdominal region covers such skin signs as new or old scars, stretch marks caused by previous pregnancies in a woman, and veins that suggest a disorder. Scars gradually change color from red to skin color over a period of about six months, and scars caused by surgery, burns, or wounds often produce rather distinct patterns that are diagnostic clues.

Jaundice: A Sign of Disease

Jaundice, a sign of liver disorder, can produce a yellowish coloration to the skin of the face and trunk, as well as to the sclera, or white areas, of the eyes. The condition, also called icterus, is caused by an accumulation of bile pigments in the tissues.

Jaundice is not a disease in itself but a sign of several possible diseases that can involve the gallbladder and blood as well as the liver. A gallstone in the bile duct, for example, can obstruct the normal route of bile pigment so that it is diverted into the bloodstream. Jaundice also can be the result of an attack of infectious hepatitis.

The yellow coloring or pigment is a substance known as bilirubin, which ordinarily is a part of the hemoglobin molecule of red blood cells. In certain types of blood disease, such as anemia, an excess of bilirubin may occur in the bile to produce the jaundice effect. Normally, the excess bilirubin is absorbed by the liver cells, but a diseased liver often is unable to absorb the yellow pigment as fast as it is produced. The bilirubin generally is distributed in tissues throughout the body, but it is more likely to be observed in exposed tissues such as the skin and other surface areas of the body. In some cases the jaundice coloration is more likely to be seen in sunlight than in artificial light. The person afflicted with an accumulation of bilirubin in his tissues may not be immediately aware of the effect because it involves a slow, subtle change in coloration.

Functions of the Liver

The liver itself is the largest gland in the body. It develops during embryonic life as a pouch or pocket on the side of the gut and gradually grows into an organ that weighs around three pounds and measures slightly less than ten inches from stem to stern. Within the massive gland are millions of specialized cells that are busily engaged in many—if not most—of the chemical processes conducted by the human body.

The liver is on the receiving end of two major blood conduits. One is the hepatic artery that provides copious amounts of freshly oxygenated blood from the nearby aorta. The other is the portal vein, which brings nutrients directly from the digestive tract that it drains. Both blood vessels divide many times within the liver to form a network of capillaries that distributes the nutrients and oxygen to as many liver cells as possible.

Nearly everything that enters the digestive tract, if it can be absorbed into the capillaries that are in contact with the stomach and intestines, is carried to the liver via the portal vein. This includes non-nutritive substances as well as nutrients that are ingested. Enzymes in the liver cells, for example, will metabolize caffeine and change the molecules into other chemicals that can be excreted quickly. Poisonous substances are neutralized by liver enzymes if the dose is small enough for the enzymes to handle. If the liver needs more enzymes to handle non-nutritive substances, more enzymes are produced. But occasionally the liver cells are overwhelmed by a nonfood item and begin to degenerate—for instance, when cirrhosis of the liver occurs from imbibing too much alcohol for too long a period of time. Then, many other substances entering the liver through the portal vein are processed more slowly. A diseased liver takes much longer to metabolize caffeine than does a healthy liver, to cite a rather simplistic example of the situation.

The liver handles nutrients such as carbohydrates, fats, and proteins in the same general manner as other substances collected through the tributaries of the portal vein. Carbohydrates that need further processing into glucose, the basic form of sugar, after being converted from starch by enzymes in the mouth and stomach, are broken down into simple glucose molecules. Carbohydrates that arrive at the liver as glucose molecules may be shunted directly into tissues where they are needed for body fuel. If the tissues already have enough glucose, the sugar units are converted to a molecule called glycogen, or animal starch, the form in which it is stored in the liver.

When the body needs quick energy and the glucose supply is low, the glycogen molecules are quickly broken down into glucose units again. This process is not easily accomplished in the body of a person afflicted with diabetes mellitus because the disorder results in a deficiency of insulin, a hormone secreted by the pancreas, another large gland in the abdomen. Insulin is necessary to build glycogen molecules from glucose sugar units in the liver cells. Without insulin, the glucose received from the portal vein or produced by the liver cells cannot be stored and is excreted in the urine.

Not all glucose is converted to glycogen for storage in the liver. An ample amount of glucose is shipped out to the muscles throughout the body for immediate use if needed. Each glucose molecule is composed of water and carbon dioxide and is held together with energy captured from the sunlight by plant cells. The glucose arrives at the liver by a circuitous route, either by a person eating plant materials, such as corn flakes with beet or cane sugar, or the meat of an animal that was fed corn or a similar grain or leafy plant product. Each glucose molecule is like a tiny time bomb waiting to release its pent-up energy in some bodily activity, like helping a muscle fiber contract.

Meanwhile, back at the chemical factory, millions of liver cells are processing fats and proteins. Actually, the proteins usually arrive at the liver in the form of amino acids, the chemical building blocks from which proteins are constructed. There are 22 amino acids utilized by the human body, some of which are essential amino acids—that is, the body must acquire them from certain foods which are the sources of those particular chemical units. Milk and eggs, for example, are sources of essential amino acids. Other amino acids are also essential for normal healthy body functions, but it isn't essential that you eat certain foods to get them into your system. This brings us to the role of the liver in the processing of proteins, because it is the liver that is responsible for building the nonessential amino acids from molecules of other amino acids received via the portal vein from the intestinal tract. The liver cells also reconstruct proteins from amino acids.

Since there are 22 amino acids to use for building human proteins, the variety of protein molecules is almost limitless. The proteins are made from strings of amino acids arranged somewhat like words formed from letters of the alphabet. But the proteins literally have a language of their own, with chains of hundreds or thousands of the basic units linked together in various patterns.

Fats also reach the liver in the form of their basic subunits, the fatty acids. Fatty acids can be converted into glucose molecules, which can be converted into glycogen, or they can be converted into free fatty acids for quick energy combustion, or they can be put into storage in cells of fat deposits. Sugars also can be changed into fats for storage, which is what happens with excess sweets in the diet. Fat is an economical way for nature to store energy for future use since one ounce of fat can hold more than twice as many calories of energy as one ounce of sugar.

Nearly all cells of the body can use fatty acids as a source of energy, except the cells of the nervous system, which includes the brain. The brain and nervous system need glucose for normal functioning. Glucose generally is preferred by the body cells as a fuel, and when glucose is available for energy fatty acids are not used. For that reason, glucose sometimes is called a fat sparing substance. Glucose also is a protein sparing substance because, in the absence of either fat or glucose, the body can digest its own protein molecules, converting them into fuel. This is what happens during a period of starvation, or even in some instances of crash dieting. If protein digestion is allowed to go on for more than a brief period, permanent damage can occur to vital organs that become stripped of their proteins.

The role of the liver in the circulatory scheme of the body cannot be underrated. There are reservoirs of blood in the liver, called venous sinuses, that can hold as much as six pints of blood in reserve for boosting the blood volume in emergencies. Special cells in the sinuses of the liver also cleanse the blood entering the liver from the portal vein. The cells trap any bacteria that may have entered the blood supply from the intestines before the blood is passed along into the general circulation.

The liver also filters out about half of the amino acids and two-thirds of the glucose running through the portal vein before returning the blood to the body's general supply. By doing so, the liver helps equalize the levels of nutrients distributed to the body cells. Otherwise, there would be great sudden increases in nutrients after a meal and inadequate blood levels of nutrients between meals.

In a similar manner, the liver manages the iron supply of the body so it is metered out only as it is needed. When the diet contains an abundance of iron, the liver transforms it into a substance called ferritin, which is stored until needed by body tissues such as red blood cells and the myoglobin of muscle fibers. Then the liver releases the stored iron in a form that can be readily used.

The liver secretes a fluid called bile, which is composed of a number of substances including bile salts, some cholesterol, and the yellowish pigment called bilirubin. The liver extracts bilirubin from red blood cells that have served their life span in the bloodstream and have been broken down into salvagable components. The only substance in the bile that enters into digestion is the bile salts, which drip back into the intestine where they act like a laundry detergent to break up the globules of fat from food being digested. Without the bile salts to break up the fat globules passing through the gut, the fats in the diet could not be digested. The bile salts do not digest the fat, but merely break up the larger fat units into smaller bits that can be digested by substances called lipases.

The rest of the components in bile have nothing to do with the digestive processes. They are waste products that are released from the liver into the bile duct to be excreted.

The liver produces bile continuously even though it is not used except during meal periods. The bile is stored between meals in the gallbladder, which can hold several ounces of bile. The inner surface of the gallbladder allows the fluid portion to be reabsorbed into the bloodstream, but not the bile salts, cholesterol, and bilirubin. After several hours the contents of the gallbladder become highly concentrated because of fluid reabsorbed from the bile. When food begins to enter the small intestine from the stomach, a very potent solution of bile is likely to be squeezed into the gut.

Gallbladder and Liver Disorders

There is a potential problem when too much fluid is reabsorbed from the bile while it is held in the gallbladder. The cholesterol portion of the bile becomes highly concentrated, along with the bile salts and bilirubin. In a single day the concentration of cholesterol can be 10 to 12 times that of the amount originally secreted from the liver cells. The cholesterol becomes oversaturated and chemically attracted to the bile salts, with the result that small crystals begin to precipitate from the fluid bile. The crystals grow and continue to accumulate, eventually forming gallstones that soon fill the entire gallbladder and obstruct the flow of bile from it—an excruciatingly painful experience.

Gallbladder Attack The pain of a gallbladder attack, sometimes referred to as biliary colic, may be triggered or aggravated by a meal rich in fats. The pain may be constant and severe, and accompanied by vomiting and fever. The fever may be due to a complication involving a bacterial infection of the gallbladder; the infection in turn may result in inflammation and an accumulation of pus along with stagnant bile in the gallbladder. If the foregoing description of biliary colic, or acute cholecystitis, seems gross, there's a good chance the reader has been lucky enough to avoid this not uncommon health problem. Those who have suffered a severe attack may feel that this description is inadequate.

The pain of biliary colic frequently begins in the epigastric region, which can be located on the tic-tac-toe pattern right above the umbilicus. In some cases the pain is relieved by one or more factors, such as an obstructing gallstone dropping away from the gallbladder opening. Or the pain may increase and spread into the right shoulder area. Jaundice frequently is a sign of gallbladder inflammation.

Treatment may consist of bed rest, antibiotics to control the infection, and analgesics to relieve the pain. Eventually, however, surgery may be advised to solve the problem of gallstones. If the gallstones are removed and the gallbladder is left in place, there is a chance that more gallstones will develop there in the future. If the gallbladder is removed with the stones, the operation will have no serious effect on the lifestyle of the patient, who is most likely to be a mature woman. Since the bile is produced in the liver and will continue to flow into the intestine and work its effect on fat globules, it just won't be stored in between meals.

A patient who has a cholecystectomy, the medical term for removal of the gallbladder, undergoes a series of X-ray examinations before, during, and after surgery. The X-ray pictures are taken after a dye is administered to the patient's digestive tract to enhance the outlines of the gallbladder and the stones that may be in it. The dye is contained in a tablet given the patient. During surgery a dye is injected through a catheter inserted into the bile duct to make sure it is not obstructed. A final X-ray is taken after surgery, again to make sure that the bile duct leading from the liver to the duodenum portion of the intestine is open, so that bile can pass directly into the gut.

For about ten days after surgery the cholecystectomy patient has a tube connected from his chest to a receptacle beside the bed. Bile flowing into the container is measured each day and the amount is recorded. After about the tenth day the tube, called a "T" tube, is removed, and the patient can resume eating regular meals.

Hepatitis Inflammation of the liver is called hepatitis, and a frequent cause is a viral infection. The early signs and symptoms of hepatitis may include nausea, loss of appetite, and abdominal pain. Jaundice almost always accompanies hepatitis as an early sign of the disease. When the examining physician checks the liver by palpation, he frequently will find signs of tenderness on all available surfaces of the organ.

There are several different types of hepatitis, including two or three kinds that are caused by viruses. One kind of viral hepatitis, sometimes identified as infectious hepatitis and at other times as hepatitis A, seems to be transmitted from one person to another through direct or indirect contact. The virus apparently is found in feces, urine, and saliva. Children and young adults are the most likely victims, and they are most likely to become infected in the fall or winter months. Infectious hepatitis takes from 15 to 45 days to develop signs and symptoms in a patient who has been exposed, and the onset of an attack can be severe or mild.

Hepatitis B, the second common type of viral hepatitis, also is known as serum hepatitis because it frequently is associated with infection by blood transfusion. It may not make an appearance as a disease in a patient until four or five months after actual transmission of the virus. Its onset is insidious and its effects can be quite severe, particularly among older persons or those already in poor health. Unlike the A form of hepatitis, the serum or B type can affect persons of any age. It can be transmitted the year around; it has no seasonal incidence like the A form.

Hepatitis patients usually are treated at home with rest and special diets. They are encouraged to drink plenty of fluids but no alcoholic beverages, particularly during the early acute stages. Most drugs also should be avoided. Meals are planned to provide abundant supplies of important nutrients, and the patient is encouraged to eat a large breakfast because nausea frequently increases during the day. Bed rest is not required but physical activity may be limited in order to avoid fatigue. If the patient's condition worsens or fails to show signs of improvement, he usually is hospitalized for more intensive treatment.

In addition to the A and B types of viral hepatitis, there are forms sometimes identified as C and D, but little is known about their role in hepatitis. There also are numerous noninfectious agents that can cause hepatitis, including industrial chemicals, metals, medications, and mushrooms. The industrial chemicals that cause hepatitis signs and symptoms generally are of the kind used in cleaning and degreasing, such as carbon tetrachloride and trichloroeythlene. Certain tranquillizers and oral contraceptives have similar effects on certain individuals.

Cirrhosis of the Liver Cirrhosis of the liver usually is marked by the death of liver cells, the development of scar tissue, and the loss of normal blood circulation to the functioning cells, along with hypertension of the portal vein. As cirrhosis develops the liver becomes enlarged, nodular, and hard. If it could be seen through the abdominal wall, the cirrhotic liver would have a tawny brown coloration. Hepatitis is a common cause of liver cirrhosis. Consumption of alcohol probably is at least a runner-up in the leading causes of cirrhosis, although experts on the subject doubt that ordinary social drinking is likely to cause the permanent liver damage found in chronic alcoholics, who have to consume the equivalent of a pint or more of whiskey per day for five to ten years in order to develop cirrhosis.

Malnutrition sometimes is suggested as a contributing factor in cases of cirrhosis in chronic alcoholics. Some studies have found that diets rich in proteins and vitamins can help improve the condition of a cirrhotic liver. But other studies have shown that heavy alcohol consumption can cause cirrhosis even when the patient consumes a well-balanced diet along with his booze.

As cirrhosis progresses, normal liver cells are gradually replaced by fibrous tissue. The fibrous tissue puts pressure on the veins distributing blood from the portal vein, forcing the blood back and producing the condition of portal vein hypertension. Eventually, the liver fails and the patient sinks into a hepatic comma, which frequently is fatal.

The Pancreas and Its Disorders

The pancreas, another gland in the upper abdomen, empties more than a quart of assorted digestive juices into the small intestine at a point a little more than an inch beyond the pylorus, the valve that empties the stomach. The pancreas is well known as the source of insulin, used by the liver to convert a basic sugar into a form that can be stored, but it also provides other important secretions. The pancreas produces at least four different enzymes that are needed to digest fats and proteins, as well as carbohydrates. It also secretes sodium bicarbonate, which mixes with the hydrochloric acid emptied from the stomach so that the acid is neutralized, and at the same time becomes sodium chloride, which is the same as common table salt. As sodium chloride the substance is less of a hazard to the lining of the intestine, and it can be dissolved in water so that its component parts can assist in several normal body fluid functions, such as helping to regulate the amount of water in body tissues.

The digestive enzymes produced by the pancreas usually are identified collectively as the pancreatic juice. The juice is manufactured in numerous small saccules that lie along a duct which runs the length of the pancreas. The duct drains the pancreatic juice into the intestine at the same place as the bile from the liver enters that part of the digestive system.

Insulin Deficiency Insulin, the hormone essential for normal carbohydrate use by the body, is produced by groups of cells called islets of Langerhans; the islets are found between the saccules, or lobules, that secrete the pancreatic enzymes. The disease known as diabetes mellitus occurs when the pancreas fails to produce insulin, a hormone that functions as a chemical messenger for the control of glucose storage. As noted earlier, the liver normally converts excess glucose into glycogen so it can be stored and converted back into glucose, the basic body fuel, when it is needed by the tissues. Glucose that cannot be stored, as in the body of a diabetic person, is excreted in the urine.

When glucose is not available to burn as a body fuel, fatty acids are stoked into the furnaces of the body tissues. However, even the fatty acids require a certain amount of glucose in order to burn completely. Otherwise, a residue of ketone bodies will accumulate in the tissues. Ketone bodies are chemicals such as acetone that are parts of incompletely burned fatty acids, and they can have a poisonous effect. When they accumulate in the body of a diabetic person, they can cause a disorder known as diabetic ketoacidosis, or acidosis, for short.

A person afflicted with acidosis may experience nausea and vomiting, air hunger, and abdominal pain and tenderness. The symptoms can be so similar to those of appendicitis that the condition sometimes is referred to as pseudoappendicitis. The patient may have low blood pressure, dry skin, and signs of mineral depletion, since sodium and potassium levels are associated with the general insulin-glucose health picture. The patient may sink into a coma that is quite similar to a different sort of problem faced by diabetics, an insulin reaction.

In an emergency, when a doctor is unable to tell immediately the cause of a diabetic's coma, he will inject a glucose solution into the patient's blood vein. At the same time a blood sample will be taken for laboratory analysis. The rationale for giving a diabetic in a coma a shot of glucose is that the glucose may help—and it is unlikely to cause any harm. If the coma is due to an insulin reaction, the patient probably will regain consciousness soon after the glucose has gone to work in his system. The procedure for treating a coma caused by acidosis may vary according to the needs of the individual patient; part of that information will come from results of the laboratory tests.

If the diabetic patient is unconscious because of an insulin reaction, the cause may be one of using too large a dose of insulin (which must be administered by injection at least once daily, and in some cases more than once a day), or waiting too long for a meal, and/or physical exertion which can alter the rate of glucose consumption by the body.

Diabetes Diabetes is an ancient and worldwide disease, described in some of the earliest Chinese and Greek medical writings, and today affecting an estimated 200 million people. There are a number of causal factors associated with the disease, including genetic factors, obesity, and drugs and diseases that affect the normal functioning of the pancreas. Among the drugs that may trigger an onset of diabetes are certain steroid hormones and diuretics. Tumors of the pancreas can destroy the insulin-producing cells, and there is evidence that virus infections may be followed by diabetes in some individuals. There are instances in which the pancreas must be removed surgically, in which case the patient becomes an instant diabetic.

Diabetes may occur in children or adolescents. The first signs are a sudden tremendous thirst and an equally abnormal need to urinate, with bedwetting problems returning to plague the youngster. The child may experience a loss of weight and strength, and become easily fatigued because of the glucose metabolism problem. Examination by a physician may reveal that the child is a victim of juvenile-onset diabetes.

Diabetes also may occur in middle age in a form called maturity-onset diabetes. The disease may be discovered during a medical examination for some seemingly unrelated problem such as skin ulcers of the feet (caused by poor circulation), visual difficulties, fatigue, loss of sensation, or urinary bladder problems. The symptoms may begin at the same time as a significant weight gain or weight loss. However, the symptoms are not as serious as those of juvenile-onset diabetes.

The patient afflicted with maturity-onset diabetes may have several advantages over the juvenile-onset diabetes patient. The person whose symptoms do not manifest themselves until later in life usually can manage without daily injections of insulin. There are several kinds of drugs called oral hypoglycemic agents available for maturity-onset diabetes patients to help them maintain rather normal levels of blood sugar, or glucose. The oral hypoglycemic agents are not a form of insulin, nor are they a substitute for insulin, which may have to be administered in the event of an attack of acidosis. The oral hypoglycemic agents help the patient by increasing the output of insulin by the islet cells of the pancreas, which generally continue to function in cases of maturity-onset diabetes, and by causing the liver to curtail its output of glucose. Maturity-onset diabetes patients frequently can control their symptoms with diet alone, and diet is a prime factor in the ability of any diabetic patient to lead a fairly normal life.

A typical diabetic diet might provide ten calories for every pound of normal body weight. For example, a woman weighing 60 kilograms, or 132 pounds, could plan meals providing a total of 1,320 calories per day. The basic diet requires one gram of carbohydrate per pound of body weight and one gram of protein for each two pounds of body weight. Fat intake is based on the number of calories still available in the daily budget after allowing for carbohydrate and protein calories. Dietitians who plan meals for diabetics recommend that the fats come from plant products rather than animal products whenever possible, because of the association between animal fats and blood vessel diseases such as atherosclerosis.

Actually, the calories in a diabetic diet can add up to a large amount in a hurry. Each gram of carbohydrate and each gram of protein is worth four calories when credited against the total of 1,320 for the hypothetical 132-pound woman patient. Nearly 800 calories, spread over all the day's meals, must be used for protein and carbohydrate foods. This amount is minimum, however; greater proportions of protein and slightly larger proportions of carbohydrates are acceptable. The number may seem large, but one ounce of cooked beef contains 100 calories and one glass of milk may add another 200 calories, as would only two tablespoons of peanut butter. Thus, a balanced diet for a diabetic patient can involve something of a juggling act.

Fortunately for patients with diabetes, good diet suggestions and detailed meal plans are available from such sources as the American Diabetes Association. Most diabetic diet plans are based on a system of exchanges offering the patient equivalent foods in each of several categories, such as milk, bread, vegetables, fruits, and fats, that provide 15 grams of carbohydrate or 12 grams of protein. One slice of bread, for example, could be equivalent to one-half cup of mashed potatoes in providing 15 grams of carbohydrate and two grams of protein. Similarly, one ounce of chicken would equal five shrimp in providing seven grams of protein and five grams of fat. Because each gram of fat adds nine calories, five shrimp would account for 28 protein calories and 45 fat calories, as would each ounce of chicken in a meal.

Since the pancreas is only about five inches long and weighs between three and six ounces, it is hard to believe it can have such an important influence on the health of hundreds of millions of persons throughout the world. Yet, it has still other effects only recently discovered, such as a hormone that can stimulate the flow of gastric acid in the stomach and under certain conditions may cause an overproduction of gastric acid in the digestive tract.

Pancreatitis Just as other glands, such as the liver, can become inflamed by an obstruction that blocks the flow of glandular secretions, so can the pancreas suffer from dammed-up accumulations of pancreatic juice. Because the pancreas

and liver both normally empty their secretions into the intestine at the same point, it is not unusual for the pancreatic secretions to be blocked by a gallstone that has been passed into the common duct from the gallbladder. The disorder is called pancreatitis.

The condition may make itself felt after a meal, with nausea and vomiting and a pain in the upper abdominal area that radiates to the back of the patient. The patient frequently is admitted to a hospital, where tests are made to determine the precise cause of the discomfort; the signs and symptoms may resemble several other conditions. A great danger in an attack of acute pancreatitis is that the pressure of the dammed-up digestive enzymes will cause a rupture. If this occurs, the enzymes that are designed by nature to digest proteins, fats, and carbohydrates may begin digesting the other organs in the abdomen. To control this complication, the patient may be given a drug such as atropine to stop the production of the enzymes by the pancreas. Pain killers and antibiotics also are administered, and an apparatus is set up to drain the enzymes from the abdominal cavity.

Chronic pancreatitis has symptoms similar to those of acute pancreatitis, with abdominal pains and loose, fatty, floating stools, the result of faulty fat digestion due to inability of one of the enzymes, lipase, to enter the digestive tract. This fat-digesting enzyme also may no longer be produced in sufficient quantities to handle fatty foods because in chronic pancreatitis fibrous tissue gradually replaces the enzyme factories in the pancreas saccules.

Cancer of the pancreas is an insidious, dangerous disease. It generally is treatable only in the very early stages when the head of the gland, usually the site of the cancer, can be excised and the unaffected portion connected directly to the small intestine. However, cancer of the pancreas produces no early symptoms; the only sign of a possible problem is the appearance of jaundice in the patient's tissues when the disease frequently has advanced to a stage that is not curable.

The Digestive Tract

The liver, gallbladder, and pancreas are only accessories to the main digestive tract, but digestion would not be possible without the contributions of these organs. As we have observed, a seemingly small disturbance in one of the accessory organs can disrupt normal eating and drinking habits for a lifetime. In some cases nearly all normal activities need to be designed to accommodate the erratic behavior of a few microscopic tissue cells in one of the organs.

Although most of the route of the digestive tract lies in the abdomen, the system actually begins in the mouth—or the nose if the sense of smell is included, which it should be. It ends at the anus, where the residue of a meal is expelled from the body.

The digestive tract has many twists and turns. The small intestine alone would stretch for some 20 feet if it were not coiled snugly in the center of the abdomen; the large intestine loops up and around the abdomen for an additional five feet of total length. And there are a series of valve-like structures that control the openings between sections of the digestive tract. Incidentally, if you wonder why the small intestine is longer than the large intestine, the explanation is that the names are determined by the size of the bore, or diameter, of the tubes; the small intestine has a smaller caliber than the large intestine.

The point is, most nutrients consumed in meals never enter the body, at least in the form in which they are eaten; the food simply passes along the digestive tube, while intestinal villi and other structures lining the tube sort out and absorb the bits and pieces of nutrients the vital organs of the body need for normal activities. A swallowed piece of vegetable, for example, might be picked clean of any protein, fat, carbohydrate, vitamins, or minerals it had originally, and the indigestible cellulose framework is excreted; seen under a microscope lens this residue resembles an office building stripped of everything except its steel skeleton.

A related point to remember is that the human body makes its own decisions regarding what it wants in the way of food. You may decide what you would like to eat, but your body may not agree. In extreme cases of disagreement, you may experience effects ranging from indigestion to malnutrition. Fortunately, for most people living in developed countries, there are adequate amounts of essential nutrients in most of the available foods, so the body is not likely to suffer more than temporary deprivations of vitamins or essential amino acids. Certain diseases and disorders of the body require special attention to the diet, as in the case of a person with diabetes mellitus or an individual with congestive heart disease or hypertension who must watch the amount of sodium in his meals. But even these problems usually can be managed with palatable meals that provide all the essential nutrients from a wide variety of meats, dairy products, vegetables and fruits, and breads and cereals.

Going outside the abdomen briefly, but remaining within the digestive system, a quick review of the events leading to the arrival of food in the stomach should begin with the mouth. In case you have been eating for a number of years without having stopped to consider how it is accomplished, you might be interested to know that there is quite a bit of muscle power involved in getting a meal in proper shape for the trip to the stomach.

The tongue itself is a flexible bundle of muscles that can move a piece of food up or down and from side to side. The tongue muscles can contract to produce a top surface that is fairly flat, a surface that is rounded at the top, or one that is concave or hollow at the center. The tongue moves the food between the different types of teeth, which are designed at the front for cutting and tearing, and at the rear of the mouth for grinding. Other species of animals have teeth that are better designed for tearing and cutting, while some have teeth that are more efficient for grinding. The cutting and tearing teeth are the canines; the grinding teeth are the molars. Humans have both canines and molars because people eat a wide variety of foods— meats, grains, etc.—that require some cutting and some grinding.

The cutting and grinding of food requires muscle power. This is supplied by groups of muscle fibers such as the temporalis, which works with the masseter muscles to raise the lower jaw and press the lower teeth against the upper teeth; the pterygoid muscles that move the jaw from side to side when grinding action is needed; and the buccinator muscles of the cheeks, which help move the lump of food around as it is being chewed.

The process of chewing food, known as mastication, molds the food into a soft plastic ball called a bolus. Moisture is provided by the secretion of saliva from salivary glands in the cheeks, under the tongue, and in the floor of the mouth. In addition to moistening the food while it is being molded into a bolus to be swallowed, the saliva contains an enzyme called ptyalin that begins to digest starches while they are still in the mouth. There are other enzymes in the saliva that help destroy bacteria which might be present in the food.

Ptyalin does not affect proteins and fats in the food, and it will aid in the digestion of starchy foods only if they have been cooked before eating. The reason is that starches in nature are enclosed in cellulose envelopes which cannot be penetrated by human digestive juices. Cooking starchy foods, however, results in breaking the envelope so that ptyalin, which is a chemical relative of the enzyme amylase, secreted by the pancreas, can split the starch molecules into smaller units. A starchy food, such as potato, cannot be digested by humans if it is eaten raw. However, some animals other than humans are able to subsist on raw starchy foods because their digestive systems secrete enzymes that break through the cellulose capsules surrounding starches in the raw.

The average human adult produces around one and a half pints of saliva daily. When the saliva is not being used to prepare food boluses to be swallowed, it washes the teeth and interior surfaces of the mouth, keeps the lips, mouth, and throat from becoming dried out, and kills some bacteria with the substance lysozyme, which the saliva contains. Although the antibacteria enzyme lysozyme can kill some disease organisms, there are others that can live in saliva. They include viruses, such as poliomyelitis and mumps viruses. The rabies virus also can live in saliva, which is why the disease can be transmitted by the saliva of a rabid animal.

After the bolus of food is ready to be dropped into the stomach, it is pushed to the back of the mouth by the tongue, which presses upward and backward against the hard palate in the roof of the mouth. At the same time the soft palate beyond the hard palate is raised to close the opening to the nasal cavity, and the cartilage lid of the windpipe, the epiglottis, closes the trachea, while the larynx shifts upward to seal the closure. All this is to prevent the food from being pushed into the trachea instead of the esophagus, which is behind the windpipe.

The Esophagus

The esophagus is a long flexible tube that takes no part in the digestion of food, but serves merely to move the food or beverage from the back of the mouth to the stomach. The esophagus is composed of two layers of muscles, one of which forms a series of circles about the diameter of the food tube; the other has fibers that run the length of the esophagus. The circular set of muscles can contract and relax to help push the bolus through the esophagus, while the longitudinal muscles alternately contract and relax to help move the food along the tube. The route of the food tube is not a straight one between the back of the mouth and the top of the stomach. The esophagus actually curves somewhat as it passes through the neck, and it bends again after reaching the diaphragm to enter the stomach, which is on the left side of the abdomen.

There is a ring of muscles near the top of the esophagus that normally holds the tube closed except when you swallow. At the lower end of the esophagus is another ring of muscle tissue, called a sphincter, that normally is closed except when food is coming through to the stomach. The lower esophageal sphincter prevents a reflux of stomach acid into the esophagus. The reflux of stomach acid, which can occur under certain conditions, produces some of the symptoms associated with heartburn.

The esophagus is somewhat unique in that it passes through several anatomical regions of the body, starting at the head, passing through the neck and chest, and ending in the abdomen. Its total length can be as much as 12 inches, and because of its twists, turns, and sphincters, it can present more than a minor challenge to a physician examining the structure. When inserting instruments into the esophagus, for example, the doctor must have a pretty good idea of where obstacles might be encountered. Also, there is no standard human esophagus; some are longer than average and some are shorter, and in some individuals the stomach is on the right side instead of the left—a condition known as dextrogastria.

Dysphagia, which means difficulty in swallowing, is a symptom of a disorder involving the esophagus. In some instances it is the only symptom of trouble in the esophagus. An obstruction in the esophagus can result in regurgitation of food and loss of weight. If the lower esophageal sphincter has become faulty or weakened, the patient may experience heartburn because of the backflow of gastric juices from the stomach.

The patient may report feeling that food becomes stuck at a point in the chest, behind the sternum, or breastbone. The swallowing difficulty may be accompanied by pain or it may be a painless symptom. Examination may reveal a dilatation of the esophagus because of an accumulation of food near the lower esophageal sphincter, or pouches may form along the route of the esophagus and become filled with food. In either type of food accumulation in the esophagus, there would be symptoms of regurgitation.

Examination of the gullet, another name for the esophagus, may begin by having the patient swallow a "barium meal," a fluid with the consistency of a milk shake but containing radio-opaque barium, which coats the inner walls of the esophagus and outlines the tube in detail for X-ray pictures. An obstruction or narrowing of the esophagus, as well as the length and route of the food tube, will show clearly on the X-ray. The X-ray picture of the esophagus, which the medical personnel may call an esophagram, also is helpful in locating a possible tumor of the esophagus. A cancer of the gullet usually begins with dysphagia and is followed weeks or months later by pain behind the sternum.

The esophagram may be followed by a direct inspection of the gullet with an instrument called an esophagoscope. This long metal tool is quite versatile in that it can be equipped with a light for viewing the interior of the esophagus, and various kinds of forceps can be added for removing foreign objects or taking biopsy tissue samples. An esophagoscopy examination is not undertaken without careful preparation and procedures. The patient is given a general anesthetic in order to obtain complete relaxation of the muscles involved. The neck of the patient must be fully ex-

tended to permit the passage of the esophagoscope through the gullet with a minimum of obstacles. Any dentures worn by the patient must be removed, and the doctor tries to avoid doing any damage to the natural teeth and gums while working with the esophagoscope. The patient is positioned on an operating table with the head extended beyond the edge of the table, and a nurse holds the head in a suitable position while the instrument is inserted and maneuvered in the esophagus.

The esophagoscopy procedure is commonly used to remove a foreign object that has been swallowed. Children frequently swallow small toys, coins, or other objects; older persons with poor teeth or dentures occasionally swallow small bones or improperly chewed pieces of meat. Because the walls of the esophagus are easily punctured, any foreign object that becomes lodged in the gullet must be removed quickly and carefully. It is hazardous for a person who has swallowed a foreign object to take anything further by mouth until the object has been removed, because the simple act of swallowing can force the foreign object to puncture the gullet wall. A tiny puncture is enough to begin leakage from the esophagus into the chest cavity, or mediastinum, causing severe inflammation that can in itself become fatal.

An inflammation of the esophagus, called esophagitis, may be the most common complaint involving the esophagus. The most common cause of esophagitis probably is reflux of gastric juices from the stomach. If the reflux of stomach acid continues without corrective treatment the lining of the lower portion of the gullet will acquire scar tissue that will cause that part of the esophagus to have a stricture, or narrowed opening. The reduced bore of the tube will result in some difficulty in swallowing.

The problem of heartburn, or gastric reflux, occurs most often in persons who are overweight and those who wear tight clothing, which can increase the pressure on the organs within the abdomen. The symptoms of heartburn frequently plague pregnant women in the third trimester of their pregnancy for similar reasons, except that in the case of a pregnant woman the symptoms may disappear after the baby is delivered. For an overweight woman who wears a girdle, the problem is not easily solved.

Older persons, whose lower esophageal sphincter muscles have become weakened, may have to find other solutions to their discomfort. One solution is to avoid situations in which gravity is allowed to aggravate the condition; sleeping with the head and chest raised will help keep the gastric juices in the stomach, and not bending over to pick up objects will have the same effect for a similar reason. The doctor may recommend the use of antacid medications to neutralize excess stomach acid. It's wise to check with the doctor before going this route because there are different formulations in various brands available and some might not agree with other medical problems or medications.

Occasionally, there is bleeding from an inflamed esophagus. Unless the patient vomits or regurgitates some of the blood, he may not be aware of the problem. Food boluses passing over the inflamed membrane will cause periods of bleeding. Eventually, the patient will experience signs and symptoms of anemia because of the blood loss. The doctor may refer to this type of blood loss as occult bleeding, not because it has anything to do with witchcraft but simply because the source of the bleeding is hidden from view.

A disorder of the esophagus that may be associated with hiatus hernia is the development of a peptic ulcer caused by irritation of the mucosal lining of the food tube by gastric juices from the stomach. The esophagus is more vulnerable to the effects of stomach acid than the stomach itself since it lacks the protective layer of mucus that prevents the stomach lining from being digested by gastric acid.

The waves of muscle contractions that push the food bolus through the esophagus is a physiological phenomenon called peristalsis. It is an unconscious act that continues to move food or its residue through the digestive tract beyond the esophagus—unconscious in that the activity of the smooth muscle fibers occurs without conscious effort on the part of the person. Swallowing food begins as a voluntary act, and there usually is a point where you still have some control as to whether or not the mouthful of food is going to be pushed into the pharynx for the trip down the food tube. But once past the stage where the muscles at the back of the throat grasp the food bolus and force it into the esophagus, the food is under the unconscious control of the digestive system.

The Stomach and Its Disorders

The stomach, if it has not received food for a while, is a narrow vertical tube with a sort of bubble, or fundus, that extends beyond the connection with the esophagus at its upper end. It is only after it fills with food and beverage that the stomach takes on the horizontal pear shape usually shown in illustrations. Empty, the stomach looks more like a flabby letter "J," with the fundus usually distended by gas.

Like the esophagus, the stomach has walls made of layers of muscles, some of which run in circles and some longitudinally, or lengthwise. However, the stomach also has a third layer of muscles which run in an oblique pattern. Because the stomach must churn and grind food, particularly pieces of food that were not thoroughly chewed in the mouth, the muscles must be able to move the stomach walls in a variety of ways.

The lining of the stomach contains some 35 million glands that secrete gastric juices of several kinds. The lining forms a number of ridges and folds, especially when the stomach is empty; the folds tend to flatten out as the stomach fills with food. When the stomach lining is flattened the numerous gastric pits are easily visible without a microscope. Gastric juice glands line the walls of the gastric pits and secrete hydrochloric acid, mucin, pepsin, and rennin into the pits, which empty into the stomach.

The hydrochloric acid secreted by the stomach glands is remarkably strong—a fact that has baffled medical scientists for generations. Theoretically, it is too powerful to be tolerated by living cells, but without the hydrochloric acid produced by the gastric juice glands, the stomach would have trouble digesting our meals.

Mucin, a slimy combination of glucose and a protein that forms the mucus, helps protect the stomach lining from being eroded by the digestive juices. Some mucin also is contained in saliva, which is mixed with the food while it is being masticated in the mouth.

Pepsin begins the breakdown of proteins into amino acids, but it takes the protein molecules only through the first stage of digestion. The subunits of proteins, called peptones, are composed of groups of amino acids that will be separated by enzymes secreted by the pancreas. Pepsin works hand-in-glove with rennin to digest milk; the rennin converts milk into curds, which are a form of casein, and the pepsin breaks the casein into peptones.

The activity of the stomach's digestive glands is controlled by several types of stimuli. One is the nervous or psychic stimulus which can cause gastric juices to be secreted by tasting, smelling, or just thinking about food. The second type of stimulus is gastric and involves the control of gastric secretions by food reaching the stomach. Certain substances in foods, particularly protein, have an indirect chemical effect by causing the release of a hormone called gastrin. Gastrin is absorbed into the bloodstream and stimulates the release of gastric juices. A third stimulus is triggered by food entering the small intestine through the pylorus, a sphincter-controlled opening between the stomach and the intestines.

Some stimuli seem to retard the digestive activity of the stomach. One is the ingestion of fats; another is the effect of anger, tension, and anxiety that can turn off the digestive system. The effect of fat ingestion, which seems to work through the small intestine as a chemical stimulus to control stomach activity, frequently is used to retard hunger pangs. Some individuals find that by including a certain amount of fat in a meal they do not get hungry again as quickly as they would if the meal contained only proteins and carbohydrates.

The most active area of digestion in the stomach is the bottom portion. The upper part of the stomach serves as a reservoir for food boluses that will gradually be squeezed into the antrum, or region along the bottom curve of the "J" shape. No solid food normally remains in the antrum after it has been churned by repeated waves of peristalsis into a fluid with the consistency of cream. When it is ready to be passed along to the first section of the small intestine, the fluid is squirted through the pyloric valve. Any bits of solid food are rejected at this point by cells of the pylorus that appear to be able to tell the difference between solids and fluids, and they cause the valve to snap shut if a bit of solid food touches the walls.

Vomiting Contrary to popular notion, vomiting does not occur by any action of the stomach, at least in adults and older children. The act of vomiting is produced by contractions of the diaphragm and abdominal muscles while the esophageal sphincters open. In other words, the stomach is squeezed by muscles that surround it while the mouth and esophagus are held open. A number of different factors can cause the onset of vomiting, including motion that upsets one's equilibrium, as in sea sickness or air sickness, emotional upsets, drugs, foods that contain toxins, or brain disorders. Drugs that inhibit vomiting work by suppressing a vomiting reflex center in the medulla oblongata portion of the brain. Ingested substances that cause vomiting also work by affecting the same reflex center. Certain brain disorders such as tumors or abscesses may affect the vomiting reflex by the pressure of their growth.

Vomiting, or emesis, is a common complaint of patients who visit a doctor about a digestive system problem. With the exception of projectile vomiting, the kind associated with brain disorders and caused by intracranial pressure, the act of vomiting usually is preceded by feelings of nausea. If the unpleasant sensation of nausea accompanies the vomiting, the patient and doctor can assume that a brain disease is not responsible, although this fact might be small comfort for a person in gastric distress. On the other hand, nausea can occur without vomiting.

The examining physician usually will want to know somewhat precisely what sort of vomiting a patient has experienced and how the vomitus appeared. Regurgitation of food without contraction of the abdominal muscles may indicate diverticula, or pouches, on the walls of the esophagus that have become filled with putrified food; an obstruction of the esophagus; or simply an enormous meal that overloaded the stomach. Another form of vomiting, retching, is marked by the failure of the lower esophageal sphincter to open, so that the contents of the stomach cannot be expelled. Still another form of vomiting is characterized by the stomach's expulsion of clear burning fluid called water brash.

Vomited blood is bright red when fresh and a brown coffee-ground color when it has been exposed to the digestive juices in the stomach. It may have been swallowed from a blood loss that originated in the nose, lungs or bronchi, or the mouth. In fact, the blood in vomitus might originate anywhere from the adenoids to the duodenum, and it is a sign of disease or injury that requires further examination and testing. The doctor may order X-ray examinations of the esophagus, stomach, and upper end of the small intestine. He may also order an esophagoscopy and a gastroscopy.

X-ray examinations of the digestive

system generally involve a radio-opaque barium meal. A general anesthetic is administered before an esophagoscopy examination, but a gastroscopy examination usually is done without a general anesthetic, which would interfere with normal stomach activity. The patient is given drugs to make him feel relaxed and to eliminate secretions that might hinder the examination. A local anesthetic for the throat is administered to prevent gagging, and the patient is forbidden to take anything by mouth for 12 hours before the examination.

The gastroscope is a long, flexible instrument that has a light and lenses at the end. It transmits pictures, via glass fibers, that can be recorded as still photographs or movies, thus giving the gastroscope a flexibility lacking in the esophagoscope. Like the esophagoscope, the gastroscope can be used to take biopsy samples of tissues while checking for ulcers, tumors, or other causes of illness.

Ulcers Peptic ulcers that develop in the stomach usually are identified as gastric ulcers. They are most likely to appear in men between the ages of 45 and 55; duodenal ulcers tend to occur most often in men in their 30's. Women develop ulcers as well as men, but during their reproductive years the chances that a woman will have an ulcer is about one-tenth that of a man.

The cause of peptic ulcers is still somewhat controversial, but it is generally agreed that overproduction of gastric juice by stomach glands is a key factor. Peptic ulcers seldom develop in persons whose stomachs are abnormally deficient in gastric acid production. There also are a number of relationships with other possible factors. Because peptic ulcers tend to occur in persons who are closely related to other peptic ulcer patients, there is a strong suspicion that ulcers may run in families. There are also a couple of clues that a tendency toward ulcers may be inherited: ulcer patients are likely to have "O" type blood, an inherited factor, and they lack an inherited blood factor that appears to protect against peptic ulcers.

Since women seem to be protected against peptic ulcers during their fertile years, it has been suggested that a female sex hormone factor may be involved. Finally, peptic ulcers seem to occur in individuals who are plagued with certain other diseases, such as cystic fibrosis, cirrhosis of the liver, pulmonary emphysema, and rheumatoid arthritis.

Whatever the exact cause, peptic ulcers begin as erosions of the membrane lining the wall of the digestive tract between the esophagus and the duodenum. Some peptic ulcers never become more than a shallow hole in the mucous membrane of the gut, but others grow bigger and deeper in a very short time. The latter eventually eat a hole all the way through the muscle layers of the digestive tract, causing blood, digestive juices, and food to leak into the peritoneal cavity, the space between the abdominal organs and the inner wall of the abdomen.

Gastric ulcers, the kind that develop in the lining of the stomach, are similar to those that occur in the duodenum. But in some ways they are more insidious because most gastric ulcers produce no serious symptoms and frequently are not discovered until doctors examine the stomach for other possible disorders, such as a cause for bleeding or perforation of the stomach wall. When symptoms are present, they may be simple complaints of nausea or gas after eating a meal, although a gastric ulcer patient also may suffer from burning or cramping pains, particularly after a meal.

Gastric ulcers generally are benign lesions, but it is not uncommon for a stomach ulcer to evolve into a stomach cancer. In some cases treatment of a stomach cancer may have been delayed because it was assumed that the cancer was a peptic ulcer. In the early stages of growth, an ulcer of the stomach may be mistaken for a cancer, or vice versa.

Treatment of a gastric ulcer may include diet, medications, and surgery. Surgery usually is reserved for the more serious cases that involve perforation, obstruction, bleeding, or failure to respond to purely medical therapy.

Treatment of duodenal ulcers is similar to that used to cure gastric ulcers, with a few exceptions. An example is the use of drugs designed to reduce the production of gastric acid without affecting the ability of the gastric juice to digest food; this technique is used for duodenal ulcers but not for gastric ulcers. Cigarette smoking and the use of caffeine beverages are prohibited as part of the healing process. Greasy, fried foods and foods that add roughage to the diet may be eliminated from the menu of peptic ulcer patients. Milk and other protein foods that have a buffering effect on gastric acid become more important to the daily diet.

Antacids may be administered after meals because the effects last longer than when they are taken before meals. The peptic ulcer patient may receive sedatives or tranquillizers on his doctor's prescription, not because they have a direct effect on the ulcer but rather because they may make the patient less tense and anxious during the healing period.

Peptic ulcers tend to develop in the same stomach areas of most patients. Duodenal ulcers almost always appear about one inch beyond the pyloric valve of the stomach. Gastric ulcers usually occur in the lower part of the organ, a short distance from the pylorus.

It is not unusual for a person to have both a duodenal and a gastric ulcer. For reasons that remain a mystery, the duodenal ulcer almost always develops first, followed by the gastric ulcer.

If the stomach is seriously diseased, surgery may be necessary to remove a part or all of the stomach. A seriously diseased duodenum also may be excised by surgeons. An operation to remove a part or all of the stomach is called a gastrectomy, which is partial or total depending upon how much is removed. A number of variations of this operation can be performed, such as cutting away the lower portion of the stomach and sewing the upper portion to the small intestine, joining the esophagus directly to the small intestine, or joining the top part of the stomach to the portion of the intestine beyond the duodenum. Still another option, depending upon the details of the patient's case, is surgery that severs the vagus nerve, which stimulates the flow of gastric acid.

Special care is required for patients who have undergone a gastrectomy, particularly during the first few weeks after surgery. Removal of the pylorus changes the way in which foods are handled by the digestive system. The patient may experience iron deficiency anemia and a vitamin B-12 deficiency, both of which can be corrected when detected. Food frequently must be taken in a series of small meals that contain a minimum of sugars and starches. Water or other beverages are taken between meals rather than with meals. Otherwise, the patient may suffer from diarrhea, gas, and feelings of nausea and distension.

Cancer of the Stomach Stomach cancer, like peptic ulcers, appears to be associated with genetic factors and food habits. Men are more likely to develop stomach cancer than women, and the incidence is highest among older persons, with perhaps 95 percent of the patients being over the age of 40. Stomach cancer is more likely to affect a person who has a close relative afflicted with the disease than an individual whose family is free of stomach cancer. Persons with "A" type blood are reportedly favored as targets of the disease. Stomach cancer is relatively uncommon in North America, compared to parts of Asia, South America, and eastern Europe, suggesting a cultural food factor as a culprit. Perhaps not surprisingly, persons with a medical history of gastritis, or inflammation of the stomach mucosa, have a better than average chance of developing stomach cancer.

Symptoms of stomach cancer are quite varied. Some patients complain of nausea, a feeling of fullness, or loss of appetite; others report severe, steady pains. Weight loss and anemia are possible signs of the disease.

As in examination for peptic ulcers, doctors may diagnose stomach cancer through X-rays, gastroscopy, and laboratory tests. But in baffling cases, a form of exploratory surgery may be required to make sure the problem is stomach cancer rather than another disorder.

The most effective treatment for stomach cancer is surgical removal of the growth, along with any nearby tissues that may have acquired some of the cancer cells by metastatis, a term used to describe the way in which malignant tumor cells migrate from one organ or body area to another by floating along in the bloodstream. A gastrectomy generally is performed to reroute the digestive system in the same kind of patterns used to repair the stomach of gastric ulcer patients. Chemotherapy and/or radiation therapy also may be administered to prolong the life of the stomach cancer patient.

Some persons with stomach cancer, as well as those who have experienced a partial gastrectomy, may be faced with a complication of achlorhydria, a medical term indicating a lack of gastric acidity. The condition can affect patients with a variety of other disorders, including tuberculosis, parasitic infections, kidney disease, and alcoholism. The signs and symptoms might be diarrhea or constipation and, sooner or later, the effects of pernicious anemia. The treatment for achlorhydria generally provides for administration of a form of hydrochloric acid with meals, plus medications to control related effects such as diarrhea.

Gastritis Stomach irritants do not always lead to ulcers or stomach cancer. The effects may be in the nature of dyspepsia, or gastritis. Alcohol, spices, hot foods, certain chemicals used in industry and in medications, and foods that are associated with individual allergies can cause acute gastritis. In some instances the substance produces inflammation severe enough to lead to internal bleeding. The gastritis of some infectious diseases, such as influenza, scarlet fever, and diphtheria, can cause erosions of the stomach lining with damage to the underlying blood vessels.

Symptoms of acute gastritis are familiar to most persons who have suffered one kind of stomach upset or another—nausea with or without vomiting, headache, dizziness, fullness or pressure in the abdominal region, and possibly exhaustion. In severe cases associated with the ingestion of poisonous chemicals, the patient may experience disturbances of the heartbeat, cyanosis or a bluish tint to the complexion because of lack of oxygen circulating in the red blood cells, severe abdominal pain and tenderness, and in some cases, extreme thirst and difficulty in swallowing.

Relief for symptoms of acute gastritis depend in part on the cause, if known. For that reason the examining doctor will want to know what substances the patient may have ingested, accidentally or in food and drink, and any history of allergies to substances consumed. He may look for signs of the agent apparently responsible for the stomach problem; these might include traces of the offending substance about the lips or mouth, or a sample of the vomitus, so it can be analyzed.

If the patient has vomited, the symptoms may become less severe. If vomiting has not occurred, the doctor may advise inducing the process of emptying the stomach, or he may recommend gastric lavage, which means simply washing out the stomach. Induced vomiting isn't always recommended, especially when the gastritis may be caused by petroleum products such as gasoline or kerosene, or corrosive acids or alkalis. Gastric lavage may be performed by inserting a tube into the stomach and flooding it with water briefly, then pumping out the water which will have diluted the offending agent. The washing and pumping may be repeated until all available traces of the substance have been removed.

If acute gastritis has been caused by bad food or the flu, the follow-up treatment may consist mainly of bed rest and a light diet of tea, bouillon, etc. When the problem is caused by a poisonous substance, immediate treatment usually consists of emergency measures such as administering antidotes and analgesics, clearing the digestive tract as quickly and carefully as possible, and giving blood or other intravenous fluids as needed to maintain normal blood circulation. If the ingested substance is a corrosive chemical, emergency surgery may be required to repair damage to the stomach and to prevent leakage of fluids from the digestive tract into the peritoneal cavity.

Chronic gastritis, a form of stomach inflammation that is less severe but continues for a relatively long period of time, may have symptoms similar to those of peptic ulcer. The patient may have some of the same conditions as those of persons with achlorhydria or pernicious anemia. An examination by gastroscopy and tissue biopsy may be required to give the doctor information he needs for a proper diagnosis. When the cause has been determined, the treatment could be like that advised for either peptic ulcer or achlorhydria patients. The doctor also may recommend a bland diet with vitamin and mineral supplements if it is necessary for the patient to give up meats or fruit juices. In most cases of chronic gastritis, the patient will have to avoid spices, alcoholic beverages, smoking, and certain medications that can aggravate an inflammation of the mucosal lining of the stomach—at least temporarily.

Persons who have been immobilized by a serious illness or injury may develop a condition called gastric dilatation, in which the stomach loses much of its muscle tone and fills with gas or fluid. The disorder may follow a serious accident involving the chest or abdomen. There may be symptoms of fullness, vomiting or regurgitation of food, severe thirst, and breathing difficulties due to distension of the abdomen to a point where the diaphragm is pushed upward against the lungs. The distension and vomiting are associated with abdominal pain. The loss of body fluids through vomiting can upset the normal balance of vital mineral salts in the tissues.

Therapy includes emptying the stomach by suction through a tube that may remain in place for hours or days, medications to help relieve the distension, replacement of fluids, and the use of intravenous solutions to replace lost minerals.

Pyloric stenosis, or a restriction of the pyloric valve between the stomach and small intestine because of a muscular overgrowth, can occur at any age but is most common among infants. Vomiting and the associated loss of weight and dehydration are among the signs of pyloric stenosis. The only cure is a special kind of surgical procedure in which the surgeon carefully separates the muscle fibers of the pylorus without puncturing the mucous membrane lining the digestive tract. Such an operation, obviously, must be approached from the outer surface of the pylorus. An incision is made through the outer coat of the pylorus and along the length of the outer muscle fibers. As the inner muscle fibers are teased apart, they lose their tight constrictive hold over the small opening through which digested food from the stomach must pass.

The Peritoneum

The abdominal cavity has a lining similar to the pleural membrane layers of the chest. The membrane that lines the inner walls of the abdominal cavity, including the underside of the diaphragm, with a second layer that covers much of the abdominal organs, is called the peritoneum. As in the chest, the membrane along the walls is called the parietal layer, and the membrane that covers the organs is known as the visceral layer of the peritoneum. However, the peritoneal membrane does not extend over the entire cavity of the abdomen. The pancreas, the kidneys and ureter, and part of the duodenum in the upper part of the abdomen, for example, are not included in the peritoneal cavity, although they are in the abdominal cavity.

Of more significance, for some doctors at least, is the fact that there are a couple of apron-like layers of peritoneal membrane called the lesser and greater omentum. The lesser omentum is so called because it has only two folds, while the greater omentum has four folds. The lesser omentum covers the stomach; the greater omentum covers part of the intestines. The membranes of the abdomen do have job responsibilities in maintaining the health of the human, as do most tissues and organs in the body; nature is seldom wasteful about the use of building materials provided, but it is quick to discard items that are not needed for the foreseeable future. In the case of the peritoneal membranes, they help suspend the viscera from the abdominal walls, and in certain emergencies they may serve as adhesive bandages. If a perforation occurs in the bowel, for example, part of the peritoneum will become attached to the area to seal the opening.

Small Intestine

The small intestine is supported by part of the peritoneum that is attached to the back of the abdominal wall, at a point about level with the belly button. It is partly because of this attachment to the membrane, called a mesentery, that enables the 20-some feet of gut to twist and turn through an abdominal cavity area that is perhaps only one foot square.

The small intestine comes in three sections, with distinctions barely noticeable to anyone other than a doctor. The first section, and the shortest, is the duodenum, which has already been mentioned as the portion that receives the creamy-looking chyme, the partly digested food from the stomach. The duodenum also receives the bile from the gallbladder and various digestive juices from the pancreas. It also is the most common location for a peptic ulcer.

The duodenum is barely a foot in length, and much of that distance is built into a curve that fits around the head of the pancreas. It has only two layers of muscles, compared to the three layers of the stomach; one inner layer runs in circles around the duodenum, and the outer layer runs lengthwise. This arrangement makes it possible for the intestine to continue the business of peristalsis, or squeezing the digested food along in snakelike wave motions. One layer of muscles contracts while the other relaxes, alternately, to produce the waves of peristalsis.

The inner surface of the small intestine resembles a carpet that has been folded in numerous small wrinkles. The wrinkles or folds are covered with intestinal villi, the "pile" of the carpeting. The many folds and hairlike villi are another of nature's tricks for covering as much area as possible in a minimum amount of space. If the inside layer of the small intestine could be spread flat the surface would cover an area of about 90 square feet—a good bit

of exposure for a tube with a length of about 20 feet.

The villi are in almost constant motion, bobbing and weaving as the digested food passes through the folds. The action enhances the exposure of the villi, which are covered with cells adapted for absorbing nutrients from the digested food. At the center of each villus is a lymph gland, called a lacteal because it frequently is filled with a milky fluid, and a network of fine blood capillaries.

In the spaces between villi are glands that secrete additional digestive juices into the small intestine. Glands in the mucosal layer of the small intestine secrete mucus which helps protect the inside of the small intestine from erosion by digestive juices, although by the time the meal has reached the lower portion of the duodenum, most of the gastric acid has been neutralized by other fluids in the digestive tract. The total daily volume of fluids secreted by the small intestine of the average adult is about three quarts, which is an amount approximately equal to the combined secretions of the saliva glands, stomach glands, liver, and pancreas.

More important, however, is the work of the small intestine in absorbing whatever passes through the myriad folds of villi. The small intestine daily absorbs nearly eight quarts of fluids, an amount that includes nearly all of the saliva and assorted digestive juices from the stomach, gallbladder, pancreas, and its own gland, plus the fluids contained in foods and beverages. Only about a pint of fluid is passed along to the large intestine, where most of it is absorbed as feces are formed.

The nutrients absorbed by the villi enter the bloodstream through the network of capillaries and are routed to the liver and other organs to be used in building, repairing, and otherwise maintaining normal body functions. Generally, the contents of a meal have been broken down into fatty acids, amino acids, sugar molecules, mineral salts, or similar basic units before they are absorbed. The villi can be quite selective about which substances are absorbed and which are not absorbed, reinforcing the law that the person selects what he wants to eat but the body makes the final decision about what it wants to keep from the meal. A bit of protein that was fried in fat, for example, may be rejected by the intestinal villi because it has been transformed into an unrecognizable chemical compound that would not yield a usable amino acid. Or through one of the body's mysterious biochemical feedback systems, the villi may have been alerted to accept no more iron molecules because the body was overstocked with them.

Carbohydrates, in the form of sugar molecules, and proteins, in the form of amino acids, are absorbed from the chyme in the intestine by being combined with a substance on the surface of the villi cells, and then are carried into the capillary network on the other side of the cell layer. Fats, however, are absorbed by a sort of diffusion process whereby the fatty acids pass through the villi walls and into the lymphatic reservoirs in the center of the villi.

After moving through the duodenum, food being digested enters the second segment of the small intestine, the jejunum. Except for the fact that the jejunum is about eight feet long, compared to only one foot of duodenum, the inside of this second segment looks like the inside of the first segment. The digestive processes in the duodenum and the jejunum are essentially the same. However, the folds of villi

gradually diminish in the third segment, the 12-foot-long ileum, and are absent entirely at the lower end of that part of the small intestine.

At the end of the small intestine, where it joins the large intestine, is another in the series of valves that control the movement of meals from the mouth to the anus. The valve separating the small and large intestines is the ileocolic valve, appropriately named because the ileum is on one side and the ascending colon is on the other. The ileocolic valve opens to allow the contents of the ileum to be swept into the colon during a peristaltic wave. The valve is designed like a floodgate that allows material to move in one direction but not in the opposite direction. Fortunately, this protects the small intestine from a backflow of fecal material in the large intestine. In fact, an enema that would irrigate the ascending colon does not get beyond the ileocolic valve.

Large Intestine

The large intestine, as noted earlier, is shorter than the small intestine; the total length from the cecum, the beginning portion, to the end is about five feet. It normally loops up along the right side of the abdomen, then crosses over to the left side along the lower edge of the stomach and liver, and drops down again along the left side before curving back toward the center to form the rectum.

Except for absorbing most of the remaining water in the digested food, the large intestine performs no digestive function. In that respect it is similar to the esophagus in merely moving along its contents to the next stage of the digestive process. Glands in the large intestine secrete mucus that serves as a lubricant to help move fecal material to the end of the line.

There are no folds or villi on the inner surface of the large intestine. However, there are bands of longitudinal muscles that draw the large intestine into pouches.

The sections of the large intestine generally are identified as the ascending colon, the transverse colon, and the descending colon, depending upon which way the gut is going within the abdominal cavity. The large bowel also is sometimes segmented into the cecum, the blind pouch at the beginning where the ileocolic valve is located; the colon, which covers most of the length of the large intestine; the rectum; and the anal canal. The large intestine is largest in the cecum and the rectum; it narrows somewhat in the middle stretch of gut.

The appendix, technically known as the vermiform appendix because it resembles a slender worm about three inches in length, extends below the cecum. The appendix occasionally may become inflamed—a condition commonly known as appendicitis. The artery supplying the organ can become blocked, as by thrombosis, causing the death of wall tissues, which may become perforated, spilling contents of the intestine into the peritoneal cavity. Such an event sometimes is described as a ruptured appendix, which can be quite serious because the intestine is a storehouse of bacteria. Leakage of the bacteria-laced intestinal contents into the peritoneal cavity produces a disorder called peritonitis, which can be fatal if not corrected as quickly as possible. Before the development of modern surgical techniques, acute appendicitis usually ended in the death of the patient.

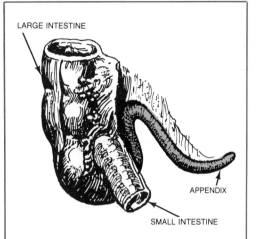

LARGE INTESTINE

APPENDIX

SMALL INTESTINE

Drawing of a portion of the intestinal tract at the junction of the small and large intestine, showing the location of the appendix in the lower right corner of the abdomen. Digested food from the small intestine passes through a valve-like opening into the large intestine. Inflammation of the wormlike appendix, resulting in the painful symptoms of appendicitis, can be caused by a bacterial infection as well as other factors. Usually, the most effective way to treat an inflamed appendix is to remove it surgically before it develops gangrene or ruptures and leaks pus and other infectious material into the abdomen.

Even today, appendicitis can be a serious problem and a doctor should be consulted when symptoms of the disorder occur. They include abdominal pain that seems to originate in the lower right side of the abdomen, followed soon after by nausea and vomiting. There usually is extreme tenderness in the region of the appendix. The patient generally has a fever with temperatures around 101 to 103 degrees Fahrenheit. The doctor examining the patient probably will recommend hospitalization and laboratory tests to check the white cell count in the blood, if time and other conditions permit. If the appendix ruptures, vomiting which may have stopped is likely to begin again, the fever may rise, and the white blood cell count will increase. Surgery is the treatment for either acute appendicitis or its sequel, the ruptured appendix.

A person who has an epigastric pain, or belly ache in plain language, should not be given a laxative if the pain is accompanied by vomiting or other signs or symptoms of acute appendicitis. The action of the laxative in producing an induced bowel movement can by itself cause a ruptured appendix.

Although the large intestine undergoes peristalsis, it is not the same as the peristaltic waves of the digestive tract on the other side of the ileocolic valve, where there may be somewhat rhythmic churning and squeezing actions. A peristaltic wave in the large intestine tends to occur at intervals when the bowel pushes a batch of fecal material into the rectum, after which there may be no peristaltic action until another batch of fecal material is ready to be swept into the rectum. The movement of feces into the rectum, a sort of holding pouch at the end of the colon, may stimulate the individual to have a bowel movement.

A band of circular muscle fibers in the wall at the end of the bowel forms a sphincter valve that normally holds the feces in the rectum until the bowel movement begins. A bowel movement involves a complex patterning of nerve and muscle actions that can be described in a rather simple manner as a combined voluntary contraction of abdominal muscles and diaphragm holding while the larynx is closed. This increases abdominal pressure on the lower end of the bowel, and the anal sphincter is relaxed to release the feces.

Intestinal Disorders

The traditional health education advice about training the bowel to move in a regular pattern is not without medical foundation. If a person develops a habit of planning a bowel movement each day at a particular time, such as soon after breakfast, the bowel adapts easily to that pattern. If the bowel is not emptied at regular intervals, however, it can adapt to the habit of holding the feces in the rectum. This is not necessarily a dangerous situation; people in some parts of the world train their bowels to go for several days between movements. But there is a risk that water will continue to be absorbed from feces held in the bowel, so that the fecal material becomes increasingly drier and less plastic. Bowel movements may become difficult and a condition of constipation can result.

A complication of constipation frequently is a swelling of the blood veins in the anal canal, a condition known as hemorrhoids, or piles. Hemorrhoids are actually a case of varicose veins in the anus, and the act of straining to have a bowel movement usually aggravates the hemorrhoid condition that may have been caused by constipation in the first place. Nevertheless, true constipation generally is a matter of individual discomfort; each person has his or her own idea of what a regular bowel movement should be, and the doctor may become involved in the problem only when the patient complains about chronic constipation, which may be characterized by symptoms of headache, listlessness, a feeling of fullness, and digestive disturbances.

An obstruction in the bowel, which can be the result of a strangulated hernia, a tumor, fecal impaction because of dehydration, or abuse of laxatives, causes chronic constipation. The condition not uncommonly occurs in some individuals whose work routine interferes with regular meals and other regularities. The danger in using laxatives is that the bowel can become "hooked" on the substances that stimulate bowel movements. When the bowel becomes dependent upon a daily dose of laxative to get moving, increasingly larger doses are needed to produce the desired results. If a patient really needs a laxative to produce a bowel movement, perhaps because of painful hemorrhoids, he should discuss the matter with his doctor because various laxatives and cathartics work in different ways, some of which may be better than others, depending upon the individual's problem.

Some people are concerned about a possible danger from bacteria and toxic substances contained in fecal material. At one time it was a popular notion that self-poisoning could occur if one did not empty the bowel frequently, using laxatives or enemas if necessary. There is little danger, however, that the toxins in feces are a threat to other tissues except in a case of accidental injury or perforation of the bowel.

Development of Pouches (Diverticulitis) Diverticulitis is a disorder of the intestinal tract that is rather common in men and women over the age of 50. It is caused by the development of diverticula, or pouches, in the wall of the intestine. A diverticulum usually develops at a point along the intestinal wall where the muscle layers have become weakened, or where a blood vessel penetrates the wall of the bowel.

Diverticula can occur without any particular signs or symptoms. There may be signs of intestinal bleeding, which results in a maroon coloration of the patient's feces. Or there may be symptoms of constipation if feces accumulate in the diverticula and become hard and impacted. Eventually, a diverticulum may become inflamed, and the inflammation may spread to other portions of the intestine. The bowel may have spasms, and the patient will develop a fever and complain of lower abdominal pain. If the bowel becomes perforated as a result of the inflammation, the condition will be complicated by peritonitis.

In many cases diverticulitis will subside with treatment that includes medications to relieve constipation and the pain of muscle spasms, and antibiotics to control bacteria involved in the inflammation process. The condition also can develop into an emergency that requires immediate surgery to correct.

Diverticula can develop at almost any point along the intestines, from the duodenum to the colon, but the pouches or herniations in the intestinal wall tend to have differing characteristics in different sections of the gut. This fact sometimes helps the doctor diagnose the source of the problem. Duodenal diverticulosis, for example, rarely produces symptoms of inflammation or abdominal pain, whereas diverticula in the next segment of the small intestine, the jejunum, can be the cause of severe inflammation, perforation, bleeding, and such complications as abscesses and leakage into the peritoneal cavity.

Other diverticula can develop in the ileum, including a type that occurs occasionally in the area of the ileocolic valve and is called Meckel's diverticulum, and in the colon. The symptoms of Meckel's diverticulum may be similar to those of appendicitis, but frequently include a sign of gastrointestinal bleeding which can be identified by its color as originating in the gut below the stomach.

Symptoms of pain and tenderness on the left side of the abdomen can suggest diverticulitis of the colon, especially in older persons. Numerous small pouches begin to develop in the wall of the colon in some people after middle age. The pouches, or diverticula, trap bits of feces and become inflamed. The inflammation can lead to abscesses and the diverticula can rupture.

Diverticulosis of the colon can be accompanied by signs of obstruction, marked by alternating periods of constipation and diarrhea, pain, and flatulence, which means excessive gas formation in the gut. The signs and symptoms are quite similar to those of cancer of the colon, so the doctor may order a barium enema administered in order that X-ray pictures can be taken of the gut. If the X-ray film indicates the presence of a diverticulum rather than a cancer, the doctor has a better idea of how the case should be handled. In either instance, surgery may be needed to correct the problem. Surgery for diverticulitis generally is directed toward removing the diseased portions of the gut and restoring the remainder of the intestinal tract so that it will function normally.

Medical treatment, which may be followed in an effort to restore normal function without surgery, usually consists of physical rest, medications including antibiotics, and diet, which can be high fiber, low residue, liquid, or some other variation including intravenous feeding, depending upon the individual case. In some instances, sedatives or tranquillizers may be prescribed. A few patients have found relief from the barium enemas used in diagnosis because the barium apparently fills the diverticula and prevents irritation by the other substances in the gut.

Twisting of the Bowel (Volvulus) Once in a while a segment of the intestine may become twisted so that obstruction occurs because of the kink or "knot" that develops in the gut. The twisted coil of intestine, called a volvulus, can be a cause of abdominal pain and constipation. When a volvulus develops in the colon, the gut becomes distended by the accumulation of food residue, the vessels supplying blood to the affected area may become occluded, and gangrene of the gut then becomes a serious complication.

For reasons unknown, volvulus of both the small and large intestine is more likely to occur in a tropical or subtropical climate than in a temperate region. If the disorder is detected early, it can be corrected in most cases by surgery to simply arrange the loop of intestine in a way that eliminates the kink and permits normal functions to resume.

Hernias A strangulated hernia involving the intestine is a common and dangerous disorder. Frequently identified simply as a hernia, or rupture, the condition involves the protrusion of a part of the intestine through the abdominal wall. The hernia tends to occur at one of the normal openings in the tissues that ordinarily hold the gut in place. Among the common sites are the inguinal canal, a small tunnel through which a man's spermatic cord passes from the abdominal cavity to the scrotum; the umbilicus; and the femoral area where large blood vessels pass between the abdomen and the leg.

Although an inguinal hernia is most likely to occur in a man, or boy, the disorder also can affect a girl or woman since the abdominal wall tissues of the area are similar, even if there is no spermatic cord involved. An inguinal hernia may appear as a bulge in the wall of the lower abdomen, on either the left or right side, or in some cases the segment of intestine may push into the scrotum. In some individuals a bilateral hernia may appear, that is, a hernia on both the left and right sides of the abdomen at the same time.

The doctor usually will look for signs of hernias during a general physical examination. A hernia in the early stage may not cause noticeable symptoms, but the problem will generally progress from minor to major in a matter of time, so it is important that the condition be corrected before the hernia becomes incarcerated, or strangulated.

A strangulated hernia is one in which the loop or portion of intestine becomes trapped in the tissue fibers of the abdominal wall. The intestine becomes pinched by the tissue and obstructed. A strangulated hernia is an emergency health problem. In addition to the serious symptoms that can include intense pain, vomiting, and shock, there is a danger that vital tissues of the organ will die as blood flow to the intestine is interrupted by swelling and inflammation.

In the early stages an inguinal hernia may be reducible, which means that the doctor examining the patient can push the gut back up into the abdomen. Also, the hernia may protrude only when the patient is standing; when he is lying on his back, the hernia will disappear as the gut drops back into the abdomen. During a general examination the doctor may put his finger against the inguinal ring and ask the patient to cough. The doctor can tell by the way the intestine pushes back against his finger during the cough whether the patient has a hernia problem and, if so, which way it is likely to protrude through the inguinal ring, or the tissue opening in the abdomen.

A femoral hernia frequently is overlooked because it usually makes a smaller bulge and often is concealed by fatty tissue in the upper leg area. Strangulation of a femoral hernia sometimes is associated with a thrombus in a varicose vein of the leg.

A hernia that has not yet reached the stage of being strangulated, or incarcerated, is easily repaired with surgery that closes the opening in the abdominal wall and reinforces or strengthens it if necessary. The operation usually requires only a brief stay in a hospital; some patients undergo surgery in the morning and return home in the evening. Either a general or a local anesthetic is administered, depending upon the patient's and the surgeon's preference.

Tumors Most tumors of the bowel occur in the large intestine. Tumors that occur in the small intestine generally are not malignant and do not produce symptoms. When they are detected, it often is in connection with some other problem involving the gut, such as an appendectomy. Small intestine tumors may be hard to diagnose and are located by detailed examination of a patient who complains of abdominal distress or experiences gastrointestinal bleeding that cannot be explained by X-rays or other usual procedures. Cancers of the small intestine are most likely to occur in patients who have been plagued by other gastrointestinal disorders, such as regional enteritis, for a long period of time.

Cancer of the large intestine, on the other hand, is relatively common and accounts for nearly as many deaths in America as lung cancer—about 40,000 each year. As with many other human health disorders, cancer of the colon can be cured if detected in the early stages. Nearly three-fourths of all the cancers of the large intestine occur in the descending colon-to-rectum segment. This portion of the bowel is rather easily examined by a doctor with a sigmoidoscope, an instrument equipped with a lens and light for viewing the inner walls of the bowel.

Cancers of the colon generally develop from glandular tissues in the mucous membrane lining of the gut. The most common signs of cancer of the colon are the appearance of blood in the feces (or stools, as the fecal deposits may be identified) and iron-deficiency anemia resulting from loss of blood. The bloody stools usually are noticed by the patient. However, if bleeding from a cancer involves the beginning portion of the large intestine, that is, on the right side near the appendix, the blood may not be as noticeable because it would have had time to become well mixed with fecal material. In cases of cancer involving the right side, or ascending colon, the effects of anemia may be the first clues that all is not well.

A general feeling of illness, loss of appetite, and a resulting loss of weight may accompany the cancer-bleeding signs. The changes in bowel habits associated with cancer involve variations in the frequency of bowel movements and the size of the stools, possibly because of a cancerous ob-

struction of the rectal area of the bowel. But there also may be a feeling after bowel movements that the bowel evacuation was incomplete.

See also Chapter 16: *Cancer.*

Nonmalignant tumors of the large intestine are generally polyps that develop in the mucous membrane and extend into the open portion of the intestinal tract. Some medical studies suggest that up to 15 percent of the adult population develops one or more polyps in the colon, although these tumors rarely produce symptoms and usually are less than a half-inch in length. Polyps that increase in diameter and produce symptoms such as bleeding should be removed because they may become cancerous. In most cases, polyps of the descending colon can be removed by an instrument inserted through the rectum, thereby avoiding the need for surgery that would require an abdominal incision.

Bowel Surgery Not uncommon as a part of the treatment of a disease or injury affecting the small or large intestine is an operation to create an ostomy, or artificial opening, between the gut and the abdominal wall. An ostomy also may be constructed between the urinary tract and the outside of the abdomen. An ostomy may be a temporary opening to drain the contents of one part of the intestinal tract while the remainder of the gut is recovering from a wound or disease. Or it may be constructed as a permanent solution to a problem involving the gut.

A colostomy is constructed as part of the treatment for a disease of the colon such as cancer. A temporary colostomy usually is constructed so that an opening in the abdominal wall is located in the middle of the transverse colon, the segment that runs horizontally across the abdomen, just below the stomach. When a permanent colostomy is constructed because the rectum must be removed, the colostomy opens through the lower left area of the abdominal wall.

A similar type of surgery performed to provide an exit through the abdominal wall for the small intestine usually is an ileostomy. An ileostomy may be constructed when both the colon and rectum must be removed from the body. However, it is more commonly used to treat inflammatory bowel disease when it is important to divert the flow of intestinal material while the remainder of the tract heals. For example, if the intestinal flow itself might aggravate the condition and delay recovery, a temporary diversion provided by an ileostomy may be needed.

In a typical ostomy operation a loop of intestine is pulled through an incision in the abdomen, and a supporting rod is placed under the loop to help prevent the bowel from slipping back into the abdomen; the bowel also is sewn to the abdominal wall. The bowel loop is cut and the upper end, called a spigot, is fitted with a faceplate and drainable bag, into which the residue of meals will drain. The lower end of the bowel becomes nonfunctional until the problem requiring the ostomy is cured, after which the two ends can be rejoined in a normal manner beneath the abdominal wall, and normal bowel functions can be resumed.

Patients with colostomies usually eat the same kind of meals that persons without colostomies eat. However, if they are bothered by odors and gas exiting from the stoma, or the opening through the abdominal wall, they quickly learn which foods to avoid. They can either eliminate the beans and cabbage, or whatever, from

their meals, or use charcoal tablets, antacids, or other easily available medications that help control the problem.

Colostomy patients learn to empty the bowel by irrigating it through the stoma with a daily enema. A cone-tipped irrigator is inserted into the stoma and about a quart of warm water is allowed to flow into the opening from an enema bag placed about shoulder high. The return flow usually comes in two stages about 30 minutes apart. After completing this routine, the patient can shower and cover the stoma with a plastic cap device designed for that purpose. He then may resume his normal activities for the rest of the day. The patient can wear a plastic bag under his clothing if he feels insecure about possible leakage from the gut through the stoma. But in most cases the colostomy patient finds that a morning irrigation routine performed each day takes care of the matter, and that a plastic cap fitted over the opening and held in place with adhesive sealant is all that is necessry.

Inflammation of the Bowels An increasingly common type of inflammation of the small intestine is known as regional enteritis, or sometimes as Crohn's disease. Originally, doctors believed it was a disorder involving only sections of the ileum, but in recent years it has been found to involve the wall of the gastrointestinal tract anywhere from the esophagus to the colon. The disease may involve all of the layers of the intestinal wall as well as the mesentery membrane that holds the gut in place and the neighboring lymph nodes. The disorder causes the intestinal wall and the mesentery to become red and swollen with fluid. In one form of the disease the neighboring coils of intestine may stick to each other and perforate, so that a fistula, or fleshy tube, connects the segments and allows the contents of one segment to mix with the other. Or the bowel may fuse with the bladder.

The symptoms have been described as similar to those of appendicitis except that the abdominal pain, nausea, fever, and loss of appetite can continue for weeks or months. Other effects may include loss of weight, intestinal obstruction, or diarrhea. Treatment varies according to the individual case but generally includes complete bed rest, especially during acute attacks, drugs to control pain, and a diet that helps maintain adequate nutrition and fluid balance.

Ulcerative colitis is a disease of the mucous membrane lining of the colon. Like regional enteritis, the specific cause of the disease is unknown, although there is evidence to support a number of theories that involve disease organisms, reactions to foods, and changes in the patient's body chemistry. The usual symptoms are abdominal pain, fever, weight loss, and bloody diarrhea. The patient may have from four or five to as many as 20 bowel movements per day. Because the disease tends to cause the walls of the bowel to become abnormally thin, perforation of the bowel is a possible complication. Both men and women of all ages, from children through the elderly population, can be afflicted with ulcerative colitis, and the disease may have particularly severe effects in pregnant women.

Treatment of acute cases requires bed rest in a hospital, where trained personnel are immediately available to help with the sometimes unpredictable effects of an attack. Regular meals may be replaced with a liquid diet, or in some cases by intravenous feedings that give the bowel a chance to rest. Drugs to control pain, diar-

rhea, and other symptoms are administered. A small percentage of ulcerative colitis patients undergo colectomy, or surgery to remove the colon, as the final solution to treatment of the disorder.

Hemorrhoids Hemorrhoids, commonly known as piles, occur as a result of the swelling of blood veins in the anal canal. They are quite similar to the varicose veins that develop in the legs of some persons. The disorder gets its medical name from the identity of the blood vein involved, the hemorrhoidal vein. Internal hemorrhoids occur in the anal canal, and external hemorrhoids are outside the anus. Both types of hemorrhoids are common and occur most frequently in persons of middle age, although they can affect children in their teens as well.

The symptoms of hemorrhoids include the loss of blood during defecation, with the result that stools and toilet tissue become stained a bright red, and the discomfort of a prolapsed vein when the enlarged blood vessel pushes through the anus. The blood loss can result in anemia and there may be other complications of thrombosis or infection.

Hemorrhoids that become permanently prolapsed or complicated by thrombosis are treated by surgery. In less severe cases the doctor may treat hemorrhoids by injecting a solution that helps shrink the swollen vein or by having the patient take sitz baths, which provide moist heat. Medications may be prescribed to soften the stools, since straining during a bowel movement tends to aggravate a case of hemorrhoids.

Tapeworm There are several kinds of worms, or helminths, that may find a temporary or permanent home in the human intestinal tract. One is the beef tapeworm, which is rarely found in North America but may be acquired by travelers in eastern Europe, Asia, Africa, and Latin America who eat meals containing raw or undercooked beef. The tapeworm embryo is contained in a kind of cyst in the flesh of cattle that have eaten vegetation contaminated by tapeworm eggs. About two months after beef containing a cyst is eaten by a human, an adult tapeworm develops in his small intestine, attached to the wall by a set of four suckers in the head of the worm. Eventually, the tapeworm may grow to a length of 15 or more feet. Symptoms include weight loss, diarrhea, and abdominal discomfort. Treatment is by the administration of drugs that kill the head of the worm, called a scolex, and destroy the segments behind the head that contain tapeworm eggs.

A similar kind of tapeworm, the pork tapeworm, enters the human digestive tract when undercooked pork is eaten. Like the beef tapeworm, the pork tapeworm attaches itself to the inner wall of the small intestine. Treatment also is by taking medications that kill the worm and its eggs, or embryos, so that they are excreted through the bowel. Prevention is fairly simple: meat should be thoroughly cooked before eating, even if the meat presumably has been inspected for signs of tapeworm cysts.

Protozoa, one-celled organisms such as ameba, also can enter the human digestive tract and produce illness. A disease called amebiasis is caused by the biggest troublemaker of a half-dozen types of ameba that may pass through the gut. In some people the presence of the parasite produces no symptoms. But it can produce diarrhea and dysentery. Loose stools containing mucus and blood may be associated with the diarrhea, along with cramps and gas. Sometimes the ameba invades the appendix and produces symptoms of appendicitis. Treatment includes medications that relieve the symptoms and kill the parasitic amebas.

The Spleen and Its Disorders

The spleen is an organ of the abdomen that frequently is ignored or overlooked, probably because it is hard to describe its size and functions, which vary according to the age of the person and other factors. At birth the spleen may be a tiny, half-ounce organ responsible for the manufacture of red blood cells. In adult life the spleen may be ten times larger than in infancy and may be involved in the destruction of red blood cells. Under certain conditions, however, the spleen may return in adult life to manufacturing red blood cells, and it may become smaller in size after late middle age.

The spleen is located between the stomach and the diaphragm at the top of the abdominal cavity. It is about four or five inches long, and is little more than an inch in thickness; the coloration is dark purple because of the numerous blood vessels on the inside. The spleen controls the red blood cells of the body by culling aged cells and helping to salvage the chemical components for new red blood cells. The spleen also has a protective responsibility as part of the lymphatic system; like the much smaller lymph nodes, its condition may reflect the general health of the individual.

However, the spleen is not a necessary part of the normal human body, and in some cases of abnormal activity that threaten the health of a patient, the spleen may be removed by a surgeon. When the spleen is taken out of the body, in an operation called a splenectomy, other organs and tissues take over the work previously performed by the spleen. The benefits of a splenectomy are difficult to predict in advance in individual cases, partly because spleen problems tend to be systemic disorders involving more than one organ or organ system, and because other body tissues may be producing the same or similar effects.

Among body disorders that may involve or affect normal spleen function are the overproduction of red blood cells, or polycythemia vera, and the excessive destruction of red blood cells, a condition known as hemolytic anemia. When there are too many red blood cells in a capillary, they tend to stick together and blood circulation becomes sluggish. In some instances red blood cells become stacked like a pile of coins in a capillary. This kind of disorder frequently occurs at a time when the bone marrow fails to produce a normal quota of fresh red blood cells, approximately one million per second, and the spleen resumes its old job of making red cells.

The cells have a normal life span of about 120 days and are destroyed at the same rate at which they are produced, or around one million per second. But if the rate of destruction falls behind the rate of production, red cells can accumulate quite rapidly. Hemolytic anemia is a sort of reverse situation in which the cells are destroyed faster than they are produced. The spleen may not be the cause of excessive destruction, but the spleen is such an important part of the red cell salvage operation that an obvious way of controlling excessive blood cell destruction is to remove the spleen. That is one reason for performing a splenectomy. A splenectomy also may be performed in a case of rupture of the spleen or the development of tumors, cysts, or abscesses in the spleen tissue.

Kidneys and Kidney Diseases

Almost everyone is aware that the kidneys produce urine, which contains various waste products of the body's cellular metabolism. But the kidneys are importantly involved in a number of other normal body functions, such as controlling the level of body fluids, maintaining a healthy acid-base balance, eliminating poisons and drugs, and helping to form red blood cells. Disorders of the body's urinary system, sometimes called the renal system, may be reflected in a variety of diseases ranging from gout to hypertension, and from skin problems to potassium depletion effects.

The kidneys produce in an average adult between one and one and a half quarts of urine per day. Much more fluid than that passes through the kidneys, which receive from 20 to 25 percent of the blood pumped from the heart every minute. In fact, it has been calculated that the kidneys filter an amount of fluid every six hours that is equivalent to the body's entire supply of water. But the kidneys release less than one percent of all the fluid they process daily; the remainder is reabsorbed as part of the organ's function of conserving the body's water supply.

Each of the two kidneys contains about one million units called nephrons. Each nephron consists of a filtering component, known as a glomerulus, and a collecting tubule, plus a tiny network of arterioles and venules for circulating blood through

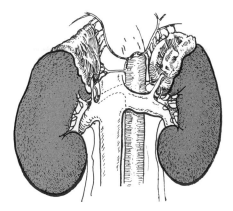

KIDNEYS

The kidneys, which lie in the back of the abdomen between the top of the pelvis and the bottom of the rib cage, literally take the blood apart and put it back together again several times each day. Through a complex filtering system, the kidneys remove excess fluid and some waste products of cellular metabolism along with certain nutrients, depending upon current body needs. Messages received from other body systems advise the kidneys about how much water, minerals, and other substances should be excreted or put back into the bloodstream for further use.

the nephron. Blood enters the kidney through a renal artery and is distributed into the system of some one million arterioles, each leading to a different nephron. The blood reaches the glomerulus, a microscopic knot of capillaries, under very high pressure. The pressure forces fluid through the membrane surface of the glomerulus into a capsule. In addition to fluid, a number of dissolved solids are leaked into the capsule, which diverts the fluid and dissolved substances into a tubule.

The tubule walls absorb most of the water and some of the dissolved materials;

other substances are not absorbed. For a person in normal health, nearly all of the glucose is absorbed and so are most of the essential minerals, such as calcium, potassium, and sodium. Waste products, including uric acid and urea, as well as most foreign substances, are not reabsorbed but are allowed to flow with some of the fluid into collecting tubules that drain into ureters leading to the urinary bladder. The fluid and absorbed substances are routed back into the bloodstream, which exits from the kidney via a renal vein. How the cells of the kidney tubules select substances to be retained and those to be excreted is something of a mystery. However, it appears that secretions of parathyroid hormone are the messengers that tell the tubules whether to absorb or excrete calcium and phosphorus at any given time.

Another hormone, the antidiuretic hormone of the pituitary gland, normally stimulates the reabsorption of water by the kidney tubules. When the pituitary gland fails to secrete enough antidiuretic hormone, such as in the disease called diabetes insipidus, too much water is released in the urine.

The antidiuretic hormone may be suppressed when you drink a large amount of water or a similar beverage. A significant increase in water intake can dilute the blood so that receptors in the brain send a message to the pituitary gland, which reduces its output of antidiuretic hormone. The eventual effect is that the production of urine is increased. This is a normal response. Another normal response is increased production of the antidiurectic hormone to conserve body water by reducing the amount of fluid in urine—for instance, when you lose body water by perspiration faster than you replenish the supply by drinking more water. The condition of increased urine production sometimes is called polyuria; the condition of reduced, or below normal, urine output is called anuria.

Polyuria or anuria can result from injury or disease involving the kidneys. Ordinarily, each of the two million nephron units in the kidneys acts independently, and the kidneys may continue to function even if a significant percentage of the nephron units are lost. Some individuals continue to lead rather normal lives after losing an entire kidney through disease or accident, or after donating an organ for transplantation. In a disorder such as nephritis, however, enough nephron units can fail so that substances normally reabsorbed by the tubules are excreted in the urine, or substances such as urea that normally are excreted are reabsorbed by the bloodstream. The patient may experience polyuria at first, then anuria, and finally develop a condition called uremia, marked by the accumulation of normally excreted substances in the blood. The patient may have convulsions and slip into a fatal coma.

Normal kidneys are not easily palpated by the examining physician in a person of normal build. Since the kidneys lie deep in the abdomen, the doctor locates them by using the fingers of both hands. He presses one set of fingers along the left or right side of the abdomen from the front, and pushes the other set of fingers at the back into the soft area between the bottom of the ribs and the top of the pelvic bones. Because the kidneys tend to move downward when the patient breathes deeply, the doctor usually asks the patient to take a deep breath. If his fingers are located in the proper positions front and back, he frequently can feel the kidneys slide into

his indirect grasp. This is accomplished more easily while examining a skinny person or a patient with large kidneys.

Disorders of the urinary tract frequently are diagnosed with the help of indirect clues. For example, a kidney stone may form because the concentration of solids in the urine becomes too great for the amount of fluid, so the solids precipitate and form a stone. The stone can damage the lining of the urinary tract and cause bleeding. The patient notices blood in the urine and consults his doctor.

A kidney stone is not the only cause of urine with a bloody tinge. The liver or gallbladder can be the source of a dark bloody color in the urine, for example, and various foods can color the urine when it is strongly concentrated. In many cases laboratory tests are needed to help identify the cause of a urine sample that appears to be discolored by internal bleeding.

If the kidney stone leaves the kidney and begins working its way down a ureter toward the urinary bladder, the stone is quite likely to scratch the inner wall of the ureter, producing blood in the urine and severe abdominal pain. The symptoms are part of a disorder frequently called renal colic, although the colic actually is in a ureter rather than in the kidney. The pain may be felt in the lower back or it may radiate to the inguinal region on the lower front of the abdomen, or even as far down as the genital area.

The pain of renal colic may be accompanied by nausea and vomiting, chills, fever, a change in the frequency of urination, and other effects. In some cases the symptoms of renal colic may mimic those of appendicitis. In other cases the patient has few if any severe symptoms. However, kidney stones are not rare; more than

100,000 Americans are hospitalized each year for this reason, and there is evidence that perhaps ten times that number have stones in their urinary tracts.

X-ray pictures usually will confirm the presence of kidney stones when symptoms might suggest other possibilities, such as appendicitis. Some stones show more clearly on X-ray film than others, depending upon their chemical composition. In most cases kidney stones contain calcium, but other substances may predominate in stones formed as a result of certain types of bacterial infections.

Treatment for kidney stones may vary according to the chemical composition of a stone, its location in the urinary tract, the size of the stone, and other factors. A small stone may be passed in the urine; a stone that obstructs normal functioning of the kidney is likely to be removed by surgery. In a few cases the stone may be dissolved in the urinary tract by special diets and medications.

The Urinary Tract

The urinary bladder usually resembles a small deflated basketball when it is empty. It has thick muscular walls and inflates to an oval-shaped reservoir when filled with urine. The amount of urine a bladder can hold is a matter that even anatomy experts may argue about, but it generally is in the neighborhood of one pint. There also is some disagreement regarding whether the male bladder is larger on the average than the female urinary bladder, partly due to the fact that the vertical and horizontal measurements may not be the same in both sexes.

The ureters leading from the kidneys enter the bladder in the lower half of the organ. The urine drains from the bladder through the urethra, which is near the bottom of the bladder. The urethra in both the man and woman begins as an opening surrounded by a ring of sphincter muscle that normally is contracted to prevent the loss of urine. Because of the differences in male and female anatomy, the urethra literally takes a different turn in the male than in the female. In the woman the urethra is rather short and direct, carrying urine downward and forward to an opening in the vulva. In the man the urethra makes a long S-shaped curve to reach an opening in the penis. There is a second sphincter in the male urethra, below the point where the prostate gland covers the urethra.

Pressure on the walls of the urinary bladder usually is translated as a message to relieve oneself, or empty the bladder. This is accomplished anatomically by contracting the muscles in the walls of the bladder while at the same time relaxing the sphincter muscles of the urethra. Normally, the act of emptying the bladder is under voluntary control and is an example of a physiological response that, as part of toilet training, one learns to control, although urination is an involuntary act for an infant. Disease, injury, or some other disabling factor, however, can cause a person to lose normal voluntary control so that urination occurs more or less automatically when the bladder becomes filled.

Loss of normal muscle contractility in later years for many individuals—an effect experienced by some persons even before adulthood—can result in the accidental loss of urine during coughing, laughing, or other actions that produce added pressure in the abdominal area. This accidental loss of urine is most likely to happen to women, and while it may be embarrassing, the event is not the same as loss of voluntary control; also, only small amounts of urine are involved.

Strictures or other obstructions in the urethra are likely to have the opposite effect, which is most likely to affect men because of the long curved path of the male urethra and the fact that it is surrounded for part of the distance by the prostate gland. Enlargement of the prostate can narrow the opening of the urethral tube, making it difficult to start and stop the flow of urine. The bladder muscles may contract and the sphincters relax, but the urine may exit in spurts or dribbles, or both, due to constriction of the flow through the urethra.

If the bladder does not empty completely, a condition that can result from a weakening or herniation of tissues in the floor of the pelvis that alters the normal position of the bladder, the stagnant urine may become a breeding ground for bacteria. The effect may be noticed in the form of painful urination or dysuria. However, there also may be other causes for pain or discomfort in urination, such as inflammation of the prostate in men. An example of an infection that can produce symptoms of dysuria is the veneral disease gonorrhea.

The urge to urinate usually occurs when the bladder reaches its normal capacity of one pint or slightly less, and this happens from four to six times per day for most people. But patterns of urination frequency are partly a matter of habit or convenience, including the urge to get up and go during the night, and it would not be wise to establish as "normal" a particular volume or frequency for persons who are otherwise in good health.

GLOSSARY

THE ABDOMEN

The following list of words defines and gives pertinent information about diseases and other medical terms relating to abdominal organs and tissues. Italicized words refer to separate entries within this Glossary.

abdomen The part of the body between the thorax and the pelvis, but including certain organs and tissues that may extend into the rib cage at the top or into the pelvic cavity at the bottom.

abdominal apoplexy A term sometimes used to indicate severe bleeding from an artery serving an abdominal organ such as the spleen or stomach. The hemorrhage usually begins suddenly from rupture of the artery.

abdominal walls The tissues, including bones and muscles, that form the shape of the abdomen. They include the lower ribs of the chest which enclose the upper part of the abdomen, the pelvic bones, the vertebrae or backbone between the chest and the pelvis, and muscle fibers that run in sheets and straps over areas not enclosed by bones.

achlorhydria An absence or lack of hydrochloric acid in the stomach. Atrophic gastritis, a digestive disorder that affects mainly older persons, is one of the medical problems associated with insufficient production of hydrochloric acid by the cells lining the stomach.

acute abdomen A term used by doctors to describe a condition marked by the sudden development of severe pain in one of the abdominal organs due to obstruction, perforation, or another cause requiring emergency surgery.

alimentary tract Another name for the digestive tract, a 30-foot-long muscular tube that extends from the mouth to the rectum and includes the stomach, intestines, and accessory organs that provide digestive secretions such as the pancreas and liver.

amebiasis An infection caused by amebas, one-celled animals that sometimes become parasites of humans. The invasion of the body by amebas, which is most likely to occur in warm, tropical climates, may be manifested as amebic dysentery, amebic hepatitis, or ameboma, a tumor-like reaction of the body to amebas in the intestines. Amebic infestation of the gastrointestinal tract frequently produces symptoms of acute abdominal pain.

amylase An enzyme secreted by the pancreas to help break down starches into simple sugar molecules which can be absorbed by the small intestine.

anal canal A short passageway between the rectum and the anus composed mainly of a mucous membrane lining and layers of sphincter muscles, which normally are contracted to prevent the accidental exit of feces from the rectum.

aneurysm An abnormal weakening and swelling of the walls of a major blood vessel. The aneurysm may appear as a ballooning of an arterial wall that may rupture if not treated at an early stage by surgery. A dissecting aneurysm is one in which the innermost wall of the artery may fail, so that blood flows between the layers of the artery wall. However, a dissecting aneurysm of the aorta as it passes through the abdomen can result in severe abdominal pain, with disruption of normal blood circulation to vital organs of the abdomen.

anorexia A loss of appetite which is a common symptom of gastrointestinal distress. Anorexia accompanied by severe abdominal pain, for example, may be associated with appendicitis. Anorexia also may be regarded as an index to the severity of an illness, being at a level somewhat below that of nausea.

Anorexia nervosa is a term used to describe a psychotic condition in which a person refuses food and suffers a severe loss of body weight and malnutrition, with possibly fatal consequences.

anuria A term used to describe abnormally small amounts of daily urine production. True anuria, which may be associated with acute kidney failure or an obstruction in the urinary system, frequently refers to cases in which urine production falls below three or four ounces per day. For purposes of comparison, the low end of the normal range of adult human urine production is about one and a half pints of urine per day, and the high end of the scale is about two quarts per day.

appendicitis An inflammation of the vermiform appendix, a short, thin tubular projection below the *cecum*, where the small intestine joins the large intestine on the lower right side of the abdomen. Appendicitis frequently begins with signs and symptoms of indigestion and/or "gas," followed by pain and tenderness in the lower right portion of the abdomen. There may be *anorexia*, nausea, and vomiting, as well as fever and occasionally constipation. The onset of intestinal discomfort and constipation as symptoms occasionally can mislead a patient to use laxatives or cathartics in an effort to produce a bowel movement, an effect which would only aggravate an already dangerous situation.

Acute appendicitis almost always requires emergency surgery to remove the inflamed appendix, which otherwise would likely develop gangrene and would rupture, or perforate, so that intestinal contents could spill into the abdominal cavity. Leakage of the bacteria-contaminated contents of the intestine into the abdominal cavity would result inevitably in *peritonitis*, which could be fatal. Before the development of modern surgical techniques and antibiotics, appendicitis frequently resulted in death.

ascaris A medical term for *roundworms*, a possible cause of intestinal obstruction, particularly in warm, tropical regions. The worms enter the digestive tract and set up housekeeping in the middle segment of the small intestine, where they multiply until they form a mass so large that the gut becomes blocked and food cannot move through the digestive tract.

azotemia A disorder marked by abnormally high levels of nitrogen compounds, such as *urea*, in the bloodstream. Azotemia usually is due to a failure of the kidneys to filter from the blood substances normally removed by their nephron units.

barium meal A solution of barium sulfate in water that is swallowed before an X-ray picture of the gastrointestinal tract is made. The barium is radio-opaque, meaning that it will form a white image on the X-ray film outlining the interior of the tube through which it passes. The barium image enables the doctor to locate such defects as tumors and ulcers in the stomach lining, obstructions in the esophagus, etc. A barium meal also can be used to help the examining physician observe the digestive actions of the stomach through the use of X-ray equipment that permits the doctor to watch the movements of internal organs.

Barium enemas may be used by doctors to study the interior of the colon, particularly in areas of the large intestine that are beyond the range of a sigmoidoscope, a device for viewing the *sigmoid colon*. In the colon the barium can show *diverticula*, tumors, or the abnormally smooth effects of ulcerative *colitis*.

benign prostatic hypertrophy A fancy medical term for a problem rather common in men over 50, an overgrowth of prostate tissues causing an obstruction of urinary flow. The signs and symptoms of the disorder include increasingly frequent urges to empty the bladder, including a need to get out of bed at night to urinate, and difficulty in starting and stopping the flow of urine. Fever with or without a burning sensation when urinating can indicate an infection associated with urinary retention. If uncorrected by medical or surgical techniques, urinary retention can lead to kidney failure or other complications.

bile A thick greenish fluid secreted by liver cells and important in the digestion of fats. Bile is composed of water, cholesterol, bile pigment, and bile salts. The bile pigment contains the waste products of old red blood cells that have become worn out and destroyed. The only significant digestive substance in bile is the bile salts, which act as a detergent in the intestine to break up large fat globules into smaller units that can be digested by enzymes. Bile is produced by the liver at a rate of about a pint a day and is normally stored in the gallbladder for release as needed to digest fats.

biliary colic The name sometimes used to identify the painful symptoms of gallstones which may become lodged in the ducts leading from the liver or gallbladder to the small intestine. The pain frequently is accompanied by vomiting, fever, and extreme tenderness in the abdomen, with pain radiating toward the right shoulder area.

bilirubin A pigment occurring naturally in the blood and bile as a breakdown product of the hemoglobin of worn-out red blood cells. Bilirubin normally is taken out of the bloodstream by the liver cells and excreted into the bile as a waste product. However, in certain cases of liver or gallbladder disease the bilirubin is deposited in tissues throughout the body and gives the skin the yellowish coloration of jaundice.

Billroth operation The name given a surgical procedure used to treat certain types of ulcers by removing the lower portion of the stomach and sewing the remaining part to the small intestine.

blackbottom sign A term occasionally used by doctors to identify a type of hematoma, or blood blister type of discoloration, around the anus that may be a sign of an aneurysm of the abdominal aorta. The discoloration is caused by blood leaking through the abdominal cavity and into the skin around the anus.

bolus The medical term sometimes used to identify a ball of food that has been swallowed, or that is ready to be swallowed.

borborygmus A medical jawbreaker for rumbling sounds in the gut, caused by gas moving through the intestines. It is pronounced "bor-bor-ig-mus."

bougie A slender flexible rod that sometimes is used to measure the bore, or caliber, of a passageway in the body, or to treat a structural problem by enlarging the passageway. Various sizes and shapes of bougies may be used in the diagnosis or treatment of body areas such as the esophagus or the urethra.

Bowman's capsule A part of the nephron, the basic unit of blood filtration and urine production in the kidneys. Fluid and dissolved substances in the blood are forced by the blood pressure through capillary membranes and into the capsule, from which they flow into tubules where part of the filtrate is put back into the bloodstream and the rest, mainly waste products, is routed into ureters to be excreted.

calculi A medical term meaning stones, as in urinary calculi for kidney stones.

cancer of the colon A common condition that can affect a person of any age, although cancer, or carcinoma, of the colon is most likely to occur in men who are beyond middle age. Nearly half of all colon cancers develop in the area of the rectum; an additional 25 percent occur in the descending segment of the colon above the rectum; thus, approximately 75 percent of all colon cancers occur in a portion of the large intestine that can be inspected by a doctor during a routine physical examination. There are several types of cancers of the colon, one of the most distinctive being a malignant stricture which develops into a tight ring around the lumen of the intestine, thereby obstructing it. As is the case of cancers developing in other areas of the body, bowel cancers begin as small local lesions and, if not treated at an early stage, spread to other organs and tissues of the body.

cast A term used to describe an object that may be excreted in the urine with the shape of a kidney tubule in which it was formed. A urinary cast may be composed of fatty, waxy, or other material. Similar casts occasionally appear in the sputum of persons who have experienced a respiratory disease, in which instance the casts will have the shape of a mold for a bronchiole.

cathartic A substance that helps evacuate the bowel. Various types of cathartics and laxatives are available to stimulate bowel movements in various ways, such as by serving as a lubricant, or by irritating the lining of the large intestine.

catheter A flexible tube that is used to withdraw fluids from the body. For example, a catheter may be employed to drain urine from the bladder when normal methods of emptying the bladder are not possible or feasible. A catheter also may be used to introduce fluids into a part of the body, or to force open a passage that has been blocked by disease or injury. Some catheters are designed with two parallel tubes, one for introducing a fluid and the other for draining the fluid.

cecum The pouch-like beginning of the large intestine. The small intestine empties into the cecum on the lower right side of the abdomen. The vermiform appendix is attached to the cecum.

celiac artery An artery that distributes blood to most of the organs in the upper abdomen, including the esophagus, stomach, duodenum, liver, gallbladder, spleen, and pancreas. Chronic pain in the upper abdominal area frequently is associated with abnormalities, such as strictures, of branches of the celiac artery.

celiac disease An intestinal disorder caused by an inability to digest glutens, or proteins present in rye and wheat flours. The mucosal lining of the small intestine undergoes changes when rye or wheat cereals are eaten. The signs and symptoms may include vomiting, abdominal distension, iron deficiency anemia, and in some cases muscle wasting with difficulty in walking. When the patient is placed on a gluten-free diet, the symptoms gradually diminish and the lining of the intestine regains its normal condition. The disease seems to be inherited, or to run in families, although genetic evidence is not complete. Small children are the most likely victims, although symptoms may develop in some individuals as late as middle age.

cholangiogram An X-ray picture of the bile ducts.

cholangitis An inflammation of the bile ducts. An inflammation caused by bacteria which may move up the bile duct toward the liver is known as ascending cholangitis. The disorder often is accompanied by gallstone obstruction and may be marked by chills, abdominal pain, nausea, and vomiting.

cholecystitis An inflammation of the gallbladder, usually involving a bacterial infection. Cholecystitis may be caused by gas-producing disease organisms which invade the gallbladder.

cholelithiasis A medical term for the small stones or concretions in the gallbladder, or simply *gallstones*.

choleretic A medical term meaning a medicine that is designed to stimulate the production of bile in the liver. An agent with a similar name, cholagogue, is used to stimulate the flow of bile into the small intestine.

chronic gastritis Any of several types of inflammation of the stomach. In older people a form of gastritis known as atrophic gastritis is associated with changes in the structure of cells lining the interior of the stomach. Symptoms may include nausea and abdominal pain and distress, especially after eating a meal.

chyme The fluid-like gruel produced in food by the digestive action of gastric juices in the stomach. After food has been churned and dissolved into chyme, it is released into the small intestine for further digestive action.

cirrhosis A disease, generally associated with the liver, that is characterized by a degeneration of the liver's normal structure and the replacement of functional cells by fibrous tissue and nodules. Cirrhosis of the liver, a common cause of death among persons beyond the age of 45, can follow infections such as hepatitis or exposure to chemicals. The disease also may be associated with a number of congenital defects. However, it is most frequently the result of the abuse of alcoholic beverages.

Treatment may vary according to the cause of cirrhosis and the condition of the patient. In a case of cirrhosis resulting from alcohol abuse, the patient may recover with rest, abstinence from alcohol, and a special diet fortified with vitamins and protein-rich foods. Cirrhosis caused by obstruction of a bile duct may require surgery to correct the problem.

colectomy The surgical excision of a portion of the colon, or of the entire colon in the case of a complete colectomy.

colitis A chronic disease involving the *colon*. The disorder may be marked by diarrhea with blood mucus being passed, loss of appetite, and loss of weight. The patient may have a fever and show signs of deteriorating muscle tone. Examination of the colon usually shows an ulcerated area, which is why the disorder frequently is identified as ulcerative colitis.

The cause of colitis is unknown. It may affect a person of any age, although the victims most frequently are young adults. Some patients recover after a single attack, while others experience such serious complications as hemorrhage or perforation of the bowel. But for most victims the disease becomes a chronic condition with a high risk of causing cancer of the colon after a number of years. Surgery often is advised to remove the affected portion of the colon, but only when the rectal area is involved. Otherwise, treatment may involve medications, diet, and rest and relaxation.

colon Another name for the large intestine which extends from the cecum to the rectum. The first segment, the ascending colon, runs uphill along the right side of the abdomen; the middle section runs across the midsection of the belly below the stomach; and the third major segment, the descending colon, runs downhill to the rectum. The general pattern of the colon resembles the sides and top of a picture frame. See *colitis; colostomy.*

colonoscope An instrument that can be inserted by an examining physician through the anal canal so that the inner walls of the colon can be inspected. Obviously, fecal material must be removed from the colon before the examination so that the physician's view will not be obscured.

colostomy A surgical technique developed in the 19th century for the treatment of cancer and other disorders of the colon or rectum. The operation involves making an incision in the abdomen so that a portion of the colon can be brought to the surface of the skin and an artificial opening, or stoma, made in the bowel. Contents of the colon then drain through the new opening rather than the anus. The colostomy can be performed as a permanent or a temporary measure. The stoma may be located at any of several points on the surface of the abdomen, depending upon the problem to be corrected. The opening is covered with a plastic cap in order that the patient may work or perform other normal functions after the operation. Most colostomy patients learn new procedures for regular emptying of the bowel through the artificial opening so that the need will not interfere with their daily activities.

constipation A term generally used to describe difficult or delayed defecation. As in urination, what is considered as a normal pattern varies with different individuals. Some people consider it normal to have more than one bowel movement per day, while others believe it is normal to go for several days without a bowel movement. A type of constipation associated with an inactive colon may develop in old persons or those who have become inactive because of serious illness. Fecal impaction may develop along with a distended bowel. Treatment requires enemas or, if that fails, physical removal of the impacted feces, which in desperate cases may involve surgery with a general anesthetic.

Crohn's disease Another name for regional enteritis, a condition in which the wall of the intestine becomes inflamed. The symptoms may include abdominal pain, fever, anorexia, nausea, and loss of weight. The walls of the intestine can become thickened and swollen from fluid retention. In one form of the disease the walls of different segments of the intestine may stick together and form a fistula, or opening between the segments, so that the contents of one part of the intestine become mixed with the contents of another portion. Treatment in early stages frequently involves only medications and diet, but in advanced stages surgery may be required.

cystitis Inflammation of the urinary bladder from infection or exposure to irritants such as chemicals. The signs and symptoms can include pain and tenderness of the bladder and urethra areas, changes in the urgency and frequency of urination, and the appearance of blood in the urine. Cystitis in both men and women is frequently due to an infection that travels upward to the bladder through the urethra. Infections due to bacteria or fungi are generally treated with antibiotics or other drugs.

diabetes A disease characterized by excessive urination. A most common form of several types of diabetes is diabetes mellitus, which is associated with a failure of the pancreas to produce sufficient amounts of insulin for the normal metabolism of carbohydrates. Insulin, a hormone, is needed by the cells of the liver in order to convert sugar molecules into glycogen for storage until the energy-rich food is needed. As a result, diabetes mellitus patients tend to excrete sugar in their urine unless they take regular periodic injections of insulin, or in the case of some persons who develop diabetes after reaching adulthood, oral medications called hypoglycemic agents, which lower the blood sugar level. Diabetes mellitus develops suddenly in childhood as juvenile diabetes, or later in life as maturity onset diabetes.

Another type, diabetes insipidus, is associated with a disorder of the pituitary gland which results in an abnormal production of a hormone that controls urine flow. As a result, the patient may produce enormous quantities of urine that is normal but very dilute. He also develops a tremendous thirst. Diabetes insipidus usually develops following a disease or injury affecting the pituitary or hypothalamic areas of the brain.

dialysis A technique for removing toxic substances from the blood of a patient with a mechanical kidney after failure of the natural kidneys because of disease or injury. Several types of dialysis systems are available for use at home as well as in a hospital or clinic. One type, known as peritoneal dialysis, or peritoneal lavage, involves the use of the patient's own peritoneal membrane, which is punctured with a catheter and then becomes a semipermeable membrane for the diffusion of electrolytes. Fluid for dialysis is allowed to flow into the abdomen to irrigate the area and then is drained out, removing molecules of waste substances such as urea that have diffused across the membrane. The treatment may last for 24 to 72 hours, depending upon individual patient factors.

Another dialysis technique utilizes a cellophane membrane on a kidney machine. Arteriovenous shunts are attached to arteries and veins in the forearm or lower leg. Tubes that run from the patient's arteries and veins circulate the patient's blood into a machine that contains sheets or tubes of cellophane, through which the waste products are diffused and the blood is returned to the patient's body. This technique, called hemodialysis, requires only four to six hours to achieve the same results as 48 hours of peritoneal dialysis in removing toxic substances from the blood.

diarrhea The rapid movement of fecal material through the bowel, usually resulting in frequent or repeated bowel evacuations with watery stools. Because excess water normally is absorbed by the intestine, the rapid movement of fecal material doesn't permit water absorption. The person afflicted with diarrhea also loses vital nutrients such as potassium which do not have time to be absorbed. A person who experiences more than an occasional attack of diarrhea may eventually suffer from dehydration and symptoms of electrolyte imbalance because of premature bowel evacuations.

Causes of diarrhea are many and varied, including emotional upsets, chemical irritants of the intestinal tract, and infectious disease agents. Treatment for most cases involves rest and relaxation, warm soap and water to clean the anal region and thereby reduce irritation and discomfort, the use of medications that relieve the accompanying symptoms of *peristalsis* and cramps. Frequent attacks of diarrhea that appear to be related to nervous tension may require psychotherapy.

digestion A simple term that covers a vastly complex series of chemical and biological processes through which a cheeseburger, for example, can be broken down into invisibly small molecules of amino and fatty acids, sugars, vitamins, and minerals for use by various body tissues as fuel or building materials.

diuretic A medicine or other substance that promotes the secretion of urine by the kidneys. There are many types of diuretics, including the caffeine, theophylline, and theobromine chemicals that occur in coffee, tea, and cocoa. Most diuretics work in one of two ways: they either increase the rate of filtration of fluid by the glomerulus portion of a kidney's nephron unit, or they suppress the normal reabsorption function of the kidney's tubules, which ordinarily recover most of the filtered fluid so that it can be routed back into the bloodstream. Either mode of action results in a greater excretion of water, which is an objective of diuretic use. In a case of congestive heart disease, for

example, a diuretic may be needed to help reduce the accumulation of fluid, or edema, in the body tissues since the extra fluid results in a heavier work load for the diseased heart.

diverticula Small pouches that poke out of the side walls of the intestine; one such is a diverticulum. Diverticula are a rather common abnormality among both men and women past middle age. In most cases diverticula produce no symptoms, but on occasion fecal material may accumulate in one or more of the side pockets. The diverticulum lacks muscle tissue so that feces deposited in it cannot be squeezed back into the mainstream of the gut. The feces may become compacted and hard, causing an inflammation called diverticulitis.

Diverticulitis may become complicated by periods of constipation or bloody diarrhea, as well as abdominal pain. Most cases can be treated medically and with diet restrictions. However, serious complications, such as perforation of the wall of the intestine, must be corrected by surgery.

drip feeding A common term sometimes used to describe the administration of fluids and nutrients to a patient by a route other than the mouth. For example, an intravenous drip of a parenteral food solution—that is, nutrients introduced outside the bowel—may be used for several days or more after surgery involving the digestive tract. The solution provides all the essential food elements in a form that can be absorbed directly into the bloodstream.

dumping syndrome A term used to cover the symptoms of nausea, weakness, sweating, palpitations, and other effects experienced shortly after a meal by patients who have undergone a partial gastrectomy. The symptoms, which are not accompanied by pain or vomiting, frequently subside if the patient lies down right away after eating.

duodenal ulcer A peptic ulcer that develops in the lining of the *duodenum*. Although the cause is not certain, it assumed that duodenal ulcers are caused by gastric acid from the stomach. Most of the ulcers occur around the area where gastric juices from the stomach hit the wall of the duodenum when the digestive substance is squirted from the stomach by the pyloric valve.

Duodenal ulcers begin as small erosions of the mucous membrane lining of that area of the intestine. The ulcers are never completely healed once they develop, but they may become covered with scar tissue and produce no further symptoms for an indefinite period. However, if the scar tissue breaks down, ulcer symptoms begin again under the stimulus of new or renewed irritants such as alcohol, tobacco, nervous tension, or similar factors that are associated with increased gastric acid production. It is for this reason that duodenal ulcers appear to go through periods of remission, when symptoms subside for months or more at a time.

Complications of duodenal ulcers include perforation of the wall of the duodenum, which would allow the intestinal contents to leak into the peritoneal cavity of the abdomen, causing the severe and potentially fatal type of inflammation known as peritonitis. In some cases the wall of the duodenum facing the pancreas becomes perforated, or the erosion affects an artery running between the duodenum and pancreas, causing hemorrhage, or heavy internal bleeding.

duodenum The first segment of the small intestine, starting at the pyloric valve at the end of the stomach. The duodenum is the shortest and widest of the three main segments of the small intestine. It is approximately 10 inches long and normally is wrapped around the head of the neighboring pancreas. The pancreas secretes its digestive juices into the duodenum, as do the liver and gallbladder, via the common bile duct, at a point an inch or two beyond the pylorus. The duodenum gets its name (Latin for "twelve") from an ancient anatomical measuring system which found that the intestinal segment was the length of 12 fingers' breadth.

dysentery A severe form of diarrhea characterized by inflammation of the intestine, usually centered in the colon, and accompanied by stomach cramps, fever, and involuntary spasms of the stomach muscles which simulate the action of a bowel movement. However, there may be little or no feces in the watery discharge from the bowel, and the feces that is passed may be marked with mucus, pus, and/ or blood. A serious consequence of the repeated bowel movements, which may total more than 30 a day, is a loss of body fluids and nutrients that normally would have been absorbed from the intestinal tract.

Dysentery can be caused by a number of different possible agents, including protozoa such as amebas (as in amebic dysentery), bacteria, viruses, worms, or chemical irritants. Viral dysentery is a common occurrence among travelers to less well-developed areas where meals may be served with raw fruits or vegetables, or with tableware that is contaminated; it usually is self-limiting and the symptoms usually subside within two or three days. Dysentery caused by bacteria or amebas may require special drugs, and in some cases administration of intravenous fluids to replenish body fluids and nutrients lost during the diarrhea attacks.

dyspepsia A common term used to describe the discomfort one may feel after a meal. The term literally means impaired digestion.

dysphagia Difficulty in swallowing, frequently a symptom of a serious esophageal disease that may be a stricture, obstruction, or cancer of the esophagus. Food may be regurgitated and the patient will lose weight. The problem usually can be diagnosed by a doctor without too much difficulty; a *barium meal* swallowed before an X-ray picture is taken will outline in rather clear detail all the normal or abnormal surfaces of the lining of the esophagus. Also, the doctor can view the inside of the esophagus directly with an esophagoscope, a long hollow tube, equipped with lights and lenses, that can be inserted into the food tube.

ecchymosis A term sometimes used to identify a greenish or yellowish discoloration of the skin caused by blood accumulation, usually from bleeding in another part of the body or from a deep organ. An ecchymosis area on the skin at the back of the abdominal area, for example, could be a sign of bleeding from the pancreas, the blood having seeped through openings in tissue layers into the abdominal cavity.

edema Abnormal fluid retention by the body tissues. The condition frequently is a sign of a heart and/or kidney problem. It usually is corrected with drugs that improve heart function or help the kidneys produce greater amounts of urine, or both.

electrolyte a vital chemical substance that is capable of carrying an electrical charge when dissolved in a body fluid. Examples are sodium, potassium, and chloride (chlorine). Electrolytes function as electrically charged ions that regulate electrochemical functions in the body, such as the transmission of nerve impulses and contractions of muscles. They also are involved in fluid balance and acid-base balance of body tissues.

enterectomy A surgical procedure in which a portion of the small intestine is removed and the two open ends are sewn together. It usually is performed to treat a problem resulting from damage to an area of the intestine by disease or injury.

enzyme test A laboratory test of the blood and urine to measure the levels of certain digestive enzymes secreted by the pancreas. Abnormally large amounts of the enzymes usually are found in cases of acute *pancreatitis*, a disorder that is marked by abdominal pains, rapid pulse, and abnormally high temperature. Since the signs and symptoms also could indicate one or more other abdominal disorders, the enzyme test may be used to eliminate other possible causes.

epigastric A word that generally refers to the upper half of the abdomen. Epigastric distress, for example, suggests a medical problem in one of the organs below the diaphragm but above the pelvic region. The term used to describe the area in the lower half of the abdomen is "hypogastric."

favism A reaction to eating fava beans, or broad beans, by persons who are sensitive to a substance that occurs naturally in the beans. Symptoms of favism include dizziness, vomiting, diarrhea, and changes in red blood cells that can lead to anemia. The sensitivity to fava beans tends to occur in families whose members have inherited digestive enzymes that are unable to metabolize the food substance.

feces The residue left from food after nutrients have been removed by the body's digestive processes, mixed with some intestinal secretions, mucus, and bacteria. The color, consistency, odor, and other factors are determined by the types of food consumed, disease conditions, etc. Cellulose from vegetables, for example, is generally indigestible and passes through the digestive tract virtually unchanged, except for being broken into small pieces. Clay-colored feces may indicate a lack of bile in the digestive tract, either because the liver fails to produce enough bile or the flow is blocked. Fatty feces may be the result of eating too much fatty food, or a sign of a disease involving the gallbladder or the pancreas. Bleeding in the upper part of the digestive tract can give the feces a black, tarry coloration; bleeding in the lower digestive tract, near the rectum, may produce a red coloration.

femoral hernia A rupture of a portion of the intestine through an area of tissue at the bottom of the abdominal cavity where the femoral artery passes from the abdomen into the leg. The disorder is corrected by surgery.

fibrocystic disease Another name for cystic fibrosis, a hereditary disorder in which the body produces an abnormally thick mucus that interferes with several normal functions, such as breathing, by obstructing passages. In the abdomen the thick mucus can obstruct the flow of digestive juices from the pancreas so that food, particularly fatty foods, is not digested properly. A small percentage of babies born with the defect also suffer from an accumulation of putty-like secretions that obstruct the intestines and must be removed surgically in order to prevent the death of the infants.

Treatment of the digestive aspect of fibrocystic disease involves special diets that are high in protein and low in fats, and meals that are supplemented with extracts of animal pancreas.

fibroscopy A term sometimes used to mean an examination of the digestive tract with a long flexible fiberscope, equipped with lights and lenses, so that the interior of the stomach or other digestive organs can be studied. The examination usually is done while the patient is conscious, but after he has been given sedatives and local tranquillizers, and after the stomach has had time to be emptied of food.

fissure in ano A lesion that can develop in the anal canal, probably due to passage of a hard stool that tears the mucosal lining of the canal.

fistula An abnormal opening or passage between two internal organs or between an organ and the skin. A fistula may develop between two segments of intestine, for example, as a result of inflammation associated with *regional enteritis.* After the walls of adjoining bowel segments stick together and fuse, an opening develops so that contents of one portion of the intestine can flow into the other.

flanks The sides of the abdomen between the chest and the pelvis. During a medical examination the doctor may palpate the flanks to determine whether fluid has accumulated in the abdominal cavity. If a patient has a large amount of fluid retention—a condition known as *edema*—the flanks will bulge outward when he lies on his back.

flatulence A Latin-derived word for excessive gas in the digestive tract. Excessive gas in the stomach usually can be expelled by belching. Excessive gas in the intestines generally is expelled through the anus, although in some cases of extreme discomfort or before administration of a saline enema, a rectal tube may be

inserted into the anal canal to aid expulsion of gas. Gas in the stomach frequently is the result of swallowing air while gulping food or drink. Flatulence sometimes can be relieved by taking activated charcoal tablets or other medications, or by changing body positions—for example, sitting upright or lying down if the discomfort is felt when the body is in another position.

food diary A record of the foods eaten by a patient, along with the date and perhaps the time of the meal. Doctors occasionally ask patients to keep food diaries so that possible food allergies can be identified. As a follow-up to the diary entries, the doctor may recommend eliminating certain foods listed in the diary, one at a time, to see if the symptoms of illness diminish when a particular food is omitted from a day's meals.

galactose tolerance test A test of liver damage due to cirrhosis or hepatitis. Galactose is injected into the patient and the time required for the liver to convert the carbohydrate into glucose is measured. If the liver is normal, the galactose will disappear quickly from the bloodstream when it is converted to glucose. But if the liver cells are damaged, galactose continues to appear in blood samples long after it should have been changed by the liver.

gallbladder A small, pear-shaped pouch beneath the liver that collects and stores bile which is produced by the liver cells. Since the gallbladder cannot store all the bile as it is produced by the liver, the cells lining the gallbladder absorb water from the bile which becomes increasingly concentrated until it finally is released into ducts that empty eventually into the small intestine.

gallstones Small stones formed in the gallbladder by deposits of cholesterol and other materials in the bile. The stones begin to form from crystals that precipitate from the bile when it becomes too concentrated because of the absorption of excess water from the bile by the gallbladder. Gallstones are treated by diet, medications, and sometimes surgery.

gangrene The death of normally vital tissues, usually as a result of an interruption of the blood supply. Gangrene in the abdominal cavity can affect the appendix, gallbladder, or intestine. It can occur in the intestine, for example, as a result of an incarcerated hernia. Gangrene is a critical problem that usually requires emergency surgery to correct.

gastrectomy Surgical excision of all or part of the stomach. A gastrectomy may be performed to reduce the production of gastric acid by cells in the lining of the stomach. The amount of stomach removed may depend upon the extent of ulceration and acid production, among other factors. In a partial gastrectomy the portion nearest the pylorus usually is removed; the remainder of the stomach is sewn to the small intestine. In a total gastrectomy the esophagus and small intestine may be joined directly; see *Polya gastrectomy*.

gastric juice Sometimes called gastric acid, it is secreted by the stomach for digestive purposes. The mixture consists of hydrochloric acid, an enzyme called *pepsin*, and a substance known as *mucin*, a sticky material that helps neutralize excess acid, among other functions. The proportions of gastric juice components frequently vary among different individuals. The greatest amount of hydrochloric acid that is considered normal, for example, is about ten times the smallest amount of acid that is still regarded as within the normal range.

gastrin A hormone that helps the stomach to produce gastric juice. The presence of food in the stomach stimulates the release of gastrin.

gastritis An inflammation of the mucous membrane lining of the stomach. The condition may be acute or chronic and may be caused by disease organisms, foods, beverages, drugs, or ingested chemicals. Corrosive gastritis is the result of swallowing strong acids or caustic chemicals.

gastro-colic reflex An automatic urge to defecate that may be stimulated by eating a meal. It is a common reflex present in humans and other animals, although most people and domesticated animals learn to override the natural urge if it is not convenient to have a bowel movement when the reflex occurs.

gastro-enteritis An inflammation of the small intestine and stomach. The stomach and intestinal linings become red and inflamed. Symptoms may include abdominal cramps, vomiting, and diarrhea. The causes may be varied and include infection by a disease organism or a food substance, or both—that is, a food that is infected by bacteria.

globus hystericus A type of *dysphagia* that usually is associated with an emotional upset. The patient may be convinced that something is stuck in the esophagus, but careful examination shows that there is no obstruction. The muscles in the walls of the esophagus may contract as a result of anxiety or tension, producing the feeling of a "lump in the throat."

glomerular disease Any of a group of disorders, including bacterial infection of the kidneys, that results in impaired function of the *glomerulus*. One effect may be the excretion of red blood cells and protein molecules in the urine because of the glomeruli's failure to prevent the loss of the substances from the bloodstream.

glomerulus A part of the basic functioning unit of a kidney. Anatomically and physiologically, a glomerulus is a tiny knot of capillaries which acts as a filter to permit water and certain chemicals to be removed from the bloodstream, while retaining larger, important substances in the blood, such as blood cells and protein molecules. Each kidney contains about one million glomeruli.

glucose tolerance test A test of blood sugar levels performed as part of an examination for the possible presence of diabetes. The patient may be instructed to consume at least five ounces of carbohydrates each day for three days before the test. Then, after a period of fasting, blood and urine samples are taken for laboratory tests of the amount of sugar present. Next, a measured amount of glucose in water is swallowed by the patient, and blood and urine samples are taken at intervals of 30, 60, 120, and 180 minutes. In an otherwise normal person, the glucose level will rise sharply, then drop off to the pretest level within three hours. A test sample showing that glucose is still in the blood three hours after it was ingested is a sign of diabetes.

gluten A protein present in wheat and other grains that is valued in bread and other bakery products because it gives dough a tough, elastic consistency. However, gluten cannot be tolerated by persons with *celiac disease* because it produces a reaction in the lining of the small intestine. Gluten is present in rye, oats, barley, and wheat. For these grains celiac patients can substitute corn, rice, and soy flour, all of which lack gluten.

glycosuria The presence of easily detectable glucose in the urine. Some glucose normally is present in the urine, but at levels too small to be measured by methods used in the diagnosis of diabetes. Glycosuria is a sign of diabetes but it also can be the result of several other abnormalities, including a benign hereditary disorder in which the tubules of the kidney nephron units fail to reabsorb glucose as efficiently as the nephron tubules of normal kidneys.

gut A common term for the intestines, although the term sometimes is used solely to refer to the small intestine.

heartburn A burning pain in the chest that may be accompanied by regurgitation of gastric contents into the esophagus and even the mouth of the patient. It usually occurs after a meal and most often while the person is lying down, which makes it easier for the offending fluid to move "uphill" from the stomach to the mouth. Heartburn often is associated with hiatus hernia, a weakened area of the diaphragm that permits a part of the stomach to poke up from the abdomen into the chest cavity. Persons afflicted with hiatus hernia may experience heartburn when bending forward or when wearing tight clothing that puts pressure on the abdomen and pushes the abdominal organs upward against the diaphragm.

helminths A medical term used to identify certain parasitic worms that may invade the human body, particularly the abdominal organs. An example is the roundworm that migrates to the liver and gall bladder, where it may obstruct the bile duct or aid in the formation of gallstones. Other parasitic worms include a liver fluke that can enter the body of a human who eats raw or improperly cooked fish, and the schistosomiasis species that can invade the portal vein leading to the liver, causing hypertension and gastrointestinal bleeding. Helminth diseases are rare in most parts of the western world where good hygiene measures are practiced, but they may be encountered by travelers who visit exotic tropical communities.

hematemesis A medical term meaning vomiting of blood. The source of vomited blood occasionally can be identified by the color. Blood that has been exposed to gastric juices of the stomach usually has a brownish "coffee grounds" color because of the action of stomach acid on the hemoglobin. Vomited blood not of that color may have originated in a nosebleed or the lungs and been swallowed accidentally. Blood that passes all the way through the digestive tract usually acquires a black, tarry appearance.

hematuria Blood in the urine. The color of the blood can vary from red to brown, depending upon a number of factors such as the acidity of the urine. Hematuria may cause little or no color change in the urine; its presence must be verified as blood cells by laboratory tests.

hemorrhoidal vessels A term that refers to the blood vessels involved in hemorrhoids, or piles. There are two sets of hemorrhoidal veins: one drains downward into the groin area; the other drains upward into the liver region. The condition of hemorrhoids, or piles, involves abnormal dilation of one of the sets of hemorrhoidal vessels.

hernia A weakening of the abdominal wall so that the intestine bulges through; see *femoral hernia; inguinal hernia; rupture; strangulated hernia.*

hydrochloric acid test A test that may be performed to determine the amount of hydrochloric acid produced in the stomach of a patient afflicted with *peptic ulcers.* A known stimulant of hydrochloric acid, such as gastrin or histamine, is injected into the patient; the hydrochloric acid resulting from the stimulus is collected by a tube and measured. If no hydrochloric acid is recovered as a result of the test, the patient is regarded as having a condition called *achlorhydria,* an abnormality associated with disorders such as stomach cancer, pellagra, and pernicious anemia.

hydronephrosis A kidney disease characterized by an accumulation of urine in the portion of the kidney that normally collects the urine from the myriad nephron units. The region at the beginning of the ureter, the tube that drains urine to the bladder, becomes distended and, if uncorrected, becomes a functionless fluid-filled pouch. The cause of the urine accumulation usually is an obstruction due to kidney stones or a tumor, although the problem also may be the result of a tissue change in the prostate, bladder, or urethra. Diagnosis of the precise cause can be made with the help of pyelography, a type of X-ray of the kidney and ureter involving the injection of a radio-opaque substance into a vein. Treatment generally requires surgery or other methods that will drain the urine, plus medications such as antibiotics to control infections that are associated with the disorder.

hyperesthesia Abnormally increased sensitivity of the skin or an organ to the pressure of external stimulus. Hyperesthesia is a common symptom of appendicitis, particularly in the skin area over the lower right quadrant of the abdomen.

hyperglycemia An abnormal increase in the amount of sugar in the blood. It is a sign of diabetes mellitus in patients who lack normal secretion of insulin, which is necessary in order to convert glucose (sugar) in the blood to glycogen, or body starch, which can be stored for later use by the body's tissues. A form of hyperglycemia can occur in infants, particularly premature infants who are given intravenous feedings; the condition leads to excess urine production and dehydration. The problem in newborn infants usually is self-correcting if normal fluid balance is maintained. Diabetes patients require insulin or oral hypoglycemic medications to control their blood sugar levels.

hypochondriac This word has two meanings. As commonly used, a hypochondriac person is one who has an abnormal concern about his health and may exaggerate trivial symptoms. But the term, hypochondriac, also refers to the upper abdominal area, the hypochondrium. Therefore, if a doctor refers to a hypochondriac problem he may be talking about gallstones, a duodenal ulcer, or a liver infection, rather than about a neurotic patient.

hypoglycemia A condition somewhat the opposite of *hyperglycemia* in that signs and symptoms of the disorder are the result of an abnormally low level of glucose in the bloodstream. There are many possible causes of hypoglycemia. An excess production of insulin and rapid absorption of glucose following a meal may occur in reaction to an overdose of insulin or oral hypoglycemic medications taken by a diabetes patient, or as a reaction to the use of certain other drugs and medications, including alcohol and aspirin, in some individuals. Vigorous exercise, fever, and pregnancy occasionally cause hypoglycemia by utilizing blood sugar faster than it may be made available to the tissues from food intake.

Symptoms of hypoglycemia may include hunger with nervousness, faintness, sweating, and palpitation. Severe attacks of hypoglycemia may be marked by headaches, visual disturbance, weakness, tremors, and loss of consciousness.

ileac abscess Occasionally, a perforated duodenal ulcer may leak contents of the intestinal tract along the right side of the abdominal cavity. The accumulation of the leakage will produce an inflammation of the ileum near the junction of the small and large intestines, where there normally is a hollow space. The inflammation can result in signs and symptoms of appendicitis, even though the basic cause of the problem is elsewhere in the abdomen.

ileitis An inflammation of the *ileum*, or the lower segment of the small intestine. The symptoms are similar to those of appendicitis, with cramping pains and tenderness in the abdomen, fever, and diarrhea. One difference is that diarrhea frequently is the first symptom. The feces may be stained with blood. Treatment usually consists of medications to relieve symptoms, diet, rest, and surgery if it is necessary to remove an obstruction associated with the problem.

ileocecal sphincter Another name for the ileocolic valve, the muscular mechanism that controls the emptying of the small intestine into the large intestine just above the cecum, or the blind pouch at the beginning of the ascending colon. An important function of the valve is that of preventing a backflow of fecal material from the colon into the small intestine.

ileostomy A surgical operation in which an artificial opening is made in the abdominal wall so that the contents of the *ileum* can be emptied outside the body, rather than into the colon through the ileocolic valve. An ileostomy may be constructed as a temporary opening to divert the intestinal flow as part of the treatment for an inflammatory bowel disease. Or it can be a permanent opening required by the surgical removal of the colon and rectum.

ileum The last and longest of the three divisions of the small intestine. Of the 20-plus feet of length of a normal adult-size small intestine, a bit more than 12 feet is the ileum, which ends at the *ileocecal sphincter*, or ileocolic valve.

infarction of bowel An occlusion or obstruction of the artery supplying blood to a segment of the bowel, usually causing pain, fluid accumulation, and gangrene. An infarction can occur as a result of a hernia or *intussusception* involving the intestine.

inguinal hernia A hernia, or rupture, that allows a portion of the intestine to protrude through the muscle layers in the area of the groin. The inguinal canal, or the normal passage through the abdominal wall for the male spermatic cord, is the point through which the abdominal contents push to produce an inguinal hernia. The intestine may follow the spermatic cord route into the scrotum, or it may produce a bulge in the abdominal wall near the ridge of the pelvic bone. An inguinal hernia almost always must be corrected by surgery in order to prevent incarceration, or entrapment, of the intestine in the opening through the muscles and fibrous tissues of the abdominal wall.

insulin A hormone secreted in the pancreas by groups of cells called the islets of Langerhans. Insulin is essential for normal human life because it enables the liver to store glucose, the basic sugar molecule derived from the metabolism of carbohydrates. When insulin is lacking in the bloodstream, the excess sugar obtained from food is excreted in the urine— one of the important diagnostic signs of *diabetes* mellitus.

insulinoma A tumor in the islets of Langerhans of the pancreas. Hypoglycemic symptoms, such as hunger, sweating, nausea, anxiety, headache, and fainting, after vigorous exercise or fasting, are associated with the disorder. Excessive insulin secretion is a cause of the symptoms and an effect of the tumor, which usually can be corrected by surgery.

intestinal polyposis An inherited disorder characterized by the development of polyps in the intestine and the appearance of pigmented brown spots, resembling freckles, on the face, hands, lips, and mouth. The signs and symptoms include anemia from bleeding of the polyps in the feces and general abdominal discomfort.

intestine For small intestine, see *duodenum, ileum, jejunum;* for large intestine, see *cecum, colon, rectum.*

intussusception A tongue-twister used by doctors to describe a condition in which one part of the intestinal tract telescopes into the adjoining portion. The *ileum,* for example, may invaginate, or push into, the *cecum* of the *colon.* The result usually is an intestinal obstruction. The disorder occurs most frequently among children in the western world, where nearly three-fourths of the cases occur during the first two years of life; however, in regions of Africa and Asia, intestinal intussusception is more common in adults. Symptoms generally include abdominal distension and pain, vomiting, constipation, and the passage of blood and mucus from the anus. The disorder generally is corrected by surgery.

jaundice A yellowish discoloration of the tissues caused by an abnormally high level of bilirubin in the bloodstream. The bilirubin accumulation results from disease or damage involving the liver cells, which normally excrete the bilirubin pigment with the bile. Jaundice also can be the result of an obstruction of the bile ducts. The yellowish tint produced by the bilirubin is most easily detected in the sclera, or white portion, of the eyeball in natural light.

jejunostomy An artificial opening made in the abdominal wall over the *jejunum* so that food can be introduced into the intestinal tract of a patient who is unable to consume food by mouth because of disease or injury. A fluid diet composed of the proper amount of calories and nutrients is poured into the jejunum through a catheter.

jejunum The middle section of the small intestine. This segment is approximately eight feet in length, compared to the ten-inch long duodenum which separates the jejunum from the stomach. The interior of the jejunum is carpeted with velvet-like villi on the surface of numerous folds of mucous membrane; the villi and folds are important in digesting food since they enable a maximum amount of intestinal surface to be exposed to nutrients mixed with the digestive juices.

kidney ptosis A term meaning a kidney that is displaced downward from its normal location at the level of the lower ribs. Normally, the left kidney is located slightly higher in the abdomen than the right kidney, but occasionally it may slip downward as far as the pelvis. The right kidney also may slip downward from its normal position.

Kupffer cells Cells in the liver that are responsible for filtering bacteria and other foreign substances from the bloodstream. Because they are efficient in trapping infectious agents, the Kupffer cells often involve the liver in diseases that enter the body.

lacteal A tiny vessel in the center of an intestinal villus. It is part of the lymphatic system and gets its name from the milky appearance of the fluid inside it. Fats pass through the lacteal vessels as part of the digestive process.

lactose intolerance A cause of gastro-enteritis among many black Americans, American Indians, and Orientals who lack an enzyme in their systems for digesting lactose, or milk sugar. Most individuals of northern European ancestry are not affected by the disorder because they inherit a gene for producing the enzyme that digests lactose. Symptoms may include *borborygmus,* or "gut rumblings," bloating, nausea, cramps, gas, and diarrhea. Although the lactose sugar molecule generally is regarded as the offending agent in the disorder, other disaccharide types of sugars also can cause similar symptoms in persons whose bodies lack the necessary digestive enzymes.

laparotomy An operation that involves an incision through the wall of the abdomen. It is a common type of operation for correcting disorders of the digestive tract or other organs within the abdominal cavity.

lavage A term meaning to irrigate, or wash out, the stomach, intestine, or another body organ or cavity. It is most commonly employed to remove swallowed poisonous substances from the gastrointestinal tract. The irrigating fluid may be water, a salt solution, a specific poison antidote, or a similar solution that is allowed to flow into the stomach through a tube inserted through the nose. The irrigating fluid is then siphoned through the tube, carrying out the diluted offending substance.

lazy colon A term sometimes used to describe a type of constipation that develops in elderly people. Feces accumulate in the rectum but there is no urge to have a bowel movement. Various reasons are found for the condition, including a long dependence upon the use of laxatives or enemas to produce bowel movements, lack of the usual stimuli such as eating and physical activity which ordinarily help in maintaining regularity of bowel evacuation, or no physical awareness of the need to have a bowel movement when the rectum is filled.

lipase One of the digestive enzymes secreted by the pancreas. It is involved in the digestion of fatty acids.

lipid An old Greek word for fatty substances. Lipids can be fats, waxes, fatty acids, and similar substances occurring in foods, the bloodstream, or body tissues. Lipid metabolism refers to the processes of the body involved in digesting and utilizing fatty acids or similar substances.

malabsorption syndrome A medical term for a condition marked by the presence of undigested fat or lactose in the stools of a patient with chronic diarrhea and malnutrition.

Markle's sign A diagnostic test sometimes used by doctors who are examining a patient with symptoms of abdominal pain. The patient is asked to stand erect with his heels raised above the floor and the weight of the body on his toes. Then he is asked to suddenly let the

heels drop so the body is jarred slightly. A pain associated with an abdominal disorder should then be felt by the patient in a rather precise location, thus helping the doctor to determine the exact cause of abdominal discomfort.

Meckel's diverticulum A duct that provides a route for the nourishment of the fetus but which normally shrivels up and disappears before birth. In a small percentage of people the duct remains attached to the end of the *ileum* after birth and becomes a diverticulum (see *diverticula*). The diverticulum may become inflamed, producing symptoms similar to those of appendicitis. In some cases, surgery is necessary to determine whether the cause of the symptoms is appendicitis or Meckel's diverticulitis.

meconium ileus A type of intestinal obstruction that may affect newborn infants. Meconium, a thick green material normally present in the small intestine of the fetus, does not move out of the bowel after birth. Signs and symptoms include a distended bowel and vomiting. Some cases of meconium ileus can be cleared up with a special type of enema; otherwise, surgery is necessary to save the life of the child. The disorder usually accompanies pancreatic disease, which is treated separately.

melena A medical term meaning black or tar-colored feces. The color is caused by the interaction of digestive juices and the hemoglobin of blood. The effect can indicate bleeding from any point between the esophagus and the *ileum*. Melena may be caused by swallowing blood from a nosebleed or blood that has been coughed up from the lungs.

mesenteric artery An artery that runs along the *mesentery* and supplies blood to the intestine.

mesenteric thrombosis An occlusion of the artery, or a portion of the artery, supplying blood to the intestine. If the blood flow through the mesenteric artery is interrupted, the tissues of the affected area of intestine will die, causing gangrene. The disorder is insidious in the onset of symptoms, which can include mild abdominal cramps and mild nausea and vomiting for several days, plus frequent bowel movements showing, in some cases, traces of blood. Fever, bowel distension, and peritonitis follow if the problem is not corrected; in cases where medical treatment is delayed too long, mesenteric thrombosis may have progressed to a point where the patient's life cannot be saved.

mesentery A fan-shaped blanket of membrane that hangs from the inner back wall of the abdominal cavity and helps support the small intestine.

micturition Another word for urination.

milk-alkali syndrome A reaction experienced by some persons who consume large amounts of milk and cream, or who take calcium carbonate antacid medications as treatment for peptic ulcers. Symptoms include nausea, vomiting, loss of appetite, headaches, and dizziness. The milk-alkali syndrone results in abnormally high levels of calcium in the blood and causes kidney damage in some patients.

mittelschmerz A term used to identify the abdominal symptoms of a ruptured ovary follicular cyst. The event usually occurs midway between menstrual periods and may be accompanied by nausea and vomiting, along with abdominal pain that sometimes suggests an attack of appendicitis.

mucin A sticky substance secreted by glands in the lining of the stomach. Mucin helps to digest food and normally neutralizes excess gastric acid in the stomach.

mucous membrane The lining of the digestive tract. Its structure varies from the mouth to the anus, depending upon the role played by a particular segment of the digestive tract. In the esophagus, for example, the mucous membrane is composed mainly of layers of cells resembling skin cells, apparently designed by nature to resist wear-and-tear by swallowed objects passing along its surface. From the stomach through the intestines the mucous membrane contains specialized cells that either secrete digestive juices or absorb nutrients from food being digested and transported along the surface of the membrane.

mucoviscidosis Another word for cystic fibrosis, or *fibrocystic disease* of the pancreas.

nausea An unpleasant sensation associated with a disorder in the gastrointestinal system that is frequently accompanied by a tendency to vomit. Nausea is believed to be a response to irritation of nerve endings in the stomach and other body organs. It can be caused by emotions and pain in other body areas, as well as by digestive disorders. The intensity of the stimulus needed to advance nausea to the vomiting stage apparently varies with different individuals, just as the stimulus that may cause nausea in one person may result only in a loss of appetite, or anorexia, in another.

nephritis A term applied to any of several types of inflammation of the kidney. A common form of nephritis is glomerulonephritis, a disease involving the glomeruli, or clusters of capillaries that filter fluids and other substances from the blood. Acute nephritis sometimes is a complication of scarlet fever or similar infections in children. Salt-losing nephritis involves a condition of abnormal sodium excretion by persons who ingest average amounts of table salt.

nephrogram An X-ray picture of the kidney.

nephrolith A medical name for kidney stones.

nephrosis A term that may be used to indicate almost any kind of kidney disease, although it is generally restricted to a degenerative condition marked by abnormal accumulation of fluid in the body. Nephrosis often develops after a patient apparently has recovered from acute *nephritis*, but the nephrosis symptoms may not appear until years later. The patient may experience the symptoms of nephrosis as a chronic condition for many years.

occult blood Blood that appears from a source that is hidden from the normal view of a patient or examining physician. Blood in vomit or feces, for example, may have originated in any one of several points in the body. Blood from the lungs can be swallowed and appear in vomit from the stomach, or be carried through the digestive tract and appear in feces. Laboratory and other tests usually are employed to locate the source of bleeding.

oliguria The production of urine in below-normal amounts. It is a sign of a kidney disorder. However, the condition is not as critical as that of *anuria*, which is the term used to indicate any amount of urine that is less than two ounces per day. Oliguria often is applied to amounts of urine that are more than two ounces but less than one pint per day.

omentum A fold of peritoneal membrane that protects the stomach and other abdominal organs. It usually contains fat deposits and serves as insulation. The omentum also helps control the spread of inflammation in some organs in the abdominal cavity.

palpation Use of the fingers and palms of the hands to determine the condition of organs and tissues beneath the skin as part of a medical examination of a patient. An examining doctor may use palpation, for example, to judge the size of the liver or to locate a displaced kidney.

pancreatitis An inflammation of the pancreas. Causes can range from infection to alcoholism; symptoms may include abdominal pain or discomfort, nausea and vomiting, diarrhea, and jaundice. In some cases, particularly chronic pancreatitis, the gallbladder may be involved. The acute form of pancreatitis may develop quite suddenly, with symptoms severe enough to produce shock and collapse.

Treatment generally is directed toward relieving symptoms and allowing the pancreas to rest and heal itself. In most cases this involves intravenous feedings to replace lost fluids and to provide adequate nutrition; no food or water are taken by mouth during the recovery peri-od. Pain-killing drugs, small doses of insulin, and other appropriate medications are administered. In severe cases where internal bleeding may have occurred, surgery may be required.

paracentesis Aspiration of the contents of a body cavity. In a case of a patient with an abdominal disorder, a needle may be inserted into the peritoneal cavity to draw out any fluid that may have accumulated as a result of bleeding from an ulcer or pancreatitis, for example, as part of the clinical examination. Paracentesis usually is performed only when other diagnostic techniques have failed to provide necessary answers to questions about the cause of a medical problem. The patient is given an anesthetic in advance of the procedure.

parietal cells The cells in the lining of the stomach that produce hydrochloric acid. Other cells in the stomach lining produce *mucin*, which helps protect the mucous membrane lining of the stomach from being destroyed by the powerful acid.

pepsin An enzyme that helps digest proteins. It is secreted by cells in the lining of the stomach and is a part of the mixture called *gastric juice.*

peptic ulcer An ulcer that occurs in the gastrointestinal tract as a result of exposure to the *gastric juice* secreted by cells in the stomach lining. Peptic ulcers that occur in the stomach sometimes are called gastric ulcers, while those that appear in the *duodenum*, the part of the small intestine just beyond the stomach, are called duodenal ulcers. Peptic ulcers also can develop in the esophagus from a reflux of gastric juice.

peristalsis A wave-like motion of the gastrointestinal tract that moves food forward while it is being digested. The waves are produced by rhythmic contractions and relaxations of the two layers of muscles in the intestines; one layer runs in circles around the lumen, or cavity, of the tube, and the other runs lengthwise. The stomach has a third muscle layer, running obliquely with respect to the other two layers, which helps to churn food while it is being digested by gastric juices.

peritoneum The membrane lining the inner walls of the abdominal and pelvic cavities. The membrane folds back in a second layer that covers some internal organs. The space between the membrane layers is called the peritoneal cavity.

peritonitis An inflammation of the peritoneum, usually characterized by severe abdominal pain and tenderness, and accompanied by fever and a rapid heartbeat. The pain generally is aggravated by any movement or pressure involving the abdomen. But specific signs and symptoms may vary according to the cause of the condition, such as disease organisms or foreign material which may consist of blood or intestinal contents leaking from a perforated ulcer or ruptured appendix.

Treatment usually is directed toward the cause of the inflammation with antibiotic therapy and surgery as needed to correct the primary and secondary factors, when the peritonitis is a complication of another health problem. Therapy also includes bed rest, intravenous feedings to help clear the digestive tract, pain-killing drugs administered by injection, and suction or other drainage methods for controlling accumulation of pus and potentially contaminating materials in the digestive tract.

piles A common name for hemorrhoids. See *hemorrhoidal vessels.*

Polya gastrectomy A surgical procedure, named for the doctor who developed the technique of removing a portion of the stomach and sewing the remaining portion directly to the jejunum, the second segment of the small intestine. The duodenum is bypassed and closed off in this type of operation, which is employed to control peptic ulcers.

portal pyemia An inflammation of the *portal vein* caused by disease organisms entering the bloodstream from the intestines.

portal vein The main vein leading to the liver from the intestine. Smaller veins which collect nutrients absorbed by the villi in the small intestine drain into the portal vein.

pruritis ani An irritation of the skin around the anus, a condition that frequently is exacerbated by scratching the area that itches. The irritation may be associated with diabetes or an infestation of fungus or worms, among other possible causes.

ptyalin A digestive enzyme that helps break down carbohydrate molecules into smaller units. Ptyalin is secreted by the salivary glands in the mouth and becomes part of the food *bolus* that enters the stomach from the mouth, via the esophagus.

pyelitis An inflammation of the kidney, often resulting from the formation of kidney stones. However, infectious disease organisms also may be a causative factor. The symptoms include pain and tenderness in the loins, an irritable bladder, diarrhea, vomiting, and the appearance of blood or pus in the urine. The disorder also may be marked by a specific type of pain that occurs when the leg is flexed. Treatment includes the administration of antibiotics and pain-killing drugs, and the patient is encouraged to increase his fluid intake in order to help maintain a somewhat normal kidney function.

pylorus The muscular valve that controls the movement of *chyme*, or partially digested food, from the stomach to the *duodenum*, the first segment of the small intestine. When the pylorus is closed, food does not leave the stomach. When the chyme is ready for the next stage of the digestive process, the pylorus squirts it into the duodenum.

Ramstedt operation A surgical technique sometimes performed to relax or open a *pylorus* that does not permit a normal flow of chyme from the stomach into the small intestine. The operation may be needed to save an infant born with a congenitally defective pyloric valve.

rectum The final portion of the large intestine situated between the *sigmoid colon* and the anus. It is about five inches long and normally has several folds in the lining. Feces, the normally solid waste products of the digestive tract, accumulate in the rectum.

regional enteritis Another name for *Crohn's disease*, an inflammation of the ileum and neighboring segments of the intestinal tract. The inflammation may affect all of the layers of the intestinal wall, resulting in the thickening of fibrous tissues as well as ulcerations of the inner lining.

renal colic A type of abdominal pain that may start in the back of the abdomen and radiate downward to the inner thighs and genitals. The most frequent cause of the pain is a kidney stone entering or passing through the ureter. In some cases the cause may be a blood clot or a foreign body being passed through the ureter.

RLQ An abbreviation for right lower quadrant, or lower right side, of the abdomen, where pain might suggest appendicitis or other possible disorders.

roundworms A cause of intestinal obstruction in some people living in Third World countries. The worms may enter the digestive tract with contaminated food and multiply in the small intestine until the mass becomes large enough to block the flow of food. The worms can obstruct the bile duct or perforate the intestine, in which case *peritonitis* would result.

rupture A common word for hernia, generally applied to a hernia of the abdominal contents through the inguinal canal, or *inguinal hernia*. A hernia involving abdominal contents also may occur at the point where the femoral artery leaves the pelvis to enter the upper leg, making the rupture technically a *femoral hernia*. However, tissues can tear or break in almost any organ to become a rupture, as in a ruptured aneurysm, a ruptured stomach, etc.

RUQ An abbreviation of right upper quadrant, or upper right side, of the abdomen, where symptoms could suggest problems involving the liver, gallbladder, or kidney, for starters.

salmonellosis A disease that has nothing to do with fish, particularly, unless the fish is involved in this type of food poisoning. Salmonella is a kind of bacteria named for Dr. Daniel Salmon, and there are many variations of the salmonella bacteria, including a strain that causes typhoid fever. Several other types of salmonella are responsible for gastro-enteritis, causing abdominal discomfort and diarrhea in people who eat spoiled food or food that has been exposed to contamination by salmonella bacteria.

salpingitis An inflammation of a uterine tube, which may be a cause of pain in the lower abdomen of a woman. When the pain, accompanied by fever and abdominal tenderness, occurs on the right side, the symptoms may resemble appendicitis.

shigellosis A gastrointestinal disease caused by exposure to an acid-producing type of bacteria called Shigella. Shigellosis causes acute inflammation of the intestines, usually confined to the colon but sometimes involving the ileum as well. Signs and symptoms include frequent bowel movements with feces marked by pus, blood, and mucus. The patient experiences nausea, cramps, and fever. The disease is rare in communities where good sanitation and hygiene measures are enforced, but it may be encountered in primitive, overcrowded areas where food and water may be contaminated or a traveler may have direct contact with an infected person.

shock (insulin) A *hypoglycemia* reaction that may occur in a diabetes patient who has taken an overdose of insulin or has not eaten enough food to utilize the insulin administered. The reaction may begin with a feeling of weakness or dizziness, or blurred vision, and result in unconsciousness if allowed to continue untreated. The treatment usually is rather simple. When the victim is given carbohydrate food by mouth, or an injection of glucose (sugar) solution if he is unable to swallow food, he usually recovers quickly. An untreated victim of insulin shock may suffer a fatal coma. Most diabetics carry small amounts of sugar or candy to eat if they feel the symptoms of insulin shock starting.

sigmoid colon A segment of the descending *colon*, which gets its name because it is shaped like the Greek letter "sigma." It is situated just above the rectum.

siphonage A term used when referring to the use of a siphon, or to siphon technique in administering gastric lavage, that is, using a siphon to drain the contents of the stomach after it has been washed out. Siphonage also can be used to drain the urinary bladder.

Sippy diet A once popular diet for peptic ulcer patients, requiring that the patient consume a three-ounce mixture of cream and milk every hour for 13 hours each day, plus antacid medications. The purpose of the diet is to counteract the gastric acid produced by the stomach. The diet was named for its inventor, Dr. Bertram Sippy.

sphincter A name given a circular muscle that contracts to close an opening and relaxes to allow fluid or other substances to pass. There are several sphincters in the digestive tract: the cardiac or lower esophageal sphincter controls the opening of the esophagus into the stomach; the pyloric sphincter controls the exit from the stomach; the ileocecal sphincter controls the flow of digestive waste products from the small intestine to the large intestine; and the anal sphincter releases feces. Other sphincters control flow from the urinary bladder, gallbladder, and pancreas.

splanchnic bed A term sometimes used by doctors in referring to the network of capillaries that supply blood to the intestine. The splanchnic bed contains so many miles of blood vessels that it would be theoretically possible for the body's entire blood supply to be swallowed up at once in the capillary network. One reason this does not happen is that tiny valves control the flow of blood so that each of the capillary branches must wait briefly for its turn in moving blood while a neighboring capillary discharges.

splenic Pertaining to the spleen. The word "splenetic" also is used at times for the same purpose.

sprue A malabsorption disorder resulting from changes in the mucosal lining of the small intestine. A nontropical form of sprue also is known as celiac disease, a familial disease marked by intolerance to proteins in wheat, rye, barley, and oats. The symptoms occur in patients who are sensitive to gluten proteins when foods containing the offending substance are eaten. Other cereals, such as corn and rice, do not produce the effects. Tropical sprue, a variation of the nontropical or celiac sprue, affects mainly people who live in the Caribbean and in southern Asia. The symptoms are similar to those of *celiac disease*, although gluten protein does not seem to be a factor. However, the mucosal lining of the small intestine is affected in such a way that malabsorption results, and the nutrients folic acid and vitamin B-12 are not utilized from food. Anemia eventually occurs unless a special diet rich in protein and supplemented with folic acid and vitamin B-12, plus other vital nutrients, is administered.

spurious diarrhea A condition that may be associated with severe constipation in which feces in the rectum have become impacted. The colon above the impacted fecal mass is unable to absorb water normally, and the fluid escapes around the impacted feces, producing an illusion of watery diarrhea. This effect is most likely to occur in an older person.

stasis Stagnation or lack of movement of a substance. Intestinal stasis, for example, suggests that food does not move along normally through the intestine, perhaps because of an obstruction.

steatorrhea A medical way of describing feces that contain abnormal amounts of fats. The condition sometimes results from a disease of the pancreas that results in a deficiency of lipase, an enzyme that normally helps digest fats. The feces have a fatty, pale appearance and tend to float. In addition to pancreatic abnormalities, other conditions that can cause steatorrhea include *sprue.*

stenosis Another word for *stricture,* although a stenosis may involve a stricture that has become obstructive. A pyloric stenosis, for example, may be a life-threatening abnormality in that it prevents food digested in the stomach from entering the intestine.

stool Another word for feces. If a doctor asks you to bring a stool sample to his office, he expects you to produce a container holding a sample of waste products from your bowels.

strangulated hernia A condition in which a portion of the intestine has become trapped in an opening in the abdominal wall and will not return to its normal position without surgical treatment. A strangulated hernia is a serious matter because the intestine most likely will be obstructed and blood vessels supplying the intestinal tissue may be blocked, resulting in gangrene, or death of the vital tissues.

stricture An abnormal narrowing of a tube in the body. A stricture in the intestine, esophagus, ureter, etc., can obstruct the flow through the passage. A stricture can be due to a birth defect, a disease, or an injury. A functional stricture is one that is due to muscle spasms rather than a true narrowing caused by changes in the tissue because of scar formation or the spread of fibrous material.

swallowing difficulty A common term for *dysphagia.*

tapeworm A worm that can enter the human digestive tract as a result of eating raw or poorly cooked meats, mainly beef, pork, or fish. Beef tapeworms, which may appear as ribbon-like creatures nearly 30 feet in length when full grown, get into the flesh of cattle as tapeworm eggs. The eggs hatch and the tiny immature larvae conceal themselves in cysts in the muscles, which later become steaks, hamburger, etc. Pork tapeworms and freshwater fish tapeworms are similar in appearance and method of finding their way into the human digestive tract, even though they are of different species. Tapeworms can occur in foods in almost any part of the world, including North America, where they are most likely to be found in such scattered regions as Canada, Florida, California, and the Great Lakes area.

thigh-rotation test A test occasionally performed by a doctor trying to diagnose the cause of a medical problem in the abdominal cavity. The patient's leg is bent at the knee so that the thigh is flexed. By rotating the leg, certain abdominal muscles are moved. This action can result in pain or irritation at the site of a disorder within the abdomen, such as an abscess or perforated appendix. The thigh-rotation test may be employed when other diagnostic techniques cannot be used or fail to provide the correct clues.

threadworms A parasitic disease similar to hookworms. The larvae enter the human body and migrate to the intestine or lungs. In the intestine the worms can produce abdominal pain and tenderness, with vomiting and diarrhea. The chances of infestation increase with unsanitary living conditions and warm climate. Treatment is by administration of "worming" medicines which are taken by mouth each day for several days.

trypsin An enzyme secreted by the pancreas to help digest protein foods. Protein digestion usually begins in the stomach where the protein is exposed to gastric juice, the pepsin and hydrochloric acid mixture which break it down into subunits called peptides. Trypsin then breaks down the peptides into the basic building blocks of proteins, the amino acids.

tube feeding A method of providing nutrition to a patient whose digestive tract is normal but who is unable to eat food safely, perhaps because of being semiconscious. A plastic tube is inserted into the stomach, and a liquid diet, prepared from such foods as milk and eggs, and providing adequate amounts of various nutrients is mixed in a blender and fed into the tube.

turista A popular name for a type of gastroenteritis characterized by abdominal cramps, diarrhea, and nausea and vomiting. The disorder is experienced occasionally by tourists consuming food or beverages in places where foods may be contaminated by bacteria or other organisms. The disease also has other names, such as traveler's diarrhea.

ulcer An open sore in the mucous membrane of the digestive tract is called a peptic ulcer. An ulcer also may occur in other body tissues, such as the skin, as a result of disease or injury. A peptic ulcer may be either microscopically tiny or rather large. It may continue eroding the tissue until it has perforated the wall of the organ, or it may quite mysteriously stop its erosive action and become covered with scar tissue. Peptic ulcers develop in areas where the mucous membrane is in contact with gastric acid from cells lining the stomach. See also *duodenal ulcer; peptic ulcer.*

ulcerative colitis An inflammatory disease of the colon marked by the appearance of countless tiny ulcers in the mucosal lining of the bowel and of diarrhea with stools containing blood and mucus. At times the stools may be watery, and at other times composed mainly of blood and pus. The disease may develop at nearly any age, but is most likely to begin around early adulthood. It may affect only a portion of the colon or the entire colon. The disease may be fatal, especially if it begins early in life and involves the entire colon. Therapy may involve medications or surgery, or both.

umbilicus The "belly button" which marks the point where the umbilical cord was attached during fetal life.

urea A waste product of the metabolism of proteins. It is formed in the liver from ammonia, which in turn is a waste product of amino acid breakdown. The amount of urea in the urine depends in part upon the amount of protein foods consumed. Other factors which may result in abnormally large amounts of urea in urine include fever and diabetes.

uremia A disease characterized by the accumulation of *urea* in the blood, usually because of the failure of the kidneys to maintain normal rates of excretion of the substance.

uric acid An acid that is the waste product of the metabolism of nitrogen compounds called purines. Uric acid crystals often are associated with kidney stones and the concretions found in tissues of patients suffering from gout. Excretion of uric acid normally increases after eating protein foods or after vigorous exercise which may involve metabolism of body tissues.

vagotomy An operation performed to cut the vagus nerve fibers that are associated with stimulation of gastric acid production by the stomach. The surgery may be done to reduce the risk of peptic ulcer development or to increase the chances of recovery from existing ulcers.

villi Tiny finger-like projections that extend from the lining of the intestine. The membrane of the inner surface of the intestine is covered with millions of villi, like a shag carpet. Each villus is composed of cells that can absorb through their walls the vital nutrients in the digested food passing over them. The cells of the villus pass the molecules of carbohydrate, amino acids, or whatever into the center of the villus, where there are blood vessels to carry the nutrients away from the intestine and into the major veins leading to the liver.

viscera A term sometimes used to refer to the abdominal organs.

vitamins Substances occurring naturally in foods in very small quantities that are essential as catalysts to help the body utilize other nutrients in the food. The absence of a vitamin from the diet can result in a deficiency disease such as scurvy, which is a vitamin C-deficiency disease marked by bleeding gums, black and blue spots on the skin, and general weakness.

void The verb form sometimes used for the act of urination, or *micturition*.

volvulus A loop of intestine that has become twisted so that the normal flow of the contents is obstructed.

vomitus A word that doctors may use to describe the matter that has been vomited.

water metabolism More than eight quarts of water are cycled and recycled through the normal intestinal tract each day, of which perhaps only three pints are introduced into the body as water or other beverages taken with meals. The remainder is from saliva and other gastric fluids. Various minerals and hormones control the amount of water that is retained or excreted, and the shifts of water from the inside to the outside of the body's tissue cells, or vice versa, by the process of osmosis. The amount of fluid consumed and the amount excreted each day can provide clues to a variety of diseases and disorders.

Whipple's disease A rare digestive disorder characterized by a failure of the intestinal lining to handle fatty acids normally. Symptoms and signs include bowel movements that yield fatty stools, loss of strength, and weight loss.

Zenker's diverticulum A pouch or sac at the junction of the esophagus and pharynx. The tissue abnormality sometimes is associated with obstruction of the esophagus.

Zollinger-Ellison syndrome A digestive system disorder marked by severe peptic ulcer attacks, abnormally high rates of gastric acid production, and tumors of the pancreas which secrete the enzyme gastrin.

QUESTIONS AND ANSWERS
THE ABDOMEN

Q: *My wife recently returned home after a kidney transplant operation. Now she is talking about having children. Is it safe for a woman to have a baby following a kidney transplant?*

A: Kidney transplants are no longer rare occurrences and perhaps hundreds of women with transplanted kidneys already have had successful pregnancies. Part of the answer to your question depends upon whether the transplanted kidney is functioning well; if it is, your wife has a good chance of delivering a normal baby. The risk seems to be more significant for women with poor kidney function.

Q: *I have read that bran cereals in the diet can prevent the development of diverticulosis. Is it true?*

A: It is true that bran tablets have been helpful in relieving the symptoms of some patients with diverticular disease. Before you add bran to your own diet, however, it would be wise to discuss the idea with your own doctor. He would be the best judge of the effectiveness of bran in your particular case.

Q: *Are you ever too young or too old to have appendicitis?*

A: No. Appendicitis has been found in newborn babies as well as in senior citizens. In fact, there is a high rate of complications in appendicitis patients over the age of 45, perhaps because they tend to delay seeing the doctor when the symptoms develop. They apparently believe they are too old to have a medical problem usually associated with young children.

Q: *My son developed diarrhea while away at college and lost more than seven pounds of body weight before a school doctor began treating him for what he claimed was fungus in the intestinal tract. Is it possible for fungus to grow in the intestines?*

A: There is a type of fungus which actually is a strain of yeast cells called Candida that may be found in the intestine of any healthy person. The yeast cells may or may not cause any symptoms. But occasionally the yeast, or fungus, cells may go on a rampage and produce symptoms of diarrhea, abdominal cramps, and other disorders. The organism can be identified by laboratory examination of a stool sample. The disorder generally responds to antifungal drugs given several times daily for three to seven days.

Q: *If you have heartburn, does that mean you also have a hiatus hernia that eventually requires surgery?*

A: Not necessarily. The sour or acid taste and the burning sensation in the chest that are associated with heartburn are due in most cases to an incompetent sphincter muscle between the stomach and the esophagus that allows a reflux of gastric acid into the esophagus. Many people manage to control the symptoms with medications and a few commonsensical measures such as losing weight and avoiding the wearing of clothing, such as girdles, that increase pressure on the abdominal organs. Medications can include antacid tablets as well as a drug that helps strengthen the lower esophageal sphincter muscle.

Q: *What kind of antacid medications should I take for heartburn?*

A: This is the kind of question you should ask your personal physician. There are many types of antacid medications on the market, and many different kinds of chemicals are used in the manufacture of antacid tablets, powders, and liquids. The various medications have different kinds of side effects for some individuals, and they also may interact with other medicines you may be taking. For those reasons, only your doctor knows for sure what kind you should take for your particular situation.

Q: *My wife had a gallbladder attack a few days after she had an abdominal X-ray which didn't show any gallstones. Could an X-ray examination miss a solid object like a gallstone?*
A: It is not unusual for an ordinary X-ray examination to miss gallstones since most are not radio-opaque, meaning they are not composed of the kinds of substances that show up on X-ray film. A special type of X-ray picture, called a cholecystogram, is used to locate gallstones. It requires that the patient, on the night before the cholecystogram procedure, take tablets that contain a radio-opaque dye, which will coat the inside of the gallbladder and the bile ducts so that abnormalities or foreign objects will be easily visible to the doctor.

Q: *Can gallstones be removed without an operation?*
A: There are drugs that have been found to dissolve certain kinds of gallstones in select patients, but this treatment is not recommended for all patients. The medication works on gallstones that are entirely or mostly composed of cholesterol. But early tests showed that it could take as long as two years for the drug to dissolve a large gallstone; small stones dissolved more rapidly. Use of the gallstone dissolving drug generally has been limited to patients with mild symptoms who might refuse or not be able to tolerate surgery. Most patients who have experienced the excruciating pain of a severe gallbladder attack would rather not wait two years to have the problem corrected.

Q: *When my doctor examined me for chronic constipation, he said I probably have a cathartic colon as a result of taking laxatives. Was he joking or is there really such a thing as a cathartic colon?*

A: Cathartic colon is a term sometimes used to describe a condition in which the large intestine, or colon, becomes dilated and loses its normal muscle tone or strength for moving fecal material. The condition usually is the result of laxative abuse. Continued use of laxatives can damage the nerve centers responsible for stimulating peristalsis in the gut, with the result that increasingly larger doses of laxatives may be taken to achieve the desired bowel movement effect. The ultimate result is the cathartic colon.

To correct the situation, a patient must withdraw from the use of irritating laxatives and try eating high-residue foods to retrain the bowel. In some cases of laxative abuse it becomes necessary to perform an operation in which the large intestine is removed and the small intestine is attached directly to the rectum.

Q: *How much fat is "normal" for a person to carry on his body?*
A: Most average adults have between 20 and 40 pounds of adipose tissue, or fat, in their bodies. However, that amount of fat is not located in one area but is scattered throughout the body. Also, the normal human body fat is not an inert mass but is constantly being mobilized for use as body fuel or being deposited again if not used. Levels of free fatty acids from fat deposits rise in the bloodstream during periods of physical activity, such as sports and work, and even while watching an exciting movie or TV show. A person who is considered to be fat, or obese, usually has at least twice as much fat in his body tissues as a "normal" adult.

Q: *Why do many doctors claim that fat babies will become fat adults?*
A: Probably because it too often is true, although preventable. One factor involved in obesity is the number of fat cells, called adipocytes, distributed in the body. These are fat storage cells. Most normal babies start life with about the same number of fat cells, and the number can increase steadily until puberty is reached. A baby or child who is overfed develops more fat cells at a more rapid rate. This

effect is not reversible, that is, the more fat cells acquired during childhood the more that remain in the adult; they do not fade away. Possessing an above-average number of fat cells makes it easier to accumulate fat as an adult, and at the same time makes it more difficult to get rid of excess fat.

Q: *Is it safe to eat freshwater fish that have been cured by smoking?*
A: The fish tapeworm that infests lakes in North America, Europe, and Japan can survive exposure to smoke that is less than 56 degrees Celsius, or 133 degrees Fahrenheit. That minimum temperature must be maintained at least five minutes to kill the fish tapeworm larvae. If you have smoked fish that may not have been cured adequately, it should be cooked before it is eaten. Or the fish should be frozen at a temperature no warmer than 14 degrees Fahrenheit for 48 hours. The fish tapeworm can live in the human digestive tract without producing serious symptoms, but it can cause anemia by absorbing the vitamin B-12 in meals consumed by the host.

Q: *My husband is recovering from an attack of viral hepatitis. His doctor wants him to get plenty of rest and eat a nutritious diet. Is it all right to include beer with his meals?*
A: A person who is recovering from viral hepatitis should not consume alcoholic beverages for a period of three to six months as a precaution against further damage to the liver. Your husband's doctor probably will advise when it is O.K. for him to begin having beer with his meals.

Q: *Should a person who is taking care of a viral hepatitis patient get a vaccination of some kind as protection against the disease?*
A: The risk of transmission of viral hepatitis depends in part on the amount of commonsensical precautions that are taken in the care of the patient, as would be true of a person infected with any contagious disease. However, there are special preparations of immunoglobulins that can be administered by intramuscular injection to increase the protection of persons exposed to either form, type A or type B, of hepatitis.

Q: *My girl friend had to quit taking antihistamines because the doctor thinks they gave her a case of hepatitis. Can this happen to anybody taking antihistamines?*
A: Your girl friend probably is hypersensitive to a substance used in the manufacture of antihistamine medications. Some people develop hepatitis from the use of barbiturates, sulfa drugs, appetite suppressants, and diuretics. Other individuals may develop a liver-gallbladder reaction to oral contraceptives or tranquilizers. One of the functions of the liver is detoxification of the blood by converting foreign substances such as drugs into less active chemicals that can be excreted—a normal function for most people—but some individuals may lack an enzyme needed to metabolize the drug, and that triggers the reaction. It is possible that no drug exists that will not produce adverse liver effects in some person. Once a reaction to a drug is suspected, one should stop using the drug until the doctor can determine whether there is a cause-and-effect relationship, and perhaps prescribe an alternative drug.

Q: *Our granddaughter developed diarrhea while staying at our home recently, and we gave her some antidiarrhea tablets from our medicine chest. The little girl acted like she was drunk after taking the tablets. Is it possible the medicine contains alcohol?*
A: You may have given the child a common antidiarrhea medication that contains a drug called diphenoxylate, which small children may not tolerate well. The drug works by depressing the central nervous system and can cause dizziness, drowsiness, and depression, much like an overdose of alcohol. In fact, it is recommended that adults refrain from drinking alcoholic beverages while taking diphenoxylate drugs for diarrhea. In a small child the drug can result in respiratory difficulty and cardiac arrest.

Q: *I have heard that a person with diarrhea should not drink milk. Could this be true?*
A: It could be true for certain kinds of diarrhea, such as diarrhea caused by a bacterial infection. The disease may deplete the body's supply of lactase, the enzyme needed to metabolize lactose, or milk sugar. A person who normally could tolerate milk would then be in a condition similar to that of one who had inherited a lactase deficiency. The milk would prolong the symptoms of diarrhea. When the infection has been controlled, milk may be reintroduced gradually into the patient's diet.

Q: *Everybody has advice for losing weight but doctors seldom have suggestions for gaining weight. Are there any drugs that can be prescribed to improve the appetite?*
A: There are a few drugs that are used to stimulate the appetite indirectly as part of the treatment for patients with serious nutritional problems, such as anorexia nervosa. If your weight is not declining and is simply on the low end of the average range of weights for persons of your height, age, and body frame, there should be no cause for concern. If you are actually losing weight, you should see your doctor. If you simply want to increase your appetite, why not try a premeal aperitif to help relax? Since eating habits are partly psychological, relaxing in the company of friends or family may do more for your appetite than drugs.

Q: *What is Bright's disease?*
A: Bright's disease is a term once used to describe a type of kidney disease that was characterized by the excretion of abnormally large amounts of albumin in the urine. The term has been replaced in most medical texts by nephritis or glomerular disease.

Q: *What is the cause of edema in the abdominal cavity and what can be done about it?*
A: Edema in the abdominal cavity is caused by leakage of fluid from blood capillaries in the neighboring tissues because of weakened heart action. The heart fails to pump the blood through the tissues properly, and the fluid portion gradually is lost from the circulatory system. The problem is rather easily corrected with medications that improve the force of the heart action and with diuretics that help the kidneys excrete the accumulated fluid.

Q: *Is there anything that can be done about gas in the stomach?*
A: The answer depends upon the source of the gas. In most cases the gas associated with belching results from swallowed air, or aerophagia. Small amounts of air are swallowed normally with food and beverages. Aerophagia also accompanies gum chewing. And some people unconsciously swallow quantities of air.
A certain amount of gas also accumulates normally in the top of the stomach. Gas can be produced in the stomach by the interaction of certain foods and hydrochloric acid in the gastric juice. Taking baking soda as a remedy for stomach gas, for example, can produce more gas in the stomach. The only lasting remedies for stomach gas are to learn to control the amount of air you swallow and to avoid foods that help produce gas in the stomach.

Q: *On a record of a kidney test, I noticed a reference to a Bun. What does this have to do with kidney function?*
A: The abbreviation you saw probably was BUN, which stands for Blood Urea Nitrogen. Urea is a major product of excretion by the kidneys, and the nitrogen portion of urea is measured in laboratory tests of a blood sample. An abnormally high BUN level indicates a kidney function disorder.

Q: *What is a "horseshoe" kidney?*
A: Occasionally, a person is born with a congenital abnormality in which the bottom ends of the two kidneys are joined together to form a horseshoe-shaped kidney. Kidney function is not hampered by the abnormality and the condition might only be discovered during an examination for an unrelated abdominal problem.

Q: *Where is the rectosigmoid in the abdomen and what is its purpose?*

A: A rectosigmoid is not actually a body organ or tissue. It is an area at the end of the colon that can be inspected by a doctor with a sigmoidoscope. It includes the anus, the rectum, and a part of the sigmoid, or S-shaped, section of the descending colon. Thus, when a doctor does a rectosigmoid examination, he is merely inspecting the approximately last ten inches of the large intestine.

Q: *Is it dangerous for pregnant women to eat clay to satisfy a pica craving?*

A: Yes. Pregnant women who eat clay also may ingest hookworms. They can also become anemic because clay prevents the absorption of iron.

6

SEX ORGANS

An examination of the abdomen would not be complete if the doctor did not check the condition of the reproductive organs, which share the space and some tissues of the other organ systems within the abdominal cavity. The genitals, or sex organs, of the human body in fact serve as abdominal landmarks for a doctor performing a general physical examination of a patient.

The sex organs also can provide important clues to the health of the body in general or of glands and tissues far removed from the lower abdominal region. The female reproductive cycle, or menstrual cycle, for example, is controlled by the pituitary gland, which is located at the base of the brain. A malfunction of the pituitary can result in a condition known as precocious puberty, which means that a girl may become sexually mature at eight years of age or a boy at the age of ten or earlier.

During the first two months of embryonic life the tissues that will develop as either the male or female sex organs grow side by side. By the 14th week, there are significant signs in the anatomy of the embryo that indicate whether the child will be a boy or a girl. If the baby is going to be a girl, the primitive genital tracts will develop into oviducts and uterus. At the same time a tissue prominence called a genital tubercle will recede to become an external fold of the labia for a girl. If male hormones are present during this period, the tissues that would develop into a female oviduct and uterus gradually disappear while the neighboring genital tract develops into a vas deferens, the tube that carries sperm from the testis. The undifferentiated gonads in the eight-week-old embryo become either ovaries for the female or testes for the male. If a male, the genital tubercle develops into the penis, and the testes migrates from a point somewhat above and behind the developing urinary bladder to a new location in the scrotum, a pouch outside the abdomen and under the penis.

Actually, the sex of the child is determined at the time of conception. At that moment a spermatozoon from the father fertilizes an ovum from the mother. Each of the male and female sex cells, also known as gametes, carries 23 chromosomes, which are a microscopic chain of genetic information that will determine hair color, eye color, and other physical characteristics of the child who will develop from the fertilized ovum.

Twenty-two of the 23 chromosomes will be essentially the same in the female and male gametes. The 23rd chromosome will determine the sex of the future child and usually is designated as either an X or a Y chromosome. The ovum always carries an X chromosome as the 23rd chromosome, but the spermatozoon, or male germ cell, can contribute either an X or a Y chromosome. If the fertilized ovum, or zygote, contains 44 regular chromosomes plus 2 X chromosomes, it will develop into a girl baby. If the combination is a total of 44 regular chromosomes plus one X and one Y chromosome, the zygote will develop into a boy baby.

Occasionally, nature makes a mistake and produces a child with only one X chromosome or an offspring with two X chromosomes and one Y chromosome. These individuals may have the general appearance of females or males, but they lack certain specific characteristics of either women or men, a factor that becomes more obvious when they reach puberty. A woman apparently needs at least two X chromosomes, for example, in order to have functioning ovaries and menstrual cycles. Thus, a woman with only one X chromosome would have nonfunctioning ovaries and would not menstruate. A man with two X chromosomes would have rudimentary but nonfunctioning testes and thus would not be able to produce sperm. He also might have enlarged, female-like breasts that could be removed by plastic surgery for cosmetic reasons.

Ordinarily, the sex of a child is obvious from the moment of birth. But it's not unusual for a baby to be born with external genitals that are neither distinctly male or female. A sample of body cells, from the inside of the mouth or from a blood sample, would then be studied under a microscope to determine if the infant had an XX or XY combination of sex chromosomes, or some other combination. In some cases corrective treatment to establish the physical characteristics of the proper sex can be started early. A child with an XY chromosome combination but without distinctive male sex characteristics, for example, can be administered male sex hormones to aid normal development.

Male Sex Organs

The external genitalia of the man includes the penis and the scrotum. The penis is formed from three columns of erectile tissue bound together by fibrous tissue. One column of erectile tissue contains the urethra, the tube that carries urine from the urinary bladder. The urethra also is the passageway for spermatozoa that are produced in the testes and contained in the seminal fluid.

Because the male urethra has a relatively long, angular path from the bladder and collects secretions from the prostate gland seminal vesicles and bulbo-urethral glands, as well as from the testes and urinary bladder, doctors sometimes take three urine samples from a male patient during an examination. The patient is asked to void into three containers, one at a time, without interrupting the flow, if that is possible. The first sample presumably flushes out any pus or organisms that may have been in the urethra, the second represents the contents of the bladder, and the third contains any pus or other substances that may have been forced out

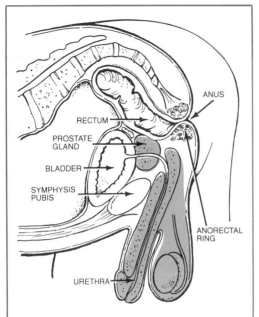

ANUS

RECTUM

PROSTATE GLAND

BLADDER

SYMPHYSIS PUBIS

ANORECTAL RING

URETHRA

Drawing shows the anatomical relationship between the male sex organs and neighboring parts of the body. Because of the thin membranes between the rectum and the prostate, the doctor often can examine the prostate gland through the anus.

the loose tissues of the penis, resulting from obstruction of the veins or the lymphatics, or from an inflammation of the penile tissues. If there has been a loss of blood as a result of an injury, the skin of the penis and scrotum will be discolored as if bruised. It is possible that discoloration from bleeding beneath the skin could occur without any symptoms of pain.

However, severe pain might accompany a fracture of the penis shaft. Each of the columns that form the shaft of the penis is composed of spongy tissue that becomes engorged with blood during an erection. Each of the two columns of erectile tissue on the top side of the penis, called a corpus cavernosum penis, is larger than the column that carries the urethra, and each carries a central artery as a source of

of the prostate and other glands. By examining and comparing the three samples, the doctor frequently can find clues to possible disorders all the way back to the kidneys.

Abnormalities of the Penis Direct visual examination usually will reveal any abnormalities of the penis. The patient may be asked to retract the prepuce, or foreskin, that may cover the glans, or head, of the penis. The doctor generally wears a rubber glove while inspecting the penis for lesions, nodules, or any other signs of disease.

A general swelling of the shaft of the penis could be due to fluid accumulation in

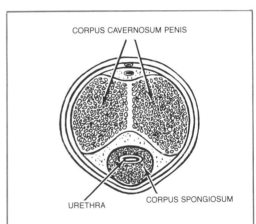

CORPUS CAVERNOSUM PENIS

URETHRA

CORPUS SPONGIOSUM

The male penis is composed of three columns of erectile tissue enclosed in fibrous tissue and skin. Two parallel columns of erectile tissue are called corpus cavernosum; the third column, which is somewhat smaller and contains the urethra, is located beneath the corpus cavernosa and is known as the corpus spongiosum. Sexual stimulation causes the erectile tissue to become engorged with blood and turgid. Otherwise, the penis is flaccid.

blood. During an erection one or both of the major columns of erectile tissue could rupture and cause a significant loss of blood within the tissues of the penis.

The penis usually is in a flaccid condition except when the male is stimulated sexually. However, there is a disorder called priapism that is characterized by a prolonged erection in the absence of sexual stimulation. The causes are varied and may include obstruction of blood vessels in the pelvic region, injury to the central nervous system, and certain malignant diseases. Priapism requires immediate treatment to prevent complications that can range from impotency to complete loss of the penis. Blood circulation in the penis is obstructed during an erection, and the effect of a persistent erection is similar to that of a thrombosis—that is, the tissues deprived of normal blood flow soon die and gangrene develops. The result in the case of untreated priapism is that the entire shaft of the penis would die and would have to be removed surgically in order to save the life of the patient.

There probably is no specific "normal" size for a penis. Size, coloration, and other features vary greatly from one individual to another. A penis may be large or small, the glans may be large or small with respect to the size of the shaft, and the foreskin may vary greatly in size.

When a penis is considered to be abnormally small, a condition known as hypoplasia, there usually are factors to explain the cause, such as castration of the boy before he reached puberty or intersexuality. Intersexuality is the result of a chromosomal or hormonal error that produces ambiguous sexual characteristics. Castration, or loss of testes, can occur as a result of disease.

The term for an abnormally large penis is hyperplasia. Hyperplasia is usually due to a disorder such as a tumor of the adrenal glands, the hypothalamus, or the pineal gland.

Perhaps 50 percent of the men of the western world have been circumcised by the surgical removal of part or all of the foreskin of the penis, usually within a few days after birth. The medical need for circumcision and, on the other hand, the need to retain the penile foreskin are still the subjects of considerable controversy among doctors. Some studies indicate that men who are circumcised are less likely to develop cancer of the penis, and their sexual partners are less likely to develop cancer of the cervix. Studies also suggest that women afflicted with a yeast fungus disease called moniliasis, or candidiasis, are more likely to become reinfected if their sexual partners have not been circumcised. And there are arguments from both sides regarding claims of increased or decreased sexual pleasure before or after circumcision.

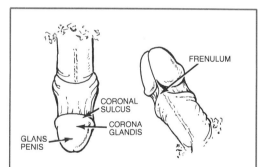

A loose fold of skin, a continuation of the skin that covers the scrotum, is attached to the base of the glans penis by a membrane called a frenulum. The skin, also known as the foreskin, may cover most of the glans penis except during periods of erection. The area where the glans penis joins the shaft of the penis, the corona, can be the site of venereal infections and other disorders of the penis.

Among problems that may be encountered in uncircumcised males, especially when the prepuce, or foreskin, has an abnormally small opening, are conditions called phimosis and paraphimosis. Phimosis is a term meaning that the foreskin fits so tightly over the glans of the penis that it cannot be retracted. This condition can be a congenital defect, that is, the person was born with the problem, or it could be the result of an inflammation that caused the foreskin to become stuck to the surface of the glans. In either case the abnormality can lead to a variety of complications, ranging from inflammation of the penis to an obstruction of the flow of urine. Phimosis also may cause "stones" to form under the foreskin from an accumulation of dirt and smegma, a mixture of dead skin cells that are shed by the foreskin and the secretion of oil glands in the area. The irritation of the glans by a phimosis condition can cause cancer of the penis.

Paraphimosis means that the foreskin is stuck in a retracted position, usually as a result of fluid accumulation, and will not slip over the glans of the penis. If the edema, or fluid retention problem, is not corrected, it can eventually interfere with blood circulation to areas of the penile shaft.

Tumors, ulcers, and other lesions of the penis tend to occur in the area where the glans joins the shaft of the penis. A syphilis chancre, for example, commonly is found at the corona of the glans or under the foreskin. A syphilis lesion may occur elsewhere on the genitals, even on the skin of the scrotum, but it is most likely to develop along the border between the glans and shaft of the penis. It may begin as a shiny elevated lesion, then erode into an ulcer that oozes a clear fluid. The ulcer is round or oval in shape and has a slightly raised border; it is usually painless.

A similar type of lesion that occurs on the penis as a result of an infection is the chancroid, or soft chancre. Caused by a bacterium, the soft chancre usually begins as a reddish papule that develops into an ulcer that is painful and discharges pus. The soft chancre may develop into multiple ulcerations, whereas the syphilis chancre usually remains a single ulcer. Athough these are different genital diseases, doctors usually test for the presence of the syphilis organism in either type of penile ulceration because chancroid and syphilis frequently occur at the same time.

Penile ulcers also can be caused by herpes virus or a venereal disease called lymphogranuloma inguinale. Genital herpes begins as small blisters, or vesicles, on the glans or foreskin that erupt and produce lesions which last for about a week. The hazard for the male with a herpes infection of the penis is that other disease organisms may enter the body through the ulcers. The lesions of lymphogranuloma inguinale are tiny sores that appear briefly on the penis as blisters or nodules, then disappear, and are followed within two weeks or less by inflammation of the inguinal lymph nodes.

Other types of lesions an examining doctor may find during examination of the penis, in addition to cancer which tends to appear near the junction of the glans and the shaft of the penis, are venereal warts. One kind of venereal wart, which goes by the medical name of condyloma latum, is a sign of secondary syphilis. Another type of wart that may appear on the glans of the penis is called condyloma acuminatum, which sounds threatening but is only a Latin term meaning a pointed lesion. It is caused by a virus and the points are villi that protrude above the skin.

Unfortunately, a cancer of the penis at first may resemble a wart, and the patient may not be aware that the growth could be a malignant tumor. The examining physician may recommend a biopsy study of the tissue to determine whether the tumor is a venereal lesion or something more serious. Any tumor, ulcer, or other lesion on the penis can be a sign of something serious and should be examined by a doctor.

Disorders of the Urethra Urethritis is the term used to identify an inflammation of the urethra. The urethral meatus, where the urine exits from the penis, may be red and swollen, and it may discharge pus if the urethra has been invaded by an infectious organism. Urination and erection usually are painful. The inflammation could be due to a gonorrheal infection, or it could be nonspecific. One of the diagnostic tests may be the examination of three urine samples discussed earlier in this chapter. The first sample should contain some evidence of the cause of the urethral inflammation.

Nonspecific urethritis, which means no virus or bacteria can be found to account for the inflammation, can be a first sign of a disorder known as Reiter's syndrome. The disorder is characterized by symptoms of arthritis and conjunctivitis; the urethritis and conjunctivitis symptoms may subside, but the effects of arthritis remain with the patient. Reiter's syndrome seems to affect only the male sex.

A couple of variations in the development of the male urethra during fetal life result in congenital abnormalities. One abnormality, identified as hypospadia, is characterized by a urethra that opens on the underside of the penile shaft. The oth-

er variation is manifested by a urethra that opens on the top side.

Another abnormality, apparently due to a fibrosis disease of the penile shaft, results in a curvature of the penis during erection. The disorder is known by a variety of fancy medical names such as strabismus penis and induratio penis plastica.

Testes and Prostate Gland The scrotum, the second external male sex organ, is a thin wrinkled pouch of skin that hangs from the root of the penis. It contains the testes, or as they are more popularly known, the testicles. The testicles are to the male what the ovaries are to a female, that is, they are the source of the gametes, or germ cells, which are needed to produce another generation of humans.

The left side of the scrotum normally is lower than the right side because the spermatic cord on the left side is longer. The scrotum also appears larger when surrounding temperatures are warm because muscle fibers in the wall of the scrotum contract when it is cold and relax when the environment is warm. This temperature response is part of nature's plan for protecting the developing sperm cells from extreme cold or warmth. The sperm cells, unlike the ova of the female reproductive organ, cannot tolerate normal human body temperatures for more than a brief period. In fact, there is evidence that sperm-developing tubules within the testicles can atrophy when the scrotum is held close to the body by tight clothing. The result is sterility.

When the testicles fail to descend from the abdomen of the developing male child—a not uncommon occurrence—the result is the same: he will be sterile, but not necessarily impotent. In some cases one testis may descend normally into the scrotum while one remains in the abdomen. Or they may descend as far as the inguinal area, near the junction of the thigh and the abdomen. The condition of undescended testes, which goes by the medical term of cryptorchidism, usually is treated surgically before the boy is five years old. If treatment is delayed beyond that period, sterility may result. An undescended testicle should be corrected by a surgeon in any case. The trapped testis is subject to inflammation from pressure by other abdominal organs, and an undescended testicle is 20 times as likely to become cancerous as a testis in the scrotum.

Orchitis, or inflammation of the testes, can result from an infection of the mumps virus in the post-puberty years. The scrotum may become very tender and enlarged by as much as three times its normal size. Only one testicle may be inflamed by the infection and may atrophy as a result. However, hormonal function usually is not affected and sterility after an attack of mumps is rather rare.

The testes contain about 1,000 tiny twisted tubules, each about 30 inches in length if they were straightened. The sperm cells, or spermatozoa, are formed on the walls of the tubules by a process in which each of the original germ cells in the testes produces four spermatozoa. The process takes about nine days to complete. However, there are millions of germ cells in the tubules and millions of spermatozoa can be produced each day—unlike the female reproductive system which usually releases only one ovum every four weeks.

The spermatozoa accumulate in the tubules and the epididymis, which is the beginning portion of the vas deferens, a tube that serves as a passage for movement of the sperm into the urethra at a point where the prostate gland surrounds the urethra at the base of the urinary bladder. The prostate, usually described as being the size of a chestnut, serves partly as a sphincter to control the flow of urine. But its chief function is to produce a thin alkaline fluid that becomes part of the opalescent white substance called semen, in which the spermatozoa are transported during ejaculation. Other components of the semen are produced by the seminal vesicles, which empty into the urethra at about the same place as the vas deferens-urethral junction. Other glands also participate in supplying a nutrient fluid for the spermatozoa on their reproductive trip.

Ejaculation means the propulsion of semen and spermatozoa through the urethra

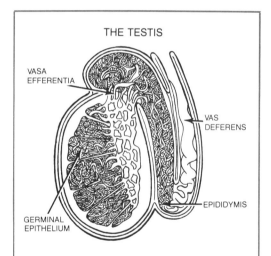

THE TESTIS

VASA EFFERENTIA

VAS DEFERENS

EPIDIDYMIS

GERMINAL EPITHELIUM

The male gonad, a testis, manufactures the spermatozoa necessary for reproduction of the human species. There are two testes normally located in the scrotum. Spermatozoa are produced from basic male germ cells in the germinal epithelium and move through the vasa efferentia into the epididymis, where they are stored in a series of ducts. The sperma eventually move into the vas deferens which terminates in the ejaculatory duct of the prostate gland.

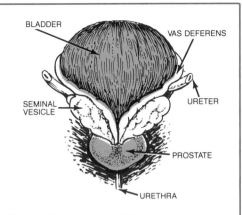

The prostate gland, one of the accessory sex organs of man, is located at the base of the urinary bladder. The vas deferens carrying sperm from the testis joins with the ejaculatory duct of the seminal vesicle duct from either side so that spermatozoa can be propelled through the urethra during ejaculation.

during the male orgasm. During ejaculation about one-tenth of a fluid ounce of semen is expelled through the urethra along with as many as 300 million spermatozoa. The amount of semen per ejaculation can vary by 30 to 40 percent, and the number of spermatozoa ejected may vary by nearly 80 percent from what is regarded as normal or average. However, if the number of spermatozoa in the semen falls below 20 percent of the average, the man may have difficulty in fathering a child.

Ejaculation is ostensibly an involuntary act, although the man has some control over the timing. It is triggered by a nerve reflex center in the lumbar, or lower back, area. A muscle that sheaths the base of the penis, called the bulbocavernosus muscle, contracts to produce the ejaculatory action. Ejaculation can occur without an erection of the penis, and erection can occur without ejaculation; but when such

events happen frequently, it usually is a sign of a disorder that warrants examination by a doctor.

Erection is accomplished by the flow of blood from the central arteries of the corpora cavernosa into the spongy tissue that forms the columns of the penile shaft. At the same time veins leading from the penis are obstructed so that blood cannot flow out as rapidly as it enters the penis. The penis thus becomes expanded, firm, and turgid. After the orgasm is reached there is a general relaxation of the muscles and the penis becomes flaccid once more.

Male Impotency

If a man is unable to begin, maintain, and conclude an act of sexual intercourse from erection through ejaculation, he is considered to be impotent. However, there are no established standards regarding the amount of time that should elapse between the start of erection and the phase of ejaculation. Younger, less experienced men may experience premature ejaculation, or ejaculation that occurs before the penis enters the woman's vagina, or shortly after. This condition frequently is a psychological problem, due to stress or anxiety. If it is a chronic problem and the cause has not been determined, the man should consult a physician.

Some drugs used for the treatment of hypertension, as well as tranquillizers, can interfere with normal sexual function in the man. Alcohol and narcotics also can hamper normal sexual potency. Diseases that can affect male potency include diabetes and progressive ailments involving the nervous system, such as multiple sclerosis. Hernias, fibrosis, and calcification of the penile tissues, as well as several hormonal and metabolic disturbances, may be responsible for failure to perform the sex act in an adequate manner.

If a man experiences a nocturnal erection, one that occurs involuntarily while he sleeps, it is assumed that his failure or inability to have an erection while awake is due to psychological causes.

Disorders of the Scrotum

Many common disorders involving the testes or scrotum can be studied by a doctor using the technique of transillumination. This means that with a good flashlight and a darkened working area, the doctor can visualize the inner structures of the scrotum by shining a light through the thin walls of the pouch. A solid body, such as the testis, will appear as a dark object or opaque shadow during transillumination, whereas a hydrocele, a rather common disorder, will allow light to pass because it is composed of clear fluid. A hematocele resembles a hydrocele in some ways, but it will not appear translucent when illuminated because of the presence of blood in the scrotum.

A hydrocele may develop as a result of injury or a disease-caused inflammation that causes an accumulation of normal fluid; it also may be due to an obstruction in a vein or lymphatic that results in poor drainage of normal tissue fluid. A hematocele, as the name indicates, is caused by an accumulation of blood within the scrotum. Most hematoceles and some hydroceles require surgical treatment.

A quite painful disorder involving the scrotal area can result from testicular torsion, which means that the spermatic cord becomes twisted so that drainage of the blood and lymphatic systems are obstructed. Fluid retention and congestion develop

and emergency surgical care may be required.

An obstruction of the lymphatic system by a tropical worm known as filariasis can result in a tremendous accumulation of fluid in the scrotum. The condition is called elephantiasis scroti. The lymphatic obstruction can affect the legs, resulting in huge elephant-like legs, which explains the origin of the medical name, elephantiasis, for this monstrous edema effect.

Disorders of the Prostate

A more common problem of the male reproductive system is prostatitis. Because of its location astride the urethra, the prostate gland may become swollen and constrict the tube leading from the urinary bladder to the penis, preventing the normal flow of urine. The prostate also is a target for cancer, infectious diseases, and the formation of stones, or calculi. In some cases the prostate may press against nerve centers to cause low back pain, which may be mistaken for symptoms of a "slipped disc." A swollen prostate can aggravate infectious diseases of the bladder, since residual urine trapped in the bladder by the prostate can become a cesspool for breeding bacteria.

Bacterial infection of the prostate may be marked by chills and fever, low back pain, and a variety of urinary disorders including nocturia, or an urge to get out of bed during the night to urinate, painful or burning sensation on urinating, increased urgency and frequency of urination, and occasionally bloody urine. Treatment depends upon identification of the bacterium responsible for the prostatitis so the proper antibiotic can be administered. Another form of prostatitis has the same symptoms as acute bacterial prostatitis, but the cause is unknown because no disease organism is found in urine samples of the patients. They are treated with medications and procedures such as the use of hot sitz baths, but no antibiotics are employed.

Cancer of the prostate probably is the most common type of cancer affecting older men. It is an insidious disease in that it can grow slowly without producing symptoms until it has reached a dangerous stage of development. The first signs and symptoms can include urinary difficulty and signs of blood in the urine. If the cancer has spread to the lower spinal column and the pelvic bones, there may be symptoms of bone pains.

Some disorders of the prostate gland can be detected in early stages during routine medical examinations since the prostate can be palpated through the anus by an examining physician. If cancer is suspected, a biopsy tissue sample is taken for laboratory tests. If cancer is confirmed as the cause of the disorder, the problem is corrected by surgical removal of the gland. Female sex hormones may be administered as part of the treatment. The hormones do not cure cancer of the prostate but they may extend the life of the patient by many years. Many men who have been treated for cancer of the prostate by surgery or hormones, or both, have had their lives extended by ten or more years.

Removal of the prostate should not affect sexual potency. Because the prostate produces only about 20 percent of the seminal fluid, the amount of semen ejaculated during intercourse is reduced only slightly. It has been suggested that because of the slightly reduced ejaculate for transporting spermatozoa, one aftereffect of a prostatectomy might be a reduced

chance that the patient could father a child by conventional means. However, if a patient whose prostate has been removed really wants to father a child, medical techniques are available to get the sperm to the woman's ovum.

Female Sex Organs

The external genitalia of the woman consist mainly of the vulva, a pair of tissue folds or lips surrounding the clitoris, the urethra, and the vaginal opening. The outer fold of tissue sometimes is called the labia major; the inner fold is known as the labia minora.

When a doctor performs a pelvic examination, which is a way of saying an inspection and palpation of the internal genital organs and surrounding tissues, he generally begins by inspecting the vulva for signs of abnormal conditions. Various lesions, papules, cysts, nodules, etc., may appear on the inner surfaces of the labia.

The examination of the female genitalia usually is done while the woman is lying on her back on an examination table. The table may or may not be equipped with stirrups to hold the patient's feet, while the knees are bent at right angles. Some doctors feel a more effective examination can be performed when stirrups are used. As an alternative, the woman may be asked to position herself so that her buttocks are near the edge of the examination table and her legs are bent so that her heels are against her buttocks. While in this position, the woman may be asked to bear down so the doctor can check for any evidence of prolapsed tissues that would bulge through the opening to the vagina. The opening to the vagina sometimes is called the introitus by doctors, but there is nothing mysterious about the word; it is simply a Latin word for entrance. The main part of the examination of the female sex organs begins with the introitus.

The vagina is inspected with the aid of a speculum, an instrument designed specifically to widen a body opening. There are different kinds of speculums for different body openings—rectal, ear, nose, etc. A bivalve speculum is used for the vagina, and its two blades are spread apart to widen the opening. The vaginal speculum usually is warmed in a water bath so it will be close to the normal temperature of the body when it is inserted. One blade of the speculum is shorter than the other so the cervix of the uterus will be easily visible when the vaginal vault, or upper surface, is raised by the opened blades. In addition to the direct vaginal examination performed with the speculum in place, the examining physician may collect samples of tissues or other materials for biopsies, laboratory tests, and a Pap test. This kind of examination generally is not done while a woman is menstruating unless there is a reason why it cannot be postponed.

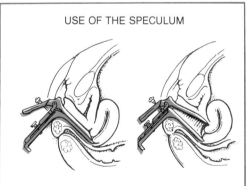

USE OF THE SPECULUM

Examination of the woman's vagina and cervix is assisted by the use of a speculum, an instrument with curved blades that can be adjusted to spread the walls of the vagina so they can be inspected; the cervix is near the end of the vagina.

Vagina Normally, the interior of the vagina has a smooth, pinkish lining of mucous membrane that may be arranged in folds. A bluish coloration to the lining of the vagina can be a sign of congestive heart disease or a circulatory obstruction caused by a tumor in the pelvis. However, the bluish signs of cyanosis of the vaginal lining also can be early evidence of a pregnancy.

Abnormally red coloration of the interior walls of the vagina could suggest several different kinds of inflammation, or vaginitis. A hot douche or a pessary, for example, can cause a diffuse red coloration. A red mucous membrane with small lesions that discharge a yellowish substance could indicate an infection of trichomoniasis. A gonorrheal infection can result in a similar kind of vaginitis but also would involve the urethra and the Bartholin's glands near the vulva. A reddened vaginal lining with white patches is a sign of a Candida infection, caused by a yeastlike fungus.

Venereal warts and ulcers that may be found in the vagina and on the vulva are quite similar to those that occur on the penis of the male. They include chancres, herpes, and condylomas, or warty growths.

When viewed from the vaginal introitus, the normal cervix appears like a button at the top of the end of the vaginal tunnel. In the center of the button is a small opening, the cervical os. (An os is a medical term for any body opening.)

If the woman has been pregnant the cervix may show signs of cuts, tears, or scars. Some damage to the cervix during birth is common, and the extent of healing of the tears or cuts can indicate how recently a baby was delivered. A bluish coloration of the cervix, as in the vagina, can be a sign of a new pregnancy—or of congestive heart disease or a pelvic tumor.

In making a Pap test smear, or the Papanicolaou cervical cancer test, the examining doctor usually wipes the area of the cervical os with a cotton-tipped applicator or with a special spatula. The loose cells wiped from the end of the cervix are transferred to a glass slide for microscopic examination. The test, which is recommended for all women over the age of 30 at least once a year, will show evidence of cancerous or precancerous tissue cells at a stage before more dangerous symptoms appear.

The doctor also will look for signs of infection or inflammation around the cervix. Signs of blood could be a danger signal, and so could the discovery of an ulceration or erosion of the cervical tissue. Cervical polyps or cervical cysts often are visible to the doctor examining with the help of a speculum. A cervical polyp could account for a discharge or bleeding from the tissues. The doctor usually will palpate the cervix with a gloved finger to determine whether it is soft or hard, and its size, shape, and position. He also may determine whether a fingertip will easily enter the cervical canal through the os.

The pelvic examination of a woman also requires a bimanual inspection, that is, the use of two hands, one the gloved hand with one or two fingers for palpating internally and the other hand for pressing into the abdomen. This sometimes is called examination of the adnexa, which means the ovaries, uterine tubes, and other organs that cannot be inspected directly through the vaginal orifice. By pressing into the abdomen with the outside hand, for example, the uterus, ovaries, and tubes can be pushed downward so they can be palpated by the fingers inside the vagina. The doctor can estimate the size, shape, and surface condition of the uterus in this manner, comparing what he feels with normal uteri he has examined directly or indirectly. Since the uterus normally can be moved about somewhat without causing pain to the patient, the doctor can check this factor at the same time. The ovaries and Fallopian tubes similarly may be palpated for signs of abnormalities in size, surface condition, or masses that might suggest a tumor.

The vaginal inspection usually is followed by a rectal examination. The rectal examination is basically the same as the rectal inspection given a male patient, except that the doctor will palpate the vaginal wall from inside the rectum of a woman; in the case of a man, he will inspect the prostate gland that can be felt through the wall of the rectum. The rectal approach to vaginal examination may have added importance if the woman has an intact hymen, the membrane that traditionally protects the vaginal orifice of a virgin. Before the hymen is ruptured, the doctor may be able to insert only one finger into the vagina for palpating the inner structures. After it has been ruptured, the doctor generally is able to insert two of his fingers. If the doctor can insert three fingers into the vaginal orifice, it may be a sign of an enlarged vaginal introitus resulting from tissue damage following one or more pregnancies.

An enlarged vaginal introitus represents an abnormal condition of the pelvic floor in most cases, and it usually is a result of childbearing stress on the tissues. The doctor may find in an inspection for pelvic floor damage evidence of a cystocele—that is, a portion of the bladder covered by vaginal lining may be seen in the vaginal introitus and may resemble a round tumor. If a portion of the rectum, covered by vaginal mucosal lining, is seen, the disorder is known as a rectocele. Some women may have both a cystocele and a rectocele.

Cystoceles and rectoceles are prolapses of the organs—essentially hernias or ruptures—usually caused by the tearing of supporting tissues during pregnancy or childbirth. When the uterus itself drops into the vaginal cavity, the disorder is called a uterine prolapse. A prolapse requires surgical repair.

Uterus The fundus, or main body of the uterus, normally lies at an angle that is about 90 degrees, or a right angle, from a line that might be drawn along the path of the vagina. Occasionally, it may become tilted at a different angle, or may even extend directly beyond the end of the vagina. Such a variation is known as a retroversion or retrodisplacement of the uterus. Retroversions are classed as first, second, or third degree, depending upon how far from normal alignment they have deviated. In some cases the cervical portion of the uterus enters the vagina at a normal angle, but the uterus itself is bent into an L- or C-shaped curve. That condition is called a retroflexion. When a displaced uterus remains freely movable, it generally does not cause any serious symptoms.

When movement of the uterus is restricted or painful, it can be a sign of a disorder such as endometriosis, ectopic pregnancy, or an infectious disease. Endometriosis is a condition caused by the development of endometrial tissue, the normal lining of the uterus that sustains the life of an embryo, in abdominal areas outside the uterus. Endometrial tissue can

occur in the ovaries, on the outside of the uterus, or even on the colon. An ectopic pregnancy is one in which the embryo develops outside the uterus, as for example, in a Fallopian tube where the fertilized egg became trapped while descending to the uterus. An example of an infectious disease that could make movement of the uterus painful is gonorrheal inflammation of the uterine tubes.

Fibroid growths in the uterus usually appear as hard nodules in the fundus of the organ. They sometimes are referred to as uterine myomas or fibromyomas. They are not unusual in women over the age of 35 and often occur as multiple tumors, causing various kinds of abnormal bleeding. Fibroids can be removed during a D & C, or dilation and curettage, procedure in which the patient's uterus is dilated and the lining scraped. The procedure is performed while the patient is anesthetized during a brief hospital stay. Any suspicious lesion found during a D & C can be analyzed by a biopsy at that time to determine whether the growth is malignant, meaning cancerous, or benign, meaning relatively harmless.

Any general enlargement of the uterus discovered during a pelvic examination could indicate a pregnancy in a woman of childbearing years. However, the uterus seldom reveals signs of pregnancy in this manner before other clues are present, such as the bluish coloration of the cervix and vagina, the softening of the cervix and fundus, interruption of menstruation, morning sickness, and so on.

A complete pelvic examination will include an inspection of the vulvovaginal glands, or Bartholin's glands, on each side of the vaginal orifice. They become prominent during a period of infection or inflammation and appear as red spots that may release pus; otherwise they are barely noticeable.

The general appearance of the external genitalia will vary somewhat with the age of the individual. Older women, for example, may have labia that normally appear shrunken and smooth, with a bright red carbuncle, or fleshy eminence, at the urethral opening.

Genital Infections There are several diseases of the genital tract that are of particular concern for women who are pregnant or who are contemplating pregnancy. Because of the potential hazard to the fetus, immediate treatment after first signs or symptoms of the diseases is warranted.

One is genital herpes infection, which usually presents symptoms within a week after exposure. The symptoms can range from mild to severe and may be marked by the appearance of small, cold sore-type blisters around the vulva, vagina, or cervix, or all of those surfaces. The vesicles or blisters become shallow, painful ulcers that heal within two or three weeks. If the virus spreads to the fetus early in the pregnancy, the result can be spontaneous abortion; late in pregnancy, the infection can be a fatality after birth due to the baby's exposure to the disease in the birth canal. There are medications that can be administered during pregnancy, and in some cases the baby may be delivered by caesarian operation to avoid exposure in the infected birth canal.

Syphilis in the mother can result in spontaneous abortion or stillbirth for the child, or congenital syphilis. Signs and symptoms of the disease include the appearance of a genital chancre within two to four weeks after exposure, and lesions of the skin and mucous membranes up to two months later. Early treatment of the mother with antibiotics, mainly penicillin, helps protect the unborn child since the disease organism rarely crosses the placental barrier before the 16th week of pregnancy.

Antibiotics also are needed to protect a fetus against a gonorrheal infection acquired by the mother during pregnancy. A whitish or yellowish discharge from an inflamed cervix may be the only clue that this infection has been acquired. If unchecked, the disease can produce serious complications, including inflammation of the amnion, the protective membrane and fluid around the developing fetus. A gonorrheal infection of the amnion can prove fatal to the unborn child. A doctor's examination at the start of pregnancy usually can detect an infection so that antibiotic treatment can begin immediately.

Other infections of the vaginal area can result in special hazards to the health of the fetus and to the health of the pregnant woman. One type of infection, candidiasis, apparently becomes an increased threat to a pregnant woman because the changes in body chemistry resulting from pregnancy make her a more susceptible host to the fungus that produces the symptoms of a thick white discharge and itching in the vulva and vaginal tissues. For another kind of infection, trichomoniasis, caused by a type of protozoa, there is a potential risk of adverse effects in treating a pregnant woman with the most effective medicine available.

The Reproductive Cycle

A woman often has her first pelvic examination either because of a pregnancy or because of a menstrual disorder. The common menstrual disorders usually include: menorrhagia, which means profuse menstruation; amenorrhea, or the absence of menstruation; dysmenorrhea, a term for painful menstruation; and metrorrhagia, which means bleeding between regular menstrual periods. These various menstrual disorders may be due to abnormal functioning of the pituitary gland, the hypothalamus, the thyroid gland, the ovaries, or the uterus.

The anterior lobe of the pituitary gland secretes three hormones that can be involved in menstrual activity. One is the follicle-stimulating hormone, often abbreviated as FSH, which starts a human ovum on its way from an ovary toward possible fertilization and life as a new individual. Before it is stimulated by the FSH, a follicle in the ovary consists of an egg cell surrounded by a layer of protective and supportive tissue cells. Each ovary contains perhaps hundreds of thousands of such follicles, each so tiny that it can be seen only with a microscope. A girl begins life with millions of follicles in her ovaries, but many—if not most—disappear during the years before puberty. For reasons equally mysterious, after reducing the number of potential ova from millions to hundreds of thousands, nature selects one each 28 days or so to be influenced by the pituitary hormone.

The egg cell becomes a primary follicle that grows into a much larger sac, known as a Graafian follicle, and fills with fluid as it increases in size. The original layer of protective and supportive cells also increases and thickens. Some cells lining the Graafian follicle meanwhile begin secret-

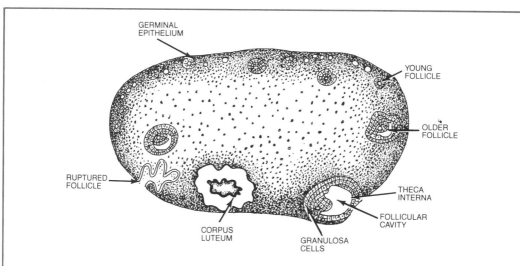

The female gonad, the ovary, contains thousands of ova, or egg cells, in various stages of development. The ovaries produce ova, at a normal rate of one every menstrual cycle, in an expanding follicle. As an ovum matures, the follicle develops a lining of special cells which become a gland secreting a hormone to support early embryonic life if the ovum should become fertilized. The temporary hormone gland is called a corpus luteum. A woman's ovary will show openings in the surface where earlier follicles have ruptured to release an ovum into a Fallopian tube where it may be fertilized.

ing another hormone, estrogen. As the Graafian follicle approaches maturation, when the ovum, or egg cell, is released into a Fallopian tube, it increases in size to about one-third of an inch.

As the estrogen level builds up, there is an increase or proliferation of the cells lining the uterus. During this proliferative phase, the uterine lining, called the endometrium, thickens and acquires deep glands along with a greater blood flow. The purpose is to make a nest for the ovum, or egg, if it should be fertilized after it is released from the ovary.

On or about the 14th day, counting from the first day of the last menstrual period, the Graafian follicle ruptures and releases the mature ovum from the ovary. Almost immediately, the fingerlike edges of the Fallopian tube trap the ovum and move it into the tube which leads to the uterus. After ovulation, the cells lining the empty Graafian follicle are transformed into a yellowish structure, the corpus luteum. The corpus luteum itself then takes on the appearance of an endocrine gland and secretes another female sex hormone, progesterone. The production of progesterone continues at an active pace for about two weeks, then diminishes if the ovum is not fertilized. During this period there also is continued secretion of estrogen and further enrichment of the uterine lining.

The reproductive cycle of the normal human female may be somewhat irregular. Although the cycle is frequently listed as 28 days, this figure is an approximate average. Many women have normal menstrual cycles that are shorter or longer than 28 days, so there is no reason to be overly concerned about a menstrual cycle that is just a few days more or less than 28. In fact, some problems in family planning can result when husband and wife rely too heavily on the expectation that the wife will ovulate on the 14th day of the cycle.

For the average 28-day menstrual cycle, however, the secretory phase usually prevails within the lining of the uterus from about the 16th through the 28th day. The glands that appeared in the early stage of proliferation swell and elongate after ovulation, the blood supply to the endometrium increases, and the lining becomes spongy and rich in glycogen, a type of sugar that can be stored in the body tissues. All this is in preparation for implantation of the ovum if it should become fertilized by a spermatozoon in the Fallopian tube.

Fertilization of the Ovum Millions of spermatozoa are deposited in a woman's vagina during sexual intercourse. But very few reach the top of a Fallopian tube and only one spermatozoon usually fertilizes the egg cell, although it is possible for more than one of the male gametes to fertilize additional ova that might be released at about the same time. That, in fact, is what occurs when nonidentical twins are conceived.

The tiny tadpole-shaped spermatozoa are produced with the help of a hormone released from the pituitary gland. The hormone stimulates one type of cell within the testes, the Sertoli cells, to produce sperm from the basic germ cells in the tubules of the testes. The basic male gametes at this stage are able to go through a series of divisions before they develop into immature spermatozoa, which are stored in the epididymis until they are potent enough to be released for reproductive duty. The pituitary hormone in the male also stimulates another kind of gonadal cell, the Leydig cells, to produce a male sex hormone called testosterone, which also helps to develop and mature the spermatozoa.

The relationship between the pituitary hormone and the development and maturation of the male sperm and the female ovum therefore is quite similar. One difference is that the male production line is more or less continuous, whereas the female production of gametes follows a pattern that takes approximately four weeks for each ovum to be formed. This four-week cycle limits the chances for a woman to become a parent to about 12 or 13 times each year during the fertile period in her life, while a man normally is equipped to become a parent on almost any day of the year. The man also retains his ability to become a parent from puberty until old age, in most cases, but a woman's ability to become a parent is ended when she reaches the menopause.

If during a normal menstrual cycle an ovum becomes fertilized by a spermatozoa in the Fallopian tube, the male and female genetic material, the chromosomes, will be joined in the beginning of a new individual. This is the moment of conception. And the new human being, which is only one cell at first and is known temporarily as a zygote, will begin almost immediately to grow by dividing in a doubling sequence of cells. In other words, the one-celled zygote will become two cells, then four, then eight, sixteen, and so on. By the time the zygote reaches the uterus it will have the appearance of a tiny mulberry. Within ten days after ovulation, the zygote usually will be implanted in the endometrium and will develop into an embryo, then a fetus, and finally a baby.

If the ovum is not fertilized or the zy-gote fails to become implanted in the endometrium, the corpus luteum formed after the release of the ovum from the ovary will quit producing the hormone needed to sustain the enriched endometrium. The endometrium will slough off and become a bloody discharge that marks the start of the menstrual period. This generally occurs around the 28th day. But it also marks the beginning of the next reproductive cycle, which will go through the same stages as the last and continue to repeat itself every 28 days or so in the normal woman, unless it is interrupted by a pregnancy or the menopause.

Menstruation Menstruation, which sometimes is known as catamenia by doctors, seems to be caused by the withdrawal of both estrogen and progesterone hormones when the corpus luteum gets the message that the ovum has not been fertilized and implanted in the lining of the uterus. Menstrual bleeding can be started or stopped by the withdrawal or administration of synthetic estrogen and progesterone hormones, which have a very similar effect on the uterus. Oral contraceptives, commonly known as "the Pill," although there are many variations or types of pills, work in a similar manner.

When an ovum has been released, the hormones secreted by the corpus luteum—estrogen and progesterone—normally suppress further follicle development until the previously released ovum has had an opportunity to become fertilized and implanted in the wall of the uterus. If pregnancy does occur, the corpus luteum continues activity in the ovary while both ovulation and menstruation are suspended for the duration of the pregnancy. An oral contraceptive has the effect of reproducing this situation artificially; the hormones in the Pill create the illusion that a pregnancy may have begun, so that development and release of the next mature ovum will be suppressed. As a result, no ovum is likely to be released at normal ovulation time and the woman cannot become pregnant.

In some cases the loss of a baby by spontaneous abortion can be prevented by supplying synthetic hormones that are needed to help maintain a favorable environment in the uterus for continuing the pregnancy.

A "normal" menstrual period may vary from two or three days to a full week, depending upon the individual and other factors. The average menstrual period lasts slightly less than five days. About three-fourths of the menstrual discharge during the period is blood; the remainder is mucus and tissue cells from the endometrium. The amount of blood loss varies from as little as one ounce to as much as four or five ounces, with an average of about two ounces. The monthly menstrual periods can gradually drain the body's stores of iron reserves, and since iron is a key mineral in the formation of red blood cells, a woman may develop iron-deficiency anemia unless she eats an adequate amount of iron-rich foods or takes iron in tablet form during her fertile years. After menopause, a woman doesn't need additional iron in her diet.

As mentioned earlier, there may be a good deal of misinformation presented in various publications about a typical 28-day menstrual cycle. Studies of thousands of menstrual cycles based on records kept by hundreds of young women have indicated that the menstrual cycle that occurred most frequently was 28 days. However, menstrual cycles as short as seven days and as long as 256 days have been reported, and more than 85 percent of the menstrual cycles fell within a range of from 17 to 45 days between the start of one normal menstrual cycle and the beginning of the next. Some women reported regular menstrual cycles of 20 days, others reported regular cycles of 44 days, and still others included in one study did not have two menstrual cycles of the same number of days during the time they were under observation.

As for predicting when ovulation will occur during any menstrual cycle—an event that theoretically happens at the midpoint of the reproductive cycle—some studies have found that ovulation actually may occur any time from two to six days on either side of the midpoint of the cycle. In only about one-fourth of the cases studied did ovulation occur on the day in the middle of the menstrual cycle. Thus, menstrual cycles and ovulation times can vary considerably and still be considered normal. This knowledge can be important in family planning and for women who may be concerned about menstrual cycles that seem to ignore the calendar.

A girl's first menstruation is called menarche. And like the several hundred menstrual cycles that normally will follow until the menopause, there are few specific guidelines about what's normal and what's not about a menarche. The average age of menarche has been calculated by some medical researchers to be about 13 years and six months. Records kept at institutions for homeless girls show that some girls began menstruating at the age of 11, but others did not experience menarche until after their 16th birthday.

The first menstruation of a girl does not

necessarily mean she is fertile. In fact, the menstrual bleeding at menarche usually is due to hormonal effects alone and occurs without the release of an ovum. The first menstrual periods generally are irregular. A predictable pattern of menstrual cycles may not be established for several years. The ovaries respond to the activity of the follicle-stimulating hormone secreted by the pituitary gland, but the mechanisms for producing mature ova usually are not in proper working order at the time of menarche. Although a very young girl occasionally does become a mother, there is ample evidence that early pregnancy is rare in cultures that permit marriage of pre-teen girls.

There appears to be no relationship between the ages of menarche and menopause despite popular belief that girls who menstruate early have a late menopause. However, there may be a hereditary pattern in the two menstrual events since daughters who begin menstruating at an early age usually have mothers who also experienced an early menarche. And mothers who reach the menopause at an earlier-than-average age usually have daughters whose menopause begins earlier than usual. The average age at menopause is about 50 years, although earlier and later ages for the change of life, or climacteric as it is sometimes called, are common. The process generally is slow and may take several years to complete. Fewer than 10 percent of menopausal women experience a sudden cessation of menstruation. Some women continue to ovulate, and may become pregnant, even after regular menstruation has stopped.

Sex Hormones Both men and women produce some of the sex hormones associated with the opposite sex, although generally not in quantities large enough to distort their sexual characteristics. FSH, the follicle-stimulating hormone in the ovaries of women, also is present in men and acts on the seminiferous tubules in the testes to produce spermatozoa. The leuteinizing hormone, LH, also occurs in men and appears to stimulate the production of hormones called androgens. The hormone prolactin, which stimulates the production of milk in the breasts of women, also occurs in men, although its function in the male is not known.

The female gonadal hormone estrogen helps determine the sexual characteristics of women, such as the growth of breasts. A male gonadal hormone, testosterone, stimulates the growth of whiskers on men. A sex hormone occasionally is used as part of a medical treatment, such as the administration of estrogen to control cancer of the prostate. Because a female sex hormone can produce secondary sex characteristics of a woman in a male patient, or vice versa, doctors exercise great caution in the use of hormonal medications. In a case of an elderly man whose life is threatened by cancer of the prostate, the use of a female sex hormone might be a worthwhile risk. But the same female sex hormone, estrogen, probably would not be used to treat acne in a young man, even though the medication might be effective in controlling an acne problem.

Hysterectomy

Except for childbearing, the uterus is not a necessary part of the body. If it becomes the site of a cancer or another type of abnormal growth, or a medical problem, the well-being of the woman can be improved by having a surgeon remove the uterus. This kind of surgical procedure is called a hysterectomy.

Removal of the uterus ends the menstrual cycles for the woman as well as the risk or opportunity for childbearing. However, it need not interfere with normal sex life after the effects of the surgery have been healed. Nor does a hysterectomy interfere with the production of sex hormones if the ovaries are not removed along with the uterus. If the ovaries are removed, the effect is similar to the change of life that occurs with the onset of the menopause, except that the climacteric begins abruptly rather than through the gradual atrophy of ovarian function.

Because the hysterectomy is a surgical procedure that cannot be undone at a later date, most doctors are reluctant to recommend the operation except when it would be important to protect the health of the woman. In some cases the problem may be the presence of fibroid tumors, nonmalignant growths that develop in the tissues of the uterus. The tumors may be small and located so deep in the wall of the uterus that they do not affect the life of the patient. Others, however, can be close to the endometrium so that they form a bulge in the lining of the uterus and cause menstrual disorders. The woman may experience spotting or bleeding between regular menstrual periods, or the menstrual flow becomes heavier than usual and lasts longer. The heavy loss of blood can cause symptoms of weakness or fatigue and anemia. A large fibroid tumor may press against the bladder or rectum, causing urinary distress or constipation.

Before a hysterectomy is performed the woman most likely would be admitted to a hospital for a D & C, or dilation and curettage procedure. The D & C may be the most common surgical procedure used for treating a variety of "female troubles." It is performed under a general anesthetic and usually requires less than one hour. The cervix is carefully dilated to admit the instruments used for curettage, or scraping of the lining of the uterus. If the fibroid tumor is easily removed by a D & C procedure, the need for a hysterectomy may be eliminated. The D & C operation also is used to remove uterine polyps.

Biopsy samples of the uterus, actually scrapings collected during the D & C, are examined microscopically in the hospital laboratory to determine whether there are any signs of cancer in the uterus. The woman may feel a vague ache in her abdomen and some minor spotting or bleeding after a D & C, but usually the cause of the uterine disorder has been corrected and the woman can go home after a brief period for recovery and observation.

If a hysterectomy is performed, the surgeon may use either of two general approaches—one through the vagina and the other through the abdomen. If there is some evidence of cancer, the surgeon may prefer to open the abdomen, a procedure sometimes called a laparotomy, so that neighboring tissues can be examined and any affected lymph nodes in the region can be removed along with the uterus. Some surgeons prefer the vaginal approach if there are no complications. The recovery rate usually is quicker when the uterus is removed through the vagina.

There are two basic kinds of hysterectomies: a total hysterectomy that involves removal of the cervix along with the rest of the uterus; and a subtotal hysterectomy that leaves the cervix intact while removing the uterus. If the cervix is removed along with the rest of the uterus, the tissues of the vagina are closed at the point where the cervix normally opens into the vagina.

Following a hysterectomy the patient spends several days in the hospital. During the first portion of the recovery period she may be required to urinate through a catheter, or plastic tube, inserted into the bladder through the urethra. When she is able to eat solid foods and move around the hospital room without assistance, she probably will be allowed to return home to continue her recovery. A return to a regular work routine and normal sexual relations may be delayed for a month to six weeks, depending upon the individual and her rate of recovery. Active participation in sports may be delayed for as long as three months.

Cancer of the Sex Organs

The risk of cancer in the female sex organs can be reduced considerably by regular examinations that include taking a Papanicolaou smear of the cervix, or a Pap test, which not only can reveal the presence of cancer cells but also of abnormal dysplasia cells which might develop into cancer. The Pap test thus is theoretically capable of detecting cancer while it is completely curable, if the woman takes the test at least once a year. If the test indicates the possibility of cancer, a biopsy is performed by removing a bit of cervical tissue for laboratory study while the patient is in the hospital under a general anesthetic.

Cancer can develop almost anywhere in the female reproductive system, from the opening of the vagina to the ovaries. Unfortunately, by the time symptoms of pain or bleeding appear, the cancer may have spread to other parts of the body. Therefore, a periodic visit to a physician, at least once a year, is the best insurance against the effects of this destructive disease.

The type of treatment employed when cancer is discovered in the female reproductive organs depends upon where the growth is found and how far it has spread. A hysterectomy is one method of controlling cancer that involves the cervix or uterus; the surgeon also may remove the ovaries and Fallopian tubes if there is a chance that cancer may spread in that direction. And in some cases it may be necessary to remove the bladder or rectum as well, if there are signs that cancer cells have spread to those tissues.

Radiation therapy may be used for treating small cancerous growths instead of surgery or in addition to surgery. Radiation, which may be generated by X-ray machines or by small amounts of radioactive chemicals placed near the tumor, can help prevent the spread of cancer cells to the lymph nodes and other surrounding tissues.

Chemotherapy, the use of certain chemicals designed to interfere with the normal functions of cancer cells, may be used in treating some cancers of the sex organs, but the technique is more effective in controlling tumors of certain organs than of others. For example, chemotherapy is more likely to control cancer in the ovary than in the cervix.

Cancer of the ovary occurs at about the same frequency as cancer of the uterus and is most likely to develop during a woman's menopausal years. There are no simple tests for detecting cancer of the ovary. The first symptom usually is that of a swelling and feeling of heaviness in the abdomen. Pain or bleeding would indicate that the cancer is well advanced.

Not all growths in the ovary are cancerous. An ovarian cyst is relatively common and may grow to the size of a baseball before causing serious discomfort. A large ovarian cyst may be found after it causes symptoms that involve surrounding organs, perhaps because of pressure on the bowel or bladder. It also may press on abdominal blood vessels to produce circulatory complications.

As the cyst grows in size, the woman may feel a swelling in the abdomen and a sense of fullness there. Some patients with a large ovarian cyst mistakenly assume that they merely are "putting on weight" and fail to report the abdominal symptoms to their doctor. Eventually, the ovarian cyst may be pulled down into the pelvic cavity by the weight of the growth. Complications can include hemorrhage, infection, or rupture of the cyst.

There are many types of cysts and tumors that can develop in the ovary. Some may begin as nonmalignant growths and later develop into cancer. Some are solid but others are filled with fluid or a gelatinous material. The growths commonly develop without symptoms of pain or bleeding. But eventually, surgery may be required, and whether part or all of the ovary must be removed depends upon the individual case. In some instances a hysterectomy is required as part of the corrective treatment, but usually a nonmalignant growth can be removed without involving the uterus or other tissues.

Ovarian tumors may be associated with abnormal production of sex hormones. A tumor of the ovary, for example, can result in an excessive production of estrogen that causes abnormally heavy menstruation or menstrual bleeding after menopause. An ovarian tumor may produce male sex hormones that cause menstrual cycles to cease and masculine body hair to develop. A disorder known as the Stein-Leventhal syndrome, characterized by loss of female fertility, development of masculine body hair, and obesity, is due to one type of ovarian tumor.

Disorders of the Breast

The female breast is associated with the reproductive function and is influenced by the same sex hormones that stimulate normal activities of the sex organs. Both boys and girls begin life with rudimentary breasts, but in the girl the breasts begin to enlarge and acquire a proliferation of milk ducts when secretion of the female sex hormone estrogen increases at puberty. The size and weight of the breasts, also known as the mammary glands, vary at different periods of life and in different women. They increase in size during pregnancy, for example, and may continue to increase after the baby is delivered. Some variation in size also may occur during the menstrual cycle, with the breasts enlarging somewhat just before menstruation begins.

The breast tissue is composed mainly of glands involved in the production of milk. The glands, or lobes, are separated from each other by fibrous and fatty tissues. Just below the center of the breast is a nipple, a small cone-shaped prominence, that is perforated by more than a dozen tiny openings into the milk ducts, which lead by many subdivisions, somewhat like the bronchi of the lungs, to the myriad lobules where milk is secreted.

During a general physical examination the doctor may examine the area surrounding the nipple, a region called the areola, which changes color normally as a result of a pregnancy. Before the first pregnancy the areola usually is a delicate pinkish color. Around the second month of a pregnancy it begins to acquire a darker color, progressing toward dark-brown or black. After the baby has been delivered and nursed, the color returns toward the original hue, although the areola never regains its prepregnancy pink coloration.

The breasts grow new glandular tissue during pregnancy and begin secreting milk when the baby is born. After the baby is weaned, the glandular tissues regress and the breasts return to a non-lactating state. The glandular tissue atrophies further during the menopause, but the fibrous and fatty tissues may remain so that the breasts retain much of their premenopausal shape.

The doctor usually examines the breasts by palpation to detect tumors. He may begin with the nipple area, palpating it for signs of tumors, tenderness, or a discharge from the nipple. Examination of the nipple area may be conducted while the woman is in a seated position.

Afterward, the woman is asked to lie down on an examining table with her arms at her side. A pillow, cushion, or other support placed under the shoulder of the side to be examined can help the doctor examine the breast for lumps, because the breast will spread more evenly over the chest wall when one side is slightly elevated.

The doctor palpates the breast with four fingers of one hand, palm down, making gentle strokes from the top of the breast toward the breastbone, or sternum, while carefully feeling the tissues underneath. Each of the imaginary four quadrants of the breast is examined in a similar manner. The doctor also will palpate the area along the chest wall and into the armpit, or axilla, to check for swollen lymph nodes. The entire chest palpation procedure then may be repeated while the woman has her arm raised above her head. The examination is conducted in the same manner for the other breast.

Besides checking for abnormal lumps or masses in the breasts, the doctor may try to detect any abnormal signs in the consistency of the breast tissue. The breasts may feel slightly lumpy or granular during pregnancy or just before menstruation, and fatty at other times. However, the breasts are normally tender for a few days just before menstruation.

A breast cancer frequently develops as a tumor in a gland or duct and then spreads into the fatty portion of the tissue. A very common symptom is a lump in the breast, which may or may not cause pain at the beginning and may or may not be associated with a reddened area of skin on the surface of the breast. The skin also may show a dimple or ulceration, or the nipple may retract and produce a discharge.

An inverted, crater-like nipple often is a developmental anomaly, meaning a mistake by nature, but a harmless mistake. However, it should be checked by the doctor to make sure there is no underlying inflammation or malignant growth associated with the anomaly. Nipple fissures, or breaks in the tissue, may be a sign of an infection. The appearance of a bloody secretion, or of any secretion (other than milk during lactation), should be checked by a doctor because of the possibility that the cause can be a tumor, either cancerous or nonmalignant.

Supernumerary nipples, or extra nipples, are not uncommon occurrences on the chests or abdomens of both males and females. They result from one of nature's many developmental errors and often are mistaken for moles. Most often the extra nipples occur along an imaginary line to the normal breasts and nipples, but they may develop in such unlikely places as the armpit, shoulder, groin, or thigh. Supernumerary nipples generally are harmless and only rarely are associated with mammary gland tissue as part of supernumerary breasts.

A scaling eczema-like lesion of the nipple can be an early sign of a disorder known as Paget's disease of the nipple. The nipple and surrounding areola gradually become inflamed and the disease eventually involves the milk ducts and the skin. A deep-seated malignant tumor usually is found to be the cause, although not all eczema-like lesions of the nipple area are signs of cancer.

The presence of nodules in the breasts may or may not be cause for alarm. In cases of chronic cystic mastitis, the doctor may detect many nodules in both breasts, and the nodules may vary in size during a menstrual cycle. But if the doctor detects only one nodule or finds several clustered in one area of a single breast, he may order special tests to determine the possible presence of a cancer.

A lump in the breast during lactation, or nursing of a baby, may be due to a condition called galactocele, or caked breasts. The cause is a cyst that results in a blocked milk duct. The disorder frequently is treated by applying a breast pump to clear out the blockage. The condition also may occur after a woman has weaned a baby.

Acute mastitis is characterized by a breast that is tender, red, hard, and swollen in one quadrant, or area. The symptoms often develop during lactation and may be accompanied by periods of chills and fever with sweating. Although the disorder is not associated with cancer, a doctor should examine the patient to be sure the symptoms are due to the mastitis and not caused by other factors.

Fibrocystic breast disease often is associated with the changes in breast tissue that occur normally during each menstrual cycle. There is an increase of breast tissue and glandular activity between ovulation and the menstrual period, after which the breast activity subsides if the woman does not become pregnant. Some women are more sensitive to these changes than others and may experience inflammation, tenderness, and the appearance of breast nodules before menstruation. After a number of years of this monthly problem, the normal breast tissue may be replaced in part by fibrous nodules and cysts. The symptoms may resemble those of cancer, and while the disease is not the same as cancer, the incidence of breast cancer is much higher in women afflicted by fibrocystic breast disease. Thus, they need to be examined carefully by a doctor at regular intervals, especially in later years.

A cyst can be removed surgically or reduced by inserting a needle that allows the fluid to be drained. The procedure followed depends upon the size of the cyst and other factors. In any case, biopsy samples of tissues or fluid are sent to the laboratory for examination to determine the possible presence of cancer cells.

When cancer is found in a woman's breast, a mastectomy almost always is recommended as the only sure cure for the disease. Radiation therapy is a possible alternative in some cases when a cancer is detected at a very early stage. However, it may not provide a permanent cure, and the radiation can alter the shape and size of the breast treated.

There are several variations of the mastectomy, and the choice usually depends upon the individual case and the surgeon's evaluation of the best way to prevent spread of the cancer. A simple mastectomy results in removal of the breast. A modified radical mastectomy removes the breast and the lymph nodes in the nearby armpit. A radical mastectomy results in removal of the breast, the lymph nodes in the armpit, and the muscle tissue underlying the breast.

Radiation and chemotherapy may be administered after surgery to control the spread of cancer to other body tissues. In certain cases there may be a need to remove the ovaries and adrenal glands to help prevent the spread of cancer cells—a process called metastasis in which cancer cells break away from the primary cancer and are carried by the lymph or blood to other organs that may be some distance away. The surgical removal of the ovaries and adrenal glands is directed mainly at premenopausal women, and is based on the theory that estrogen supports the growth of cancer cells so its sources need to be eliminated. Ironically, in older postmenopausal women, large doses of estrogen have been found to relieve the symptoms of breast cancer.

Men also experience breast cancer, but the disease in men occurs at a rate of about one percent that of the incidence in women. In men the cancer may be detected more easily as a hard, painless lump or nodule because it is less likely to be masked by the mass of fat and glandular tissue that forms the female breast. Treatment of breast cancer in men is quite similar to that used in female cases. One difference is that instead of removing the ovaries to help control the spread of cancer, the male testes are removed.

Some other breast problems of women also can afflict the male of the species. Acute mastitis, for example, can occur in the male breast, usually as a result of irritation from clothing or working gear that rubs against the breast. Fibrocystic nodules also can develop in the male breast. Under certain conditions the male breast can enlarge and become functional on both sides or on only one side of the chest. The condition is called gynecomastia and is associated with hormonal disorders, diseases ranging from leprosy to leukemia, the use of certain medications, and the body's immobilization in plaster casts.

See also Chapter 13: *Pregnancy and Childbirth.*

GLOSSARY
SEX ORGANS

The alphabetized entries below of common and medical terms relate to the anatomy and disorders of the human sex organs. Words in italicized type refer to other entries in this Glossary.

acute epididymistis An inflammation of the epididymis, the storage tubes for spermatozoa produced in the testes.

acute orchitis An inflammation of one or both testes, usually as a result of an infectious disease such as mumps. The testes may be swollen, tender, and painful. In some cases there may be edema because of the accumulation of fluid.

adnexa The accessory organs of the uterus, such as the ovaries and Fallopian tubes.

adrenal glands Two small glands, weighing perhaps one-sixth of an ounce each, which are located atop the kidneys; they are the source of many hormones that stimulate various bodily functions. The adrenals sometimes are described as actually being two endocrine glands enclosed in a single capsule. One of the two glands within a gland, the cortex, produces aldosterone and hydrocortisone, hormones involved in water and electrolyte balance and in making nutrients available to the tissues. The adrenal cortex also produces androgens, or male sex hormones, and some estrogen and progesterone, the female sex hormones. The second glandular portion of the adrenals, the adrenal medulla, produces adrenalin, or epinephrine as it is also known, and noradrenaline, or norepinephrine; adrenaline stimulates and noradrenaline relaxes the heart, blood vessels, and muscles, among their other functions.

adrenarche A medical term sometimes used to indicate the beginning of puberty, or sexual maturity, as characterized by signs of increased adrenal gland activity in a child. In a girl the adrenarche is followed sometime later by the *menarche*, or first menstruation, which is a sign of increasing activity of the ovaries.

alveolar glands A technical term for the milk-producing glands in the breast.

amenorrhea An absence of menstrual activity. If a girl has not started to menstruate at an age when the event normally would begin, the condition is called primary amenorrhea. If menstruation fails to occur, in the absence of pregnancy or a similar obvious reason, after the menstrual cycle has been established, the condition is called secondary amenorrhea. Amenorrhea usually is the result of a failure of the ovaries to produce a mature ovum, or it is the hormonal system's failure to build up the endometrial lining of the uterus, which is the source of the menstrual bleeding.

ammoniacal dermatitis A form of skin inflammation caused by urine. It may be the cause of skin irritation around the genitalia of small children.

atrophy A decrease in size or function of a previously normally developed organ. An atrophied testis, for example, is one that has become smaller or less functional after an injury, or because of inflammation from a disease such as mumps, or following surgical repair of a nearby hernia.

azospermia A complete absence of sperm in the semen and a cause of infertility in the man. The cause often is an obstruction or absence of openings in the epididymis or vas deferens which normally permit the movement of spermatozoa from the testes to the urethra. In many such cases the problem can be corrected by surgery.

balanitis An inflammation of the glans penis. The cause may be an infectious organism, exposure to an irritating chemical, or an injury. The inflammation may involve only the glans of the penis, or the foreskin as well as the glans. Erosive balanitis is characterized by the appearance of small ulcers that erode the skin of the glans.

bartholinitis An inflammation of the Bartholin's glands, which are located in the vulva and secrete mucus. The glands can become involved in infections of the vagina.

benign prostatic hyperplasia A long medical term meaning an abnormal increase in the tissues of the prostate gland. The condition is most likely to occur in older men, perhaps as a result of hormonal changes in later life. While not cancerous, the growth can cause problems, mainly by obstructing the flow of urine through the urethra, which the prostate surrounds. Surgery usually is recommended to correct the situation and prevent loss of normal muscle tone in the bladder, which becomes dilated when not emptied at regular intervals.

bimanual pelvic examination A technique used by doctors in examining the female sex organs by inserting the fingers of one hand into the vagina while pressing with the fingers of the other hand on the surface of the abdomen. The bimanual technique permits the examining physician to locate and palpate the body of the uterus, the ovaries, Fallopian tubes, and other neighboring organs and tissues. This method helps the doctor to find possible abnormal conditions that might otherwise require exploratory surgery or X-rays.

breast axillary tail A portion of the breast tissue that extends from the top outer part of the breast toward the armpit.

breast self-examination A simple technique recommended for women to examine their own breasts thoroughly once a month for signs of abnormal lumps. Because of breast changes during the menstrual cycle, the Breast Self-Examination (BSE) should be done after the menstrual period when the breasts are less likely to be swollen or tender. Women who are going through the menopause or who have completed the menopause should do the BSE on the same day of each month.

BSE involves three basic steps: (1) Stand before a mirror and check both breasts for any puckering, dimpling, scaly skin, or nipple discharge; then lean forward to check for any abnormalities in shape. (2) While in a standing position, raise one arm in the air and, using two or three fingers of the other hand, gently explore the opposite breast, feeling for any unusual lump under the skin; then do the same thing to the other breast. (3) Finally, while lying flat on the back with one arm raised beyond the head, repeat the fingertip palpation of the breast tissue while the breast is spread against the chest muscles.

cancer A general term for a large number of different diseases that are characterized by a wild, uncontrolled growth of cells. The resulting wild cells, which may form a tumor, can invade and destroy surrounding normal tissues. Cancer cells also can migrate from the original tumor or source and spread (metastasize) through the blood or lymph system to start new cancers in other parts of the body. The original cancer may be identified as a primary cancer; cancers caused by metastasis are called secondary cancers. A breast cancer, for example, can metastasize and produce secondary cancers in the lungs or bones. See also Chapter 16: *Cancer.*

carcinogen A substance or agent that causes or incites cancer.

carcinoma A type of cancer that begins with epithelial cells, the type of tissue cells that form the external and internal surfaces of the body. Most cancers of the skin, breast, and uterus are carcinomas.

cavernositis An inflammation that may develop in one of the corpora cavernosa, the columns of spongy tissue that help form the shaft of the penis. The inflammation may be caused by an infection or injury. It might be marked by the appearance of an irregular hard mass. The disorder frequently is accompanied by *priapism* or *edema.*

cervix The lower, narrow portion of the uterus, sometimes called the neck of the uterus. The cervix extends into the vaginal canal and has an opening that communicates with the vagina. Spermatozoa deposited in the vagina during sexual intercourse can enter the uterus, and the Fallopian tubes beyond the uterus, by passing through the opening, or os, of the cervix. The menstrual blood and cellular debris, as well as a baby and placenta, likewise pass through the cervix when leaving the uterus.

chancre A lesion, or sore, that occurs most commonly on the glans area of the male penis as an early sign of a syphilitic infection. Although a syphilis chancre can occur on other body surfaces, it is rarely observed beyond the genitalia. The chancre usually begins as a painless, silvery pimple and gradually erodes into an ulcer with a smooth, hard border. The ulcer discharges a fluid containing the syphilis organism, Treponema pallidum.

chancroid Sometimes called a soft chancre, this kind of sore is caused by a bacterial infection and may appear on the penis or other genital surfaces. A soft chancre generally begins as a small red pimple that becomes enlarged and filled with pus; it then forms an ulcer with a grayish base and discharges pus. A chancroid usually is painful, and the infection can spread to the lymph nodes in the groin, causing them to become swollen and tender. Although a soft chancre is not the same as a syphilis chancre, chancroids frequently are transmitted by persons infected with syphilis, so doctors often advise patients with soft chancres to be tested for the presence of the syphilis organism.

chemotherapy The treatment of diseases with drugs (chemicals), as opposed to treatment by surgery or radiation. Chemotherapy is often used to treat diseases of the sex organs.

chorionic gonadotropin A hormone that is secreted in large amounts by the placenta during pregnancy. It can be detected in the urine of pregnant women about a week after the first missed menstrual period, and doctors verify its presence to confirm that a woman is pregnant. The hormone also is used to treat underdeveloped gonads.

clitoris A structure of the female genitalia that is similar to the penis of the male. It is composed of two columns of corpora cavernosa erectile tissue enclosed in a fibrous membrane and of a rounded extremity known as the glans clitoridis.

colpocele Another word for vaginal prolapse, in which the walls of the vagina protrude through the vaginal opening.

condyloma acuminatum A medical term for a venereal wart which may occur as a single growth or as a group of warts. A venereal wart occurs most frequently on the corona, the crown formed by the rim of the head of the penis, or in the sulcus, the groove immediately behind the corona. A condyloma acuminatum is distinguished by villi that project from the surface of the wart; another kind of venereal wart, a condyloma latum, has a flat surface. The venereal wart is a benign growth that can be transmitted by sexual contact. Some condylomas resemble cancers, in which cases biopsies are needed to rule out that possibility.

cord A word frequently used when referring to the spermatic cord, a cord-like structure that suspends the testes in the scrotum. The spermatic cord contains the vas deferens, plus blood and lymph vessels and nerves supplying the testes.

corpus luteum A yellowish mass that forms in the follicle of the ovary after an ovum has been released. It becomes a gland that secretes the hormone progesterone until the outcome of a possible pregnancy has been determined.

cowperitis An inflammation of the Cowper's glands, or bulbo-urethral glands, which are located near the male prostrate gland and secrete a substance that helps lubricate the urethra.

cyanosis A bluish tint in the skin or mucous membrane, usually due to a lack of oxygenated blood in the tissues. The vagina and cervix may show cyanosis as a sign of pregnancy, a tumor, or congestive heart disease.

cyst A sac that contains a liquid or semisolid material in an abnormal lump, which may be benign or malignant—for example, cysts in the breasts.

cystocele A medical term for prolapse of the urinary bladder. This kind of disorder may occur as a result of damage to pelvic tissues during childbirth. When a woman with a cystocele stands or strains, a portion of the bladder, covered with the lining of the vagina, may be visible through the vaginal opening.

deferentitis An inflammation of the vas deferens, the duct within the spermatic cord that provides a passageway for spermatozoa moving from the testes to the urethra.

displacement A term used by doctors to refer to a uterus that is not in proper alignment with the vagina and other structures in the pelvic region. For example, the uterus may be bent upon the cervix, a type of displacement sometimes called retroflexion. If the uterus remains straight but the whole organ is tilted, the condition is known as retroversion.

dysmenorrhea A medical word for painful menstruation. The pain may occur in the form of abdominal cramps, backache, or other kinds of discomfort.

dysuria Difficult urination marked by hesitancy in starting the flow of urine and/or straining to maintain the flow. The cause may vary from a nervous disorder to an obstruction in the urinary tract.

ectopic pregnancy A pregnancy that develops outside the uterus. The problem usually develops in one of the Fallopian tubes; a tubal pregnancy can result in a ruptured Fallopian tube.

edema Fluid accumulation in a loose tissue area of the body. Causes can include inflammation or injury resulting in fluid leakage from the capillaries, poor lymphatic drainage, or congestive heart disease. Edema can be a cause of general swelling of the penis.

endocervicitis A disorder of the cervical canal marked by the discharge of mucus or pus, or both. The lips of the cervix may be inflamed or eroded by the inflammation. The cause may be an infectious disease or the result of wear and tear on the tissues from pregnancies.

endometriosis An abnormal condition of the uterine wall or the ovaries marked by internal bleeding. The condition may develop because endometrial tissue, the type that forms the lining of the uterus, may occur outside the uterus, developing, for example, on the organ's outside wall. Endometriosis is stimulated by the same hormones that cause the menstrual flow from the uterus each month and may produce bleeding effects on a similar timetable. However, while menstrual blood and tissue debris can be expelled through the vagina during a menstrual period, the endometrial residue may be trapped inside the abdominal cavity, producing irritation and scarring of abdominal organs, as well as other problems.

endometritis An inflammation of the *fundus*, or body, of the uterus that is similar to the effects of *endocervicitis*, which usually is limited to the cervical area of the uterus.

epididymitis An inflammation of the epididymis, a common cause of pain, swelling, and tenderness in the scrotal area. The disorder can result from injury or infectious disease, such as gonorrhea. Epididymitis frequently is caused also by vigorous exercise such as sports activities.

epispadia A congenital defect in which the urethral opening occurs on the top of the penis instead of at the end. The opening may develop on the top side of the shaft of the penis or on the top of the glans; in some cases the mislocation may be so slight that it will go unnoticed until examined by a doctor.

Fallopian tubes Fleshy tubes that connect the ovaries with the uterus. An ovum released from the ovaries travels down one of the Fallopian tubes toward the uterus and, if fertilized by a spermatozoon in the tube, it will become implanted in the uterus and will develop into a fetus.

fertilization The union of the nucleus of a spermatozoon and the nucleus of an ovum to form a new individual, the zygote. Each gamete—that is, the male's spermatozoon or the female's ovum—contributes 23 of the 46 chromosomes needed to form a new human during fertilization.

fetus The unborn offspring that develops in the mother's uterus following fertilization of the ovum. Technically, the developing child is considered an embryo for the first seven or eight weeks following fertilization. After the embryonic period of development and until delivery, the unborn child is considered a fetus.

follicle The chamber within the ovary in which a germ cell develops into an ovum under the influence of the follicle-stimulating hormone (FSH) secreted by the pituitary gland. A girl begins life with millions of germ cells, but only a dozen each year ripen after puberty and develop into an ovum within a follicle of the ovary.

folliculitis An inflammation of the hair follicles, or shafts from which body hair grows. Folliculitis can occur in the pubic hair.

foreskin The layer of skin that extends from the shaft of the penis and covers a portion of the glans penis.

fracture of the shaft A bit of medical terminology meaning the rupture of one or both of the corpora cavernosa, or columns of spongy tissue forming the shaft of the penis. This severely painful condition can result from injury, especially during an erection, and usually requires immediate surgery.

frenulum A piece of tissue that attaches the foreskin to the head of the penis on the underside of the penile shaft.

fundus The body of the uterus, or the main portion above the cervix.

genital herpes Also known as herpes genitalis or herpes progenitalis, this virus disease is similar to the herpes simplex that causes cold sores on the lips. But genital herpes is a different strain of virus that is transmitted sexually and produces herpes lesions on the genital surfaces.

genital warts Caused by a virus that generally is spread by sexual contact, genital warts thrive on warm, moist skin surfaces of the genitalia. They are identified medically under the name of condylomata, or condyloma.

gonadotropins Hormones that control the gonads, or sex organs. The follicle-stimulating hormone (FSH) in women is a gonadotropin.

gonads The organs that contain the sex cells, or gametes. They are the testes in men and ovaries in women.

gonorrheal vaginitis A severe inflammation of the vaginal lining and nearby surfaces as a result of a gonorrheal infection.

Graafian follicle Another name for the ovarian follicle which develops into a cyst and ruptures to release an ovum during a menstrual cycle.

granuloma inguinale A sexually transmitted disease that causes painless red nodules on the skin around the genitalia of both men and women. The lesions commonly occur on the penis or scrotum of men, or the vaginal area of women, but they also can be found in some cases on the thighs, groin, or buttocks. The cause of the disease is a bacterium that favors sex life in tropical regions and is rarely found in northern climates. If neglected, the sores gradually spread, but treatment can be provided by the administration of antibiotics.

gumma A soft, gummy tumor that is a sign of an advanced stage of syphilis. A gumma may develop in the scrotum, covering the testis with a hard, smooth surface and causing it to lose its sensitivity to pressure.

gynecography An examination procedure used sometimes to check the condition of a woman's ovaries. A gas is injected into the abdominal cavity to help produce a proper shadow contrast of the ovaries when X-ray pictures are taken. The gas, usually carbon dioxide, is injected with a needle after a local anesthetic has been administered to the patient.

gynecomastia A condition in which enlarged, and sometimes functioning, breasts develop on a man's chest, usually as a result of a tumor that produces a gonadotropic hormone.

hematocele A testicular swelling similar to that of a *hydrocele*. When examined by transillumination, a hematocele produces an opaque image of the mass, indicating that the fluid responsible for the swelling was blood, rather than clear fluid as in a hydrocele. A hematocele may be the result of an injury. In some cases the problem is corrected by aspirating, or draining, the fluid from the tunica vaginalis, or the outer membrane covering the testis.

hematoma A localized mass of blood beneath the surface of the skin or other tissues. It is sometimes called a "blood blister" but also appears as a bruised area. A hematoma may occur on the genitalia of either a man or woman, usually as a result of an injury to the area.

hematuria A condition caused by the presence of red blood cells in the urine. The concentration of red blood cells may be great enough to color the urine red. There are numerous possible causes, such as an injury to a kidney, a tumor, or kidney or bladder disease.

hemoglobinuria A disorder which, like *hematuria*, can produce urine with red coloration because of pigment from red blood cells. The difference is quite technical and depends in part on laboratory tests of freshly voided urine to determine possible sources.

hirsuitism A medical or scientific term for hairiness. It frequently is used to describe the abnormal condition in women who have an overabundance of the type of body hair associated with male virility. The condition is related to an imbalance of male-female sex hormones.

hormone A chemical substance secreted in tiny amounts by one of the body's endocrine glands, such as the pituitary or adrenal glands, or the gonads, to produce a physiologic activity in another part of the body. For example, the follicle-stimulating hormone, secreted by the pituitary gland in the head, is carried by the bloodstream to the ovaries where it orders the development of a mature ovum within a Graafian follicle.

hydrocele A testicular swelling caused by an accumulation of fluid in the tunica vaginalis, a double-layer membrane that surrounds most of a testis in the scrotum. A doctor may use the technique of transillumination to diagnose a hydrocele because the mass appears translucent when viewed against a light source such as a flashlight in a darkened room.

hypogonadism A failure or reduced activity of the normal functions of the gonads so that growth and sexual development may be retarded. The cause can be a disorder of the pituitary gland or of the gonads.

hypospadia A congenital abnormality in the male penis which has a urethral meatus, or urinary opening, on the underside of the shaft of the penis. A variation of the abnormality is *epispadia*. In either case, the abnormality may be so slight as to go undetected until discovered during a careful medical examination.

impotence A term used to describe a condition in which a man is unable to achieve normal sexual intercourse because of an inability to begin or maintain an erection of the penis. The cause may be due to the effects of alcohol or drugs, mental illness or psychological problems, or a disease such as diabetes mellitus. If the man is able to achieve a nocturnal erection, that is, during sleep, the problem is considered to be psychological, rather than due to an organic disorder.

infertility The failure of the man or woman to produce offspring, despite efforts through sexual intercourse. Male infertility frequently is due to the lack of adequate numbers of spermatozoa in the ejaculate, an inadequate volume of semen to transport the sperm, or a disorder called retrograde ejaculation, in which the spermatozoa are diverted into the bladder instead of through the urethral meatus, the opening in the glans penis. An inadequate volume of semen can result from frequent sexual intercourse or diseases of the prostate or the seminal vesicles. Absence of spermatozoa may be due to obstructions in the route from the testes to the urethra, poor nutrition, injury or disease such as the mumps, or excess heat applied to the scrotal area from hot baths, etc.

Female infertility can be caused by hormonal disorders that interfere with normal ovulation processes, obstructions that interfere with the movement of ova or spermatozoa through the Fallopian tubes, poor health in general, an infection of the reproductive tract, and in some instances an imperforate hymen.

inguinal canal An opening in the tissues of the pelvic cavity for passage of the spermatic cord between the scrotum and the junction with the urethra, near the prostate gland. A portion of the gut or other abdominal tissues may push through the opening to cause a rupture, or inguinal hernia.

intersex A disorder characterized by the failure of an individual to develop physical traits that are distinctly male or female. The person may have ambiguous genitalia, which often can be corrected by plastic surgery, plus the administration of sex hormones when feasible.

interstitial cell stimulating hormone Sometimes abbreviated as ICSH, this hormone controls the activities of the sperm-producing cells in the male testes. A by-product of this activity is the manufacture of a second male sex hormone, *testosterone.*

intertrigo The medical name for a type of skin inflammation that may develop in folds of skin that are likely to have a warm, moist environment, such as the skin of the genital area. Friction produced by the skin surfaces rubbing

against each other usually contributes to the condition, which generally is exacerbated by obesity and hot, humid weather.

karotyping A procedure employed in analyzing the sex chromosomes of an individual to determine whether the person has the XX chromosome pattern of a female or the XY chromosome pattern of a male. The procedure may be done when there is a question of the sexual identity of a child, as in an intersex problem. It is now conducted routinely in some athletic contests where entrants in women's events are suspected of actually being males.

Karotyping also may be used to resolve questions of features or functions of persons who may have some unusual combination of chromosomes, such as XO or XXY. A person with a chromosome combination of XO, for example, may have basic physical features of a woman but would not ovulate or menstruate because of the missing X chromosome.

Klinefelter's syndrome An abnormal chromosome condition characterized by a karotype of XXY. The individual develops the physical features of a tall man with long legs, scanty body hair, and small fibrous testes which do not produce spermatozoa. Male sex hormones sometimes are administered in an effort to correct some of the abnormal physical traits associated with the disorder. The individual may develop enlarged breasts, which can be removed by plastic surgery.

lactogen A female sex hormone that stimulates the enlargement and functioning of the breast tissues during pregnancy. Lactogen is produced by the placenta.

lactogenic hormone Also called prolactin, this pituitary gland hormone stimulates and sustains milk secretion in the breast.

luteinizing hormone Sometimes identified by the initials LH, this hormone is secreted by the pituitary gland and is involved in the development of the Graafian follicles of the ovary which produce a mature ovum during each menstrual cycle. It also is responsible for development of the *corpus luteum* after the ova has been released from the follicle; the corpus luteum then becomes a small endocrine gland in the space previously occupied by the ovum and secretes the female sex hormone progesterone.

lymphogranuloma venereum Sometimes abbreviated as LGV, this is a contagious venereal disease caused by a virus. Small pimple- or ulcer-like lesions appear on the genitals in about one to three weeks after exposure to the virus. The lesions may disappear and the virus spreads to the lymph nodes in the inguinal area. The infection may be accompanied by a variety of symptoms, including fever, chills, headache, abdominal discomfort, joint pains, loss of appetite, or a combination of complaints. The genitalia may become swollen because of fluid accumulation. The infection may affect the lower digestive tract, resulting in strictures or abscesses of the rectal area. Treatment involves the administration of sulfa drugs or oral antibiotics.

mammotropic hormone Another name for *lactogenic hormone*, or prolactin.

menarche A Greek word for "the beginning month," meaning the time of a girl's first menstrual period.

menopause Another Greek word meaning menses, or monthly, cessation. It generally marks the end of a woman's fertile years, although she may continue to ovulate and could possibly become pregnant after her regular menstrual periods have ceased to occur. Actually, menopause rarely occurs in an abrupt manner and is more likely to evolve gradually over a period of many months during the late 40s or early 50s of a woman's life.

menstrual cycle A span of days usually timed from the beginning of one menstrual period to the start of the next menstrual period. An average menstrual period frequently is given as 28 days in length, but individual menstrual periods may vary from as short as 17 days to as long as 44 days without being considered ab-

normal. Ovulation usually occurs at the midway point of an average menstrual cycle.

mineral corticoids Hormones that control the metabolic balance of minerals, such as sodium and potassium, in the human body. They may be produced by cells in the adrenal glands,. the same glands that produce sex hormones. But they have different physiological targets in the body.

nodular prostate A prostate gland that shows signs of nodules when palpated during a medical examination. The nodules may be evidence of several possible disorders, including carcinoma, stone formations, or tuberculosis.

oligospermia A term used to indicate a less than normal number of spermatozoa in a sample tested for evidence of male infertility. Normal sperm counts range from 40 to 200 million per 1.5 milliliters of semen.

orchitis An inflammation of a testis, usually caused by an infectious disease such as mumps, although the infection can be due to venereal or other diseases. The inflammation is marked by swelling and signs of tissue damage in the walls of the scrotum. The patient experiences pain and fever. A severe infection can result in atrophy of the testis. The treatment usually consists of bed rest, treatment of the infectious disease, and the application of ice bags to help relieve the pain and swelling.

ovary A female *gonad*, a rather flat oval-shaped organ about one inch long, located above and attached by a ligament to the uterus. There normally is one ovary on either side. The human ovaries at puberty contain probably several hundred thousand primary ova or germ cells, but only about one in 1,000 develops into a mature ovum; some ripen partially, then degenerate. Most primary ova remain dormant throughout the life of the woman.

ovulation The release of a mature ovum, or egg cell, from a woman's ovaries. The ovum develops in a *Graafian follicle* which grows rapidly from a microscopic pinpoint to a cyst perhaps one-third of an inch in diameter within a short period of time. The follicle ruptures when the ovum is ready to be released, and the egg cell drops into a *Fallopian tube,* which leads to the uterus. Ovulation occurs about halfway through a typical 28-day *menstrual cycle.* There is some evidence that in shorter or longer menstrual cycles about 14 days will elapse between ovulation and the start of menstruation, regardless of the number of days that a nontypical menstrual cycle may take.

Generally, only one ovum is released during each normal menstrual cycle. But occasionally two or more ova may be released at the same time, and if they are fertilized, multiple births such as fraternal twins will result. Identical twins develop from a single fertilized ovum that divides into two equal parts before continuing the cell division process leading to embryonic life. During an average reproductive life period, a woman's ovaries will release a total of perhaps 400 ova.

oxytocin A female sex hormone produced by the pituitary gland for two separate functions in the reproductive process. One is to stimulate contractions of the uterus at the time of birth, thereby helping to move the baby through the birth canal. The second is to promote the release of milk from the mother's breasts by stimulating contractions of the muscles that control the milk ducts.

paraphimosis Failure of the foreskin to return to its normal position over the glans of the penis after it has been retracted.

pediculosis pubis A fancy medical term for crabs, or an infestation of the pubic hair by the crab louse. The disorder is often but not always transmitted by sexual contact with a person infested with the lice. While the crab louse usually thrives in hair of the anal-genital area, it may be found on other body areas, particularly among individuals who have a lot of body hair.

phenotype A term sometimes used to classify the physical traits of an individual as male or female. The classification often is used during examination of a newborn child.

phimosis An inability to retract the *foreskin* from the glans of the penis.

pituitary gland The "master gland" of the body, which is located in the brain tissue, next to the hypothalamus. It is composed of two parts, a posterior lobe and an anterior lobe, which develop separately in the fetus and fuse into a single organ. The pituitary gland secretes a number of hormones, including a growth hormone, the follicle-stimulating and luteinizing hormones, a hormone that stimulates development of sperm in the male testes, lactogenic hormone or prolactin, hormones that control the thyroid and adrenal glands, a hormone that controls urine production, and oxytocin, the hormone that contracts the pregnant uterus and helps produce milk from the breast.

plastic induration of the penis Also known as Peyronie's disease, this condition is marked by fibrosis of tissues of the sheath of the penis and the occurrence of firm nontender plaques in the corpora cavernosa. The condition is of concern to the patient because it may result in a curvature of the penis during erection, making normal sexual intercourse difficult.

precocious puberty The attainment of puberty at an earlier than normal age. In either sex, precocious puberty may occur before the age of ten. In some cases, particularly among boys, precocious puberty may be a sign of a tumor that stimulates the production of sex hormones.

premenstrual tension A condition marked by the occurrence of a variety of physical and mental symptoms just before the onset of a menstrual period. The complaints may include migraine headaches, depression, irritability, fluid retention, weight gain, and swollen and tender breasts.

priapism A prolonged erection of the penis in the absence of sexual stimulation. The condition can be painful and frequently requires immediate medical treatment of the cause, which may be thrombosis or hemorrhage in the penis, a tumor, inflammation of the penis, a lesion in the spinal cord, or in some cases a blood disease such as sickle cell anemia.

prolactin A name for a lactogenic hormone of the *pituitary gland* that helps to produce secretion of milk in the breast.

prostatic calculus The formation of stones, or concretions, in the prostate. The disorder can be painful and pain symptoms may radiate to the genitals.

prostatitis An inflammation of the prostate gland by one of several possible disease organisms. The disorder may be marked by *hematuria*, or bloody urine, and accompanied by high fever, chills, low back pain, and a frequent urge to urinate although urination may be difficult. Hospitalization frequently is required to insure proper treatment of bed rest, analgesics, and special medications. If the inflammation results in obstruction of the bladder, a urethral catheter or similar measure would be needed to drain the bladder.

puberty The period of life when children begin to develop their adult sexual characteristics. Girls usually reach puberty around the ages of 11 to 13 and boys attain puberty about two years later, although there are great individual variations. Puberty in a girl is marked by the widening of the hips, development of adult breasts, appearance of pubic hair, and *menarche*. Male puberty is characterized by the appearance of pubic hair, growth of facial hair, a deepened voice, and development of an adult penis and scrotum.

renal calculus The formation of kidney stones, a condition which, like *prostatic calculus*, may produce pain that is felt in the testes.

scabies A parasitic infestation of the skin by the scabies mite. The waistline, thighs, and genital areas frequently are involved, as well as the hands, wrists, and armpits.

spermatozoa The singular is spermatozoon and both are commonly referred to as sperm.

Spermatozoa develop from primordial germ cells that line the seminiferous tubules of the testes. A primordial germ cell goes through a number of cell divisions and growth periods before emerging as mature spermatozoa. During the cell division process, a sperm reaches a stage in which it acquires half the chromosomes of the parent cell. A similar event occurs in the development of a female ovum. Thus, when a spermatozoa fertilizes an ovum, the full set of 46 chromosomes—23 from the sperm and 23 in the ovum—is given to the newly formed zygote.

Stein-Leventhal syndrome A disorder related to the development of enlarged cystic ovaries and accompanied by the appearance of male facial hair, or *hirsuitism*, in the woman. Obesity and infertility also are among the characteristics of the disease.

teratocarcinoma The name of a malignant tumor that may involve a testis. Surgical removal of this type of tumor, followed by radiation treatment and chemotherapy, may be necessary. Some types of testicular tumors, such as seminomas, may respond to radiation therapy alone, so that surgery is not necessary. Any hard, painless lump that appears in the scrotum should be examined by a physician to determine whether or not it may be a tumor.

testes The male *gonads*. The testes develop high in the abdomen during fetal life and normally descend into the scrotum before birth. During early childhood the testes are quite small, but they grow to adult size during puberty. The bulk of a testis is composed of the seminiferous tubules in which spermatozoa are produced.

testicle A common name for a testis.

testosterone A male sex hormone produced by the Leydig, or interstitial cells, of the testes. At puberty a hormone secreted by the pituitary gland signals the start of testosterone production in large quantities. Testosterone in turn helps in the production and maturation of spermatozoa.

tinea cruris Also known as jockstrap itch or dhobie itch, this is a type of ringworm or fungal infection that may involve the moist, warm skin areas of the anal-genital area. The condition usually is aggravated by warm, humid weather and tight clothing that may rub against the inner thigh areas.

torsion of the testis A painful condition resulting from the rotation of a testis from its normal position in the scrotum. The rotation puts a twist in the spermatic cord that in turn causes a blockage of the blood and lymph vessels which supply the testis from the abdomen. The disorder can occur in an undescended testis as well as a testis in the scrotum. In a person with testes in the scrotum, torsion can occur during vigorous physical exercise or, occasionally, simply by making a sudden change in body position. Immediate surgery usually is needed to reposition the testis; otherwise, gangrene may develop in the testis because of the interrupted blood supply, and the testis would have to be amputated.

trichomoniasis An infection caused by a parasitic organism that usually is transmitted during sexual contact. In women the infection, also known as trichomoniasis vaginalis, produces a nonbloody, whitish discharge from the vagina. The discharge also may be identified as leukorrhea.

Turner's syndrome A karotype abnormality in which a person is born with one sex chromosome missing. The individual has the general body features of a woman, but the ovaries do not function and menstruation does not occur, making the person sterile.

urethritis Any infectious inflammation of the urethra. The cause of the infection may be a venereal disease, such as gonorrhea. However, urethritis can also be caused by a wide variety of pathogenic organisms, and many of the disease organisms, although not ordinarily venereal, can be transmitted by sexual contact.

vaginitis A general term applied to any of several forms of inflammation of the vagina. The disorder usually is characterized by itching and a nonbloody discharge from the genital tract. Common causes may be infections by bacteria, trichomonads, or the yeastlike Candida. Senile, or post-menopausal, vaginitis sometimes is accompanied by a bloody discharge. Most forms of vaginitis are corrected with proper hygiene measures, such as regular washing of the area, and the use of appropriate medications.

varicocele A varicose vein that develops in the spermatic cord and produces a "bag of worms" swelling in the scrotum. It may be caused by a tumor that obstructs normal flow in the blood vein or by faulty return flow of venous blood toward the abdomen.

vasectomy A method of rendering a man infertile by surgical incision that cuts the vas deferens, or results in removal of a portion of the duct, which provides a passageway for spermatozoa that normally would be transported from the testis to the urethra. In some operations the lower portions of the vas deferens from the right and left testes are tied together. A vasectomy is a common birth control technique, but sometimes it is done in connection with surgery of the prostate gland, which is the site of the terminal end of the vas deferens.

venereal disease A disease that usually is transmitted by sexual contact. The term, through a bit of irony, is derived from the name of Venus, the goddess of love. There are more than a half-dozen common venereal diseases, including gonorrhea, nongonococal urethritis, syphilis, chancroid (soft chancre), lymphogranuloma venereum, granuloma inguinale, genital herpes, and venereal warts. Some venereal diseases have become widespread because infected individuals often are unaware that they carry the disease organism, victims sometimes delay effective treatment in the early stages as the result of a false sense of modesty, and the development of strains of the disease agents that are resistant to medications formerly used to control their spread.

virilism Masculine physical and mental traits, normal in men but abnormal in women.

Wassermann test A laboratory test for the presence of the syphilis disease organism in the blood of a patient. Technically, the test is identified as a serologic test for syphilis (STS) and may employ any of a wide variety of proce-dures, rather than the original Wassermann test named for the German bacteriologist who developed the technique more than a half-century ago. In addition to blood antigen tests for syphilis, doctors may use dark-field microscope examinations, spinal fluid tests, and X-ray examinations in diagnosing cases of syphilis infections.

QUESTIONS AND ANSWERS

SEX ORGANS

Q: *Is there an antibiotic you can take for a genital herpes infection?*
A: No. Herpes Type 2 is a viral disease and viruses generally are not affected by even massive doses of antibiotics. But a Herpes Type 2 infection is even more serious since it is one of a few viral venereal diseases that cannot be cured by any remedy available at this writing.

Once a person has acquired the genital herpes infection, he or she can experience recurrences from time to time for the rest of his or her life. In addition to the severe pain of these periodic attacks, a woman who is infected has an increased risk of developing cervical cancer, and if she becomes pregnant her baby may become infected during the birth process and suffer mental impairment or death.

Q: *What are the chances of catching a herpes infection by having sexual relations?*
A: The chances probably are pretty good if you aren't well acquainted with your sex partner, or at least well enough acquainted to be quite sure that he or she is not infected. There are an estimated five million persons in America alone who carry the Herpes Type 2 virus because of sexual contact with an infected person. That's an average of about one in every 40 persons; the ratio would be much closer if children and grandparents were eliminated from possible infected persons and the pool of five million was properly narrowed to include mainly sexually active teenagers and young adults.

Q: *How can you tell if somebody has a Herpes Type 2 infection?*
A: You can't unless you happen to see the fluid-filled lesions, which resemble "cold sore" blisters but are not exactly the same since they are caused by a different virus than the cold-sore virus, Herpes Type 1. The Herpes Type 2 sores appear around the genital area and occa-

sionally on the thighs or buttocks. The sores may appear from about two to ten days after a person becomes infected, but then the sores may vanish for a while and erupt again some time later. During an attack the infected person may have a fever, muscle aches, swollen lymph glands, and other general symptoms of illness. But like some other venereal diseases, such as gonorrhea and syphilis, the disease organism may be present even though the infected sexual partner does not show any obvious signs of infection.

Q: *Can cancer of the breast be inherited?*
A: The best information to date indicates that parents do not pass cancer on to their children. However, it is not unusual for both a daughter and mother to develop cancer of the breast or cancer of the uterus, or for the same type of cancer to occur in other female members of the same family.

Scientists who have studied the problem have suggested other possible answers. Women in the same family may have similar lifestyles that increase the risk of breast cancer; they may eat the same foods, live in the same environment, or share some other possible risk factor. In other words, the cancer may appear to be inherited but could actually be the result of two or more women of different generations being exposed to the same factors that increase the chances of developing cancer of the breast, uterus, or some other body organ.

Q: *My wife had an ovariectomy recently because of a tumor. Is it still necessary to use contraceptives, or would the operation make a woman sterile?*
A: The answer would depend upon what was removed during the surgery, among other factors. Theoretically, at least, a woman who is of childbearing age can become pregnant as long

as she has a uterus and one functioning ovary and Fallopian tube. By a similar measure, a man with only one testicle can become a father if the testicle and attached tissues are in normal functioning condition.

Q: *I recently became pregnant and have made an appointment for a pelvic exam by an Ob-Gyn specialist. Is it all right to tell him about the medications prescribed by my psychiatrist?*

A: By all means, you should tell your Ob-Gyn doctor about any and all drugs you may be taking, including nonprescription drugs. There are many substances, in addition to drugs, that can have a teratogenic effect on a child developing in the uterus, especially during the first trimester, or first three months. Teratogens are substances that can cause birth defects in the embryo or fetus. Some drugs are incompatible with certain medications used in managing delivery of a baby. Still another reason is that occasionally a doctor will prescribe a medication that is the same as or similar to a medication that already has been prescribed by another physician, because the patient failed to tell each doctor what medicines he or she already was taking. If you aren't sure of the names of the drugs you are using, bring along the vials or containers for the Ob-Gyn specialist to check.

Q: *My daughter began developing adult breasts when she was 11 years old and pubic hair before she was 12. However, she has not had her first menstrual period yet and she is 13. Is there possibly something wrong that has interrupted her puberty?*

A: Actually, it appears that your daughter may be perfectly normal. Breast development and pubic hair normally occur two or three years before the menarche, or the first menstrual period. Delayed puberty might be a possibility if no signs of breast development or pubic hair appeared before the end of the 13th year, and menstruation for many girls does not occur until they are around 16.

Normally, there is a spurt of pubertal growth, as characterized by the development of breasts, followed by a pause before menstruation begins. It generally takes about three years for a girl to pass through the various stages of puberty. Some girls, of course, begin pubertal development before the age of nine, and precocious, or early, puberty may unfortunately be accepted as what is normal when perhaps it is not.

Q: *Is precocious puberty a sign of a tumor or disease?*

A: True precocious puberty in girls, which is more common than precocious puberty in boys, sometimes is associated with a disease such as encephalitis that may involve the brain. But in most cases no specific disease can be identified as a possible cause. Precocious puberty in boys, however, often is linked to a tumor or a neurological or brain disorder. Early puberty in a boy may not be true precocious puberty if a tumor of an adrenal gland or a testis is involved. When early puberty is associated with a testicular tumor, for example, one testis may appear to be an enlarged adult testis while the other remains infantile. Or a boy may have most of the usual adult sexual characteristics, except that the testes remain in the prepubertal stage. Normally, boys do not complete their growth spurt until after the genital changes have nearly completed their transition to the mature stage.

Q: *My son has an undescended testicle. Will that make him sterile or cause delayed puberty?*

A: Generally, only one normal testis is required for normal sexual development of a male. However, there are other reasons why it would be a good idea to have the abnormality corrected at the earliest opportunity. One is the increased risk of cancer that is associated with an undescended testicle in a young man.

Q: *Is surgery needed to correct problems of delayed puberty?*

A: Only when it may be necessary to correct an obstruction or a similar type of difficulty in order to increase the chances for fertility. True delayed puberty usually can be treated by sex hormone replacement therapy. Boys may be given intramuscular injections of a testosterone preparation every two or three weeks, or a testosterone tablet every day. Girls can be given a daily oral medication containing female sex hormones.

Q: *Why would a doctor use a flashlight to examine the scrotum when the problem is a hernia?*

A: Perhaps the doctor wants to determine if the inguinal hernia has penetrated the scrotum. Since the walls of the scrotum will transmit light, the interior can be studied for the presence of objects other than the testes. An inguinal hernia will show up as an opaque shadow when the scrotum is illuminated in a darkened room with a flashlight. Tumors also will appear as opaque shadows, but a fluid accumulation, such as from a hydrocele, will produce a translucent reddish glow when the scrotum is examined in this manner—a procedure called transillumination.

Q: *I am worried about having a prostate examination as part of a physical checkup. Is it painful?*

A: A simple examination of the prostate gland and the seminal vesicles, which lie alongside the prostate, should be painless. Both organs can be palpated through the anus and both normally are what medical personnel consider as nontender, meaning they should produce no pain when palpated.

You may find the examination more comfortable if you remember to urinate before the prostate examination because pressure on the gland from palpation may trigger an urge to urinate. Also, some patients are apprehensive about having a doctor or nurse insert a gloved finger into the anus, and they react by tightening the anal sphincter muscle, thereby making entry a bit difficult. The patient, therefore, may be asked to bear down as if moving his bowels so the anal sphincter will be loosened for the prostate examination.

Q: *Is it true that a man can lose the entire penis if he has an erection that continues too long?*

A: You probably are referring to an abnormal condition called priapism in which the erection occurs without sexual stimulation and may persist for 24 hours or more. This condition results in obstruction of the normal flow of blood through the tissues of the penis—erection occurs because blood flows in faster than it returns to the abdomen. The effect of priapism is similar to that of thrombosis or an infarction, when tissues die because of obstructed blood flow. If tissues of the penis are allowed to die, gangrene develops and the entire shaft of the penis can be lost. A priapism often requires emergency medical treatment to prevent loss of the penis.

Q: *I have been taking medications for high blood pressure and plan to marry for a second time in the near future. Would oral contraceptives interfere with the treatment for high blood pressure?*

A: This is a question that only your doctor can answer for your individual case. Generally speaking, oral contraceptives are known to increase the risk of high blood pressure. However, the women most likely to be affected, according to published medical studies, are those who are older or overweight, or who have a medical history of hypertension or come from families with members known to suffer from high blood pressure.

Q: *I have heard that IUDs can cause an increase in menstrual blood flow. Is there any truth to it?*

A: There is some statistical evidence to support the notion that menstrual blood loss may increase as a side effect of using the intrauterine contraceptive device. This effect has been a reason given by many women who have quit using IUDs. The reason for the effect is unknown and there have been many efforts to reduce the problem of excessive and prolonged menstruation by changing the design of the device. Some success has been reported in the development of IUDs that do not increase menstrual blood loss by using different materials in the manufacture.

Q: *What is cystic breast disease? Is it a cause of breast cancer?*
A: Cystic hyperplasia, or mammary dysplasia, is a condition that makes the breast lumpy and tender, especially during the premenstrual phase of the menstrual cycle. In some cases there may be cystic masses that change in size from time to time. This is perhaps the most common disorder involving the breast; women between the ages of 30 and 50 are the most likely to be affected. It is believed to be the re-

sult of an imbalance of female sex hormones. The condition eventually can lead to an increase in connective tissue in the breasts and the formation of obvious cysts.

Another kind of benign breast disease is fibroadenoma, which affects mainly young women and adolescent girls. It is characterized by the appearance of firm, painless nodules, some of which can become quite large.

While cystic breast diseases generally are not a cause of breast cancer, there is evidence that women who are afflicted with cystic breast disease are more likely than others to develop breast cancer later in life.

7

BONES AND MUSCLES

Your medical records may refer to the bones and muscles of your body as a musculoskeletal system. For purposes of medical records, the musculoskeletal system also includes the nerves, blood vessels, joints, and other tissues that are vital for normal functioning of the spine, limbs, and other structures needed for locomotion and body support.

Doctors, as well as medical records, may refer to both arms and legs as limbs or extremities. Since an extremity usually is defined as the terminal portion of an object, it may seem confusing to a patient to think of a hip or shoulder as being the terminal portion of anything. But medical terminology often seems obscure to patients, and many doctors try to bridge the gap of understanding by using words like "upper extremity" when referring to an arm and "lower extremity" when discussing a leg.

A doctor usually examines a limb in a systematic manner, beginning at the very

extremity of an extremity—the fingers or toes—and working upward toward the shoulder or hip. The examining physician inspects one limb at a time, checking the condition of the skin, muscles, joints, and blood vessels by direct observation and palpation. The inspection will include an overview of the shape of a limb, in the event an unusual contour or angle might indicate a deformity caused by injury or disease.

Joints may be checked by asking the patient to make a tight fist, then spread the fingers and move them apart as widely as possible. The patient may next be asked to make a fist again and roll the hand at the wrist, first in the direction of the thumb and then in the direction of the little finger. These seemingly meaningless exercises may indicate the conditions of the joints in those areas; the doctor will watch for any signs of stiffness, tenderness, swelling, or inflammation about the hands. He may even hold the patient's hand while it is being moved in various directions.

Flexing, bending, rotating, or extending movements may be followed all the way up to the shoulder as the doctor checks the muscles, bones, and joints by observation and palpation. Any scraping or grating vibrations noted at a joint, particularly at the shoulder, can be a sign of an abnormal condition. Palpation of the muscles can give an indication of their firmness and strength. The doctor also may watch for any signs of tremor when an arm is extended in an otherwise steady position.

Similar inspections of the lower limbs begin with the feet and ankles and work up through the knee and hip joints. In addition to checking the health of the joints

from hip to toe, the examining physician may watch for signs of varicose veins and edema, or fluid accumulation, in the lower extremities. If the doctor can indent the skin by pressing a finger into the skin of the feet or ankles, it often is a sign of a condition called pitting edema. Edema also may appear as hard, woody tissue under a thin layer of bluish or colorless skin. Edema and varicose veins tend to occur in the lower extremities because of the pull of gravity on the fluids and, in the case of varicose veins, of failure of the valves that normally prevent a backflow of blood returning toward the heart. A doctor may check the femoral pulse by pressing firmly on the femoral artery, the main artery supplying tissues in the leg that is located

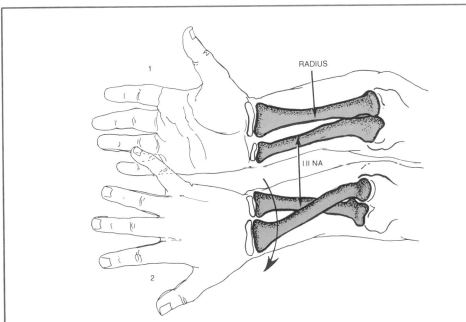

A pivot joint at the elbow allows a person to turn the hand palmside up or down. When the palm of the hand is up, the radius and ulna, the two bones of the forearm, are parallel. The radius crosses over the ulna, as shown in the diagram, when the palm of the hand is turned downward.

slightly inside the midline of the leg where it joins the pelvis.

Doctors sometimes divide the skeleton into two major sections. The bones of the skull, the spinal column, and the rib cage comprise the axial skeleton. The rest of the bony portions of the body, the extremities plus the shoulder and the pelvis bones, make up what is known as the appendicular skeleton.

The appendicular skeleton features some of the body's most interesting arrangements of bone-to-bone joints. The hip and shoulder joints, for example, are ball and socket connections not unlike the linkages found in modern mechanical equipment. Knees, elbows, and fingers function as hinges or simple levers. Curved surfaces of facing bones in the wrists and ankles allow angular flexibility, while the unusual pivot-joint arrangement of the wrist and elbow permit the radius and ulna, the two long bones of the forearm, to cross over when the palm of the hand is turned downward. This action is independent of the lever action of the elbow, that is, the hand can be rotated at the wrist regardless of whether the arm is straight or bent at the elbow—a minor engineering miracle that most people take for granted.

All such movements of the bones are made possible by muscle contractions. The muscles that move the bones, however, do not come in direct contact with the bones. Muscles are attached to tendons or, more likely, the ends of muscles become tendons that are connected to rough surfaces at the ends of bones. The fibers are twisted into very strong cables of tissue. Tendons do not stretch or tear under normal or even greater than normal stress or strain; as a result, it is not unusual for the muscle or bone to be damaged, rather than the tendon, when a tremendous amount of pressure is applied to a joint.

Ligaments, on the other hand, serve a similar function, but ligaments usually contain elastic fibers which allow them to give a bit under pressure. Ligaments connect one bone to a neighboring bone rather than bone to muscle, or vice versa.

Your fingers are moved by tendons that are connected to muscles in the forearm. You can feel the tendons at work if you grasp one forearm above the wrist and flex the fingers of the arm being held. The tendons pass through protective sheaths in the wrist and hand, but they can be felt nevertheless.

Bones and Bone Tissue

Approximately one-fourth of all the bones in the human body are located in the feet. The normal adult complement of bones totals 206, which is considerably fewer than the 270 bones an average individual possesses at birth. We lose 64 bones while growing up because many of the separate "baby bones" fuse into larger adult bones. Of the final total, each foot requires 26 bones to maintain the two natural arches that span the space from heel to toe. One arch, a longitudinal arch, supports the length of the foot, and the other, a transverse arch, supports the width of the foot. The arches were designed by nature millions of years ago to help support the upright human animal, and they are virtually identical with arches built by engineers to support bridges, aqueducts, and vaulted buildings since the dawn of civilization.

The bones that form the arch of the foot need to support a sizable amount of human body weight, even if the person supported is small and skinny, when the support is calculated in pounds per square inch and is subjected to perhaps 70 or more years of daily wear and tear. Generally, human bone is rated at the strength of cast iron; however, it is several times lighter than cast iron and is much more flexible. Even more startling is the fact that your bones are composed of living tissue that is constantly undergoing changes in structure and composition. For example, calcium, one of the minerals that gives bone its strength and light weight, may be eroded from the bones when it is needed by other body tissues for such tasks as maintaining muscle contractions or the ability of blood to clot. But calcium also is replaced daily by supplies of the mineral absorbed from the intestinal tract and transported by the bloodstream to bones needing calcium replacement.

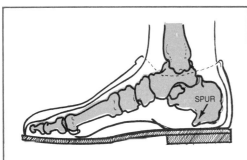

Illustration shows how a bone spur can develop from the heel bone. The spur presses into soft sensitive tissues of the foot, especially when the weight of the body adds to the pressure. Treatment is by surgical removal of the spur.

Bone tissue of a living human is about 20 percent water; the remainder is a mixture of about two-thirds mineral compounds of calcium, phosphorus, mag-

nesium, and other elements, and about one-third organic materials that may be quite similar to the fibers that form tendons. The outer walls of a long bone such as the femur, the bone that runs between the hip and the knee, may be quite solid—solid enough to withstand pressures of 1,200 pounds per square inch. But the inside of the bone at the ends is a meshlike network of spongy, or cancellous, bone. The shaft of the bone may be filled with yellow marrow, and the spongy bone spaces may contain red marrow. The patterns of the relatively thin walls of the spongy bone network are not distributed by nature in a random manner; instead, they show the lines of stress that are likely to occur when the weight of the body is shifted about during movement such as walking or running. The stress patterns are transmitted to the thicker layers of compact bone along the walls of the bone shaft.

The knobs and ridges at the ends of certain bones are designed to accommodate joints with neighboring bones, or to serve as attachments for muscles and tendons. If you ever have a chance to inspect the skeleton of a gorilla in a natural history museum, you may see that the larger muscles of the animal are provided with bigger areas of muscle attachment ridges at the ends of the long bones, as compared to similar areas of human bones.

As living tissue, bones contain several types of living cells that are nourished by blood vessels permeating the bone tissue. One special type of bone cell is an osteoblast, which has the job of building and repairing bone tissue. Another kind of bone cell is an osteocyte, which maintains the bone tissue surrounding it. A third special type of bone cell is an osteoclast, a cell that seems to have the unique responsibility of making sure that no bone contains more material than is absolutely necessary to maintain normal form and function. After a broken bone has been set, for example, a thick callus forms around the surface of the bone at the broken edges. The callus helps hold the broken ends together while the healing process goes on.

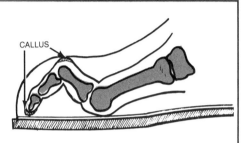

A callus can form as a localized thick layer of horny epidermis at a point where there is friction between the inside of a shoe and the skin of the foot. As indicated in the drawing, calluses can occur from wearing shoes that distort the position of the bones of the toes.

But as the broken bone heals, the callus gradually loses its thickness as the osteoclast cells shave away excess bone matrix that is no longer needed to protect the broken ends.

A tough membrane covers the surfaces of the bones except at the ends that are covered with cartilage. The membrane, called the periosteum, is united with tendons and ligaments that may be attached to the bone. The periosteum also carries nerves and blood vessels that feed into even seemingly solid walls of bone through tiny tunnels. If a bit of periosteum is peeled away from a bone surface, a number of bleeding points marking the passageways for blood vessels entering the bone will appear. The cartilage layers at some bone ends provide cushions of gristle which not only absorb some of the shock of actions such as walking or jumping, but permit some twisting and turning of the bones without the hazard of bone rubbing or grating against bone. The latter effect is experienced by some older individuals who suffer from osteoarthritis after a loss of cartilage cushions at weight-bearing joints.

Cartilage cushions also separate the stack of vertebrae that forms the spinal column, which helps to support the head and trunk of the body. The spinal column, which protects the spinal cord, is composed of 26 vertebrae in an adult and 33 vertebrae in a newborn child. Five original vertebrae fuse into a single sacrum bone and four fuse into the coccyx, at the bottom of the spinal column—thus accounting for the loss of seven of the 64 bones that gradually vanish as one grows older.

A typical vertebra, or unit of the backbone, is a cylinder of bone with spiny processes that extend behind the cylinder and form an open circle of bone. The spinal cord runs through the open circle, extending downward from the brain and sending out branches through openings in the sides of the vertebrae. The spinous processes of the vertebrae provide attachments for numerous groups of muscles. Twenty muscle groups are attached to the two vertebrae at the top of the spinal column, and 35 muscle groups are attached to the other vertebrae.

An important segment of your musculoskeletal system is your head, which also accounts for many of the bones and muscles of the body, including some of the tiniest bones and muscles. The skull contains 22 separate bones, plus a bone at the root of the tongue known as the hyoid bone, and the tiny bones of the middle ear, the ossicles, that transmit sound from the eardrum to the inner ear. Thirty-five different muscle groups can be found under the skin covering the skull, including six muscles needed to move each eyeball in various directions (but not including the small ciliary muscles that control the size of the pupil at the front of the eye).

Skeletal Muscles

Muscles of the musculoskeletal system, usually called skeletal muscles to distinguish them from other types, such as the cardiac muscle in the heart or the smooth muscles of the blood vessels and digestive tract, work in teams. One skeletal muscle group moves a bone or joint in one direction, and the opposing member of the team moves it back again. The skeletal muscles move joints and bones only by contracting; they never push, they only relax while the other team pulls. For example, to bend your elbow the biceps muscle is made to contract. To straighten the elbow again, the triceps muscle on the other side of the arm is made to contract while the biceps relaxes.

Muscles also may be identified as flexors or extensors, depending upon whether they flex, or bend, a joint, or whether they extend, or straighten, a joint. To flex or extend a part of the body, a skeletal muscle generally needs one bone as an anchor. In the case of both the biceps and the triceps, the muscles are anchored at the shoulder. The point where a muscle is anchored may be identified as the origin of the muscle; the other end, called the insertion, indicates the bone that is moved. The insertion of the biceps is on the lower end of the forearm, near the thumb side of the

wrist. The insertion of the triceps also is at the lower end of the forearm, but on the side of the little finger.

Each muscle has a name and a specific function. The quadriceps is so named be-

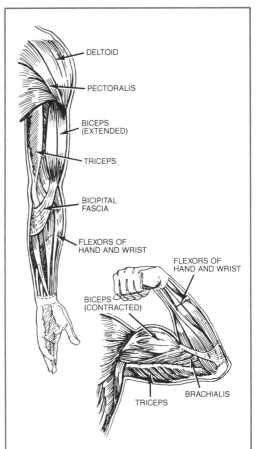

Muscles of the arm demonstrate how muscle groups work in opposition to each other. When the triceps is contracted, the biceps is extended in order to straighten the arm. To flex the biceps, that muscle must contract while the triceps becomes extended. Hand and wrist muscles similarly work as opposing pairs in extending the fingers or making them into a fist.

cause it consists of four separate muscles extending from the shoulders to the hips that work together in tasks such as kicking a football. The deltoid muscle, on either shoulder, is a more or less triangular-shaped muscle which gives the shoulder its rounded appearance and is needed to raise the arm to the side. At the top of the back is the trapezius, which resembles an inverted trapeze and lifts the shoulders when it is contracted. Since there are more than 600 muscles in the human body, it would take an entire chapter just to list and explain each of them. However, since mention was made earlier of one of the smallest muscles in the body, credit also should be given to one of the longest mus-

cles, the sartorius, which extends along the inner side of the leg and is used to pull the thigh into the lotus position for yoga exercises.

Skeletal muscles are known as voluntary muscles because the individual usually has voluntary control over their action, although there are exceptions such as reflex responses. Smooth muscles and cardiac muscle tissue, on the other hand, are considered involuntary, or autonomic, because they function without conscious control. Heart contractions, respiratory movements, digestion, or contraction of the pupil of the eye in bright light normally occur without our thinking about it. Exceptions might be cited, of course, in instances of biofeedback types of manipulation of involuntary muscle actions.

Both voluntary and involuntary muscle contractions require stimulation by a nerve impulse, a brief electrical charge that travels along the pathway of a nerve fiber at speeds of as much as 100 yards per second in a thick nerve fiber, but at slower speeds in a thin nerve fiber. The target of the nerve impulse is the junction of the nerve fiber and the muscle fiber. The muscle fiber reacts to the nerve impulse by contracting to as much as one-third to one-half its relaxed length. At the same time, the fiber becomes thicker. Because a contracted muscle becomes shorter and thicker, the effect often is visible as a bulge in the muscle. What happens at the microscopic level of muscle tissue when fibers contract is that the fibers, composed of tissue filaments that lie in alternate parallel paths, slide together when the nerve stimulus is received and are held in that position like magnets of opposite polarity until released by a message to relax.

Some muscles can remain in a condition

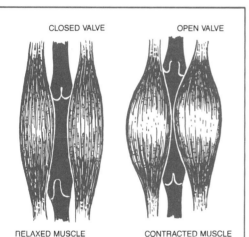

CLOSED VALVE   OPEN VALVE

RELAXED MUSCLE   CONTRACTED MUSCLE

Muscles of the legs have a secondary function of helping to pump blood from the feet to the heart. When the muscles contract they expand in width and squeeze the vein between the muscles, pushing the blood up the leg. When the muscles are relaxed, valves in the veins close to prevent a backflow. People who stand or sit still for long periods may eventually develop circulatory problems in the legs.

of partial contraction for very long periods of time. The muscles that hold your jaw closed and your head erect, for example, are in a constant state of at least partial contraction whenever you are awake. This is another exception to the rule that voluntary muscles require voluntary control. It also is an example of muscle tone, with some fibers taking turns automatically in contracting and relaxing.

Skeletal muscles can increase in size as a result of physical activity, and those that are not exercised can shrink in size. Exercise can mean repeated hard contractions just for fun or because of a work task that requires use of the muscles. Generally, only those muscles that are exercised will increase in size; part of the increase is in muscle tissue and part is due to a gain in blood capillaries and nutrient stores in the muscle tissue. Muscle tissue that has improved through exercise needs to be maintained in a healthy state of conditioning. Muscles that are not used tend to atrophy, or degenerate; the muscle tissue is reduced and some muscle fibers are replaced by nonelastic fibrous tissue.

Muscular Disorders

A muscle or group of muscles that may be used in continuous or endurance-type effort can develop a condition identified as muscle strain. In most cases of strain the muscles and tendons ache for a while but recover after a period of rest, frequently recovering overnight. However, a strain also can be severe enough to cause bleeding, swelling, or muscle spasms. A strain can result in a rupture of muscle tissue, with the muscle tearing away from its connection with a bone. The injury can be quite painful and result in impaired muscle function.

A sprain usually involves injury to a joint and may involve abnormal stretching or rupture of ligament fibers. Like muscle strain, there are various degrees of sprains, ranging from pain and tenderness with little or no loss of normal motion of the joint or limb, to a complete ligament rupture and obvious loss of normal use of the joint or limb involved.

Muscle cramps are usually caused by cold or fatigue and will respond to massaging of the muscle or moving the affected arm or limb to help relax the muscle. A muscle cramp often begins suddenly and is accompanied by a symptom described

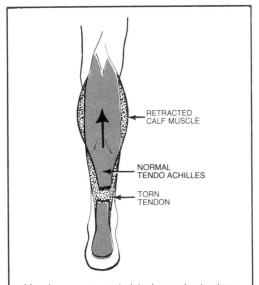

RETRACTED CALF MUSCLE

NORMAL TENDO ACHILLES

TORN TENDON

Muscles are connected to bones by tendons, which are bands of strong, white, fibrous tissue. An example is the tendo Achilles, better known as the Achilles tendon, which connects the triceps muscle of the leg to the heel bone. Tendons seldom rupture but a powerful contraction of the calf muscle may tear the Achilles tendon, particularly in an athlete who skips warm-up exercising before a sports event.

by some patients as feeling like the muscle is tied in a knot by an extremely powerful contraction.

Bursitis may occur in certain joints that are cushioned by a fluid-filled sac called a bursa. The bursa may become irritated and inflamed because of overactivity of the joint. Bursae are located in many parts of the body where friction might occur because tissues rub together. Among the more important locations for these sacs of slippery fluid are the knee, hip, elbow, and shoulder.

In body areas where tendons rub against each other or against bone or cartilage, protection is provided by enclosing the tendons in lubricated sheaths. Muscle fibers, groups of fibers, individual muscles composed of groups of fibers, and groups of individual muscles also are enclosed in protective membranes to help reduce friction of fiber rubbing against fiber, muscle against muscle, and so on.

Sensory and Motor Nerves

It has been estimated that the average adult human body contains about six billion muscle fibers, each about the thickness of a hair but much stronger and more flexible than a human hair. Although that number may seem enormous, it pales in comparison with the number of nerve cells and fibers in the same human body. The brain alone, for example, contains perhaps 12 billion nerve cells. And a major nerve trunk might contain as many as 25,000 separate nerve fibers that carry sensory messages to the brain and motor nerve messages outward to the body's muscle fibers.

Sensory nerves transmit information about conditions affecting various body tissues, including muscles. They may advise the body's control centers about pain, temperature, pressure, and the position of a part of the body—a sensation that helps people move about when they are blind or unable to see clearly because of darkness.

The nervous system messages that move the muscles are known as motor nerve impulses. They travel along different but somewhat parallel sets of nerve fibers. In some situations the sensory nerve fiber may carry a message all the way to the brain, which will evaluate the input and send back an appropriate message to a muscle unit, or several muscle groups, advising what action to take. If the situation requires immediate action, the messages follow a preprogrammed response route, a reflex arc to the spinal cord and back again.

The difference between the two kinds of nervous system direction for muscle activity might be illustrated by a person smelling smoke that comes from the kitchen. He reacts to the odor of smoke by getting up and walking to the kitchen to investigate the source of the smoke. If he is concentrating on an interesting television program when the smoke signal reaches the olfactory portion of his sensory nerve system, it may take a moment or two for the message to get through to the brain for evaluation and to instruct the muscles needed to move the body from the easy chair to the kitchen door.

After arriving at the kitchen entrance, the subject of the illustration observes that his dinner has started to burn because he forgot to turn off the fire under the pot when he started watching television. He reaches for the pot to move it off the fire, but the pot is too hot, and he jerks his hand away in a fraction of a second. Because of the intensely painful input of heat from the hot pot, the man's nervous system produced an immediate response and caused the arm muscles to contract and jerk the hand away from the source of the heat. The body made its own decision to react without waiting for the message to travel to the brain for an evaluation and a decision about whether some muscle action would be required.

It is possible occasionally for a person to learn to control a set of muscles so that a natural reflex action can be inhibited. Zen masters and Yogis are able to control sensory inputs that ordinarily would result in reflex actions. Other examples can be shown in biofeedback control of bodily functions, and even such basic activities as toilet training a child or housebreaking a pet in which conscious control of normal reflex actions is achieved.

Doctors often check the nervous system condition by testing a patient's reflexes. A common test of this sort is the patellar, or knee jerk, reflex test. The test may be conducted with the patient seated so that the lower legs hang freely and the knees are bent at right angles. With the legs in this position, the doctor will tap or strike a tough cord, or tendon, that is located just below the knee cap, or patella. Normally, the tapping or striking of the tendon will result in the foot automatically jerking forward. The doctor may perform the knee jerk reflex test on both the right and left legs for comparison.

Doctors have known for many years that nerve fibers on the right side of the brain cross over to the left side of the body and vice versa, so that signs of left-sided paralysis or other abnormal muscle activity can be a sign of disease or injury involving a motor nerve center on the opposite, or right side, of the brain.

Many of the motor nerve tracts that control various muscle activities have been mapped, as have the sensory nerves from the same muscle areas. Sensory nerves running between the limbs and the brain, for example, pass along the left center portion of the spinal cord if they carry messages about temperature or pain, but nerve messages relating to the sense of balance travel along the left outer edge of the cord.

Another example of the close relationship between the nervous and musculoskeletal systems can be found in the doctor's use of the Babinski response test, or plantar reflex test. The test requires only that the doctor scratch the outer edge of the sole of a patient's foot. The big toe of a normal person flexes downward in response to the stimulus. But if the patient has a lesion in a motor nerve cell in the brain, the big toe will flex upward. Thus, a doctor can literally diagnose a disorder in the brain by observing the contraction of a muscle in the foot, at the opposite end of the body.

Locating Musculoskeletal Sources of Pain

When a patient experiences a pain in a limb, or perhaps another body area composed mainly of muscle and bone, the examining physician may try to determine whether the source of the pain is actually in the bone, the muscle, a nearby joint, or possibly some other part of the body. A gallbladder disorder, for example, can produce a referred pain in the shoulder area on the right side of the body, while pain in the left arm can be a sign of a myocardial infarction, or heart attack. However, a pain in the right shoulder also can simply be the result of a disorder of the right shoulder, and a pain in the left arm can quite easily be due to an inflammation of muscles or tendons in the left arm.

The doctor often can distinguish muscle pain from either joint pain or neuritis, another possible cause, by testing the tenderness of the muscle. This may be done by gently squeezing the muscle mass; if the muscle is tense or firmly contracted it will feel harder than normal. Muscle pain is likely to increase if the affected limb is moved. Movement also increases the pain of a limb if the source of the problem is in a joint.

The doctor checking for causes of musculoskeletal disorders may find some clues in sounds made by the joints. Loss of cartilage in the knees or hips, for example, may result in creaking sounds. Roughened surfaces of joint membranes rubbing together can produce a vibration known as bony crepitus that the doctor can detect while palpating the limb.

During the examination the doctor probably will palpate the entire region of bone and muscle, using firm fingertip pressure. The source of the pain, which may be identified as the trigger point, often is found some distance away from the area where the pain is observed by the patient. To test the apparent trigger point located by palpation, the doctor may inject a solution of an anesthetic drug at that point; if his diagnosis is correct the referred pain will disappear within a few minutes.

Musculoskeletal Disorders

Musculoskeletal disorders may be associated with loss of muscle tissue which can result from injury or disease involving the muscle or motor nerves, or simply the failure to use the muscle enough to maintain normal function. In some cases the muscle degenerates to a short hard cord with restricted movement. A larger than normal muscle mass can simply be the result of physical exercise or, occasionally, one of several congenital disorders. An abnormal tissue mass in a painful muscle may be the result of a herniated muscle which may have ruptured through its sheath, or a hemorrhage in the muscle tissue caused by a tumor, a bony deposit in the muscle, or another factor. If the lump or abnormal mass moves freely when the muscle is relaxed but does not move easily when the muscle is contracted, chances are that the mass is in the muscle tissue.

Bone pain often is referred to a nearby joint. Careful examination usually is required to determine that the source of the pain actually is in the bone rather than the joint or the overlying muscles. An X-ray of the bones may be necessary to verify the source of the problem. The bone pain may be accompanied by tenderness and swelling; the symptoms may increase in intensity at night or when the offending limb is moved or is subjected to weight-bearing.

When X-ray examination fails to indicate a cause for the pain, laboratory tests may be ordered to check, among other factors, abnormal levels of bone minerals in the blood or urine.

Osteoporosis Bone pain often is the only symptom of a disease called osteoporosis, in which there is a demineralization, or loss of minerals, of the bones. The bones become thin and fragile and may break under pressure of ordinary movements in the average day's activities of a normal person. Among the several causes of osteoporosis are simple disuse of the limbs that results in a lack of stimulus for the body to deposit minerals needed for normal stressful activities of the limbs, excessive loss of vital minerals from the body stores, and failure to include sufficient bone-building minerals in the daily diet. Signs of the disease, besides spontaneous fractures of weight-bearing bones, include the collapse of vertebrae and demineralization of bones of the skull.

Treatment for osteoporosis depends upon the precise cause of the disease for each individual. Diets rich in proteins and calcium, hormone therapy, and physical activity geared to the abilities of the patient are among steps recommended to aid recovery.

Brittle Bones Spontaneous bone fractures also may occur in persons afflicted with a genetic disease sometimes identified by a medical term, osteogenesis imperfecta, and more commonly by the name of brittle bones. This congenital defect is marked by the development of bones that are harder but more brittle than normal bones. The persons affected by the disease tend to be of shorter than normal stature and may have a skull shape that is not normal. But otherwise the individuals do not show the signs of abnormal bone conditions found in patients with osteoporosis.

Osteomalacia Osteomalacia is still another bone disease that may be characterized by pain and tenderness, and result from failure of new bone to develop normally. The disease is similar to rickets, a vitamin D deficiency disease that can affect the development of children's bones before closure of the epiphyses, the ends of the long bones that fuse with the shafts when skeletal growth ends. In osteomalacia the problem develops after the epiphyses are closed—in other words, after normal growth of the bones is completed. There is inadequate intake of calcium or phosphorus, or the minerals are excreted

faster than they are consumed in food. The bones appear in X-ray examinations much like those of osteoporosis patients.

The bones of osteomalacia patients may fracture spontaneously, that is, with little or no stress, and may be slow to heal because of the body's inability to form a normal bone mineral matrix. Bone pain, low back pain, and muscle weakness characterize the disorder. Treatment of osteomalacia is similar to the therapy used in treating rickets and is based on supplying adequate amounts of vitamin D along with foods that provide the necessary amounts of calcium and phosphorus for normal bone development.

Vitamin D is required for the absorption of calcium and phosphorus, the key bone minerals, from the intestinal tract into the bloodstream, and for utilization of the minerals by the cells that assemble bone tissue from available nutrients. Rickets can develop in otherwise healthy and well-nourished children who are deprived of vitamin D. Their bones are relatively soft and easily deformed; legs and arms may be bowed.

Bone Cancers Bone pain occasionally may be due to cancer that develops in the bone marrow or results from the metastasis of cancer cells that travel in the bloodstream from a malignant tumor in the breast, prostate, lung, stomach, or other part of the body. Cancers that are found in the bone marrow, called multiple myelomas, may be difficult to diagnose without special tests. Clues other than the symptom of bone pain may be anemia or X-ray pictures that show "holes" in the bone due to erosion by the cancer growth.

Osteosarcoma, another type of bone cancer, affects the bone-forming cells and causes the bone to become soft and gelatinous. An osteosarcoma will spread eventually to the surrounding muscles and tendons. The bone pain may be accompanied by fever and a swelling of the tissues in the area, so the disease may be mistaken for arthritis or a muscle strain, and treatment can be delayed by the patient who attempts to relieve the symptoms with home remedies.

Chondrosarcoma is similar to osteosarcoma in signs and symptoms, although it originates in cartilage tissue rather than the bone-forming or blood-forming tissues of the bone. However, both chondrosarcomas and osteosarcomas generally spread into the bone marrow.

Treatment for bone cancers may include radiation therapy, chemotherapy, and surgery. Surgery involves amputation of a limb at the joint above the cancer. Radiation and/or chemotherapy may be administered in addition to surgery because, just as cancers can spread to the bones from other organs, bone cancers can metastasize to soft tissue organs.

Arthritic Diseases One of the more common disorders of the musculoskeletal system is rheumatoid arthritis, which can affect any person of either sex or any age, but develops most frequently in women between the ages of 35 and 45. The synovial membranes, double-layered membranes of fluid-secreting connective tissue lining the joints, are involved initially. Although the exact cause is unknown, the onset of rheumatoid arthritis usually is marked by an increase in the number and size of the synovial membrane cells. Tongue-like projections of synovial tissue may extend into joint cavities.

Rheumatoid arthritis symptoms may begin suddenly, with inflammation of several or more joints at about the same time.

There may be pain, stiffness, and difficulty in moving the joints. The stiffness may be more noticeable in the morning after a period of bed rest, or after a period of inactivity. Spasms of muscles around an inflamed joint can occur and the joint may become deformed. Low-grade fever often accompanies the symptoms, and nodules may develop under the skin.

There are nearly a dozen different signs and symptoms of rheumatoid arthritis, including laboratory test findings. Because a person may have several signs or symptoms without actually being afflicted with the disease, the doctor's diagnosis depends upon an evaluation of a combination of the clues and the length of time the effects have been observed. A person may experience what appears to be morning stiffness and pain in a joint, for example, but if the symptoms do not persist for several weeks, usually along with signs that can be verified by an examining physician, the cause of the complaints may be traced to some other disorder. Joint pain and swelling sometimes is found to be due to German measles, a salmonella infection, fungal infections, mumps, or drug reactions, to cite a few alternative causes of the symptoms.

When rheumatoid arthritis has been verified, the course of treatment may include complete bed rest during the most painful stages of the disease, administration of medicines to relieve pain and inflammation, special diets that insure proper nutrition, and exercise or physical therapy to preserve a range of motion that is as normal as possible. Surgery may be recommended in severe cases to relieve pain or to enable the patient to move about when the hips, knees, or other weight-bearing joints are affected.

Osteoarthritis probably is the most common of all disorders of the bones and joints, especially among persons of middle age or older. It results from degenerative loss of the cartilage cushions in the joints and the growth of bone tissue in the joints. The disorder may be accompanied by inflammation of the synovial membranes.

Unlike rheumatoid arthritis, osteoarthritis symptoms develop gradually and may be limited to a very few joints, usually those subjected to wear and tear from many years of weight-bearing. The patient may experience some stiffness after a period of inactivity but the stiffness lasts only a few minutes. There can be pain and tenderness in the affected joints, and the doctor probably will detect the sounds or vibrations of the worn joint surfaces rubbing against each other. When the knee or hip joints are involved, the patient may walk with a painful limp. In addition to the limbs, the disease can affect the spinal column and limit motion that requires movement of the lower back, or lumbar area, or of the neck and shoulder region.

A common cause of muscle pain and stiffness among individuals of middle age or older is known as polymyalgia rheumatica, which also is called senile arthritis or anarthritic rheumatoid disease. The disorder often begins with sudden muscle pains in the neck, shoulders, and upper arms. It may be associated with fever, weight loss, and loss of appetite. The muscles may appear to be normal and show no signs of weakness or atrophy. The joints may appear to be normal. There may or may not be evidence of tenderness in the affected muscles.

The source of the discomfort in polymyalgia rheumatica often is found to be a form of arteritis, or an inflammation of the arteries. Any or all of the arteries except the arterioles, the small branches leading to the capillaries, may be involved in the condition. The disorder usually is self-limiting and symptoms recede over a period of several years. In the meantime, treatment generally consists of corticosteroid medications given in doses that gradually are reduced as the symptoms disappear.

Gout Gout is a form of arthritis that usually involves the peripheral joints of the body, such as the toes or fingers, and is marked by deposits of urate crystals in the affected tissues. The urate crystals result from an abnormal accumulation of uric acid in the body, although one factor does not necessarily lead to the other. Some individuals have high levels of uric acid in their blood but do not develop gout symptoms. And gout occasionally occurs in persons who are not regarded as hyperuricemic, that is, persons with high levels of uric acid.

The typical gout patient experiences an onset of symptoms rather suddenly, after an injury to the foot, hand, or another joint, or perhaps following an emotional upset, fatigue, surgery, or excessive consumption of rich food or alcohol. The affected joint may feel warm and tingling, burning, or numb. Next, there is a rapid swelling and painful tenderness. The pain may be so severe and the joint so sensitive to pressure that the patient cannot tolerate even the weight of a blanket over the inflamed joint. Laboratory tests during the period of a gout attack usually show a high blood level of uric acid. The attack may last only one or two weeks, even if untreated in many cases, but other attacks will follow later.

Treatment generally includes the administration of medicines that relieve the symptoms and lower the level of uric acid in the blood, abundant fluids to prevent dehydration, abundant rest, and some changes in lifestyle, with emphasis on a diet that excludes foods rich in substances called purines if the doctor feels that such foods, including organ meats, sardines, and anchovies, may be a causative factor. Since the excessive uric acid that leads to gout may be a cause of kidney stone formation, part of the gout therapy is directed toward preventing kidney stones as well.

Pseudogout, also known by the medical name of chondrocalcinosis, has symptoms similar to those of true gout, and similar signs include deposits of crystals in the affected joints. However, the crystals are not salts of uric acid but of a calcium compound. And a medication commonly used to control true gout, colchicine, does not relieve the symptoms.

Pseudogout tends to occur in the knee or wrist, with sudden swelling and pain accompanied by a feeling of heat and a fever that may reach as high as 103 degrees Fahrenheit (39.4 degrees Celsius). The symptoms may last for several days, then gradually subside. Treatment may be limited to corticosteroid or other medications, although in severe cases the synovial membrane of the affected joint may be drained of fluid. Chances for recovery are very good. The attacks do not lead to a disabling form of joint disease.

Backaches Backaches that involve the spine generally occur in the area of the neck, involving the cervical vertebrae, or in the lumbar, or low back, area. Pain in the lumbosacral, or sacroiliac, section of the spinal column often follows the sciatic nerve down one or both legs and is commonly called sciatica. Sciatic pain may be felt all the way down to the sole of the foot and often is aggravated by movements of the legs that stretch the nerve. Low back pain, with or without sciatica, can be caused by a prolapsed intervertebral disk, or "slipped disk," by sacroiliac or lumbosacral strain, and by arthritis of the lower spinal column, among various possibilities. X-rays and palpation of the lower back are needed for diagnosis in most cases.

See also Chapter 19: *Arthritis: The Great Handicapper.*

GLOSSARY

BONES AND MUSCLES

This list of entries defines and describes the common and medical names of disorders, anatomical features, and other terms that relate to bones, joints, and muscles. Italicized words in the individual entries refer to separate entries in this Glossary.

acetabulum The bony socket in the pelvis that is part of the hip joint. The head of the *femur*, the long bone of the upper leg, fits into the acetabulum socket.

Achilles tendon The thickest and strongest tendon of the human body. It connects the two major muscles of the lower leg, the soleus and the gastrocnemius, with the heel bone, or calcaneus. The Achilles tendon is easily torn, or ruptured, when vigorous physical exercise is begun after a long period of sedentary activity. If the tendon becomes torn, the person cannot rise up on his toes, and walking generally is impossible because of the excruciating pain in the lower calf muscle resulting from the injury.

Achilles tendonitis An inflammation of the *Achilles tendon*, caused by an injury. The Achilles tendon is particularly vulnerable to stress or injury because it does not have the protection of a synovial sheath, which surrounds other tendons.

acromioclavicular joint A medical term for a part of the shoulder girdle that includes the shoulder blade. The joint often is the site of shoulder pain and a cause of stiffness that limits motion of the shoulder.

adhesive capsulitis A medical term meaning a "frozen" shoulder. The condition may be associated with a variety of causes and conditions, including a fracture, immobilization of the shoulder for a prolonged period of time,

and tendonitis. Motion is limited, and severe pain is felt in the deltoid muscle.

Adson's test A medical examination test for a disorder in which there are symptoms of pain, numbness, or tingling in an arm or hand. The cause of the disorder is the compression of an artery between two muscles in the shoulder area. To take Adson's test the patient sits with his chin raised and head turned in the direction of the shoulder that may be involved, while the doctor checks the pulse in the affected arm. If the pulse diminishes or disappears, it is evidence that the blood flow to the arm has been interrupted by compression of the artery.

arteritis An inflammation of the wall of an artery. The disorder sometimes causes a thickening of the artery walls so that blood supply is restricted. The disease also may be the cause of pain and other symptoms resembling arthritis or rheumatism. Some forms of arteritis involve the arteries of the head, especially in older persons, producing severe headaches and damage to nearby tissues.

arthritides The plural of arthritis, a medical term applied to diseases of the joints. See *osteoarthritis*.

arthrodesis A surgical procedure in which a joint is artificially locked or immobilized in order to relieve discomfort. The operation may be performed, for example, to reduce hip pain when other medical or surgical measures have failed to solve the problem.

atlas The vertebra at the top of the spinal column and the bone upon which the skull rests. The atlas was named for the mythological strong man who carried the earth on his broad shoulders.

autonomic nervous system A part of the nervous system that is not generally under voluntary control. Impulses of the autonomic nervous system fibers travel through the spinal cord and brain stem in much the same way that the sensory and motor nerve fibers carry messages between the skeletal muscles and the central nervous system. However, the autonomic nerves are primarily involved in activities of the smooth muscles and internal organs of the body.

The autonomic nervous system is divided into two parts: the sympathetic and the parasympathetic systems. The sympathetic nerves are associated with smooth muscle functions required for action, such as increased heart and lung activity, and constriction of blood vessels of the skin and of the muscles of the bladder and rectum. The parasympathetic nerves control the opposite, or vegetative, activities of the smooth muscles, lowering the rate of breathing and heartbeat, relaxing sphincter muscles, and so on. The autonomic nervous system ordinarily coordinates its activities with those of the sensory and motor nerves serving the skeletal muscles—for example, increasing oxygen and blood supply when the skeletal muscles are actively engaged in an athletic contest.

axis The second vertebra from the top of the spinal column. It has a toothlike upward projection, called the dens or ondontoid process, which fits into a facet, or notch, in the atlas above. Normally, the joint formed by the atlas-axis combination permits the head to be turned about 45 degrees to the left and 45 degrees to the right. Flexibility of other tissues in the spinal column allows additional head movement to the right or left without moving the rest of the body.

axon The shaft of a nerve cell and the portion of a neuron, or nerve cell, that is identified as the nerve fiber. The axon is attached to a cell body which serves as a sort of relay station for nerve messages. Axons always carry nerve impulses away from the cell body; shorter fibers, called dendrites, carry impulses or messages toward the cell body. Axons range in length from a fraction of an inch to three feet or more for nerve fibers extending from the spinal cord to the muscles of the foot.

Babinski reflex A medical examination test for a possible lesion of a motor nerve cell in the brain. The test is conducted by scratching the outer border of the sole of the foot. If the reflex response is normal, the large toe will flex upward. If there is a motor nerve cell disorder, the large toe will bend backward and the smaller toes will fan outward.

Baker's cyst A cyst that can form in the knee joint, causing pain and discomfort when walking. The problem usually is corrected by surgical procedures.

benediction hand A hand deformity in which the little and ring fingers are flexed but the other fingers can move normally, so the hand has the appearance of a clergyman's while giving a blessing. The cause can be a disorder involving the ulnar nerve of the arm or a degenerative disease of the spinal cord.

biceps Literally, a muscle with two heads. The term usually is applied to the biceps brachii muscle of the upper arm, which flexes the arm and forearm. The muscle's two heads begin at separate points in the shoulder area but unite in a long tendon that crosses the elbow joint and inserts into the radius, a bone of the forearm. In addition to raising the forearm, the biceps is used to turn the palm of the hand upward.

brachial plexus A group of nerves that pass from the spinal cord near the shoulder and extend to the hand. Abnormal compression of the nerve plexus can produce feelings of pain and numbness in the fingers, hand, forearm, or shoulder area. The little finger and ring finger can be the sites of referred pain from compression on the plexus, which actually is located near the top of the rib cage.

brachialis Also known as the brachial muscle, a muscle that lies alongside the *biceps* and *triceps* and has the job of helping to bend the elbow.

brain stem The extension of the spinal cord into the brain tissue. The upper portion of the brain stem is called the midbrain, a message-coordinating center for the central nervous system; it contains the nuclei, or cell bodies, for many of the sensory and motor nerve fibers of the cranial nerves.

bunion A lesion that may appear as a bony swelling, usually at the base of the large toe. The lesion often is accompanied by an inflammation of a bursa in the joint of the toe, and by a deformity in which the tip of the large toe is forced against or under the adjacent toe. The condition usually is the result of wearing tight shoes with pointed toes.

bursa A medical term derived from the ancient Greek word for wine pouch and used to identify one of the many saclike cavities of the body that contain synovia, or lubricating fluid, to reduce the friction of tendons, muscles, bones, or other tissues rubbing against each other when skeletal muscles contract or relax.

calcaneal pad Another name for heel pad, which is composed of fatty and fibrous tissues that form a cushion to absorb shock when walking. The heel pad can develop pain and tenderness as a result of inflammation or irritation. It loses its cushion effect for many people in later years of life, and others suffer pain while standing or walking because they were born with an inadequate layer of protective tissue in the calcaneal pad.

callus An area of thickened skin that may develop on the foot, usually in the sole areas under the heel or toes, as a protective mechanism against pressure on the tissues beneath the skin. When a callus appears elsewhere, it usually is a sign of excessive pressure against the skin in that area. Calluses generally cause no pain.

carotenoderma A yellow coloration of the skin, usually in the palms and soles, that results from deposits of excessive carotene in the diet. Carotene-rich foods generally are those with yellow coloring, such as oranges, carrots, and apricots. The skin coloration also can result from diseases, such as a liver disorder in which carotene in the diet is not converted to vitamin A—a normal liver function.

carpal tunnel syndrome A disorder of the fingers marked by a feeling of numbness and tingling. It is felt in the first three fingers, often during the night when the patient is awakened by the sensation. It is caused by compression of a nerve that passes under a tunnel of carpal ligament that is located at the wrist. The tunnel also contains the flexor tendons of the fingers. The examining doctor may test for the cause by having the patient flex the wrist as far as possible for one minute; if there is carpal tunnel compression of the nerve, this test will produce pain that is quickly relieved by extending the wrist.

carpometacarpal joint A medical way of saying the base of the thumb. This joint is one of the areas of the musculoskeletal system most commonly affected by degenerative joint diseases such as arthritis. The disorder can affect young people, particularly women, producing pain, stiffness, tenderness, and sounds of bone edges rubbing together in the carpometacarpal joint. Use of the thumb and hand may be impaired. Therapy includes injections of steroid medications, rest, and surgery.

cartilage A gristle-like substance that covers the ends of bones and serves as a component of the joints. There are several types of cartilage. One form, *fibrocartilage*, forms the disks that separate the vertebrae in the spinal column; it is different from the *elastic cartilage* of joints. Still another kind of cartilage develops in advance of bone formation and is gradually replaced by the mineral deposits of bone tissue.

cervical A term that refers to the neck. Cervical vertebrae, for example, are vertebrae in the portion of the spinal column that passes through the neck area.

cervical spondylosis A medical term for a type of headache that begins at the back of the neck and spreads up over the back of the head and occasionally as far as the forehead. The pain often is described as nagging or wearing. The condition is most likely to affect persons after middle age. The cause is unknown.

claudication A painful disorder of the lower legs caused by an inadequate blood supply to the muscles of the calf, ankle, and foot. The symptoms develop while the person is walking but subside within a few minutes after he stops walking. The muscle cramps may begin again when the person resumes walking. Claudication is derived from a Latin word for limping, which is what the patient with this disorder often does.

cockup splint A device used to immobilize the wrist during treatment of *tennis elbow.* Although the pain and problem of tennis elbow is associated with the elbow, it is motion of the wrist that can trigger the symptoms.

collagen A type of connective tissue found throughout the body. It consists mainly of whitish fibers that are bound in bundles for great tensile strength.

collateral ligaments Ligaments of the knee joint that may be torn or injured during athletic events in which the athlete's leg is twisted while running or jumping. Similar injuries to the ligaments can occur in nonathletic activities, such as walking. Ligament strains and tears usually heal with rest and proper medical care.

corn A growth of normally thin skin into a thick layer, similar to a callus except that the thickened skin evolves into a cone of keratin that points into the structures beneath the skin and produces pain there. The cone also has a central core. Some corns are hard corns and some are soft corns, which undergo maceration because of exposure to moisture and disease organisms.

cruciate ligaments A pair of ligaments in the knee joint that connect the *femur,* the upper leg bone, with the tibia, one of the lower leg bones. The ligaments help prevent damage to the knee joint by shearing the forces that would move the upper leg and lower leg in different directions.

curvature of the spine See *scoliosis.*

deltoid ligament A ligament that helps hold the tibia, one of the bones of the lower leg, to the ankle.

deltoid muscle A large triangular, or delta-shaped, muscle in the shoulder that is used to raise the arm to shoulder level, draw the arm forward or backward, and rotate the arm inward or outward.

demyelination The loss of myelin, a fatty protective substance that surrounds the nerve fibers of the brain and spinal cord. When myelin is lost, the nerve fibers lose their ability to conduct impulses, and paralysis or other neuromuscular effects can result, depending upon the function of the nerve fiber, or *axon,* affected. Multiple sclerosis is an example of a demyelination disease.

dendrites Short nerve fibers extending from the nuclei, or cell bodies, of nerve cells. Nerve impulses travel toward the nerve cell body along dendrite fibers, and move away from the cell body on the longer axons.

denervation A surgical technique for relieving pain by blocking or cutting a sensory nerve that is responsible for the sensation of pain. The technique sometimes is used in treating pain associated with problems of the hip joint or other limb disorders.

differential spinal block A technique for relieving back pain by injecting an anesthetic into the area where the patient appears to feel the pain. The doctor usually "maps" the tender area first by palpating or pinpricking the skin, while the patient advises the doctor whenever he touches a particularly sensitive spot on the back.

disk Sometimes spelled disc, this is a pad of *hyaline cartilage* that separates two adjacent vertebrae in the spinal column. The disk is composed mostly of fluid at birth, but it gradually loses water during adulthood while becoming more fibrous and inelastic. See *herniated disk.*

dislocation The displacement of a bone from its normal position in a joint. Dislocations probably occur most often in the shoulder and knee joints. The shoulder joint is the most vulnerable joint because it is held loosely in place by ligaments and muscles. The knee is relatively stable for such purposes as walking, running, standing, and swimming, but it is easily dislocated by the twisting and turning maneuvers of a contact sport such as football.

disseminated sclerosis Another medical term for multiple sclerosis. The word "disseminated" is used to indicate that the areas of *demyelination* are scattered throughout the central nervous system.

drop attack A common term for a symptom of a type of epilepsy in which the legs are involved. During an attack of this form of epilepsy, the patient may lose control of his legs and fall to the ground without losing consciousness.

dura mater One of the three layers of membrane that separate the brain and spinal cord from surrounding bone. The dura mater is the outer layer and is the toughest of the three protective membranes.

dystrophy A term sometimes used to indicate a wasting and weakness of muscle tissue. There are several types of muscular dystrophies, such as dystrophia myotonica in which the muscles not only lose strength but fail to relax normally after contracting. The patient

affected by this disorder may grasp an object but have difficulty in releasing his grip afterward. See also *muscular dystrophy.*

elastic cartilage Smooth cartilage of the type that covers the ends of bones and serves as the facing surfaces of joints.

electromyograph Also called electromyogram, this is a recording similar to an electrocardiogram except that it records the contractile activity of a muscle after it has been given a mild electrical stimulation. Electromyography can be used to diagnose a disorder such as *carpal tunnel syndrome,* or to help a patient learn to relax a muscle that is painfully contracted because of tension.

epidural block A type of spinal anesthesia procedure in which the anesthetic is injected into the epidural space of the spinal cord, or the space outside the *dura mater.* An anesthetic injected between the dura mater and the next protective membrane of the spinal cord is called an *intradural block.*

extra-articular A term meaning "outside a joint." An extra-articular pain might occur because of inflammation of a bursa beneath the skin but actually outside a joint. Housemaid's knee is an example of an extra-articular disorder involving a bursa between the *patella,* or knee cap, and the tip of the tibia, or lower leg bone; the bursa is subjected to pressure and irritation when the body is in a kneeling position.

extracranial A term referring to muscles, blood vessels, and other tissues of the head that are outside the skull. An extracranial headache, such as certain migraine headaches, for example, may be related to the vessels and muscles of the scalp rather than to intracranial tissues.

fascia Connective tissue sheaths or membranes that protect other tissues. A muscle group is covered with fascia to separate it from neighboring muscle groups. The walls of the fascia usually are lubricated by a fluid that reduces friction when the muscles are moved.

fascitis An inflammation of the *fascia.*

fat pads Closely packed fat cells that are found in various parts of the body, particularly the joints. Fat pads serve to lubricate and cushion parts of the joint.

femoral A term that refers to the thigh bone, as in femoral artery or femoral nerve.

femur The thigh bone, or the bone of the upper leg.

fibrocartilage The type of cartilage in the intervertebral disks. It is so named because the cartilage contains compact parallel bundles of collagen fibers.

foramen magnum A Latin-derived term literally meaning "big hole." The term is used by medical personnel to identify the opening at the base of the skull through which the spinal cord passes from the head into the top of the spinal column.

frozen shoulder A condition in which there is limited motion of the shoulder joint.

gait The pattern of walking as characterized by the rate, rhythm, and other aspects of foot locomotion. The gait of an individual varies from normal to waddling as in the case of patients with *muscular dystrophy* who must twist the pelvis and walk with a wide base, or spastic as in the gait of a paraplegic who pulls the knees together and sways his body with each step, or propulsive as in the gait of a victim of Parkinson's disease who takes short shuffling steps and may increase his speed of walking to avoid falling forward.

ganglion A mass of nerve tissue, composed mainly of nerve cell bodies, located outside the brain or spinal cord.

glenohumeral joint The joint formed by the humerus, or upper arm bone, and the glenoid cavity, or socket, of the shoulder blade. Injury, abuse, or degenerative diseases of this joint are responsible for most of the pain, discomfort, and disability that are associated with the shoulder.

Guildford brace A brace designed to immobilize the head and neck during therapy for a neck injury. The brace consists of a chin rest and occipital (back of the head) pad attached to metal bars, front and back, which are affixed to a chest pad that in turn is held in place with shoulder and chest straps. A Guildford brace can be used instead of a plaster cast to prevent flexion or rotation of the head, and it can be removed easily for other types of therapy during the patient's rehabilitation.

hallux A medical word meaning "big toe." Hallux rigidus refers to an immobilized big toe; hallux varus, to outward displacement of the big toe; and hallux flexus, to *hammertoe.*

halo brace A body jacket brace that is used sometimes to immobilize the neck. It is one of the most restrictive types of neck braces and is used in the treatment of serious orthopedic and neurological cases of neck injury.

hammertoe A deformity in which the toe is fixed in a flexed, or bent forward, position. The deformity can be congenital or acquired. Calluses usually develop at points where the tip of the toe and the flexed joint rub against the inside of the shoe. Surgery usually is required to correct the problem.

hamstring muscles A set of three muscles that run down the back of the thigh from their attachment to the ischium, a part of the hip bone. The hamstrings flex the leg and rotate it inward and outward. The muscles also are used to draw the trunk of the body backward when raising it from a stooping to a standing position.

hand-shoulder syndrome A complication of shoulder disorders in which the hand, which is dependent somewhat on the shoulder for its own functions, becomes limited in use. Edema, or fluid accumulation, may follow, and the hand may become painful and useless until the problem is corrected by medications, surgery, exercise, or a combination of therapies.

heel pain Pain in the area of the heel often is due to changes in the tissues behind and under the calcaneus, or heel bone. The heel pad, or *calcaneal pad*, a cushion of fatty and fibrous tissue under the calcaneus, can atrophy with advancing years or become inflamed. A spur may develop on the heel bone. Or there may be inflammation of the tendon that connects the heel bone to the base of the toe bone, a condition that often is followed by development of a heel bone spur.

herniated disk A term often used interchangeably with slipped disk or ruptured disk to explain a degenerative condition in which an intervertebral disk, one of the cartilage cushions that separates the bones of the spinal column, becomes extruded or bulging and presses on a nerve. The disk in a normal condition—or more accurately, at birth—is a sort of capsule containing mainly water. During the aging process the fluid content is lost faster than it is replaced, and the disk becomes increasingly a wedge of fibrous tissue that tends to bulge beyond its original limits; in some cases the bulge may become calcified, or bony. When the bulge finally pushes into a nerve root of the spinal cord, which the vertebrae were designed to protect, severe and often disabling pain results. The pain may be felt anywhere from the buttocks to the toes. The exact area of pain helps identify the nerve root that has been pinched by the extruded disk, or by vertebral bones brought closer together by herniation of the disk.

The onset of herniated disk pain may be abrupt and associated by the patient with pressure on the spinal column from running, jumping, lifting heavy objects, and so on. However, in most cases the conditions leading to a herniated disk involve repeated pressures over a period of time, while the fluid-filled disk is gradually losing its fluid.

hinge joint A joint that works like a hinge—for example, the elbow.

housemaid's knee Inflammation of a bursa near the *patella*, or knee cap, usually due to irritation or pressure from kneeling.

humeroulnar joint A joint formed by the humerus, the upper arm bone, and the ulna, one of the two bones of the forearm. It permits flexion and extension of the elbow and may be involved in certain kinds of elbow pain.

hyaline cartilage The type of homogenous matrix cartilage, usually quite flexible, that forms in the limbs and other areas of the body during fetal life. It is gradually replaced by bones that reproduce the general pattern of the hyaline cartilage templates.

hyperesthesia Increased sensitivity to pain or pressure on limbs or other body areas because of irritation or damage to sensory nerve fibers.

immobilization Restriction of movement of a portion of the body while an injury to bones or muscles is being treated. *Tennis elbow* and *whiplash* are examples of injuries that may require immobilization during the healing process of the muscles, bones, and joints involved.

intercellular Tissues or substances that are outside the cell walls of other tissues or organs. Connective tissue such as collagen fibers may be identified as an intercellular substance.

interdigital neuritis A disorder involving nervous tissue that may develop between two digits, or the toes or fingers. An example is Morton's neuroma—or Morton's toe, as it is better known—which causes a painful burning sensation between the third and fourth toes, counting from the large toe. The pain is caused by pressure from the metatarsal heads, or knobby ends of bones forming the toe joints, on branches of a nerve that pass between the bone processes. The problem apparently is not encountered by people who do not wear shoes, and it is aggravated by wearing shoes that squeeze the toes together, thereby putting pressure on the nerve branches.

intervertebral disk The cartilage cushion that separates neighboring vertebrae of the spinal column.

intra-articular injection Injection of an anesthetic or other substance into a joint.

intradural block A spinal anesthesia injection in which the drug is released on the inside of the *dura mater*, the protective membrane that surrounds the spinal cord and brain.

joint The point at which two separate bones come together. There may be cartilage, connective tissue, or other tissues in or around the joint, as well as on the facing surfaces of the bones. The joint may or may not have a movable function. Some bones of the skull, for example, are separated only by a membrane and do not flex or extend. Other joints, such as the facing surfaces of pelvic bones, may be slightly movable. Freely movable joints include the shoulder, elbow, hip, knee, etc. See also *carpometacarpal joint; glenohumeral joint; hinge joint; humeroulnar joint.*

kinesiology The name given the study of bones, muscles, nerves, and related tissues involved in body movements.

kinetic pain A term sometimes used by doctors to identify pain that is associated with movement of a body part. The term is used to distinguish pain of movement from static pain in bones and muscles that is experienced when there is no stress or pressure from movement of the body. A kinetic pain in the leg, for example, would occur as a result of walking, running, or other activity, while a static pain would be experienced when standing, sitting, or lying down.

lateral capsular ligaments Heavy fibrous ligaments that are lined with *synovial membranes* and located at various body joints, for example, the knee joint.

lateral collateral ligaments Ligaments connecting bones of some joints, such as the knee and ankle, to provide additional stability. Lateral collateral ligaments of the ankle usually are involved when a person sustains a sprained ankle by twisting the joint in a way that makes it unstable.

ligament A band of tough tissue connecting the ends of bones to form joints. See *carpal tunnel syndrome; cruciate ligaments; deltoid ligament; lateral capsular* and *lateral collateral ligaments; nuchal ligament.*

longitudinal arch The arch formed lengthwise, from the heel bone to the toes, by the bones of the foot.

low back pain Pain and discomfort associated generally with the lumbar portion of the spinal column, consisting of the first five vertebrae above the sacrum. The lumbar vertebrae differ from those farther up the spinal column in that they permit bending forward and arching backward, but their design prevents rotation or movement of that part of the spine to the left or right. As a result, most of the stress involved in back-bending occurs in the sacral-lumbar area of the back.

lumbar plexus A group of nerves that supply the hip joint and the muscles of the hip joint.

manipulation A technique used in physical therapy to aid the rehabilitation of a musculoskeletal disorder by forcefully moving a joint beyond its usual limits of motion. Manipulation sometimes is used in the treatment of *tennis elbow*, except when the problem involves the belly of the muscle.

march fracture A fracture of a toe bone that is discovered after a long period of walking, or marching, although no particular injury was involved. The fracture may be only a hairline break, and the appearance of a bone-healing callus about the fracture line may be the only physical evidence of a broken bone, although the patient may complain of pain in the area of the break. Treatment may require a plaster cast or simply avoidance of weight on the foot while it heals.

meniscus A curved wedge of *fibrocartilage* material in the knee joint.

metatarsalgia A painful condition involving the bones of the feet that face the sole. The cause of the disorder is a failure of the arch of the foot to support the weight of the body. The arch becomes depressed and the bones that normally do not touch the ground become weight-bearing structures. The remedy often includes the use of pads inside the shoe to restore the normal arch of the foot.

motor neuron A motor nerve that transmits a stimulus resulting in a muscle action. A motor neuron usually consists of a nerve cell body located in the brain or spinal nerve root and a long axon that extends to a muscle.

muscular dystrophy A term used to identify a group of several different diseases marked by a wasting of muscle tissue. The diseases are inherited. One form of muscular dystrophy affects some sons—but not all—of a mother who carries the genetic disease. The boys develop what appear to be very muscular legs, but the tissue is found to be not muscle but fat and connective tissue. Other muscles of the body gradually degenerate, and death often occurs after the respiratory muscles fail to function. Another form of muscular dystrophy affects only the muscles of the shoulders and pelvis; while it may be disabling, the disease merely restricts normal adult life and does not lead to death at an early age.

myalgia Tenderness or pain in the muscle tissue; sometimes called muscular rheumatism.

myasthenia gravis A disabling disease of the nerves and muscles caused by a failure of the nerve impulse to produce a proper muscle contraction. The disease may affect only certain muscles, such as those involved in vision or breathing. The impulse failure is due to a lack of acetylcholine at the junction of the nerve and muscle; acetylcholine is a chemical needed to translate the nerve impulse into a muscle contraction. Treatment involves admin- istration of a substance that prevents destruction of acetylcholine by other chemicals in the body.

myoclonic jerks The sudden violent, jerking movements of one or both arms, or of the legs, by an epilepsy patient during an attack. If the legs are involved, the patient may experience a *drop attack* and fall to the ground without losing consciousness.

navicular bone One of the bones of the foot which form the instep and the longitudinal arch of the foot.

neuraxon Another name for *axon*, the long nerve fiber that carries impulses from a nerve cell body to a muscle.

nuchal ligament A ligament attached to the cervical vertebrae, which form the neck bones.

obturator The name of a nerve and of a muscle of the hip joint. The obturator nerve and/or the obturator muscle may be involved in a painful disorder of the hip joint.

osteoarthritis A medical name for degenerative joint disease, the wearing away of cartilage layers on the facing surfaces of a joint. It is the most common type of arthritis and presumably affects every human who lives long enough to experience the effects of wear and tear on knees, hips, and other joints. Most patients are past middle age when symptoms or signs of osteoarthritis occur, usually as a result of a previous injury or disease involving the joint. Obesity, congential defects, misalignment of a joint because of rickets, diseases such as rheumatoid arthritis, fractures, and torn menisci are among the factors, in addition to aging, that may contribute to or aggravate osteoarthritis.

osteochondritis An inflammatory disease of the bone and/or joint. One form of the disorder, osteochondritis dissecans, is caused by a piece of cartilage or bone breaking loose in a joint. Osteochondritis juvenilis, which affects children, is characterized by the softening of a bone, usually the femur, which becomes deformed while in the softened state.

osteophyte An abnormal outgrowth on a bone. The presence of osteophytes is a sign of a condition called osteophytosis.

osteotomy A surgical procedure that involves cutting through a bone. An osteotomy may be performed to correct a disorder of the hip joint, to eliminate a problem of knock-knee, or to treat other musculoskeletal conditions.

palmar plate A plate of fibrous cartilage material that helps protect the palm side of the hand bones.

patella The knee cap; a small flat bone held by the tendon of the quadriceps muscle, a group of four muscles that begin in the area of the hip joint. The tendon is attached at the lower end to the shaft of the tibia, one of the bones of the lower leg.

pelvic traction The name used to identify any of several contrivances used in hospitals to treat disorders of the back. The devices are designed to pull on the legs or pelvis of the patient with weights and pulleys, and the objective is to hold the spinal column in a normal posture.

periarthritis Inflammation of an area surrounding a joint. The term sometimes is used to describe the pain from a *frozen shoulder* or similar joint disorders.

piriform pain A type of low back pain that can be caused by compression of the sciatic nerve by the piriform muscle, which extends from the pelvis to the femur, or upper leg bone, and rotates the hip.

plantar fascitis Inflammation of a tendon on the sole of the foot that connects the heel bone to the toes. The disorder is marked by pain and tenderness beneath the heel, where the tendon is attached. If untreated, the disorder can eventually develop into a heel spur.

plantaris tear A painful disorder caused by strain or tearing of the plantar muscle or its tendon, which extends for most of the length of the leg. The pain usually is felt in the calf, which may become quite tender. Because the muscle and tendon are located near the *Achilles tendon* and a couple of larger calf muscles, an examining doctor may test the various muscle and tendon functions of the leg and foot in order to find the injury. The problem most often results from strenuous physical activity involving the legs.

polymyalgia rheumatica A disorder involving pain in the muscles of the neck and shoulders, back, and pelvic region. The disease most often affects women who are of middle age or older. It is treated with corticosteroid drugs. Because the symptoms are similar to those of muscular dystrophy and several other diseases, a careful medical examination usually is needed to determine the cause and treatment.

quadriceps rupture A not unusual problem for men of middle age or older because of degeneration of the tendon which carries the action of the quadriceps muscle across the knee joint. The tendon may tear or pull loose from its lower mooring as a result of a sudden contraction of the quadriceps. An injury to the patella that fractures the knee cap may result in rupture of the quadriceps.

Quervain's disease A disorder of the tendons that move the thumb. Movements of the wrist and thumb can be painful, particularly activities that stretch the tendons, such as making a fist. The cause frequently is an accumulation of fluid in the tendon sheath that restricts movement of the tendon. Treatment generally consists of injections of medications to relieve the symptoms and immobilization of the thumb and wrist. Surgery may be advised in severe cases.

radial nerve A nerve that passes along the radial (radius) side of the forearm to the thumb and index and middle fingers, as well as part of the ring finger. The radial nerve can be the source of various aches and pains involving the arm and hand, resulting from playing tennis, using a screwdriver or hammer, and other activities for which the arm muscles are not in condition to tolerate. The radial nerve also can be pinched or compressed by muscles and joints on its way down the arm.

radiohumeral joint The elbow joint formed by the radius of the forearm and the humerus bone of the upper arm.

radius A slender bone of the forearm that attaches to the thumb side of the wrist. When the palm of the hand is held upward, the radius is parallel to the other bone in the forearm, the ulna. When the palm is turned downward, the radius crosses over the ulna.

Raynaud's phenomenon A condition marked by pain and abnormal skin coloring, ranging from pallor to cyanosis, in the extremities, particularly the fingers. The cause usually is a spasm of small blood vessels, triggered by exposure to cold. However, similar effects can be produced by compression of a nerve or blood vessel, an inherited abnormality, or the use of machinery or equipment that produces severe vibrations.

referred pain Pain that is felt at a point some distance from the source of the irritation. The hand, for example, may be the site of pain resulting from a problem in the shoulder joint, and a pain in the shoulder can be caused by a disorder involving the heart or the gallbladder.

replacement arthroplasty A technique for treating damaged joints of the hip, knee, or other areas with artificial parts. For example, a hip joint that is no longer functional because of the loss of natural tissues may be rebuilt with a plastic socket in the hip bone and a metal head in the femur, or upper leg bone.

rheumatoid arthritis A disabling inflammation of the joints, which may or may not be caused by an infection. The *synovial membrane* of the joint affected by rheumatoid arthritis becomes thickened by effects of the inflammation. This may be followed by erosion of the cartilage and possible destruction of the bone surfaces. Inflammatory nodules may form under the skin and tendons may rupture to complicate the disorder and aggravate the deformity of the joint inflammation. Although any joint may be affected, those of the extremities are the most frequent targets.

Young persons and middle-aged adults are most often the victims of rheumatoid arthritis. The disease may subside after an active period of months or years. But there usually is permanent damage to the joints affected, and they may be further eroded by *osteoarthritis* after being weakened by the rheumatoid variety of arthritis.

rotator cuff A term used to describe the action of a series of muscles in the shoulder joint. They form a cuff and rotate the head of the humerus.

sciatic nerve The great sciatic nerve is one of the longest and thickest nerves in the body, starting at the sacrum, at the lower end of the spinal column, and extending branches to the soles of the feet; it measures three-quarters of an inch in width at one point. The muscles of the back of the thigh, the leg, and the foot are supplied by the nerve. A small sciatic nerve sends branches to the skin along the back part of the leg and thigh. The sciatic nerve is responsible for a major share of pain involving the lower back and the legs.

scoliosis A medical term for lateral curvature of the spine. The person with scoliosis usually has a spine that makes an S-shaped curve down the back. The cause may be congenital, paralysis of the back or abdominal muscles, or other factors. Other types of abnormal curvature include lordosis, in which the back appears concave in the lumbar region, and kyphosis, in which the spinal column is flexed forward in the thoracic region. Persons with scoliosis and kyphosis may experience heart and lung problems because of the distortion of the space inside the chest.

sensory nerve A nerve that detects information about the position and environment of the body and transmits the information to the central nervous system for evaluation. Various sensory nerves, with special sensory endings, report on joint positions and movements, as well as temperature, pain, pressure (from touch), odors, etc.

Simmonds test A medical examination test for the condition of an *Achilles tendon*. Squeezing the normal Achilles tendon should produce an ankle reflex action, but the flexion should not occur if the tendon has been torn. The test also helps distinguish other possible causes of pain and discomfort, such as plantar muscle damage or *Achilles tendonitis*, which can present similar symptoms.

static pain Pain that occurs in a limb or joint when no movement is involved. Static ankle pain would be felt when a person simply stands naturally.

synovial membrane A thin membrane of connective tissue found in all freely movable joints of the body.

tabes dorsalis The medical name for a neuromuscular condition that is associated with an advanced stage of syphilis. Because of destruction of sensory nerves by the disease, the patient experiences a loss of sensations relating to temperature, position of body areas with respect to the environment, and touch. The patient may slam his foot on the ground when he takes a step because he has difficulty in determining the distance between the foot and the ground, and the inability to feel the normal contact sensation of his feet on the ground.

talus The keystone of the foot structure. It is a wedge-shaped bone that forms a joint with the tibia, one of the bones of the lower leg. The talus transmits the body weight from the leg to the rest of the foot bones, including the heel bone, or calcaneus, situated directly beneath the talus.

tarsals The tarsal bones are the middle segment of the foot structure, linking the toe

bones with the *talus* and calcaneus, which are the bones directly under the leg bones.

tennis elbow The common name for epicondylitis. Actually, the elbow joint itself may not be affected by the condition, which is marked by pain and tenderness involving the muscles that extend the forearm. The cause generally is severe strain or perhaps partial rupture of muscle fibers, with a pain trigger point over the area of the elbow joint known as the lateral epicondyle. Although the symptoms may occur after a fast game of tennis, other activities involving the extensor muscles of the forearm can produce the same effect.

tone Firmness and resilience of a tissue. Muscle tone may be defined as a natural resistance to the stretching of a relaxed muscle.

torticollis A Latin-derived word which means, more or less literally, a twisted neck. It may be used by doctors to identify a type of stiff neck, or wry neck, that causes the head to be tilted to one side. The causes of the disorder range from spasmodic muscle contractions to visual difficulties that may result in the patient tilting his head to one side or the other.

transverse arch The arch of the foot that runs at right angles to the longitudinal arch that extends from heel to toe.

triceps A muscle that runs from the humerus, or upper arm, to the ulna, one of the bones of the forearm, and has the job of extending or straightening the elbow joint. The triceps works in tandem with the *biceps*, which is the main muscle used to bend the elbow.

ulna One of the bones of the forearm, attached to the wrist on the side of the little finger.

ulnar nerve The nerve that extends down the arm at the side of the ulnar and supplies fibers to the side of the palm and the fourth and fifth fingers, counting from the thumb. Numbness or other abnormal sensations felt on the little finger's side of the hand often are due to compression or other injury to the ulnar nerve.

vertebral A term that refers to a vertebra, one of the 26 bony units that form the spinal column. The vertebral canal is the open space in the vertebral column, or spinal column, through which the spinal cord passes. A vertebral body is one of the bony cylinders that form the spinal column, with cartilage disks above and below to separate the vertebral bodies.

whiplash A common term applied to a type of injury that involves the cervical vertebrae of the neck and the spinal cord that passes through openings in the cervical vertebrae. The injury results from a shearing action in which the head and upper neck vertebrae are jerked forward or backward, while the lower neck vertebrae and body trunk remain relatively stationary. Whiplash injuries are associated primarily with the rapid deceleration of the body in automobile collisions, although similar effects can be produced by any sudden acceleration that propels the body forward.

white fibers The fibrous connective tissue of tendons.

writer's cramp A condition caused by spasmodic muscle contractions involving the arm, wrist, and fingers. The muscles may contract but fail to relax in a normal manner. The condition is temporary and responds to a rest cure.

yellow fibers Connective tissue fibers that are elastic. The yellow coloration comes from substances that give the fibers their elasticity. Yellow ligaments are composed almost entirely of yellow elastic fibers.

QUESTIONS AND ANSWERS
BONES AND MUSCLES

Q: *My doctor has advised a procedure called chemonucleolysis as a treatment for sciatic pain. What is it and how does it help the pain?*

A: Chemonucleolysis is a substance that can be injected into a troublesome intervertebral disk to dissolve it or reduce its size by removing the fluid in the disk. When the disk has been deflated the pressure on a neighboring nerve root is reduced and the pain subsides. The procedure is done under an anesthetic and with the use of X-ray equipment to help the surgeon inject the chemical substance into the right spot. It is recommended for certain types of back and sciatic pain, such as pain due to a herniated disk.

Q: *After I took up jogging for exercise I began to develop muscle cramps. My doctor suggested that I drink milk to see if that would correct the problem. I have always been told that milk is for kids and you don't need it after you have reached maturity. True?*

A: False, as far as adult need for calcium is concerned. But true if you are thinking only in terms of fluid milk, which is the most convenient way for most Americans to get calcium in their diets. Because calcium is needed for normal muscle tone, people who are physically active are prone to develop muscle cramps if they neglect calcium in their meals. Adults who neglect their normal daily needs for calcium can develop osteomalacia, a condition in which the bones become soft and possibly deformed, and osteoporosis, a disease marked by loss of calcium from the bones, which can become so brittle that they break from the slightest pressure on a limb.

Q: *Is a plantar wart the same as a callus?*

A: A plantar wart can be hard to distinguish from a callus, especially if the wart does not project beyond the skin surface, which is typical of a plantar wart. A callus occurs only at points where the skin is subjected to more or less continuous pressure, whereas a plantar wart may develop anywhere on the sole of the foot. However, a plantar wart usually is quite tender and has a typical wartlike appearance, but a callus has a surface that blends in with the surrounding skin.

Q: *My son has flat feet. Should I buy arch supports for his shoes?*

A: Generally speaking, wearing arch supports for flat feet can be compared to wearing an arm in a sling because of weak arm muscles. The condition, commonly called flat feet, and technically known as pes planus, is a rather common disorder in which the longitudinal arch which runs the length of the foot is in closer contact than normal with the ground. The cause can be congenital or it can be due to paralysis, but most frequently the problem is the result of weak foot muscles. Children are born with flat feet; the arch develops during childhood in most persons, but the pes planus condition may persist into adult life for some individuals.

An orthopedic surgeon should be allowed to examine the boy's feet to determine the extent of the condition. He may recommend a course of exercises to strengthen the muscles and perhaps advise the use of arch supports if the exercises fail to help and the condition produces symptoms of pain or discomfort.

Q: *Is there a part of the body called the "snuff box"? A neighbor who went to the doc-*

tor for a sore wrist said she was told the problem was tendonitis of her snuff box.

A: Yes, there is an area of the wrist that sometimes is described as the snuff box. It is a hollow area on the thumb side of the wrist that appears when the thumb and forefinger are extended. Several tendons and blood vessels are located under the snuff box, which is a site of pain when the scaphoid, one of the wrist bones, is fractured. Tendonitis of the snuff box is a more colorful name for the disorder than the medical term of Quervain's disease.

Q: *What is the difference between lordosis and kyphosis?*

A: Both are terms used to identify abnormal curvature of the spine, or scoliosis. Generally, kyphosis is any curvature that produces a forward concavity of the spinal column and may include such effects as an adolescent slump, a dowager's hump, or a hunchback appearance. Lordosis is characterized by a convex curve in the lumbar section of the spinal column that makes the shoulders appear to be thrown back farther than is normal. Kyphosis and lordosis can occur in the same spinal column, one the result of trying to compensate for the other.

Q: *Is golfer's elbow the same as tennis elbow?*

A: Not quite. Tennis elbow involves the arm muscles on the outside of the elbow. Golfer's elbow is caused by strain or injury to the muscles on the inside of the elbow.

Q: *Is it possible to have both tennis elbow and golfer's elbow at the same time?*

A: Yes. And the combination probably is the most ancient of elbow problems since it seems to be associated with throwing spears or javelins. In fact, it sometimes is identified as javelin elbow.

Q: *Everybody on our company softball team seems to have a different idea about what a "charleyhorse" is. Can you settle the argument?*

A: It's true that the word "charleyhorse" has been used over the years to identify a wide variety of muscle aches, pains, and injuries. Even in recent years some coaches and trainers have applied the term to leg muscle spasms and bruised thighs. However, doctors who specialize in sports medicine have tried to agree on standard names for sports injuries, and most now agree that the term "charleyhorse" should be used to identify soreness and stiffness of the quadriceps, a thigh muscle, due to strain or injury. The disorder often occurs as a result of overuse of an undertrained muscle.

Q: *What about "shin splints"?*

A: Shin splints is a common name for a strain of the flexor muscle that moves the tendons of the toes. Like tennis elbow, the condition is named not for the affected muscle but for the part of the anatomy where the pain is centered, in this case the shin bone, or tibia.

Shin splints can occur as a result of almost any kind of vigorous activity involving the legs, from playing basketball and football to walking and cross-country running.

Q: *Is a shin bone bruise the same as shin splints?*

A: No. Whereas shin splints involves a leg muscle, a shin bone bruise probably is characterized by bleeding under the periosteum, the membrane covering the shin bone, after the bone was injured. The medical name of the shin bone is the tibia. The muscle involved in shin splints lies near the shin.

Q: *I have read that intermittent claudication is like angina pectoris except that it involves blood vessels of the legs instead of the heart. Is this correct?*

A: It is correct in that the painful condition is related to a reduced caliber of the arteries, so that the muscle tissue cannot get enough fresh blood to sustain normal activity. The result in both disorders is a kind of painful cramp that restricts physical activity. In the case of intermittent claudication, painless walking is restricted.

There usually are no symptoms when the patient is resting. But pain or weakness develop in the calf muscle after the individual has walked a certain distance without resting. If he stops walking for a few minutes, the symptoms disappear as the blood supply catches up with the demands of the leg muscles. Then walking can be resumed for a similar distance before the pain or weakness returns.

Q: *For the past several years I have had a crackling in my hips and knees when I walk. Does this mean I am susceptible to arthritis?*
A: Since you did not reveal your age, it's a bit difficult to guess the source of your problem. If you are of about middle age or beyond, it would be a safe guess that the crackling sounds are indications that osteoarthritis already has developed.

This is not the most disabling form of arthritis, but is a rather common result of growing old enough to have the signs and symptoms of joint wear and tear. However, there are some precautions that should be taken to prevent the osteoarthritis from developing into a more serious problem. One is weight control; every pound within reason that you can take off the weight-bearing joints of your legs will help to make your life more pleasant in future years. Some gentle exercise and application of heat to the joints, plus a nutritious diet, also can make the symptoms of osteoarthritis more tolerable.

Q: *Is a pulled muscle the same as a torn muscle?*
A: Yes. A pulled muscle usually is marked by sudden pain in the area of the tear. The muscle

fibers usually tear because more tension is applied than the muscle can handle. The cause may be an accident that puts a sudden strain on a muscle, such as stepping in a hole while running, or, in the case of a pulled muscle during a sports event, failure to warm up properly before an event. In some cases there may be other factors involved, such as muscle imbalance, in which a muscle that straightens a joint is more powerful than the opposing muscle that flexes it, or vice versa.

Any pulled or torn muscle should be immobilized as quickly as feasible. Continuing to use a torn muscle will tend to increase the rupture. Medical attention should be sought immediately for proper care of the damaged tissue.

Q: *What could cause a pain in the shoulder and upper arm that only occurs when the arm is partly raised? I can hold my arm over my head without pain, but when I lower it to shoulder height the pain becomes terrific, and then it stops again when I lower the arm further.*
A: What you have described sounds like a condition called painful arc. It could be caused by a calcified deposit in a shoulder muscle, a torn muscle, bursitis, tendonitis, or a fracture of the humerus, or upper arm bone. All of these disorders can produce the strange symptom of arm movement that is restricted in the middle range of action, although the arm can be moved freely and painlessly at the upper and lower extremes of the range.

8

HOW TO USE BASIC HEALTH MONITORING EQUIPMENT

Self-care is a relatively new term for an old tradition of learning to take your own body temperature and pulse, checking your weight, and generally examining the body areas for signs of injury or disease. Mothers have been monitoring the health of their children for generations, watching for strange signs or symptoms that can be reported to the family doctor.

What may be new about self-care is that more people are learning to use stethoscopes, otoscopes, and sphygmomanometers. Some doctors have expressed concern about laypersons "playing doctor" with real medical equipment. But the effect generally has been quite beneficial since the use of basic medical equipment by ordinary people for checking blood pressure, examining their children's ear canals, or listening to internal body sounds has made those individuals more health conscious.

Many doctors now encourage a certain amount of do-it-yourself health monitoring. The increasing involvement of patients in their own health care helps the patient to understand the procedures and objectives of professional medical thera-

pies. It also gives the physician more time to help patients who have serious medical problems or who are more dependent upon guidance from the physician. Actually, it has been said by no less an authority than the American Medical Association that if every person consulted a physician for every sneeze, sniffle, cut, cough, or other minor discomfort, doctors would be unable to cope with the overwhelming tide of complaints and effective medical care probably would cease to exist. Thus, a little do-it-yourself diagnosis, if done properly, can benefit both the patient and the doctor.

Taking the Pulse

It is easy to learn how to perform some basic diagnostic procedures. Perhaps one of the most simple of the tests is that of taking a person's pulse. The only equipment required is a rather accurate watch with a second hand. In fact, the pocket watch that counts seconds as well as minutes and hours was originally a medical instrument. After it was invented by an English physician named John Flory, in the early 18th century, a watch with a second hand was called a "physician's pulse watch."

Before the invention of the "pulse watch," doctors sometimes carried tiny glasses of sand, like egg timers or hour glasses, but calibrated to measure the flow of sand by the minute. If a doctor did not have a minute glass, he would estimate the pulse rate against the ticks of a pendulum clock. Neither method was satisfactorily accurate or convenient. Most children today have better equipment for measuring a pulse than did some prominent doctors of the 18th century.

There are several points on the body where the pulse can be detected easily. The results are likely to be the same at any of the points where an artery is close enough to the surface to show a pulse beat, since all the arteries pulsate at the same rate as the heartbeat. The most common site for counting the pulse rate is the point where the wrist and forearm are joined, on the thumb side. Here the radial artery not only lies close to the surface, but it lies against a bone so that it can be easily palpated with gentle finger pressure.

Other points where the pulse is relatively easy to find include the tibial artery, on the inner side of the ankle; the temporal artery, in the temple area of the head; and the facial artery, on the lower jaw. The pulse sometimes can be seen in the carotid artery, running from the neck and over the edge of the jaw, but it should not be used as a routine pulse-counting site because pressure on that artery can have adverse effects.

When the radial artery in the wrist is palpated, or pressed gently, the pulse may be felt as a tap or throb that occurs at regular intervals. The throb is caused by a wave action produced by a contraction of the left ventricle of the heart. It is not, as commonly believed, caused by a surge of blood rushing through the artery. The wave action is something like a shock from a pounding action, transmitted along the artery.

The pulsations can be counted for 60 seconds, or counted for 30 seconds if the number is multiplied by two, to give a count of pulses per minute. Any number less than 60 per minute may be regarded as a slow pulse rate; an abnormally fast pulse is represented by a count of more than 100 beats per minute if the person is sitting or lying quietly while the pulse is counted.

The normal pulse rate of a small child is much higher than for an adult. During the first year of a baby's life, the infant may have a pulse rate of as much as 140 to 170 beats per minute without being ill. The pulse rate for an infant also may be as slow as 70 or 80 beats per minute. The child's pulse gradually slows after the first year, and by the age of four years it may average between 70 and 115 beats per minute.

For a normal adult the usual pulse rate when the person is resting is around 70 per minute. The pulse rate in trained athletes frequently is slower, perhaps 60 or 65 pulsations per minute. The reason usually is that the heart of a person in top physical condition is likely to be more efficient and produces a greater volume of blood for each contraction.

Emotional excitement, strenuous physical activity, and diseases accompanied by fever are common factors causing above-normal pulse rates. After strenuous exercise the pulse rate of a normal adult may rise to 170 or more beats per minute. An abnormally high pulse rate in the absence of fever, exercise, or emotional upset can be a sign of hemorrhage and shock. An abnormally slow pulse rate may be a sign of heart block.

When a physician takes your pulse, he does more than count the rate of pulsations per minute. He also may make mental notes about whether the pulse of a patient seems hard or soft. In certain patients he may note an abnormal pulse rhythm—for example, two pulsations followed by a pause, or three pulse beats followed by a pause, before the next set of pulsations. The wave of pulsations may appear as slow or rapid with respect to each beat rather than the rate per minute. Or the pulses may alternate: a large volume pulse followed by a small volume pulsation, then another large pulse, and so on. The pulses in some persons may vary in volume and speed depending upon whether one is inhaling or exhaling.

The variations in volume, strength, and other pulse factors are not what the layperson might notice while taking his own or another person's pulse without having a bit of experience in taking pulses. A doctor, however, would be aware of such differences because of his years of training and experience in comparing the pulses of perhaps thousands of persons, both healthy and sick.

Sphygmomanometer for Measuring Blood Pressure

A medical instrument that more recently has moved from the office of the doctor to the home of the layperson is the sphygmomanometer, the device commonly used to measure blood pressure. A sphygmomanometer needs four separate pieces of equipment to produce meaningful information for either the doctor or the patient:

a pressure cuff, an air bulb with hose, a stethoscope, and an instrument that translates the blood pressure information into an easily read set of numbers. All of the separate pieces of equipment must be in good working order and properly coordinated to yield useful blood pressure information.

The pressure cuff is a sort of folded fabric bag that fastens around the arm above the elbow. The bag is rubberized or otherwise fashioned to be airtight. It should be the correct size for the arm to be used; a cuff that is too large for a small arm, like that of a child's, or too small for an obese person can be responsible for misleading

THE SPHYGMOMANOMETER

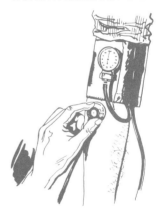

When using a sphygmomanometer, the bell, or microphone-like part of the stethoscope, should be placed over the point on the arm where a pulse can be detected. Usually, nothing will be heard until the pressure cuff around the upper arm has been inflated above 200 (millimeters of mercury) on the instrument gauge. Continue inflating the cuff until the sound of blood pulsing through the artery in the arm can be heard no more. While watching the gauge carefully, release the air in the cuff slowly. The reading on the gauge at the instant the first thump of blood pulsation is heard should be recorded as the systolic blood pressure. When the last thump is heard as air continues to be released from the pressure cuff, the reading should be noted as the diastolic blood pressure.

information about one's blood pressure, causing readings to be as much as ten points too high or too low.

The air bulb and hose attach to the pressure cuff. The bulb has a valve that can be opened or closed to control the amount of pressure resulting from air that is pumped into the cuff when the bulb is squeezed repeatedly.

The traditional instrument for translating the blood pressure information has been a column of mercury with numbers along the side, much like the numbers along the side of an outdoor thermometer. Recently, spring dial gauge instruments and devices that display blood pressure readings on small electronic screens have become available.

All sphygmomanometers made for home use work in the same general manner. The pressure cuff is wrapped around an arm of the person to be tested and is inflated by use of the air bulb. Blood pressure is indicated on the dial, electronic readout, or alongside the column of mercury, which is connected to the pressure cuff by a small rubber hose.

The fourth part of the equipment for reading blood pressure is the stethoscope, the proper use of which can be quite critical in obtaining accurate readings. The stethoscopes used today have earpieces that should fit snugly but comfortably, and rubber tubing that runs from the ear pieces to a Y-shaped connector that is attached to a diaphragm or bell-shaped chest piece. The latter term may be a bit of a misnomer when the instrument is to be used for checking blood pressure, but historically the stethoscope was developed for listening to chest sounds. In fact, its name is derived from the Greek word *stethos*, for chest.

The word "sphygmomanometer" is de-

rived from an old Greek word, *sphygmos*, meaning "to stop the pulse," plus "manometer," for pressure gauge. This is essentially how a sphygmomanometer is used to measure blood pressure: by stopping the pulse. The purpose of the stethoscope is to help the doctor, nurse, or other person checking an individual's blood pressure to hear the pulse while it is being stopped, and started again, by controlling the pressure cuff.

When the airtight pressure cuff has been fastened about the arm and inflated, it has the effect of a tourniquet that would be used in a real emergency to prevent a fatal loss of blood by stopping the flow in a major artery. A sphygmomanometer does not directly restrict the flow of blood like a conventional tourniquet, but it applies air pressure in the rubberized cuff to restrict indirectly the flow of blood in the artery being used to check blood pressure. The amount of air pressure in the cuff that is required to hold back the flow of blood in the artery is translated through the sphygmomanometer into blood pressure measured in millimeters of mercury on the scale beside the glass tube, or its equivalent on a spring dial gauge or electronic digital readout.

The diaphragm of the stethoscope is placed over the artery between the pressure cuff and the bend of the elbow, on the inside of the elbow joint, and the air pressure in the cuff is pumped quickly to a reading that is 20 or 30 millimeters above the point where the last pulse sounds are heard. At that point the pulse presumably has been stopped. Then the valve on the air bulb is loosened slightly so that the air from the cuff is released slowly. The procedure must be followed rapidly and carefully because interrupting the blood flow in the artery with a pressure cuff can be both painful and dangerous for the patient.

As the reading on the pressure gauge drops at a rate of about two or three points, or millimeters, per second, a dull thumping sound will begin when blood once again starts surging through the artery. The point on the manometer, or pressure gauge, where the pulse sounds first appear, should be recorded as the systolic blood pressure, which is produced by the contraction of the left ventricle of the heart. The pressure recorded at a particular point along the route of the systemic, or general body, circulatory system may be modified by various factors along the route. Blood pressure measured on the right arm, for example, often is different from blood pressure measured on the left arm. The facts and figures of blood pressure variations usually are evaluated by an examining physician in making a diagnosis that involves a patient's circulatory system.

As the pressure cuff is further deflated, at about the same rate of two or three millimeters of pressure per second, following location of the systolic blood pressure level, the person listening with the stethoscope will observe a point where the sounds of blood pulsation disappear. At that point the pressure gauge measures the diastolic pressure, the pressure of blood flow when the heart is relaxing briefly between contractions. At readings lower than that the blood flow is no longer restricted, and the pulse sounds heard while the pressure cuff was partly inflated will not be detected.

The sounds of blood pulsating through the artery may be called Korotkoff sounds, named for the Russian doctor who discovered that a stethoscope could be used for studying body sounds in areas beyond the chest. There are electronic sphygmomanometers that do not require the use of a stethoscope because they have sensors that detect the Korotkoff sounds and translate the information directly into systolic and diastolic blood pressure readings.

Blood pressure readings usually are recorded as the systolic number, followed by a diagonal line separating it from the figure for the diastolic reading. For example, if your own blood pressure happened to be 140 systolic and 90 diastolic, the doctor would write it on your records as "140/90," and he would verbally express the data as "140 over 90."

The systolic and diastolic readings represent the maximum and minimum ranges of blood pressure in the artery at the time the measurements were made. The systolic is the maximum pressure exerted by the contraction of the heart muscle; the diastolic is the minimum level of pressure between contractions.

Blood pressures of between 110/60 and 140/90 are considered in the normal range. But a single blood pressure measurement is only one small piece of the picture of a person's true average blood pressure. Blood pressures vary with the patient's age, sex, weight, emotional state, and other individual factors. A younger person is likely to have a lower range of blood pressures than an older individual. Blood pressures of women before menopause may be as much as ten points lower than of men of the same age, but after menopause there often is very little difference. Readings may be different in the morning than in the evening. After a meal, systolic pressures may be higher, and diastolic pressures may be lower.

Doctors who suspect a blood pressure

abnormality in a patient may take a series of readings over a period of several weeks and evaluate the pattern, if any, in the different readings. Readings that are consistently above 140/90 for a young person, or higher than 160/95 for an older individual, could be signs of hypertension.

A person who is not a member of the medical profession may need some professional advice in selecting a sphygmomanometer. Since some doctors encourage the practice of laypersons taking blood pressures at home, they will offer suggestions about buying a sphygmomanometer and in some instances may give brief instructions on its use.

Generally, the mercury column devices are most likely to give accurate readings. Gauges with a spring dial tend to lose their accuracy gradually over a period of five to ten years, so they should be checked at least once a year against a mercury column sphygmomanometer. The accuracy of battery-powered electronic blood pressure instruments usually depends upon the condition of the batteries.

Mercury column sphygmomanometers should be inspected and checked periodically to make sure of their accuracy. Their vulnerable areas are usually associated with places where air might leak and result in false readings. The rubber tubing, for example, may deteriorate and crack, or the fittings may not be secure. One way to test the integrity of the air supply routes of a sphygmomanometer is to fasten the pressure cuff—without an arm inside—and inflate it until a high reading on the pressure gauge is reached. Then close the valve tightly on the air bulb and watch the reading on the pressure gauge. If the fittings are secure and there are no leaks in other parts of the system, the reading on the pressure gauge should hold steady.

If the readings fall slowly, it can be assumed that there is a leak in the system.

Stethoscope

Stethoscopes also should be examined at regular intervals. Although the stethoscope is a relatively simple and durable piece of equipment, the diaphragm and rubber tubing can deteriorate and crack. The rubber tubing should be of the correct length, not only for the convenience of the user, but because the tubing length can affect the quality of the sounds detected with the device. The ear pieces should be fitted so that the openings are aimed at the eardrums.

While most of the inexpensive sphygmo-

USING A STETHOSCOPE

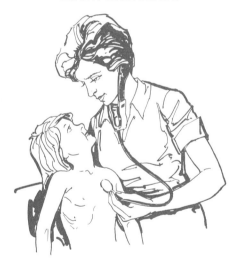

Parents can learn to use stethoscopes and sphygmomanometers so that the health of children and other family members can be monitored. Many doctors encourage their patients to learn how to check their own blood pressure, which requires both a stethoscope and sphygmomanometer, or blood pressure gauge. However, equipment should be checked occasionally for inaccuracy due to leaks in rubber tubing, faulty valve screw, or size of pressure cuff for patient's arm.

manometers available to laypersons come packaged with a stethoscope, the buyer should be aware that apparently minor differences in the design and construction of the devices can alter their effectiveness. For that reason, many doctors and other health professionals prefer to select a stethoscope that is, in effect, tailored to their personal satisfaction. "Tailored" is the appropriate word in this instance because a tall person with a short stethoscope might find it awkward to use the device.

Clinical or Fever Thermometers

Fever thermometers of the traditional design, a small glass tube filled with mercury, are found in most homes. But newer devices spawned by space-age technology are also available for home use, and in some instances they may prove to be more convenient, particularly in households with small children. The newer types of fever thermometers measure body temperatures with electronic thermistors or liquid crystals imbedded in plastic tape strips.

A thermistor is a device that measures temperature changes through variations in electrical resistance of different metals. An electronic thermometer may utilize the thermistor principle to measure body temperature and produce a direct digital readout. The sensor for such a device is enclosed in a small plastic tip attached to a wire leading to the battery-powered unit that shows the body temperature either in Fahrenheit or Celsius degrees, or both. The plastic-covered thermistor can be inserted in the mouth, rectum, or armpit to sense body temperature. The battery used to power the electronic thermometer is a nine-volt transistor radio battery.

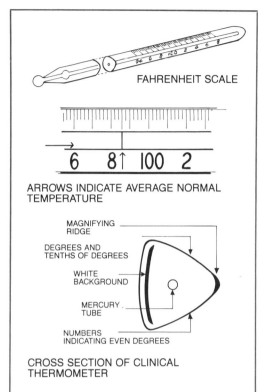

FAHRENHEIT SCALE

ARROWS INDICATE AVERAGE NORMAL TEMPERATURE

MAGNIFYING RIDGE

DEGREES AND TENTHS OF DEGREES

WHITE BACKGROUND

MERCURY TUBE

NUMBERS INDICATING EVEN DEGREES

CROSS SECTION OF CLINICAL THERMOMETER

Reading a fever thermometer is easy once you learn how to do it. Thermometers are designed like long, thin magnifying glasses so they can be read accurately by viewing the numbers along the magnifying ridge. A light background on the opposite side provides a visual contrast so that numbers and mercury level are easily visible. Illustration shows average normal body temperature in Fahrenheit scale, which would be 98.6 degrees by mouth and about one degree higher when taken with a rectal fever thermometer. On a Celsius scale fever thermometer, an average normal human body temperature would be approximately 37 degrees.

Besides being easier to read than an old-fashioned mercury fever thermometer, the electronic thermistor device has an advantage in a family with children in that the patient is not exposed to the risk of breaking the glass with his teeth and swallowing the mercury contents.

The liquid crystal thermometer consists simply of a small strip of plastic in which liquid crystals, sensitive to temperature changes of one degree Celsius, are encapsulated. Some liquid crystal strips change colors—say, from red to blue—as temperatures rise. The basic liquid crystal fever indicator, placed on the skin of the patient, will display a letter "N" for normal or "F" for fever.

The liquid crystal fever indicator strips are not as precisely accurate as the old-fashioned mercury thermometers that are still used by most doctors and hospital nurses. The mercury fever thermometer usually is calibrated to read a range of temperatures between 94 degrees and 110 degrees Fahrenheit, or from 33 to 44 degrees Celsius. Markings on the glass tube indicate temperature changes of as little as 2/10ths of a degree. An additional line often is engraved at the point considered to be normal human body temperature, that is, 98.6 degrees Fahrenheit or 37 degrees Celsius.

Normal body temperatures actually vary about one degree on either side of 98.6 degrees Fahrenheit during the day. In fact, some healthy individuals seldom have a temperature of 98.6 degrees except when they are ill; their own normal temperature is a bit higher or lower than the standard figure.

Rectal or oral temperature readings are considered the most accurate and consistent indicators of fevers or other health changes that result in alterations of body heat. Skin temperatures can be very misleading since layers of fat or blood circulation patterns can account for variations of as much as ten degrees below what is considered to be normal.

Fever is a symptom or sign of a disorder, and there is no simple yardstick for determining whether an increase in an individual's body temperature constitutes a fever. For a person who is confined to bed because of illness or injury, any oral temperature above 98.6 degrees Fahrenheit might be considered a fever. In other instances, a fever might be considered as a body temperature above 100 degrees Fahrenheit. For people whose normal body temperature is something other than 98.6 degrees, an increase of two degrees Fahrenheit above their usual body temperature is a fever. Age also is a factor; infants and small children often show body temperatures that for an adult would be considered feverish.

Most fever thermometers manufactured for home and professional use are designed for easy reading, although a person who does not understand the design may be a bit baffled during a first attempt to find the mercury column. A cross-section of a mercury fever thermometer could be said to resemble a slice of a pie. It is rounded on one side and has two sides that are flat and taper toward a narrow edge opposite the round side. The purpose of this design is to shape the glass tube containing the mercury column like a long narrow magnifying glass so that the numbers appear enlarged when viewed from one side. Also, there usually is a reflective surface painted behind the mercury column to help the user locate the nearest fractional degree line at the top of the column of mercury.

Otoscope for Checking Ear Canal

Families with small children sometimes find an otoscope an asset in checking the condition of their ears. An otoscope is a device about the size of a pocket flashlight that consists of a battery-powered light, a lens, and a speculum. When the speculum is inserted into the external ear canal, which leads to the outer surface of the eardrum, the light illuminates the walls of the canal and the lens magnifies the image so that the viewer can observe any signs of irritation, accumulation of cerumen (earwax), or any foreign object that might be lodged in the ear canal.

In a normal, healthy external ear, the viewer will see smooth pinkish walls along the inside of the fleshy tube, and at its end a white disc, the eardrum. Any accumulation of earwax will appear as a yellow to brown colored mass in the ear canal.

The otoscope, like any medical equipment used at home, must be handled with care. The instrument must be inserted into the ear canal very slowly and cautiously in the event there is a foreign object or painful accumulation of earwax that could be pushed against the eardrum. The external ear should be held back gently to help provide a straight and direct pathway into the ear canal.

When working with a small child, a second adult may be needed to hold the child's head steady. If the child struggles, the otoscope could injure the ear canal or eardrum.

Obviously, the parent should consult the family doctor about any signs of disease or foreign bodies observed in the ear canal, just as the doctor would be consulted about an apparently abnormal pulse, blood pressure, or body temperature.

Keeping Records and Accurate Measures

When checking temperatures, pulses, and blood pressures of patients, keep a pencil and pad of paper handy so you can jot down the numbers. Don't rely on your memory when giving the doctor the data you have collected. When possible, use the same system of units as the doctor in keeping health records, such as pulse rate per minute, blood pressure in terms of systolic/diastolic, temperature in degrees and fractions of degrees Fahrenheit or Celsius, and so on.

If the doctor recommends a liquid medication, make sure you have handy in your household armamentarium the accurate measures for teaspoons, tablespoons, or metric measures. Remember that all teaspoons are not alike; some tableware teaspoons are five times as large as the smallest teaspoons, and a true teaspoon measure is somewhere near the middle, or about five milliliters in size. A medication taken from a two- or ten-milliliter teaspoon would not be what the doctor ordered.

QUESTIONS AND ANSWERS
HEALTH MONITORING EQUIPMENT

Q: *Is there any particular advantage in using a special fever thermometer to measure a child's temperature?*
A: Several, in fact. One is that the fever thermometer, which also is known as a clinical thermometer, is made so that the mercury shows the highest temperature registered until it is shaken down. An ordinary thermometer would fluctuate in readings, and by the time you took it out of a child's mouth to examine the reading it would not give a true reading but probably would have dropped a couple of degrees or more. Also, a clinical thermometer, by spreading a range of about 20 degrees over the entire column, allows much better accuracy in indicating changes of less than one degree Fahrenheit.

Q: *Can you use any fever thermometer in either the mouth or the rectum?*
A: The rectal thermometer is intended primarily for small children, or unconscious or delirious patients, and is different in design. It has a stubby bulb at the end. A rectal thermometer, of course, should be lubricated with petroleum jelly, cold cream, or some other nonirritating lubricant before it is inserted into the rectum. When retrieved, after a period of about three minutes, the reading probably will be about one degree Fahrenheit higher than the temperature that would be taken by mouth in the same patient.

Q: *Is it O.K. to clean a fever thermometer in hot water after it has been used?*
A: No. It should be cleaned with soap and cold water, and rinsed under cool running water. Putting a clinical thermometer in hot water, or even storing it close to a heat source, can ruin it.

One other point about the care of fever thermometers: always shake down the thermometer before and after using it. To shake down a thermometer, point it toward the floor and shake it vigorously a few times to make sure the mercury drops below 95 degrees on a Fahrenheit scale, or about 35 degrees on a Celsius thermometer. Since the mercury otherwise remains at the highest temperature registered, it could give a false reading the next time it is used.

Q: *Will an oral temperature reading be accurate if you have been eating or drinking something hot?*
A: Any hot or cold food or beverage in the mouth will cause the fever thermometer to give a false reading. Always wait at least 15 minutes after food or beverage has been consumed before taking an oral temperature.

Q: *Does it make any real difference in the pulse reading if the patient is sitting or lying down?*
A: For ordinary home monitoring of a patient's health it doesn't matter. Body positions might be important factors in checking the circulation of a patient suspected of having an abnormality or health problem, but the effect wouldn't alter the wrist pulse significantly.

Q: *Is there any particular way the pulse should be checked?*
A: There is one way that is better than other possible methods. That is to place the tips of the first three fingers lightly on the artery that can be felt on the inside of the patient's wrist, just below the thumb. The forefinger should be placed between the tendons and the wrist bone. The patient should be in a comfortable position, and his wrist should be held so the thumb is up. The person checking the pulse should not use his or her own thumb in feeling for the patient's pulse. There is a pulse in the thumb it-

self that might distort the feel of the patient's pulse.

Q: *Is it safe for an ordinary person to use an otoscope?*

A: A layperson must be very careful about using this piece of equipment for examining the ear canal. And most doctors would advise against use of the equipment by any untrained person, even though you don't have to be a licensed physician to purchase one.

One hazard is that the patient, particularly a child, might move his head and the instrument could then damage the ear canal or the eardrum. When doctors examine the ear canal of a child, a parent usually is asked to hold the child and his head still. Also, the doctor learns through his training how to hold the otoscope so that if the child's head moves the otoscope moves with it.

A doctor's otoscope usually is equipped with different sizes of specula, designed to fit different sizes of ear canals. A layperson may try to examine ear canals of different sizes with a single-size speculum, which usually would not be life-threatening but could result in damage to the ear.

Q: *I have read that blood pressure cuffs need to be the right size for the patient's arm in order to give an accurate reading. Are there cuffs small enough for checking the blood pressure of children?*

A: As a matter of fact, yes. There are special pediatric blood pressure cuffs that can be attached to a sphygmomanometer.

Q: *Is there a special position for the patient's arm to be held when his blood pressure is checked?*

A: For an accurate reading, the patient's forearm should rest on a flat, level surface, with the elbow nearly straight and the palm facing upward. Then find the pulse inside the elbow by palpating the skin with your finger. When you find the pulse, you will know where to place the bell of the stethoscope before inflating the cuff.

9

HOME HEALTH CARE

Nearly everyone can expect to spend at least one period of home confinement because of illness or injury. In one recent year, according to a study by the U. S. Public Health Service, more than 22 percent of the population received home health care that was serious enough to warrant direct or indirect supervision by a physician or other health professional such as a member of the Visiting Nurses Association. During the same typical year, many millions of persons were treated at home for various infections and minor injuries that were serious enough to disrupt work or school routines, although not serious enough to require professional medical care. In the same year, more than 35 million Americans were discharged from hospitals, and most required at least a short period of convalescence at home before returning to normal daily activities.

There are certain obvious advantages to home care for persons whose health needs do not require the immediate availability of the staff and facilities offered by a modern hospital. One advantage is the financial one; hospital care can be fairly expensive, even when essential costs are covered by insurance policies. Another is that many individuals seem to recover from illness or injury more rapidly when in their own home. Hospital routines may be efficient and wholesome, but they are not necessarily comforting for the patient.

The extent of home care required for a person who is chronically ill or is convalescing from surgery or injury should determine your plans for equipping or staffing a room or portion of a room in the home for the purpose of giving the patient the nursing care needed to speed recovery. The mother, wife, or other member of the family should not be expected to provide around-the-clock nursing care for the patient in addition to other household responsibilities. It may be more feasible to hire a licensed practical nurse or other trained professionals to help care for the patient.

Always consult the physician who directed the care of the patient before and during the hospital stay regarding the type of home care that should be provided. It's a good idea to ask the doctor about

TAKING THE PULSE

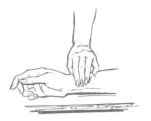

The patient's pulse and temperature should be taken at least once a day and the information recorded along with the time in the event it is requested by the patient's doctor. A most convenient place for checking the pulse of most patients is at a point just above the wrist and on the thumb side. Use the fingertips to feel the pulsations of blood being thrust through the artery beneath the skin. It may be necessary to press the artery against an underlying bone in order to make the pulse felt.

specific recommendations relating to diets, medications, the amount of activity that should be permitted, and so on.

For most ill or convalescent patients, only a relatively few inexpensive items may be needed to make home health care easier for both the patient and the members of the family providing temporary nursing care. A small intercom system that requires no special wiring because it operates on wiring already in the house, for example, can be installed to permit the patient to communicate with other individuals in the kitchen, living or dining areas, or elsewhere in the home. A bedside telephone also could be provided at small cost if it is not already available. The home care patient usually feels more secure when family members or friends are only an intercom call or telephone call away. The bedside telephone also may allow a home-bound patient to summon assistance in the event of an emergency when family members who ordinarily provide care are not at home.

Danger Signals for Alerting the Doctor

Ordinarily, a patient who is able to manage well enough to be discharged from a hospital may not require continuous care. But the home nurse should be alert for conditions that could signal the need for consulting the doctor. For example, a significant change in the patient's appetite, which might be either a complete loss of interest in food or a sudden excessive hunger or thirst, should be brought to the attention of the patient's physician.

Another signal might be mental changes, such as temporary blackouts, excitability or excessive talking, crying spells, or destructive acts.

Nausea or vomiting not due to dietary indiscretions or food sensitivities can be a danger sign. Severe forms of vomiting can indicate a disorder of internal organs or the brain. Vomiting that is particularly forceful or projectile-type vomiting can be a sign of a medical emergency. Even mild vomiting that persists or occurs frequently should be brought to the doctor's attention.

Bleeding, of course, should be a major cause for concern. Bleeding that is marked by spurts of blood is a sign of a broken artery and is a true emergency. However, bleeding in which blood flows slowly for more than five minutes also can be a symptom of a serious disorder and should not be ignored simply because the blood does not appear to come from a severed artery. Signs of blood in the urine or feces indicate possible internal bleeding; blood from the upper digestive tract gives the feces a black, tarry appearance, rather than the reddish stain associated with bleeding from the lower digestive tract. Unusual menstrual bleeding should be noted for the doctor's assessment: this includes prolonged or heavy bleeding, and loss of blood between menstrual periods or after menopause.

Blood in the patient's sputum should be brought to the attention of the doctor. Blood that is coughed up by a patient could come from several different possible sources because of the various common pathways between the top of the nasal cavity and the trachea and esophagus.

Bowel changes are another key sign of possible problems that should be reported to the physician. Since almost everyone experiences occasional variations in bowel movements, such changes may not be a cause for alarm. But the doctor probably would like to know about changes that include persistent diarrhea or constipation, or diarrhea that alternates with constipation, or feces that are black and tarry, or pale, and fatty or watery.

Urinary changes that should be noted by the person in charge of home nursing care include significantly increased amounts of urine, increased frequency of urges to urinate, a sudden need to urinate during normal sleep periods, pain or discomfort associated with urination, and production of urine that is bloody, smoky, or otherwise strangely discolored.

Muscle symptoms, including spasms, twitching, unexplained stiffness, cramps, or weakness, may be signs of nervous system disorders as well as of muscle disease. Some muscle symptoms may be due to a patient sitting or lying in one position too long; they may be relieved simply by a change of body position. However, any signs of stumbling, trembling, fumbling, tripping, dropping things, or inability to coordinate hands or feet in a normal manner could indicate something more serious is involved.

Unusual swellings, lumps, and sores that have not been noted by the doctor since the start of a period of home health care should be discussed with him. Severe pains, fever, hoarseness, headaches, digestive disturbances, dizzy spells, and numbness, tingling, or loss of sensation are other signs and symptoms of problems that could be beyond the ability of an ordinary home nurse to handle.

Beware of Home Remedies and Unauthorized Medications

Home remedies or over-the-counter medicines should not be given a person recovering from a serious illness or injury without first consulting the doctor. The nonprescription remedies might interfere with the effectiveness of drugs prescribed by the doctor. Another reason to be cautious about administering home remedies or O-T-C products without first asking the doctor is that the symptoms to be treated might mark the onset of a serious complication, and proper treatment could be delayed by the use of ineffective medications. In some cases, a home remedy or O-T-C medication may be given the go-ahead by the physician, who may recommend the size and frequency of the dose, and request that the doctor receive a report on whether or not the nonprescription remedy relieved the symptoms.

Selecting and Equipping the Sickroom

If the home care patient is likely to be confined to bed for a long period of time, a well-planned sickroom arrangement will save a lot of wear and tear and time for both the patient and the person or persons who will care for the patient. Ideally, the patient should be located in a room that is close to a bathroom and within easy access to the kitchen and other areas of the house. If these rooms are on the same floor, stair climbing can be avoided.

Patients who can get out of bed to use the bathroom or move to other areas of the home should have a low bed that is easy to get into and out of with perhaps the help of a small stool. A patient who is unable to leave the bed often but needs quite a bit of bedside care should have a high bed that permits the home nurse to attend to the patient without a lot of unnecessary bending and stooping. If the bedbound patient needs to be lifted occasionally, a high bed makes it more convenient for the home nurse to handle such tasks. A hospital-type bed with railings that can be lowered or raised as needed will satisfy the needs of a seriously ill or disabled person.

The mattress for the bed should be smooth and firm, and in many cases reinforced with a bed board or a sheet of heavy plywood cut to fit the bed area. The mattress should be covered with plastic or rubberized sheeting if it is necessary to protect the surface. Protective pads also can be used under the bottom sheet.

The bottom sheet should be kept smooth and clean. Wrinkles and food debris may contribute to the development of bed sores or skin irritations. If possible, the sheets should be changed daily. Fitted sheets that have strips of elastic sewn into the contoured corners may prove more comfortable for the patient than standard flat sheets. The contoured sheets are less likely to pull loose from the mattress corners and develop wrinkles when the patient changes positions in the bed. If a waterproof sheet is used and the patient complains that it results in discomfort, try placing the waterproof sheet under the

mattress pad to reduce the amount of reflected body heat.

Precautions for the Home Nurse

Before and after changing sheets, or otherwise caring for the home-bound patient, the person who serves as nurse should wash the hands carefully. Both patient and nurse can be more vulnerable than usual to infectious agents when the resistance of the patient is lowered by illness or injury. Therefore, the home nurse should try to keep the hands, including the fingernails, as clean as possible, using warm running water and lots of soap lather. If the hands that nurse the patient tend to become chapped as a result of all the hand washing, they should be given whatever special care is needed with creams and lotions.

Drying the hands well after each washing, with paper or cloth towels, will help prevent chapping. Soiled paper towels should be discarded, and cloth towels placed in a special receptacle for laundering.

The wash basin or sink used for hand washing should be rinsed to make sure that any contaminated water has been washed away. The bar of soap used should

GIVING LIQUIDS TO A HELPLESS PATIENT

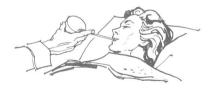

Water and other fluids can be given a helpless patient by inserting a glass or plastic tube into a drinking glass so the patient can sip the beverage through the straw.

be rinsed so it will be clean for the next use.

The home nurse should wear some kind of protective apron while in contact with a sick person. The apron should be large enough to cover any part of the nurse's clothing that might touch the patient or the bedding. The coverall apron could be a pinafore dress or an oversize man's shirt that can be slipped on backwards; that is, it can be worn with the front side on the back and vice versa. The apron should be kept in or close to the sickroom; an ideal location is a hanger attached to the door of the sickroom.

How to Bathe the Patient

When the patient needs to be bathed, which may be daily—except for elderly sick persons who are particularly sensitive to loss of natural body oils during bathing—the bath can be done efficiently while the patient is lying in bed. But the procedure requires a bit of advance planning and organizing the supplies to be used.

The nurse should arrange to have a cotton blanket, two large bath towels and one face towel, a washcloth, a basin of warm water, an extra supply of hot water nearby, and soap. The cotton blanket is used as a temporary substitute for the regular heavier blanket, which should be removed during the bathing process. One large bath towel is placed on top of the cotton blanket and tucked around the shoulders and under the chin of the patient, like a large bib. The second bath towel is placed under the patient's head. The bath towels help to prevent the patient's bed linens from becoming damp as a result of the bath.

The washcloth is moistened with warm

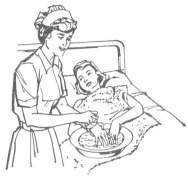

SOAP, WASH, RINSE

The home care patient can be bathed regularly in bed, using a basin of warm water, soap, and a wash cloth which can be carried to the bedside. The patient should be protected by a series of bath towels which can be placed over exposed areas of the body and the sheets and blankets. Bathing should begin with the face and head areas and progress down the body. The soapy water should be discarded and replaced at regular intervals during the bathing procedure.

water, then wrung out to prevent dripping. It can then be folded like a mitt around the nurse's hand to apply warm water and soap to the patient's skin. The extra container of hot water can be used to change the water in the basin when it becomes dirty or soapy.

Washing the patient's face, beginning in the area of the eyes and forehead, should be done with gentle outward curving motions. The washing strokes should move from the areas of the nose and mouth toward the edges of the face, rather than toward the nose and mouth. After the soap and warm water have been applied in washing, the same surfaces should be rinsed. Finally, the face areas should be dried with the face towel.

The rest of the bathing procedure should move downward to the chest and abdomen, followed by the arms and hands, and after that, the legs and feet. When bathing the chest and abdomen, the large bath towel that was under the patient's head at the beginning can be moved down to the chest, then placed under the arm or leg that is being bathed. The cotton blanket and bath towel that originally covered the chest can be moved downward as the bathing continues in that direction.

The back of the body, from the neck to the buttocks, can be bathed after the patient has been turned on the side so that the back is to the nurse's side of the bed. While washing the back, the nurse should check the skin surfaces for signs of irritation or bed sores. After bathing, the back should be rubbed to stimulate blood circulation in muscles that have been under constant body pressure. A skin lotion or hand cream can be applied to the skin. Sometimes the back rub can be applied more easily if the patient lies on his stomach. If for some reason this is not feasible, the back rub can be managed with the patient in the same position used for bathing the back—that is, with the patient lying on his or her side.

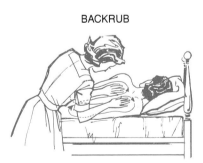

BACKRUB

After bathing, a patient should be given a backrub. Rubbing alcohol, cocoa butter, or similar skin refreshing substances can be applied. The nurse's hands should be placed flat against the skin and rubbing should follow a circular pattern, using firm kneading strokes.

The external genitalia should be bathed last. If the patient is able and prefers to handle that part of the bathing process himself, the wash basin of warm water, soap, and a towel can be placed within easy reach. A bath towel should be provided to protect the bed in the area under the buttocks.

While bathing the patient, any body areas that are not exposed for washing should be covered with the cotton blanket and/or the large bath towels to prevent chilling.

The hair and the fingernails and toenails may need special care as part of the daily bathing routine. The patient may be able to comb and brush his or her own hair. Otherwise, the nurse should provide this additional measure of personal hygiene. If the nails are tough and cannot be trimmed easily, let the fingers or toes soak in warm water for a few minutes.

Any unusual signs of health concern such as red spots on the skin or abnormally thickened nails should be brought to the attention of the doctor.

How to Change the Bed Linen

The home nurse may find the bathing period the most convenient time to change or adjust the bed linen. The fresh linen can be organized before the start of the bathing process so that it will be easily available for making a quick change.

A laundry bag or newspapers should be used to collect the soiled linen. The newspapers can be spread on the floor beside the bed to receive the used bed linen and the washcloth and towels used for bathing as well. The pillowcases, blankets, mattress pad, sheets, and other bedding materials should be removed carefully and kept away from contact with the nurse's face and clothing. To reduce the chances of contact with the soiled surface of a pillowcase, it can be removed by turning it inside out while pulling the case away from the pillow.

Similar procedures should be followed in placing fresh linen on the bed. For example, a fresh pillowcase can be turned inside out. Then, with the hands inserted through the length of the inverted pillowcase and with the end seam grasped with the fingers, the pillowcase can be pushed over the end of the pillow. After the case has started to cover the pillow, the hands can be slipped out of the pillowcase and the corners pulled down to complete covering the pillow. Whenever possible, the nurse should avoid direct contact with materials used by the patient because of the risk of disease organisms being transmitted from one individual to the other. Since the nurse usually has contact with individuals outside the home, infections could be brought into the sickroom at a time when the patient is especially vulnerable as a result of his or her weakened condition.

When the patient cannot leave the bed because of his illness or injury, the bed linen must be changed while the patient is in bed. This can be accomplished by working from the head to the foot of the bed, loosening all the bedding at the sides so it can be removed with less effort. If there is a bedspread, it can be removed first and folded neatly. The blanket under the spread can be kept in place while the top sheet is removed. If the patient is unable to hold the top edge of the blanket while the top sheet is carefully pulled toward the bottom and out from under the blanket, the blanket usually can be tucked under the shoulders of the patient to hold it in place.

If possible, the pillows should be re-moved and the pillowcases placed with the other soiled linen in the laundry bag or on the newspapers spread on the floor.

The most difficult part of changing bed linen while the patient is in bed is that of changing the bottom sheet. This can be managed by having the patient roll onto one side while the bottom sheet is gathered lengthwise and pushed next to the patient's back. The clean bottom sheet is then placed lengthwise and folded alongside the soiled sheet, and the outer edges of the clean sheet are tucked or fitted under the mattress, after the mattress pad has been smoothed to remove any wrinkles.

HOME CARE—BED MAKING

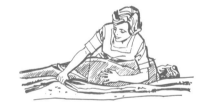

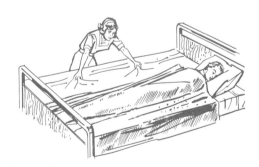

It is not difficult to change sheets on a patient's bed if the sheets are changed while the patient is rolled on his side to one edge of the bed. The unoccupied side of the bed is made, then the patient is rolled back onto that side while changes are made on the other side. If patient is able to help, he can hold edge of blanket while soiled sheets are pulled out the bottom edge of the bed.

The patient next is moved onto the part of the bed covered with the clean sheet. The soiled bottom sheet can then be removed from the bed, and the new bottom sheet can be spread over the mattress pad. Finally, the patient can be allowed to roll onto his back with the clean bottom sheet in place. The top sheet can be replaced while the blanket is removed briefly; to prevent chilling, the patient usually can be kept covered with the blanket during most of the sheet changing routine.

Blankets or other top coverings should be used as the climate of the sickroom and the condition of the patient demand. To protect a patient from drafts, a heavy cord such as a clothesline can be strung above the head of and along one side of the bed, and a light blanket draped over the line to stop the flow of cold air.

If the pressure of top coverings causes discomfort for the patient, a clothesline can be strung from above the head of the bed to the foot, and blankets or other coverings draped over the line to form a protective tent.

Ways To Make the Patient Comfortable

When the patient is able to sit or stand, he should be allowed—and even encouraged—to do so. If the bed used is a conventional type that cannot be adjusted like a hospital bed, there are many ways in which the patient can be propped up to make sitting in bed comfortable. Sometimes all that may be needed is a collection of cushions or pillows. In some instances a heavy piece of plywood can be fitted at an angle against the head of the bed to help support the patient's back. It is even possible to use an ordinary kitchen type of chair turned upside down so that the back

of the chair becomes a back support for the patient sitting up in bed. A pillow between the back of the patient and the back of the chair would be needed for comfort in most cases.

When a patient is sitting up in bed, it often is helpful to provide a pillow under the knees. Some patients are more comfortable lying in bed with a cushion or similar support placed under the knee joints.

BED CRADLE FROM CARDBOARD CARTON

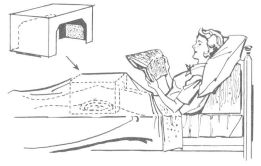

A patient who must spend a considerable amount of time in bed may experience discomfort from the weight of blankets on the feet and legs. The problem can be solved easily by obtaining a large cardboard carton and cutting holes in two opposite sides so the legs can slip through and the carton top can support the blankets. The patient also may appreciate the placement of a pillow beneath the knees so they can be supported in a flexed position.

A patient may complain about the pressure of coverings on the feet, or the inability to move his feet and legs about easily when the sheets and coverings at the foot of the bed are tucked in tightly. This problem can be solved quite easily by placing a firm cardboard box, with one side open, at the foot of the bed, and draping the top sheet and coverings over the box, so that the patient will be able to move his feet freely inside the box.

Preventing Accidents in Bed

Children, who may be the most restless of home care patients, often need to have added protection against accidentally falling out of bed. Some protection can be provided if the bed is placed against a wall and that part of the mattress on the opposite side of the bed is propped up with pillows or other supports so that the bed surface is tilted slightly toward the wall. If there is a tendency for the youngster to roll to one side, chances are he will roll toward the wall, rather than to the open side of the bed.

The open side of the bed also can be guarded with a line of chairs, which may have to be tied together or otherwise anchored so they cannot be pushed aside easily. The backs of the chairs thus form a barrier that can be moved or removed by the nurse when it becomes necessary to feed, bathe, or otherwise care for the young patient.

Still another technique is to run a folded sheet at right angles to the length of the bed over the chest of the child and under the mattress on both sides. The cross sheet should not be tight enough to cause discomfort, but it should fit snugly enough beneath the mattress to prevent the child from rolling and falling out of bed.

The same techniques for preventing a patient from falling out of bed can be used for older persons, such as patients who may suffer from senility or other mental disabilities, or persons who may have suffered a stroke and lack the normal use of their arms or legs for support.

Serving Meals

Meals for the home nursing patient may require special arrangements, particularly if the patient suffers from a serious illness. To help keep the system of feeding the sick patient as simple as possible, the patient should have a special set of dishes and tableware. The sickroom dishes could be of a different color or pattern from those used by other members of the family. The patient's dishes should be washed separately, if necessary; in most cases ordinary dish-washing methods will be adequate if plenty of hot water and soap or detergent are used.

If the doctor has prescribed a certain diet for the patient, questions about substituting other foods should be referred to the physician. The diet recommended may provide a minimum of sodium or fat, or a greater than average amount of high quality protein. Unless the meals are prepared at home from basic ingredients or

BED TABLE FROM CARDBOARD CARTON

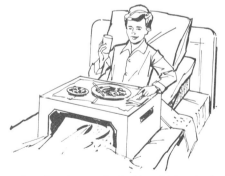

A cardboard carton can be fashioned into a bed table for a sick person in an emergency. The same carton may serve as a bed cradle to help provide space for moving the feet and legs under the blankets.

FEEDING THE HELPLESS

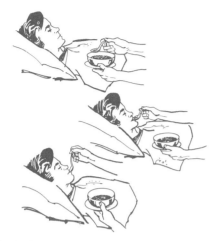

To feed a helpless patient, partly fill a spoon with food, making sure none is dripping from the bottom. Place the edge of the spoon between the lips of the patient. Then tip the spoon upward so the food drains between the lips into the patient's mouth. Be sure the patient is awake and able to swallow without choking on the food. A towel should be tucked under the patient's chin to catch any spilled food that otherwise might soil the patient's clothing or bed linen.

dietetic foods, it is wise to read the labels of packaged foods carefully. Carry-out foods from delicatessens or fast-food restaurants may contain more salt (sodium) or saturated fats than the doctor would approve.

Food served to persons who are seriously ill should be seasoned lightly. Cooked food should be served warm but not too hot; cold foods should not be too cold for comfort when served. The foods should appear attractive in order to help stimulate the patient's appetite. The meals should be served on some sort of regular schedule for the benefit of both the patient and the home nursing staff.

The patient should be allowed to sit up for meals, if possible. Bedding can be protected with towels and/or napkins or a

bib, depending upon the age and condition of the patient. If the patient is paralyzed or not fully awake, or if he has a disorder that interferes with normal swallowing, he should be offered a sip of water first. This is to make sure the patient is not likely to choke on food or beverage, or allow it to enter the windpipe by mistake. If the patient shows difficulty in swallowing normally, that fact should be reported to the doctor.

Hot foods, such as soups and beverages, should be temperature tested before serving them. This does not mean the nurse should sip the soup or tea or whatever from the patient's spoon, but a couple of drops on the nurse's inner wrist will indicate whether the fluid is too hot to be served immediately. The spoon used to serve fluids from a cup or bowl should be filled about two-thirds full and should be free of drops on the bottom. The spoon should be presented so that the edge of the spoon between the tip and one side should touch the patient's lower lip. Then tilt the spoon so that the fluid runs into the patient's mouth. And give the patient

SUPPORT OF HEAD

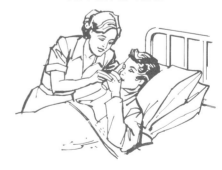

A patient who has difficulty in raising his head to sip fluids can be helped by placing several pillows under the head and holding an arm under the pillows to provide further support for the patient's head.

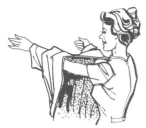

SLIP THE ARMS INTO A PINAFORE APRON WITHOUT
TOUCHING THE INSIDE OF THE GARMENT

A person who serves as a nurse to the home care patient should have a pinafore-type apron available to
wear while in contact with the patient. The home nurse
can slip the arms into the apron without touching the inside of the garment. This will help protect the nurse's
street clothes from being a source of disease organisms from the outside to which a weakened person
might be vulnerable.

time to swallow one spoonful of food before offering the next spoonful.

If the patient is able to drink from a
cup, the nurse may help hold the patient's
head with one hand behind the pillow, and
the other hand poised to help balance the
cup, if necessary. If the patient takes fluid
through a straw or glass tube, the nurse
may help hold the tube in place and the
container of fluid at a level that will keep
the liquid flowing without allowing air
bubbles to enter the tube or straw.

A record should be kept of the patient's
meals, including types of foods served,
amounts consumed, and information
about the patient's appetite.

After each meal the food not consumed
by the patient should be discarded, and
the eating utensils washed and rinsed in
scalding water. Discarded food should go
directly into a garbage disposer, or be
wrapped in a plastic bag for the incinera-
tor or garbage can. Dishes from the sickroom can be washed in an automatic
dishwasher; in fact, some doctors may recommend its use in order to apply water at

a temperature much higher than would be
tolerated by human hands washing dishes.
If the patient suffers from a serious infection, the doctor may recommend that eating utensils used by the sick person be
boiled after each meal.

Supervising Physical Activity

Most doctors advise that patients who
have been confined to bed for even a brief
span of days try to maintain some degree
of physical activity. Moving about not only
is good for the morale of most patients,
but it helps stimulate muscle tone, blood
circulation, appetite, normal functioning
of the digestive system, and the ability to
sleep without the help of medicines.

Getting out of bed, or learning to sit up
in order to leave the bed, may take a bit of
training for a person who has been lying
on his back for several days or more. The
nurse can assist the patient by helping
him to flex his knees and bend the elbows
to support his back in moving toward a sitting position. After the knees are flexed
and the elbows bent, the patient can extend an arm to push against the mattress
for additional support in straightening the
back while bending the hip joint. Next, the
other arm should be straightened so that
the patient is in a sitting position, with the
arms straight behind him and the palms of
the hands flat against the mattress.

The patient can return to his original position by reversing the procedure, that is,
slowly flex the elbows one at a time and
straighten the knees and hips, while holding the head slightly forward so it won't
fall flat against the mattress suddenly
when he returns to the supine position—
which means lying on the back with the
face turned upward.

The patient who is not used to standing

MOVING FROM BED TO WHEELCHAIR

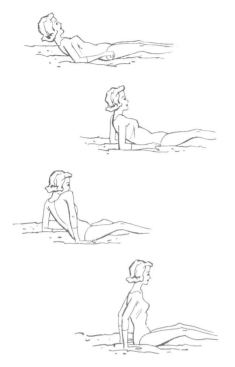

A person who has developed weakened muscles as a result of illness or injury often can learn to become more self-sufficient by raising the body from a supine (on the back) position in bed to a sitting position. The steps involve moving first one elbow, then the other, backward until the upper arms will support the top of the body. Then extend the arms and lock the elbows, one at a time, to push the body into a sitting position. The body is lowered back onto the bed by simply reversing the steps.

should first sit on the edge of the bed for a few minutes. Moving directly from a supine to a standing position can overtax the patient's circulatory system and cause him to faint; the same effect can occur occasionally in normal individuals. If the patient is a child whose legs don't touch the floor, a cushion, stool, or solid wooden box can be placed alongside the bed for him to step on, so that the move from bed to floor is done literally in a series of steps.

The nurse should assist the patient in moving from a seated to a standing position by grasping him under the armpits, if the patient needs that sort of help. Once the patient is in a standing position, he may need help in walking to a nearby chair or perhaps the bathroom. The nurse may have to walk backwards, carefully, while helping the patient to a chair. For any greater distance, it is safer to walk alongside the patient with another person helping on the other side, if necessary.

An alternative way of moving a patient from a supine position in a sickroom bed to a seated position in a chair is to place an armchair next to the bed. If the chair is located near the center of the bed, with the seat facing the foot of the bed, the patient usually is able to maneuver himself from the bed to the chair while the home nurse holds the chair steady. The patient can support himself by placing one hand on the mattress and one hand on the outside arm of the chair while moving to or from the bed.

This technique also is helpful in moving a disabled person from the bed to a wheelchair, or vice versa. The nurse holds the wheelchair steady while the patient shifts his weight from the bed to the chair, or from the wheelchair to the bed. If the wheelchair has removable arms, the arm on the side of the bed can be removed temporarily and a board placed between the seat of the wheelchair and the bed. The patient can then slide his weight along the board, while the wheelchair is held steady, from the bed to the wheelchair, or back again.

If the household does not have a wheelchair, an ordinary chair with casters might be substituted. Or an ordinary chair

USING BOTH ARMS TO SIT UP OR LIE DOWN

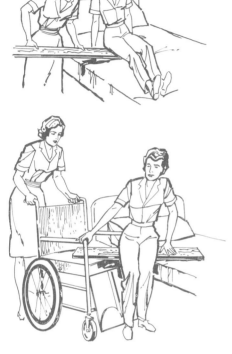

A sturdy plank placed between the bed and a chair or wheelchair will help a disabled person move from bed to chair or vice versa. The home nurse should stand by to make sure the move is carried out without a mishap.

straight back also could be used to provide support for the patient learning to move his own weight from a seated to a standing position.

When the patient is able to be moved from the bed to the bathroom, he may be able to bathe or shower in the bathtub. During the first stage of this transition, it may prove helpful to provide a waterproof tub seat or stool to sit on while he moves gradually from a wheelchair or an assisted walk to the water-filled tub. The water should be temperature tested in advance,

BATHTUB EQUIPMENT

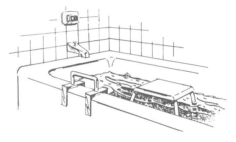

When a sick or injured person is sufficiently ambulatory to bathe himself, the tub can be equipped with a slip-proof rubber mat, a stool that may be used for taking a shower while seated or for tub bathing without lowering the body all the way into the tub, and grab bars that permit the patient to enter or leave the tub with added safety.

placed on a "dolly" or mechanic's "creeper" might be an effective device for moving a sick or injured person.

Before the patient walks much on his own, he should be encouraged to practice moving from a seated to a standing position without assistance. Sometimes this practice can be accomplished by placing a chair near the foot or head of the bed, if there is a headboard or footboard to provide support. A heavy chair with a

and the tub should be equipped with a slip-proof rubber bathmat and handholds for safety.

If the patient prefers to take a shower, which benefits the home nurse who does not have to clean the tub afterwards, the showering can be done with the patient seated on a stool. But the shower should be started before the patient enters the tub, to be sure the water temperature is adjusted properly.

Providing Basic Necessities

The bedside area of the sickroom should be equipped with some basic necessities for a person who may be very much alive despite a temporary confinement. The necessities can include a radio or television set that can be controlled from bedside, a box of facial tissues, reading and writing materials, and a container of fresh drinking water, fruit juice, or other beverage. If possible, the patient should have a window that permits a view of the outside world. A wastebasket or grocery sack within reach of the patient can be used to collect used tissues or other waste paper.

ACCESSORY BAG

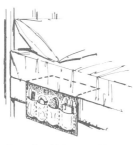

An accessory bag should be provided for the patient who is able to read, comb his hair, and do other small self-sufficient tasks. The bag, which can contain pockets for comb, hairbrush, glasses, note paper, or other personal items, can be held firmly between the mattress and box springs of the bed.

A bedside table can be used to hold or store some of these items, in addition to a fever thermometer, medications, a telephone or intercom unit, and other helpful objects.

Giving Medications

Being a home nurse often entails more than simply feeding and bathing the patient, and changing bed linen. If the doctor has prescribed a medication, it becomes the responsibility of the home nurse to make sure the patient takes the medicine according to the doctor's orders.

Some medicines are designed to be used at certain times, such as before meals, with meals, or after meals. Because of the way in which the body tissues metabolize the chemicals in a medicine, it may be important that the drug be given at certain regular intervals such as once every four hours. The drug must be taken in the size of dose prescribed; if the patient takes two tablets every eight hours instead of one every four hours, the original purpose of the treatment may be defeated.

It is important that an entire course of medication be followed, unless the doctor advises otherwise. Often, a patient or the home nurse may discontinue a medicine just when the drug is beginning to relieve the symptoms. The reasoning seems to be that if the symptoms are disappearing the medication can be discontinued. What may happen is that the patient may suffer a relapse, the symptoms may return, and if the disease organism has not received the knockout blow intended by the doctor's orders, the germ may develop an immunity to the medicine and come back stronger than ever.

Handling Bedpans

The home nurse also may be expected to handle bedpans and give enemas. In place of a bedpan, a bedside commode or a camper's portable toilet may provide the same function if the patient is able to move from the bed but cannot easily reach the bathroom. For a small child, the problem of emptying the bowels or urinary bladder may be handled with a child's potty chair placed near the bed.

When a patient uses a bedpan, the bedding beneath should be protected with a rubber or plastic sheet, or a sheet of oilcloth. The bedpan should be warmed to room temperature. The patient should be given a supply of toilet paper and whatever privacy is needed if he can manage to use the bedpan without help.

After the bedpan has been used, a cover made of newspapers or a grocery sack can be slid over the bedpan while it is carried to the nearest bathroom. The nurse should look at the contents because of the possibility that abnormal signs, such as blood, might appear with the urine or feces.

A male patient may not need a bedpan in which to void urine. A urinal usually can be used for that purpose. If a urinal is not immediately available, an empty waxed cardboard milk or fruit juice carton could be substituted. The carton, of course, would be discarded after it has been used as a urinal.

The patient should have blankets and other bed coverings arranged so that privacy and warmth are assured without the risk of soiling the bed clothes while he uses a bedpan or urinal. And the patient should be allowed to wash his hands afterward.

QUESTIONS AND ANSWERS
HOME HEALTH CARE

Q: *How does the home nurse avoid picking up germs in the sickroom of a person with a contagious disease?*
A: What you suggest—that it's almost impossible to avoid contact with one or more contaminated objects in the sickroom—is true. However, there are a number of precautions that can be taken to reduce the risk. For example, the home nurse can avoid direct contact with many objects in the room by using paper tissues when touching objects used by the sick person. The home nurse also must remember to wash his or her hands thoroughly with hot running water and plenty of soap before and after caring for the sick person.

Special care also should be used in cleaning the patient's room, using a damp cloth or oiled mop whenever possible to avoid stirring up the dust which may be contaminated with disease organisms.

Q: *What do you do with the paper tissues that have been used to handle the patient's objects, such as a comb or hairbrush?*
A: They can be dropped into the paper bag that might be attached to the edge of the patient's bed to collect the patient's own paper handkerchiefs or other items to be thrown away. The paper bag should be collected at least once a day and burned or enclosed in a sealed plastic bag if there is no safe way to burn paper on the premises.

Q: *Is it okay to measure medicines with the kitchen measuring spoons and cups?*
A: Yes, if they are accurate measures. As noted earlier, most silverware is designed to be attractive first and functional second, but rarely is it designed to be accurate as a measuring device. Measuring devices made of plastic can be obtained at many drugstores. An alternative source might be a photographic supply store;

people with home darkrooms may be more precise about measuring chemicals for a developing tank than in measuring a dose of cough medicine for a child.

In an emergency, a kitchen measuring cup might fill the bill. But be sure to measure the container at eye level and be sure it is level when being filled.

Q: *What should a home nurse do if she discovers she gave a sick person the wrong size dose of medicine?*
A: First, try to contact the doctor for instructions. If the doctor is not available, call the pharmacist who filled the prescription or who supplied the medicine given. It's possible that nothing serious will happen as a result of a mistake. But the doctor might recommend some way to compensate, like changing the amount of medicine in the next dose given. In case of a very serious mistake, it may be necessary to administer an antidote the same as if the person had been poisoned. But the doctor or druggist should be able to give you proper advice.

Q: *How long is it safe to keep medicines after the patient has recovered?*
A: Unless the doctor advises otherwise, any leftover prescription medicines should be flushed down the toilet. As for nonprescription medicines, it's generally wise to get rid of any products that have been on the shelf of the medicine cabinet for quite a while without getting much use. Replace them with fresh supplies if they are the standard standby types of O-T-C products, such as aspirin. Aspirin, incidentally, begins to smell a bit like vinegar when it loses strength; the acetic acid, which is a part of the aspirin molecule, is released as the medicine deteriorates.

Q: *When the doctor tells you to use "dry" cold on a patient, is that the same as dry ice?*
A: Certainly not! Dry ice is frozen carbon dioxide which would cause serious tissue injury if applied to any human body, healthy or sick. "Dry" cold probably is an unfortunate misnomer for ordinary "wet" ice that is placed in an ice bag or similar container, rather than giving the patient an application of "wet" cold in the form of a cold, wet compress. Even when ordinary crushed ice is placed in an ice bag, the bag must be wrapped in flannel or similar material and should never be applied directly to the skin. Also, it should not be left in place continuously because the cold temperature can impair circulation.

Q: *The doctor has recommended that my father take sitz baths because of a bladder infection. Does this require special equipment in the house?*
A: No, a sitz bath simply is a hot water bath in which the patient is immersed to the level of the hips. It often is recommended to relieve pain and discomfort of hemorrhoids, infections in the pelvic cavity, or following surgery in the lower abdomen. The temperature of a hot sitz bath may start at around 95 degrees Fahrenheit, with gradual increases to a level of 105 to 110 degrees Fahrenheit.

A sitz bath, however, can be somewhat hazardous for a person in poor health, so the patient should be watched carefully for signs of fatigue or collapse. Cool drinks should be made available and a cold compress might be placed on the patient's head while he is in the bath.

Q: *Is there some way to wring out a hot compress without burning your hands?*
A: In the old days, women used to use a device made out of a square of canvas or muslin, about 12 inches on each side. They sewed a wide hem on two opposite sides, then inserted a wooden spoon or stick through each of the two ends. This simple device made a very efficient wringer for getting excess moisture out of a hot pack without actually touching it. The wringing action was provided by twisting the two sticks or spoons in opposite directions. You might have to make your own because they probably don't sell hot compress wringers in the five-and-dime.

Q: *My mother is coming home from the hospital soon and may be an invalid for some time. She has been sleeping in a big queen-size bed at home, but my husband thinks it would be too much trouble to care for her in a big bed. Does it really make much difference about the bed size?*
A: Based on the experience of other people who have been confronted with the same situation, it would appear that your husband is right. It's much easier to care for a patient in a single bed. There probably will be times when your mother will have to be lifted or moved, and two people can't handle that task adequately from either side of a queen-size bed. When a helpless patient is in a large bed, you often need two or three home nurses on the same side to lift the head, hips, and legs at the same time. With an ordinary single bed, one person on each side can work together to move the patient.

Q: *Do you have any advice about controlling odors in the sickroom? The disinfectants on the market can smell worse than the sickroom odor.*
A: Try one of the newer deodorants which are designed to mask the odor of the sickroom but have no smell of their own. Also, try to get as much sunshine and fresh air into the room as possible without adding to the discomfort of the patient. And, of course, don't allow soiled dressings, used clothing and bedding, uneaten food, or other items to accumulate in the room.

10

WHAT TO EXPECT AT THE HOSPITAL

If you haven't been a hospital patient since you left the maternity ward as an infant, you may be a member of a minority group whose ranks are thinning daily. About 10 percent of the population enters a hospital each year for medical or surgical care. This is an increase of nearly 25 percent over the past decade, and the rate seems to be growing slowly but steadily.

This does not mean necessarily that the human race is in declining health. One reason that hospitalization is becoming more and more common is that diagnosis and treatment of medical problems have become increasingly sophisticated. Some serious injuries and diseases that might have been incurable or untreatable a generation ago are becoming virtually routine procedures. Transplants of hearts and other organs, microsurgery to rejoin severed arms and legs, "test tube baby" implants, and radiation and chemotherapy treatments for cancers are among the feats of medical magic available to almost anyone today, but these were beyond the reach of the wealthiest and most powerful individuals of the past.

As one grows older there generally are more reasons for a trip to a hospital. Older people are susceptible to chronic and disabling illnesses which were not easily treatable or curable for their own parents and grandparents. In fact, the growing population of older men and women is testimony to the effectiveness of modern medicine in prolonging life.

Types of Hospitals Available

There are literally thousands of hospitals available and all offer the same basic services. As defined by the American Hospital Association, these services are (1) an organized medical staff; (2) permanent facilities that include inpatient beds; (3) medical services; (4) continuous nursing services; (5) diagnosis and treatment, both surgical and nonsurgical, for patients with a variety of medical conditions.

In addition to health care institutions that fit this definition, there are myriad related establishments that offer similar services. A nursing care institution, for example, provides almost identical services with the exception that it admits only patients who are chronically ill and do not require surgery. There also are clinics, infirmaries, facilities for alcoholics or the physically handicapped, and so on. The U. S. Veterans Administration operates nearly 500 general hospitals, psychiatric hospitals, nursing and domiciliary homes, and clinics for military veterans.

Hospitals vary somewhat according to their ownership. They may be operated by a government body such as the state, county, or city; by a church or other religious group; by an industrial corporation or labor union; or by a profit-making corporation or partnership.

Most hospitals are general hospitals; that is, they handle general medical and surgical patients. There are special hospitals for maternity cases, geriatric patients, and patients with tuberculosis; eye, ear, nose, and throat hospitals; children's hospitals; and so on. There also are general hospitals that may have special facilities for diagnosing and treating certain disorders such as cancer.

Hospital Admittance Procedures

In an emergency, such as a highway accident far from home, you may find yourself in a hospital that is not of your choosing. If you enter a hospital for elective surgery, chances are you will be admitted to a neighborhood hospital where your doctor has "privileges," which means that he has staff status. In either situation, you will be asked a number of questions for the benefit of the attending physician, the hospital staff, and yourself. Because the hospital records generally are quite extensive, the questioning may go on more or less simultaneously with the taking of blood and urine samples, X-rays, temperature and pulse recording, and other procedures.

CHILD SHOULD BE TOLD
WHAT TO EXPECT

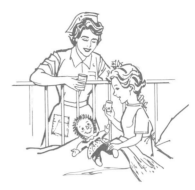

When a child must enter a hospital, the parents should discuss the situation openly without frightening the youngster. Adults should not show any fear of the hospital setting and should explain why the child will be a hospital patient. Most hospitals with facilities for handling children are stocked with books, games, and toys to keep the child entertained when he is well enough to use them. The child should be told to expect that nurses and other people will take good care of the young patient, serving his meals and giving him medicines that will help make him well.

When a patient is admitted for elective surgery or a similar nonemergency situation, a good deal of the information can be compiled a few days in advance of the date for entering the hospital. If X-rays, medical history, some blood and urine chemistry data, or other parts of the admission routine can be handled on an outpatient basis, one or more days of the hospital stay and associated expense can be avoided. If a person plans to undergo hernia repair on Monday morning, for example, he may not have to leave home for the hospital until the evening before the surgery if preliminary matters have been completed in advance. Otherwise, the patient might have to enter the hospital on the previous Friday and spend the weekend as an inpatient taking certain tests.

The information required by the hospital for its own records includes the patient's name, age, sex, address, name of the doctor, the reason for entering the hospital, previous illnesses and hospitalizations, family information, and a system history, which means a record of previous problems associated with different body parts or systems. The records also will include information about any allergies or medications used by the patient. Information about medicines used regularly by a patient can be important because of the possibility that they might interact with anesthetics or drugs administered by the hospital staff and could produce adverse effects.

The patient should be quite frank about the use of any stimulant or depressant, such as caffeine or alcohol, because the hospital diet is likely to contain very little caffeine and no alcohol. The sudden change in beverages after admission to a hospital is not likely to cause any dramatic effects if the patient has not become a heavy consumer of stimulant or depressant drugs, but an occasional patient may discover how dependent he was on such drugs after his supply is curtailed.

Entering the Hospital

After passing through the admissions routine, a patient usually is taken by wheelchair—regardless of his ability to jog all the way—to his ward or private or semiprivate room. In a typical general hospital, patients usually are assigned to floors or areas of floors where other patients with the same or similar conditions have been placed as inpatients. Maternity patients will be located in rooms with, or next to, those of other mothers-to-be, children will be placed in pediatric sections, and so on.

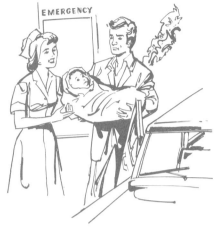

If it is necessary for a member of the family to make an emergency trip to the hospital and the hospital is close to home, it often helps to notify the family doctor of the problem. In most instances, the doctor can arrange to meet you in the emergency room and provide direct care or direction for treatment based on his experience with members of your family as patients.

Patients often are allowed to bring their own pajamas or nightgowns to wear, at least for the beginning and final days or nights of a hospital stay, although they may be asked to don hospital gowns for days during and immediately after surgery. Patients are usually allowed to bring their own bathrobes, toothbrushes, slippers, and other personal items as long as they are not likely to disrupt normal hospital routine or disturb other patients. A tape deck loaded with rock and roll tunes, for example, would not be considered an essential personal item.

After the patient is settled in the room or ward that will be the home-away-from-home for several days, one or more nurses and perhaps a staff doctor will pay visits to begin compiling temperature and pulse data and other information pertinent to the treatment of the particular case. If the purpose of the hospitalization is for corrective surgery, the anesthetist who will be responsible for the administration of drugs and gases used, and for maintaining life support systems that may be needed, will arrive to conduct his own physical examination.

The examination by the anesthetist usually is not detailed, but it may include a check of the heart and lungs so that he can obtain information needed for safe and effective use of anesthetics and related drugs. A patient who is taking medications for a chronic problem should advise the anesthetist in the event the medicines are of a type that interact with the anesthetic drugs. Certain types of eye drops for glaucoma patients, for example, can interact with anesthetics to cause heart arrhythmias, unless the dosage is adjusted before surgery. Information about medicines being used may be in the doctor's and hospital's records, but there's always the possibility that the anesthetist is not aware of the patient's medications.

The anesthetist sometimes is called an anesthesiologist, depending upon local custom. And the person who administers local or general anesthetics, which may also be called anesthesias in some hospitals, can be either a physician or a nurse. Nurses who administer anesthetics are identified as nurse-anesthetists.

Hospital Meals

As should be expected, hospital meals are carefully planned according to the needs of the individual patient and are generally adequate and nourishing, although seldom exciting. The dieticians, sometimes called food service managers, often display a considerable amount of expertise in creating a meal that is a palatable combination of a day's normal requirements for proteins, fats, carbohydrates, vitamins, minerals, and total calories.

The patient should not add anything to the hospital menu without first consulting the doctor in charge. Well-meaning friends during visiting hours may provide chocolate milk shakes or a cheeseburger with French fries from the neighborhood fast-food restaurant. But for a patient who is supposed to be on a low-fat or low-sodium diet during diagnostic tests or treatment for a medical problem, the goodies could destroy the purpose of the hospital stay. For similar reasons, a patient on a low-sodium diet should not borrow the salt from another patient's food tray in an effort to improve the flavor of his own salt-free meal.

Patients scheduled for surgery on the following day often are not allowed food or beverages after the evening meal. This usually is interpreted as "nothing by mouth" after a certain hour, ruling out the consumption of goodies that may be supplied by visitors. The rule, of course, varies according to the type of surgery planned but if there is any question about interpretation of the rule, it's better to ask the doctor or nurse.

Surgical Pre-op Procedures

For some types of surgery, a patient may not be allowed solid food for several days before the operation. Antibiotics may be administered for several days before surgery if the operation involves the intestinal tract. A patient may have to enter a hospital nearly a week before an operation if the surgical pre-operation, or pre-op procedures, as they are called, require a special effort to get the person in proper condition for a major operation.

For many kinds of surgery, however, the pre-op procedures are limited to cleaning and shaving the site of the incision and the surrounding skin surfaces. For an operation in which the incision is to be made in the lower abdomen, a nurse or intern may shave the body hair from the belly button down to and including the genital area. It's important that the entire skin surface of the region be shaved and scrubbed because one bit of hair slipping into the incision could start a serious infection.

Whether or not the pre-op phase requires the administration of a laxative or an enema to clean out the intestinal tract depends upon the type of surgery to be performed. Whatever is included usually is done for a specific reason, even though the pre-op procedures may seem baffling to the patient. For an operation to patch a ruptured eardrum, a nurse or other member of the hospital staff may shave and scrub a portion of the thigh or abdomen; this may startle the patient a bit unless the doctor has explained that the new eardrum will be fabricated from a piece of skin taken from another part of the body.

Before leaving the room or ward for the operating room, a nurse or other responsible person will collect the patient's watch, jewelry, money, or other valuables and place them in a safe location to prevent their disappearance. Theft is always a possibility in a large hospital where visitors or itinerant workmen may be wandering through the corridors. Any artificial devices—dentures, hearing aids, etc.—must be removed, as well as anything usually worn for cosmetic purposes such as a wig or false eyelashes. Such items not only are not needed by an unconscious patient on

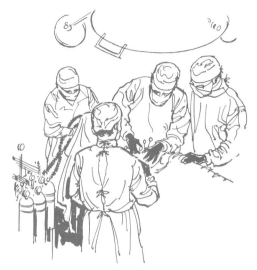

More than a million Americans every month undergo surgery in a hospital. Because surgery can save and extend the lives of people threatened with the most common causes of mortality, such as heart disease, cancer, and accidents, nearly everybody today can expect to enter a hospital operating room at least once in a lifetime. Even multiple trips to a hospital for various types of surgery are no longer uncommon. Improved surgical techniques and recovery procedures of recent years have shortened the amount of time most patients need to be hospitalized for operations.

an operating table, but they can be downright dangerous by interfering with critical efforts by surgeons and assistants in maintaining life systems while vital tissues are being removed or reorganized.

Before being moved to the operating room, the patient usually has a bonnet placed on his or her head to protect the surgical area from any disease organisms that may be present in the hair. The patient probably will be given sedatives to help him relax and perhaps may feel a bit sleepy by the time he reaches the operating room.

In a typical operating situation where a general anesthetic is administered, a tube is attached by a hollow needle to a vein in the patient's arm. The other end of the tube is connected to a bottle of intravenous fluid that will drip into the vein. The anesthesiologist may inject a drug such as sodium pentothal into the patient's vein, and that is about the last thing he will remember until he wakes up in a recovery room.

Post-op Therapy

Awakening in a hospital recovery room after being unconscious in an operating room can be a startling experience since the room may be filled with other patients in various stages of recovery from the effects of anesthetics. However, the recovery room sometimes is described as that part of the hospital where nursing care is most abundant and intensive. Nurses and other medical personnel, including doctors, watch each patient very carefully for signs of the gradual return of normal body functions. Patients who have been breathing anesthetic gases usually are given oxygen masks and asked to breathe deeply for a short while to help their lungs resume normal functioning. Oxygen mask breathing also helps prevent the risk of pneumonia by opening the alveoli, or tiny air sacs, at the ends of the air passages in the lungs.

As soon as the patient appears out of danger, he is returned to his ward or room. Depending upon the type of surgery, the patient may still be attached to a bottle of IV (intravenous) fluid, or a catheter may be connected to the urinary bladder so that urine can be collected and measured during the early period of recovery. Post-operative, or post-op, procedures generally are tailored to the needs and condition of the patient, but for the first day following surgery most patients are mainly interested in a little food and a lot of rest. There may be symptoms of nausea and some pain or discomfort that gradually diminish with the help of time and medications.

After the first day or so, the rate of recovery and the amount of additional time to be spent as an inpatient vary with the general health of the individual patient. Some patients may be able to get out of bed and walk around the room, or walk to the bathroom unassisted, within hours after leaving the recovery room. Others may have to wait a couple of days or more before they feel capable of sitting up and dangling their feet over the edge of the bed to help the circulation in the legs.

A certain amount of pain and discomfort, fatigue, and loss of appetite can be expected by most patients who have undergone surgery or treatment for a serious illness or injury. The hospital nurses should be advised of any problems that may require sleeping pills, pain killers, an ice bag, or a visit by a physician. In most hospitals, nurses or other personnel keep a close watch on patients in their charge, and through years of practice they often learn to anticipate patient needs. Even though a nurse may appear rather casual about her contacts, she probably is making continuous mental or written notes about each patient's condition—whether he is unusually restless, whether he has a good appetite and a normal fluid intake, and so on. The nurse may offer suggestions for ways to position the body in order to relieve cramps, give pain killers shortly before an exercise period so that the exercise will not aggravate the pain, or show a patient how to wiggle his feet in bed to prevent the development of thrombophlebitis.

Leaving the Hospital

Except for major operations such as intestinal surgery that requires an ileostomy or coronary bypass, an average hospital stay for surgical reasons is less than two weeks. A typical ordinary hernia operation, a simple appendectomy, a simple mastectomy, or a hysterectomy may require approximately one week of hospitalization. The total amount of time needed for hospital recovery may vary because of a number of factors, not all of them related to the health of the patient. Some people who apparently enjoy being cared for in a hospital prefer to stay as long as their hospitalization insurance policy pays the bills. Others will leave at the earliest opportunity, pretending to be in healthier condition than they actually are in order to be released.

If the reason for hospitalization was the delivery of a baby, the departure of the mother usually is coordinated with that of the child, unless the child was born prematurely or with an abnormality that requires additional hospital care. If the mother requires additional days, perhaps for minor corrective surgery of problems associated with childbearing, the baby probably will remain in the maternity ward until the mother is ready to go home.

A patient may leave the hospital room or ward the same way he entered—that is, in a wheelchair pushed by a member of the hospital staff.

Hospitalization of Expectant Mothers

Women who enter hospitals for the delivery of babies—and most still do go to hospitals despite growing interest in the use of midwives and home delivery of babies—generally face a different sort of routine from that of the patient admitted to a hospital for elective surgery, diagnostic tests, or for immediate care of serious injury or illness.

The expectant mother works toward a target date when the birth of the child is expected and, like the elective surgery patient, usually has most of her preadmission medical information on record with the doctor or hospital, or both. When the time approaches for delivery, as indicated by such traditional signs as the frequency of uterine contractions or the loss of amniotic fluid, the woman is rushed to the hospital's maternity ward. But after the expectant mother is assigned a bed, she may not see her obstetrician for hours, and possibly not until the following day. While she waits for labor to actually begin, the mother-to-be will depend upon nurses for her care. The reason she may not see the doctor right away is simple: the doctor is not actually needed until labor has really started. It would not be feasible for the doctor to pace the floor with the expectant father for perhaps 24 hours, just to be near the mother when the hour of delivery finally arrives.

A hospital with good obstetrical services can be expected to have trained nurses who are experienced in watching pregnant women for signs that labor has started. Some modern hospitals have fetal monitoring equipment that will alert the staff if problems threaten to develop before delivery begins. The obstetrical nurses know when it is time to call the doctor to attend the delivery, and they give the obstetrician an adequate amount of time to travel from his home or office to the delivery room, regardless of the hour of day or night.

Periods of Recuperation

After release from a hospital, arrangements are made with the doctor in charge for follow-up examinations and treatments, if needed. The doctor will advise about such matters as when normal routines can be resumed. The amount of time needed to recuperate after surgery before returning to work can vary from as little as a couple of days following a vasectomy to perhaps six weeks after a coronary bypass operation or surgery to create an ileosotomy in the intestinal tract. Around two weeks of absence from work should be planned for a hernia operation, an appendectomy without complications, or a cataract operation. Time lost from work for a simple hysterectomy or mastectomy averages about three weeks. However, the exact time periods will vary with individual patients, depending upon their general health and the type of work performed, among other factors. A patient recovering from an inguinal hernia repair operation or a hysterectomy, for example, should not be expected to perform strenuous physical labor until two or three weeks after surgery.

Paying the Hospital Bill

Many hospitals expect that arrangements will be made to pay for the hospital stay before the patient is officially discharged. Actually, most hospitals obtain some guarantee of payment before the patient is admitted, especially if the case involves elective surgery or a similar nonemergency situation. The hospital accounting department in most instances will accept evidence of hospitalization insurance coverage, such as Blue Cross/Blue Shield,

major medical policies, or Medicaid or Medicare. Although the matter of hospital bills is a frequent source of jokes and complaints, hospitals have their own bills to pay—salaries, supplies, utilities, equipment, etc.—and the amounts collected from patients' bills usually fall short of actual operating costs. This is particularly true for the nonprofit or voluntary hospitals operated by religious groups or community organizations.

One of the reasons for increased hospital costs is the number of hospital employees per patient. The ratio of full-time hospital employees per patient has doubled since the end of World War II and now averages about three and a half employees per patient. During the same period, medical care price increases have more than tripled, exceeding the total U.S. Consumer Price Index for the past quarter of a century.

Airing Complaints About Hospital Services

What can you do if you are not satisfied with the care given during your hospital stay? The first person you might complain to is the doctor in charge of your case. If you feel the doctor in charge failed to provide satisfactory care, there are several ways of expressing your dissatisfaction—including the obvious one of finding another doctor.

Most hospitals also have chains of command that include the chiefs of services, the hospital administrator, and the board of directors of the hospital, or a similar governing board if it is operated by a city, county, or state. There also are peer review groups made up of physicians who monitor the performance of other physicians. Some communities have organizations called Professional Standards Review Organizations and Experimental Medical Review Organizations, as well as a Performance and Evaluating Procedure for Auditing and Improving Patient Care (PEP).

In addition, most hospitals have their own review committees, such as a Tissue Committee which is responsible for examining surgical specimens to determine whether an organ or piece of tissue removed from a patient actually was diseased and required surgical excision.

Because of legal and other pressures, most hospitals try very hard to maintain high-quality patient care with a highly qualified medical staff. The numerous examination procedures, X-rays, EKGs, laboratory tests, and consultations that are involved in seemingly ordinary medical and surgical cases are indications that doctors and hospital staff members try to make sure that nothing goes wrong with any case admitted to the hospital.

GLOSSARY

HOSPITAL TERMS

The most familiar hospital terms are defined in the alphabetized list below. Words in italics refer to other entries in this Glossary.

accreditation A voluntary system in which hospitals are evaluated by an independent agency to make sure they meet certain standards of patient care. An accrediting body for hospitals is the Joint Commission on Accreditation of Hospitals, made up of representatives of the American Medical Association, the American Hospital Association, the American College of Physicians, and the American College of Surgeons. Accreditation, like a driver's license, must be renewed periodically and can be cancelled if a hospital fails to meet standards established by the commission.

admissions Patients accepted for inpatient service in a hospital.

allied health personnel A term sometimes applied to hospital workers who help physicians treat and care for patients.

ALOS An abbreviation for Average Length of Stay, a term used by hospitals and insurance companies to estimate the number of days a person may be a patient.

ambulatory care Another term for outpatient care, or medical care that does not require admission to a hospital as an inpatient. Ambulatory care may be provided at a clinic, at a doctor's office, or in the outpatient department of a hospital.

ancillary charge An item that may be included in a hospital bill for such services as X-rays, laboratory tests, use of an operating room, etc.

assignment of benefits An arrangement whereby a patient agrees to have his insurance company pay the hospital directly, rather than reimburse the patient or his family for hospitalization expenses.

auxiliaries Volunteers, such as "candy stripers," who donate their time to help a hospital with various jobs that do not require special medical training.

back-up hospital A term sometimes used to identify a hospital that is affiliated with a neighborhood health center. The neighborhood health center provides routine outpatient care but directs a seriously ill or injured person to its back-up hospital.

Blue Cross An independent nonprofit corporation that functions like an insurance company in providing protection for a patient by covering part or all of his or her hospital expenses. Blue Cross programs may vary somewhat in their operation in different regions because of state laws. In some states, for example, their operations are regulated by state insurance departments and rate increases are not granted without public hearings. However, Blue Cross contracts with hospitals generally limit the amounts that can be charged patients who belong to Blue Cross plans.

Blue Shield An independent nonprofit corporation that offers patient protection for costs of surgery and certain other types of medical care. Although Blue Shield and *Blue Cross* are technically independent organizations, they generally work together in providing comprehensive benefits covering hospital costs and some physician fees.

CHAMPUS An abbreviation for Civilian Health And Medical Program of the Uniformed Services, which provides medical care for dependents of soldiers, sailors, or other servicemen with funds provided by the U.S. Department of Defense.

chaplaincy service A department found in most hospitals that provides religious counseling for patients and their families.

closed panel A term meaning that a doctor may care only for patients on his "panel," which may be composed of patients belonging to a prepaid group practice program or a Health Maintenance Organization.

closed staff This refers to members of a hospital staff and means that only the physicians who have been accepted as members of the medical staff are permitted to admit patients for hospital treatment.

coinsurance A type of hospital insurance plan in which the patient and insurance company share the costs of treatment in an agreed upon ratio. For example, the insurance company may pay for 75 percent of the costs while the patient or his family pays the difference.

comprehensive care A program of health care that covers a wide variety of services, usually directed toward preventive or rehabilitation medicine and supervised by a group of physicians.

controlled substance A term usually applied to *narcotics* or other habit-forming drugs that may be obtained only by a physician's prescription or order. The term is derived from a federal government classification system for various kinds of medications and drugs of abuse. The system may not only require a physician's prescription for obtaining a controlled substance, but may restrict the number of times the prescription can be refilled.

cooperative hospital A hospital that is controlled by members of a group medical practice program. Cooperative hospitals often provide comprehensive health care to members who pay a fee in advance for the services offered.

dietary services Another name for the hospital department that prepares meals for pa-

tients. The department usually operates the hospital cafeteria or restaurant, in addition to caring for the nutritional needs of hospital patients.

dispensary A word once used to identify the department of a hospital that handles outpatient health care problems. While outpatients at some hospitals still may be referred to the dispensary, the department today is more likely to be called the outpatient department or ambulatory care service.

elective admission A person who enters a hospital for elective surgery or a similar non-emergency health problem that can be postponed is classified as an elective admission. Higher priority is given to emergency admission patients.

extended care services Health care programs offered patients who require a certain amount of regular nursing or medical care for a health problem that does not require hospital inpatient status. A patient in a nursing home or rehabilitation center receives extended care services.

FMG An abbreviation for Foreign Medical Graduate. FMGs are allowed to serve as interns or residents at some hospitals if they pass special tests given to assess the quality of their training in another country.

formulary A list of medications usually available at the hospital pharmacy. The list includes drugs approved by members of the staff for hospital use and may be identified by generic names rather than brand names.

full-time staff Medical personnel who work full-time for the hospital. The full-time staff usually does not include physicians who provide care for patients in their private practices.

grace period This has nothing to do with prayers before meals but refers to a limited period of time during which a person's hospital insurance policy remains in effect even if the premium was not paid by the due date. If the premium is not paid before the end of the grace period, the policy may be useless to the patient.

hospital service charge The basic daily rate charged by a hospital for use of the facilities, including bed, meals, and standard nursing care. Any special use of the facilities such as diagnostic or treatment techniques may be listed on the bill as an *ancillary charge.*

housekeeping department The hospital activity involved in cleaning floors, removing trash, and similar custodial work.

house staff Members of the hospital medical personnel who are in training as interns and residents.

ICU An abbreviation for Intensive Care Unit, the hospital department that provides emergency care in life-threatening cases.

intern A medical school graduate who has earned his doctor's degree and is serving a period of additional training in the care of medical and surgical patients.

laboratory Hospitals often have several different kinds of laboratories for helping in the proper diagnosis and treatment of patients. An anatomical laboratory may be used to perform autopsies. A clinical laboratory is equipped to analyze blood, urine, feces, and other substances. A special laboratory may be employed to study samples of bone and other body tissues.

layperson A person who is not a professional. In the medical world, a layperson is someone who is not a doctor. In a different occupational arena, a physician may be regarded as a layperson.

malpractice A legal term that may be used to charge a member of the medical profession with responsibility for an injury, damage, or loss because of negligence or improper use of diagnostic or therapeutic techniques. A malpractice case, for example, might involve a high school football player whose leg had to be amputated because hospital personnel failed to give proper care to broken bones in the leg.

multiple coverage A patient might have more than one insurance policy to cover the costs of the same medical or surgical problem. The practice usually is frowned on by insurance companies because multiple coverage places the patient in a position in which he can make a profit from an illness or injury.

narcotics Drugs that are central nervous system depressants used to produce loss of consciousness or sensibility when administered by a doctor. Narcotics usually are habit-forming and are listed as *controlled substances*, available only with a doctor's prescription.

nutritionist Another name for a dietitian, the individual responsible for planning patients' meals for a hospital's *dietary services.*

open staff A hospital staff that opens its membership to any licensed physician who wants to admit a patient to the hospital and care for him at that hospital. Most hospitals have a *closed staff* arrangement, but they may extend courtesy staff privileges to a doctor who is not a regular member of the staff but wants to use the facilities occasionally for the care of a patient.

patient's chart This refers to the medical records of a patient. The patient's chart usually is retained by the hospital after the patient has been discharged.

primary care Health care provided by a primary physician, that is, the doctor who generally is directly responsible for diagnosing and treating a particular patient. The "family doctor" or generalist, or sometimes a specialist, who usually treats a patient is the primary care physician. Secondary care may be provided by the staff of a general hospital, and tertiary care by personnel of a special hospital or health care facility.

progressive patient care A program that may be used by doctors and hospitals to plan the recovery and rehabilitation, if needed, of a seriously ill or injured person. An example might be the case of a heart attack victim who enters a hospital's Coronary Care Unit (CCU) and gradually improves over a period of months, moving into self-care, extended care, and finally home care.

radiology Another term for X-rays and other types of radiation used in diagnosis and treatment.

referral What happens when a primary care physician sends a patient to another physician, usually a specialist, who assumes primary responsibility for the care of the patient.

rounds Physician visits to the bedsides of patients in a hospital to check on their condition.

self-pay patients Hospital patients who pay directly for medical costs without resorting to the use of insurance coverage.

surgicenter A name used for outpatient facilities that provide surgery for conditions that do not require overnight hospitalization.

triage An old military medical term for a procedure in which patients are more or less sorted into categories as they arrive at a health facility so that priority can be given to the most serious cases. At clinics or other health care agencies where patients may drop in off the street without appointments, a triage procedure helps screen the patients so that each gets adequate and appropriate treatment with a minimum of confusion, lost time, and effort.

upper limits coverage The maximum amount an insurance company will provide in a policy to pay for hospitalization costs.

waiting list A list of patients waiting for admission to a hospital. The list is used mainly for *elective admissions*.

waiver A statement in a health insurance policy whereby the insurance company exempts from coverage a disability that normally would be covered by the policy.

walk-in patient A patient who arrives at a hospital emergency room, clinic, or other health facility without prior notification of his health care needs. See also *triage*.

ward clerk A member of the hospital staff who handles patient charts and other paperwork required at the ward's nursing station.

Workmen's Compensation A state supervised program of payment for injuries that occur in connection with a person's job. The benefits are financed by employers through private insurance companies or through a state fund. The benefits may be paid in cash, or as payment for medical and hospital expenses, and/or to finance rehabilitation if needed, and to compensate for loss of wages resulting from an on-the-job injury. The patient does not have to prove the employer negligent in order to collect Workmen's Compensation benefits.

QUESTIONS AND ANSWERS
HOSPITALS

Q: *Who owns the patient's hospital records?*
A: Generally, the records of a patient's hospitalization are kept on file by the hospital, although some of the information may be released to doctors or other qualified medical personnel when the need arises. The practice may vary in different communities and with individual cases. A U.S. District Court ruling has challenged an earlier decision that a patient could obtain copies of his own medical records by filing a written request. Doctors had objected on the grounds that the patient's medical records are not actually the property of the patient, that the average patient would not understand the information, and that the information could be detrimental to the patient's own well-being.

Q: *My son is going into the hospital for eye surgery in a few weeks. Will I be allowed to accompany the boy into the operating room?*
A: Various hospitals have their own rules about whether a parent can observe an operation, even through a window from outside the operating room, but generally they are discouraged from becoming that closely involved in the procedure. Some hospitals, however, do provide facilities for parents to accompany a child to a waiting area just outside the operating room where the parents can be with the youngster until he falls asleep.

Parents usually can be more helpful by reassuring the child that he is in good hands and under the care of competent medical professionals, and that it's not necessary for mother or father to become involved. The child may sense the parents' feelings of fear and distrust, and become more apprehensive than necessary if mom and pop get into the act.

Q: *Can any veteran of U.S. military service use Veterans Administration hospital services?*
A: Veterans Administration hospitals are intended primarily for persons who require treatment for service-connected disabilities, including those who have been transferred from military hospitals and those whose medical condition may not be service-connected but was aggravated by military duty. Other veterans who require treatment for nonservice-connected conditions should be veterans who served during wartime and are unable to pay for private care. Persons applying for admission to a VA hospital usually are required to sign a statement with an affidavit stating the reasons they believe they should receive Veterans Administration care, and include a personal financial accounting. More than two-thirds of the patients in U.S. Veterans Administration hospitals are from families considered to be below the nation's economic poverty level.

Q.: *What is a "block appointment" for outpatient medical care?*
A: The term, block appointment, generally refers to a system whereby a group of patients is asked to report to the outpatient department at the same time, which usually is the time the department begins taking patients for the day.

Q: *Why are there fewer hospitals in America today than there were in the 1960's?*
A: A lot of new hospitals were built after World War II when there was a high occupancy rate and a need for more hospital space. There was a "baby boom" then, and many patients with mental illnesses were being admitted to hospitals for new types of treatment.

Because contraceptives and other techniques, such as vasectomy and abortion, have become popular, the birth rate has declined sharply and fewer beds have been needed for obstetrical patients. Many mental patients were able to be released from hospitals because of the effectiveness of new psychotropic drugs. And most of the common types of disease and surgery that previously required long periods of hospitalization can now be treated effectively with medical and surgical techniques that shorten considerably the number of days of hospitalization per patient. For example, bacterial pneumonia, which at one time required extensive hospital treatment for many patients, can now be cured in a few days with antibiotics and good care at home.

Q: *Is a hospital legally responsible if a surgeon removes some body tissue from a patient without obtaining permission from the patient?*
A: That probably depends upon a large batch of factors which need to be sorted out by lawyers, juries, and judges. In an emergency accident that renders the patient unconscious and in danger of death, the medical personnel of the hospital might feel justified in doing whatever is necessary surgically in order to save a life. In a case of elective surgery, the patient should discuss such details with the surgeon in advance of the operation, and the hospital generally requires that a consent form be signed outlining the procedure to be followed in the operating room as further assurance that the patient understands what tissues may or may not be removed.

If a patient feels his body has been damaged or his life or health threatened because of something that was removed without his authorization, he should first ask for an explanation from the administrator or governing board of the hospital. The governing board of a hospital has the ultimate authority for the operation of its hospital and for providing competent medical care, even though it may delegate responsibilities to the medical staff.

Q: *Will Medicaid pay for outpatient X-rays and laboratory tests?*
A: X-rays and laboratory tests for outpatients are included in some Medicaid programs, but the details vary from state to state. States that participate in Medicaid programs are required to provide certain basic services in order to receive a share of federal matching funds, but the states are given options as to how the programs may be carried out locally.

Q: *When my husband was injured in an automobile accident and was taken to the hospital emergency room, he had to wait nearly two hours for treatment while other patients who arrived later got immediate attention. Who or what decides medical care priorities in an emergency room?*
A: One problem with hospital emergency rooms, from the point of view of medical personnel, is determining which cases really require immediate care. An auto accident victim may have cuts and bruises but appear alert and in no immediate danger of collapse, so he may be watched for signs of internal injuries that may occur later. In other words, the auto injury patient is not being ignored, but rather is being observed while medical care activity is directed toward treating patients who may have more life-threatening problems. An emergency room is not like a meat market where the customer takes a number inside the door and waits his turn.

If you are injured or stricken with a sudden illness at home or close to home, you can help expedite your immediate care by calling your doctor and asking him to meet you in the hospital emergency room. Your own doctor can concentrate on your problem in a hospital setting, while the emergency room staff goes about its first-priority system of focusing attention on the more serious cases that come in off the street.

11

DRUGS
PRESCRIPTIONS AND
NON PRESCRIPTIONS

It's doubtful that anyone will ever know why or how humans began using substances found in their environment to relieve pain, heal wounds, or treat digestive upsets. Ancient clay tablets unearthed by archeologists in the Middle Eastern "cradle of civilization" bear inscriptions that describe how to prepare medications from plants and other natural substances, indicating that doctors some 5,000 years ago had a rather well-organized science of pharmacology as a healing resource.

Ethologists, the scientists who study the natural behavior of wild and domestic animals, suggest that there may be something instinctive about the urge to seek medical cures from substances in nature. Dogs, one of the more easily observed animals, will forage for certain plants when they are ill; a common type of grass eaten by dogs with digestive problems is popularly known as "dog grass." Other animals, particularly those living in the wild state, also seem capable of finding natural medications which they administer to themselves. The evidence suggests that humans probably acquired some knowledge about botanicals, and perhaps minerals and other substances, with health benefits at a very early stage in their evolution.

Ancient Egyptian medical schools went deeply into the use of herbs for treating various ills; at least one of their colleges featured a rather large herb garden as part of the campus. At about the same time that early Egyptians were recording their knowledge of medicine formulation, Chinese doctors were doing the same thing. One ancient Chinese Pen-ts'ao, or pharmacology text, compiled around 3,000 B.C., listed more than 300 medicines that could be prepared from herbs, plus about 55 other medications that could be made from animal tissues or minerals.

Old Drugs That Are Still in Use

The old Pen-ts'ao suggested, for example, that rhubarb could be used to treat constipation because of its natural laxative properties. The early Chinese also used a plant substance for treating congestion that doctors thousands of years later identified as a source of ephedrine, which still is used as a pharmaceutical agent. Nearly 2,000 years ago, doctors in India added castor oil to the list of cathartics. And for countless generations Hindus in India used a substance extracted from snakeroot to treat mental illness, but only in the past few decades have modern pharmacologists determined that the substance in snakeroot that controls high blood pressure and certain mood disturbances is rauwolfia, from which the drug reserpine is derived.

In the past the use of medicines to treat illness competed with religion and superstition. Substances derived from nature were apt to be regarded as some tool of witchcraft if they produced significant physiological changes in people. An example was the use of digitalis to treat congestive heart disease. At one time, if a person suffered from dropsy, the common name for the edema or fluid accumulation caused by congestive heart disease, it was necessary to obtain a potion prepared by witches. These strange ladies called witches had simply carried on through the Dark Ages and the Renaissance the ancient tradition of maintaining herb gardens and the recipes for preparing curative potions with the herbs.

An English physician curious to learn what magic the witches possessed that could produce relief from congestive heart failure discovered the magic was contained in the leaves of the purple foxglove plant. Once removed from the mystical setting of a witch's garden, digitalis became an important drug that makes the heart pump more efficiently for millions of people around the world today. However, modern pharmaceutical research has resulted in a medication that is somewhat improved over the drug contained originally in a witch's brew. Laboratory experiments have resulted in a few improvements, including variations in the original molecule so that different plants can be used as sources for somewhat different kinds of digitalis needed for various patients.

Acetylsalicylic acid, better known as aspirin, has evolved through somewhat similar steps since days of yore when the bark of willow trees was ground and boiled as a herbal tea to reduce pain and fever. It also was known to relieve some of the symptoms of rheumatism and arthritis. Later research found the active ingredient was salicin, which also is available from other sources such as the poplar tree, although the botanical name of the willow, *Salix*, remained to identify the chemical. Since modern pharmaceutical chemists have mastered the salicylic molecule, aspirin can be made today in various forms without using willow trees and without producing some of the irritating effects of the original substance.

Colchicine, a drug obtained from the autumn crocus, was discovered long ago to have the ability to reduce the pain of gout. It still is the favored drug for that purpose and is so efficient in turning off the agonies of gout that colchicine also is used to diagnose the arthritic disorder. If colchicine doesn't help, the pain probably isn't caused by gout.

Modern Synthetic Drugs

By taming and converting the molecules produced naturally by plants, pharmacologists have been able to create in the past few decades a world of synthetic medicines that often are more effective than the original forms—and much less expensive. An example are the steroid hormones used for a variety of human problems ranging from rheumatoid arthritis to the control of fertility. Before the late 1940's, hormone substances were exceedingly rare and expensive; the supply depended mainly on the availability of animal glands from slaughterhouses. But experiments with chemical components of Mexican yams led to a process whereby hormones that then cost more than $3,000—a respectable annual salary in those days—an ounce could be produced for pennies. Today, more than 50 million women around the world use oral contraceptives made synthetically from what were originally plant substances.

Americans alone spend about $11 billion a year for drugs, an average of only about $50 annually per person. This is a fair price for a virtually endless variety of antibiotics, vitamins, vaccines and serums, tranquillizers, painkillers, replacement hormones, drugs for infections and for cardiovascular, respiratory, gastrointestinal, muscular, neurological, genito-urinary, and skin problems, as well as remedies for snakebites, insect bites, cancers, parasites, toothaches, poisoning, etc. Drugs also have made possible a number of surgical procedures that have extended the lives of hundreds of thousands of people. Surgical transplants, for example, would be futile without drugs to control the natural tendency of the body's own tissues to reject any foreign substance that contacts the tissue cells.

A certain amount of the knowledge of drug effectiveness is empirical; that is, it has been accepted as a therapeutic tool mainly because it has been around a long time, and it works without causing too many side effects, even though doctors and pharmacologists are not really sure how it works. Aspirin is such a drug.

Antibiotics

When the mode of action of a drug is understood, doctors usually can make even more effective use of it. Antibiotics once had some limited use, dating back to pre-Columbian times in Latin America when Mayans used a fungus produced on green corn to treat infections. But after the development of controlled production of penicillins and semisynthetic antibiotics in our century, therapy with such medicines expanded rapidly. Medical scientists learned, for example, that penicillins can destroy bacteria because they interfere with the construction of cell walls by the disease organism. Tetracyclines are among a group of antibiotics that destroy bacteria by preventing them from synthesizing proteins needed for their normal functioning. Actinomycin belongs to a type of antibiotic that kills bacteria by altering the DNA molecules in the nuclei of the invaders so that they are unable to reproduce their own kind of disease germs.

With this kind of knowledge, doctors have learned to apply a specific antibiotic to a certain type of disease organism or condition, according to the most appropriate battle plan. The physician does not make random use of antibiotics when he knows the identity of the germ and where it is most likely to be vulnerable to attack. Some patients still experience undesirable side effects from antibiotics, some strains of disease organisms have become resistant to the drug, and still other microorganisms cannot be controlled by antibiotics. However, by applying what has been learned about antibiotics and how they attack diseases, doctors have been able to extend their battle against infections to most bacteria, as well as to protozoa, fungi, most types of worm infestations, and a few viruses with substances quite similar to the green corn mold once used by the Mayans.

Although antibiotics can affect a few viruses, most viruses still defy the effects of most anti-infectious agents. Viruses consist of DNA molecules and nucleic acids, surrounded by a protein coat. The usual modus operandi of a virus is to attach itself to a living cell and break down the cell wall. Once inside the cell, the virus captures the metabolic and reproductive apparatus, and in effect makes the cell a slave that produces more viruses which invade more cells.

Medical scientists have directed efforts toward developing drugs that interfere with the viral mechanism, instead of drugs that simply kill viruses. By blocking viral replication processes, a virus disease can be stopped. In the meantime, however, medicines that can be used against virus infections are mainly vaccines prepared from either live or dead viruses that need to be administered before onset of the infection. The vaccines must be injected into the body tissues to produce a relatively mild form of the disease that generally results in some degree of immunity to that particular virus. If a new strain of the virus develops, however, as occurs frequently in influenza, a new vaccine must be administered.

Hormones

Hormones are the chemical messengers that stimulate certain life processes, including growth, reproduction, secretion of milk in the breasts, production of urine in the kidneys, and certain intellectual and behavioral effects. Some hormones influence protein, carbohydrate, and fat metabolism, or the way the body uses calcium and phosphorus to build bone. A hormone deficiency, like a vitamin deficiency, can manifest itself as a serious disease or abnormality. Because of a hormone imbalance, a person can be a dwarf, mentally retarded, or sterile.

There are many different kinds of hormones in the human body, so many that medical scientists aren't really sure of the total. Each of the endocrine glands, the usual source of hormones, seems to produce more than one kind of hormone. The adrenal glands alone produce no fewer than 25 hormone substances, each of which has a different chemical formula and physiological function. The hormones of certain animals are the same as or closely similar to human hormones, so that in treating a case of hormonal deficiency, doctors often can give a patient a medication that is derived from an animal hormone. Insulin is an example of a hormone that is derived from the pancreas of a cow or pig and modified for human use.

Many hormones are produced in such small amounts that they can virtually be measured in molecules. To extract these substances from livestock glands and convert them into medications for humans can be quite costly. During the 1940's one large pharmaceutical company was able to produce from hundreds of livestock carcasses each year only enough cortisone—actually 400 grams, or less than one pound—to treat fewer than a dozen patients suffering from rheumatoid arthritis. The way to go, obviously, was to produce synthetic hormones, for with synthetic steroid hormones it was possible to provide relief for a dozen million, rather than just one dozen, rheumatoid arthritis victims. Eventually, this became possible through an investment of more than $25 million in research over a period of more than a decade.

The universally popular birth control pills, or oral contraceptives, evolved in a somewhat similar manner over a period of many years of study and experiments. Originally, oral contraceptives were not intended to prevent conception but to aid infertile couples to have children. The first fertility control medications were substances extracted from animal glands and modified in the laboratory for injection into women. The process was difficult, painful, and expensive, but as the medical researchers learned more about the molecular makeup of the hormones and their effects on human menstrual physiology, they were able to create effective synthetic hormones that could be taken by mouth instead of by injection.

Prostaglandin Drugs

Hormones themselves are affected in turn by a group of newer drugs called prostaglandins that are produced by a number of living things, including tissue cells throughout the human body. Like quite a few other medications, such as salicylic acid, prostaglandins are named for one of the original sources of the substances. They were first isolated from semen and prostate glands of animals. There are at least a dozen prostaglandins, identified by letters of the alphabet and numbers, such as A_1, A_2, etc., through F_3, after the initials, PG. PGE_2 is a form of the drug that lowers blood pressure, while its chemical cousin, PGF_2, raises blood pressure in some animals. Prostaglandins also stimulate smooth muscle activity of the uterus and other organs and are used to induce abortions. The prostaglandin drug is injected into the amniotic sac and uterine contractions begin within a day, making the substance an effective agent for producing therapeutic abortions in cases involving the death of a fetus that is retained in the womb.

Drugs for Cardiovascular Disease

Drugs for the control of cardiovascular disorders form a large category of medications. Anticoagulants, such as heparin, are administered to prevent coagulation of blood clots; some prevent, others retard or limit the formation of new clots. Enzymes can be injected soon after a clot has formed when it is important to dissolve the clot. Coagulants may be administered for the opposite effect, that is, to prevent excessive bleeding during surgery.

Vasodilators used to increase the size of blood vessels include amyl nitrite, which may be supplied in ampules that can be crushed to release the drug's fumes, and glyceryl trinitrate (nitroglycerin), which comes in tablets to be placed under the tongue that prevent or relieve attacks of angina pectoris. Vasoconstrictors, such as epinephrine or ephedrin, are prescribed to stimulate heart action and increase blood pressure. Digitalis-type drugs, which also may be known by such names as digitoxin and digoxin, strengthen the heart muscle to improve heart contraction effectiveness and the reduction of edema, or fluid accumulation in the tissues, as a result of congestive heart failure.

Still other cardiovascular drugs may be

ordered by the doctor to control abnormal heartbeats. One type of arrhythmia drug, quinidine sulfate, reduces the number of times per minute the atria will contract, therefore slowing a rapid heartbeat. Procainamide hydrochloride also may be used to control atrial fibrillation, but it is more likely to be administered for premature ventricular contractions.

Diuretics

Diuretics are prescribed to increase the flow of urine. They also may be used to lower the amount of sodium in the body or to reduce blood pressure in conjunction with the effect of increased urine production. Various kinds of diuretics do their work in different ways. Osmotic diuretics, which may include potassium salts and urea, pull water that ordinarily would be reabsorbed by the kidney into tubules that lead to the ureters. Another kind, sometimes identified as carbonic anhydrase inhibitors, prevents the formation of carbonic acid in the blood from carbon dioxide and water, the waste products of cellular metabolism. This effect, caused by somewhat complex chemical maneuvering by the body tissues, results in the loss of sodium, and when sodium is lost, water is excreted. Thiazide diuretics, one of the more common kinds of prescription diuretics, use a combined approach utilizing both the carbonic acid inhibition method and a means of diverting water into the collecting tubules leading out of the kidney. Some diuretics cause a loss of potassium along with sodium, but others do not. Some are prescribed to work hand-in-hand with other medications designed to control glaucoma, heart disease, etc. Doctors have more than 20 generic types to choose from, each with its own advantages or disadvantages for individual patients.

Drugs for Controlling Cancer Growth

Drugs designed to control cancer growth often are identified as antineoplastic medications. They work by several different methods. One kind is known as an alkylating agent. It "poisons" the cancer cell by attaching itself to protein molecules in the tumor so that the cell cannot function normally. Since the malignant tumor cell grows faster, reproduces more often, and has a higher metabolic rate than neighboring tissue cells, it is more sensitive to agents that interfere with its activities. Nitrogen mustard, used in treating some cases of Hodgkin's disease and lymphosarcoma, is a cancer drug of this type.

A second kind of cancer drug is an antimetabolite, such as methotrexate, which interferes with a particular stage of tumor cell functions. Methotrexate interferes with the formation of folic acid. Other antimetabolites interfere with the formation of purine components in the cancer cell's genetic material or other essential functions of the cancer cell nucleus.

Radioactive chemicals sometimes are used to destroy tissue cells in a small, well-defined area where cancer is active. The radioactive isotopes usually are inserted in the tumor in pellets or needles. The radiation approach may be used to shrink the size of a tumor before it is removed surgically.

Drugs for Digestive Disorders

Drugs available for treatment of digestive tract problems include laxatives, antidiarrheals, antinauseants, antacids, and digestants. Antacids neutralize or absorb stomach acid, thereby rendering it inactive. Calcium carbonate antacids neutralize the acid while aluminum hydroxide gels absorb the acid; other antacid medications work in the same or a similar manner. The home remedy of baking soda, or sodium bicarbonate, neutralizes the acid but also produces a rebound effect in which the stomach simply secretes more acid to compensate for the baking soda effect. Digestants, which might include malt extract, pepsin, bile salts, or hydrochloric acid, are prescribed for people who have a stomach acid deficiency.

Over-The-Counter Drugs

Drugs generally are available to the public either as O-T-C (for over the counter) or nonprescription medications, or with a doctor's prescription. Although there is a small gray area between the definitions of certain prescription and O-T-C medications—as in the case of a cold remedy that may be sold as either an O-T-C or prescription product—prescription drugs usually are substances that are considered potentially risky for general public access.

Many prescription drugs, for example, contain "controlled substances," a federal government label which means that they probably are addictive. A controlled substance might be codeine, a chemical cousin of morphine and a narcotic, which could be contained in a cough medicine or in a pain-killing tablet that might be provided by a dentist.

An O-T-C product could be aspirin, an antacid, or something similar that would be obtainable in a drugstore, discount house, or supermarket. The fact that an O-T-C product is available without a doctor's prescription should not be construed as meaning the drug is harmless. An O-T-C medication could be more dangerous than a prescription drug, depending upon the individual user's sensitivity and how it is used.

Doctor's Prescription

A doctor's prescription usually is quite specific about how a medication is to be used. It includes directions to the pharmacist and directions to the patient. The directions often are written in a kind of physician's Latin shorthand, but sometimes they may be written in ordinary English. The pharmacist who fills the prescription translates the doctor's directions

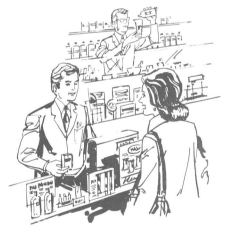

A pharmacist often helps a patient who may have prescriptions given by more than one doctor in case the prescriptions duplicate each other or contain chemicals that might interact to produce adverse side effects. Because of his knowledge of relationships between generic drugs and brand-name drugs, a pharmacist also is in a position to advise doctors and patients about possible substitutions. However, a pharmacist generally is responsible for providing whatever drug is specifically ordered by the doctor.

to the patient, and that information usually is typed clearly on the label of the medicine container.

The directions to the patient may state such things as "three times daily," "by mouth," "after meals," "at bedtime," etc. In the doctor's Latin message to the pharmacist, the same information would appear as "t.i.d.," "per os.," "p.c.," and "h.s."

The total written prescription includes several specific parts, including the traditional "R_x"—which means simply "Take thou." It also should include the date, the name of the patient, the patient's address, the signature of the physician, the physician's address (which usually is printed on the prescription form), and his registry number.

The rest of the prescription is divided into three parts—which the patient may not be aware of—called the inscription, the subscription, and the signa. The R_x might be included as a fourth part, called the superscription. The inscription tells the pharmacist the identity and amount of each drug component that goes into the prescription if the medicine is to be compounded by the pharmacist; otherwise, it may simply identify the generic or brand name of the medicine to be dispensed.

The subscription tells the pharmacist how the medicine should be prepared or dispensed—for example, as capsules, elixir, tablets, or whatever. And the signa tells the pharmacist the instructions to the patient to be typed on the label.

HOW TO READ YOUR DOCTOR'S SHORTHAND

Abbreviation on Prescription	Means
a.	before
$\bar{a}$., or $\bar{aa}$.	of each
a.c.	before eating
ad lb.	as desired
b.i.d., or b.d.	twice a day
b.i.n., or b.n.	two times at night
c., or c	with
elix.	elixir
ext.	extract
fl.	fluid
gtt.	drops
h., or hor.	hour
h.s.	at bedtime
noct.	at night
o.d.	right eye
O.D.	once a day
o.n.	once a night
o.s.	left eye
o.u.	each eye
p.c.	after eating
p.o.	by mouth
p.r.n.	as necessary
q.h.	every hour
q.i.d., or q.d.	four times a day
Rx	take
$\bar{s}$., or s.	without
s.o.s.	if necessary
$\bar{ss}$.	one-half
sig., or s.	signature
t.i.d., or t.d.	three times a day
t.i.n., or t.n.	three times a night
tinct., or tr.	tincture

Prescription Drugs for Specific Purposes

Each medicine is prescribed in a specific way for a particular purpose. Capsules are powdered drugs or liquids placed in a gelatin container. Suppositories are drugs mixed with a substance such as cocoa butter so that the mixture can be molded into a shape convenient for inserting into the rectum or vagina. Tablets and pills may look alike but technically are different; tablets are powdered drugs pressed in a mold to form a certain shape, while pills may be mixed with a syrup or other substance to help hold the drug particles together. A lozenge or troche is made by mixing the medicine in a mixture of sugar and mucilage, or a fruit base. An elixir may contain the active drug in a solution of water, alcohol, and sugar. A fluid extract is prepared by percolating an alcoholic extract of a drug, derived from a plant product, so that each milliliter of the extract contains one gram of the drug.

Regardless of how a drug is packaged—and often the purpose of dispensing it as an elixir, lozenge, capsule, or whatever, is to make it easier to swallow—the drug must eventually be dissolved and absorbed to be effective, unless it is administered by injection. Even a drug taken orally in liquid form must cross at least one membrane, the lining of the gastrointestinal tract, to reach its target. Depending upon how the drug is intended to affect the body or an organ system, it may be prepared as a weakly acidic or weakly alkaline substance. Acidic drugs, such as aspirin, are absorbed through the wall of the stomach; alkaline drugs are absorbed through the lining of the small intestine. Drugs that are designed for sustained-release action may be coated with a wax that dissolves slowly, or they may be mixed with substances that reduce the absorption rate.

Drugs may be prescribed to be taken before, during, or after meals, depending upon how the medicines are intended to be absorbed. A drug that works best by passing rapidly through the stomach could be less effective, and might even be destroyed, by becoming trapped in a highly acid environment with a meal that takes a long time to digest.

Doctors sometimes speak of the bioavailability of drugs. This refers to the concentration of a drug in the bloodstream, or other body fluid, or to the effect produced at a target organ. For some drugs it is necessary to maintain a certain concentration of the chemical in the bloodstream to achieve the desired effect. When a doctor has a choice of two or more versions of the same drug, he may recommend one particular form of the medicine because of its bioavailability. In other words, two or more drugs may contain the same chemicals in the same dosage, but for various reasons, including those briefly mentioned above, one of them may actually be more therapeutically effective for his patient than the others.

In addition to the bioavailability of a drug, the way in which individual companies formulate a medicine can affect the stability of a drug. Depending upon a doctor's familiarity with stability plus bioavailability, he may prescribe a medicine according to its proprietary, or brand, name rather than its generic name.

Generic Drug Names

The generic name of a drug identifies its chemical or pharmacological relationship in a group of drugs. A generic drug usually has a chemical name which is determined by rules of the American Chemical Society and an international organization of chemists. The trade or proprietary names of drugs are registered with the U.S. Patent Office as trademarks.

The chemical names for certain drugs can be quite long and cumbersome to memorize. For example, there is a commonly used local anesthetic that dentists often use with the generic name of procaine hydrochloride. It is manufactured under at least 27 different trade names, including novocain. The preferred chemical name is 4-aminobenzoic acid 2- (diethylamino) ethyl ester hydrochloride, and there are two equally long alternative chemical names. One drug reference book commonly used by doctors lists close to 10,000 generic names, each with one or more chemical names and an average of five trade names.

No doctor has to keep in mind 10,000 generic names and 50,000 trade names in writing prescriptions. In fact, the majority of common patient complaints probably require a current acquaintance with only a small fraction of the vast variety of substances that have been tested, tried, and accepted for use in treating all known human ills. But even with a couple hundred or less drug names to remember, a doctor may have his reasons for recommending a particular brand of a diuretic with the generic name of furosemide. Most of the drug's 23 brand names are easier to spell, and few primary care physicians would ever remember that it's really 5- (aminosulfonyl) -4-chloro-2 (2-furanylmethyl) amino) benzoic acid.

GENERIC NAME	BRAND NAME	PURPOSE	SIDE EFFECT
Acetazolamide	Diamox	Diuretic	Mild numbness
Aminophylline	Mini-Lix	Bronchodilator	Dizziness
Amitriptylene	Elavil	Antidepressant	Drowsiness
Bacitracin	Baciguent	Antibiotic	Nausea
Betamethasone	Celestone	Anti-inflammation	Itching
Calcium Carbonate	Dicarbosil	Antacid	Constipation
Carisoprodol	Soma	Muscle relaxant	Drowsiness
Chlorpropamide	Diabinese	Oral hypoglycemic (pill for diabetes)	Diarrhea
Diazepam	Valium	Tranquillizer	Fatigue
Digoxin	Lanoxin	Cardiotonic (heart stimulant)	Blurred vision
Ergotamine Tartrate	Ergostat	Migraine	Itching
Furosemide	Lasix	Diuretic	Dehydration
Hydroxyzine Hydrochloride	Vistaril	Tranquillizer	Dry mouth
Ibuprofen	Motrin	Arthritis relief	Heartburn
Imipraime Hydrochloride	Tofranil	Antidepressant	Blurred vision
Kanamycin	Kantrex	Antibacterial	Nausea
Levopropoxyphene Napsylate	Novrad	Cough remedy	Headache
Meclizine Hydrochloride	Antivert	Antihistamine	Drowsiness
Medroxyprogesterone Acetate	Provera	Amenorrhea	Weight change
Oxytetracycline Hydrochloride	Terramycin	Antibacterial	Skin rash
Pemoline	Cylert	Stimulant	Insomnia
Pentobarbital	Nembutal	Sedative	Difficult breathing
Reserpine	Serpasil	Anti-hypertension	Nasal congestion
Spironolactone	Aldactone	Diuretic	Fatigue
Triamcinolone	Aristocort	Allergy relief	Muscular weakness
Trifluoperazine	Stelazine	Tranquillizer	Nasal congestion

GENERIC AND BRAND NAMES OF DRUGS

A generic drug may appear in the marketplace under a variety of brand names. A generic prescription drug also may have more than one medical effect and numerous side effects. The names and effects listed above are examples selected from the published medical literature.

Risk of Drug Interactions

Because many patients receive more than one prescription drug occasionally, if not regularly, the doctor often has to be concerned about possible drug interactions. The risk can increase substantially when the patient self-administers one or more nonprescription drugs while taking the prescription drugs. Aspirin is a common drug interactant, and so are laxatives, certain antacids, and even alcoholic beverages and foods that contain tyramines, such as cheeses.

Any patient who receives a doctor's prescription for a medication would be wise to ask whether it might interact with any other substance being used. Or if a patient taking a drug prescribed by the doctor decides to do a bit of self-medicating with O-T-C products, the prescribing doctor should be queried about a possible interaction. A patient who is treated by more than one physician during the same period should advise each about any medications prescribed by the other doctors. There have been occasions when a patient visiting the offices of several different specialists acquired more than one prescription for the same problem. Any patient is free to visit as many physicians as he or she pleases, but if there is any reason to keep the information away from the other doctors, the patient should have all the prescriptions handled by the same alert pharmacist. He might notice, for example, that the patient would be taking three different diuretics at the same time.

QUESTIONS AND ANSWERS
DRUGS

Q: *What does it mean on a doctor's prescription when a patient is allowed to have aspirin "PO 5-10 gr q 3-4 hr"?*
A: That should be translated as "by mouth 5 to 10 grains every 3 to 4 hours." That would be a typical safe dose level for most adults taking aspirin for a headache or similar health problem.

Q: *How much aspirin is it safe to take during the day for rheumatism?*
A: If you are thinking of aspirin for rheumatoid arthritis or osteoarthritis, your doctor might recommend from 40 to 80 grains a day, divided into perhaps four equal doses. Actually, your doctor probably would want to check your daily intake of aspirin and find out whether that amount might be too much or too little for your personal benefit.

Q: *How can you tell if you are taking too much aspirin?*
A: If you develop a ringing in your ears, with other disturbances in hearing and vision, dizziness, sweating, diarrhea, and/or nausea and vomiting, it's time to cut back on your use of aspirin. If the adverse effects are mainly gastrointestinal, like nausea that can result from irritation of the stomach lining, take an antacid with the aspirin.

Aspirin is rarely a cause of adult fatalities. But it is a common cause of poisoning among children who may be tempted to O.D. on flavored aspirin tablets.

Q: *Is it true that you shouldn't drive a car after taking antihistamines for an allergy?*
A: Yes. It is particularly dangerous to drive a car at night when taking antihistamines. The chemicals in this drug can make you very drowsy and relaxed, the reason they sometimes are used in antimotion sickness reme-dies; and at one time they were a main ingredient in O-T-C tranquillizers.

Q: *Insulin is sold in containers marked U 40 and U 80. Are these different kinds of insulin?*
A: The U 40 means there are 40 units of insulin per cc (cubic centimeter) or ml (milliliter). U 40 and U 80 are the most common insulin strengths prepared, and both are sold in the same size container, usually a 10 cc vial.

Units as a measure of potency of insulin is based on the fact that the hormone is derived from animal glands. The strength of the substance varies according to the source, production conditions, and other factors. So the strength of the insulin is tested and measured in units rather than ounces, grains, milligrams, or the other standard ways of indicating drug doses.

Q: *How can you tell if it's O.K. to use a medicine that has changed color?*
A: It depends on the medicine. The label should tell you whether a change in color will affect the quality of the medicine. Otherwise, dump it down the toilet. Don't take any chances with a medicine that may have deteriorated.

Q: *Is it true that some drugs can cross the placenta in a pregnant woman?*
A: Most drugs can cross the placental barrier and may affect the embryo or fetus. The effects can be most serious during the first three months of pregnancy when vital organs are forming. A woman who is pregnant or is planning to become pregnant should avoid all pharmacologically active substances unless her doctor thinks the benefits outweigh the risks. To be on the safe side, the woman should not even use nonprescription drugs during the pregnancy period.

Q: *What other drugs will aspirin interact with?*

A: More than a dozen commonly prescribed drugs will interact with aspirin. They include steroid hormones, antidiabetic agents, sulfa drugs, and anticoagulants. In some individuals, aspirin may interact with ethyl alcohol to increase the risk of gastrointestinal bleeding, particularly in ulcer-prone people.

Q: *Will caffeine interact with any medicines?*

A: Caffeine is known to interact with monamine oxidase inhibitors to cause hypertensive crises. MAO inhibitors are administered to elevate the mood of depressed patients. Caffeine also can interact with Darvon to cause convulsions. Both of these drug interactions occur when large doses of the drugs are involved.

Q: *Are there any general signs or symptoms that give an early warning of drug allergies or adverse effects?*

A: The only general effect might be skin eruptions, itching, and redness, but this does not apply to reactions from all kinds of drugs.

12

BABIES
BY CHOICE

Marriage partners of the current generation are the first in the history of the human race to have virtually complete control over planning for the birth of their offspring. Never before have women, and men, had access to so much knowledge about human fertility patterns and methods of turning off or on nature's own time-tested techniques for helping the species to survive through the ages. A sexual partnership today has multiple options for preventing conception and terminating pregnancy if a baby is unwanted. Also, it is possible to determine whether a developing embryo or fetus may be normal or abnormal by the technique of amniocentesis, the analysis of the amniotic fluid from the sac enclosing the fetus.

Contraception Is an Old Idea

Although family planning has become so effective only recently, the idea behind that goal is hardly new. There is evidence that contraception is older than ancient civilizations. A cave once inhabited by Cro-Magnon cavemen in Les Ezyies-de-Tayac, France, displays a wall painting of a man and woman engaged in coitus while the man is wearing a penile sheath, or condom.

The Ebers papyrus, the medical handbook of Egyptian doctors who practiced some 3,600 years ago, contains several recipes for pessaries, or vaginal suppositories, that could be used to block the path of the male spermatozoa. One of the recipes recommended a mixture of crocodile dung and honey to be inserted into the vagina before copulation. Another recipe required a mixture of honey and parts of a mimosa plant. These pessaries apparently were intended as barriers rather than as devices that could kill the spermatozoa, although some recipes contained botanical materials that would be effective spermicidals, such as sources of lactic acid or tannic acid. Some spermicidal pessaries also contained salt or alum. Pessaries were concocted from figs, snake fat, lizard ashes, and pomegranate, which might suggest a bit of witchcraft rather than good medical judgment. But the materials did provide absorptive and binding properties that allowed the pessaries to be shaped for easy insertion into the vagina and to be used without falling apart. Ancient Egyptian pessaries were designed to include a piece of string for removing the device after use.

One producer of vaginal pessaries offered a money-back guarantee if one of his contraceptives failed, an offer not matched by any modern manufacturer. However, records fail to reveal whether any early Egyptian customer ever tried to collect on the guarantee.

Onanism is a term that suggests to some that another form of contraception, coitus interruptus, was known in biblical days. The 38th chapter of Genesis describes how Onan, who was instructed by Juda to marry his brother's widow, "knowing that the children should not be his, when he went into his brother's wife, spilled his seed upon the ground, lest children be born in his brother's name." In the same chapter, the story is told that after the death of Juda's wife, Juda was reunited with his daughter-in-law, who bore him twins. "The woman therefore at one copulation conceived," says the Bible, indicating that the ancient Hebrews were well aware that pregnancies could be controlled.

Although the spermatozoa were not observed until after the development of the microscope in the 17th century and the human ovum was seen for the first time many years later, early peoples obviously knew that semen containing a male genetic component of some kind could begin a pregnancy in a woman unless the semen was diverted, as by coitus interruptus, or obstructed by a pessary. They also understood that a woman's menstrual periods stopped when she became pregnant, even though the reasons were rather vague. Early Hindu and Hebrew writings suggested that the embryo might be formed

of menstrual blood and semen. One author calculated that the menstrual blood formed the skin and flesh of the child, and the semen became the brain and bones; a third source, God, contributed the behavioral qualities of the child.

In some primitive cultures women seldom had a chance to menstruate. They were betrothed before puberty and bore children almost continuously until they died. Menstruation became a part of superstition and folklore, and the mine of misinformation associated with it continued into the last century. Because some animals are most fertile when menstruating, Hippocrates believed that couples who wanted to avoid additions to the family should limit sexual intercourse to the days about halfway between menstrual periods. Those days, of course, fall in the part of the reproductive cycle when a woman is likely to be ovulating and thus most vulnerable to pregnancy.

Early Contraceptives

Since Cro-Magnon man left only cave-wall graffiti to show his knowledge of condoms, we may never know how they were manufactured. But there are records of ancient Romans fashioning condoms from the bladders of goats and other animals. Early Egyptians used penile sheaths, although some medical historians contend these were not contraceptive devices but garments worn to protect the penis from insects and parasitic worms. In the Orient penile sheaths were made of a silk paper. Gabriello Fallopio, the 16th-century Italian physician for whom the Fallopian tube is named, recommended a penile sheath made of linen. Sheep intestines, soaked in lye, then scraped and dried, were a source of condoms sold in Europe. Then, as now, condoms were promoted as a means of preventing the spread of venereal disease.

Condoms made of sheep intestines gained popularity during the 17th-century reign of Charles II, who reportedly retained an English physician, a Dr. Condom, to develop a more effective penile sheath that would permit his sexual indulgences without adding to the roster of children claiming the king as their father. Proper Englishmen purchased the devices in white or blue envelopes and called them French letters, but Frenchmen identified condoms as English ridingcoats or English hoods.

The Rubber Condom

The invention of condoms manufactured from vulcanized rubber resulted in a rapid decline in the popularity of the sheep intestine models. Rubber condoms, known popularly as rubbers, are made from thin rubber latex and sold in a single standard size at modest prices, ranging from about 25 cents to over $1 each, depending upon such factors as whether or not they are lubricated or have a reservoir at the tip.

Manufacturers of rubber condoms advise against lubricating the plain kind with petroleum jelly or other materials that may cause the rubber to deteriorate, but it may deteriorate anyway over a period of time if it is not used. Like old medicines, old condoms should be discarded and replaced with new ones. Condoms should not be tested before using by filling them with water or inflating them with air; although the user may be reassured that the condom is safe from leaks or tears, the testing itself can damage the condom.

A fresh new condom when properly used to cover the penis during sexual intercourse is not the perfect contraceptive, but it has a pretty good track record that may explain why it has remained one of the favored methods of birth control for several generations. The risk of pregnancy from a defective condom is only about one in 300. The condom also provides the greatest protection to both the man and woman against venereal disease. Such protection is greater for gonorrhea than for syphilis and herpes genitalis, both of which can be transmitted by contact of skin surfaces not covered by the condom.

Most complaints about the use of condoms involve contact dermatitis-type allergies to chemicals used in their manufacture, lack of sensitivity because of the thin rubber barrier between the penis and the vagina, and the loss of momentum in the sex act because of the need for time out to put on the condom. For those who are allergic to one brand of condom, there are alternative models made from animal membranes. Some lubricated condoms are designed to overcome the penile sensitivity complaint. And the loss of momentum can be avoided by having the woman fit the condom over the penis.

Cervical Caps and Diaphragms

Before the development of the oral contraceptive, there was hardly any birth control device available to men and women that had not been used in some variation since the earliest civilizations or before. The cervical cap and diaphragm, for example, had their forerunners in fruit rinds. Writings of more than a thousand years ago describe methods for fashioning contraceptive cups from pomegranates or citrus fruits. European women in the old days melted beeswax into a disc, then molded the wax disc to form a barrier over the

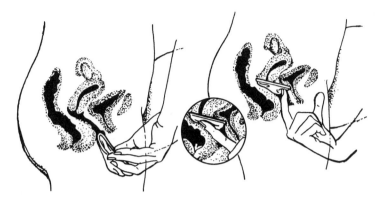

INSERTING THE DIAPHRAGM

The second most popular barrier device for birth control, after the male penis condom, is the diaphragm, which usually is obtained by a doctor's prescription and carefully fitted to insure effectiveness. A spermacide, or contraceptive jelly or cream, is applied to the surface of the diaphragm, which is then inserted into the vagina and pushed upward so it completely covers the cervix.

cervix. Chinese and Japanese women at one time formed cervical caps from oiled silk paper.

Although cervical caps that fit snugly over the cervix are still available, they have been replaced in popularity by other devices such as the rubber diaphragm, which does essentially the same job in providing a barrier between the sperm and the entrance to the uterus, but with less risk of slippage and difficulty in fitting. A typical diaphragm is simply a small rubber hemisphere with a thin metal spring enclosed around the edge to help the device hold its shape. Unlike a condom that comes in a standard size, each diaphragm is custom-fitted for the individual woman user. A doctor or a qualified member of an authorized health agency measures the area of the vagina in which the diaphragm will be fitted and writes a prescription for

a diaphragm of the appropriate size. Since the walls of the vagina will help hold the diaphragm in place while it is being used, the proper fit is very important.

The usual procedure involves an inspection by a doctor to make sure that the diaphragm fits properly and that the woman understands how to insert the diaphragm. The fitting often can be arranged to coincide with a regular vaginal or pelvic examination.

A number of factors can alter the size of diaphragm required. A diaphragm that may have been of proper size for a honeymoon may no longer fit correctly after a period of intercourse and childbearing. Actually, a diaphragm should be replaced about every two years because it gradually loses its original shape and may develop cracks or leaks.

The diaphragm itself is not the complete

contraceptive package. A jelly or cream containing substances to kill any elusive spermatozoon should be placed on the diaphragm's surface facing the cervix before it is inserted for purposes of sexual intercourse. The jelly or cream also should be put along the rim of the diaphragm to block sperm that might slip around the edge. However, applying too much jelly or cream may make the diaphragm slippery so that it will not stay in place during intercourse. The jelly or cream should be applied no more than two hours before the diaphragm is to be used because the spermacide, the name of the substance put in the jelly or cream to kill sperm, loses its effectiveness after about two hours.

While not as foolproof as the oral contraceptive or the intrauterine contraceptive device (IUD), the diaphragm fills an important role in birth control since it provides an alternative for women who may not be able to use the other methods. For a woman approaching menopause the use of oral contraceptives can be risky, and although her natural fertility may have decreased, she still could become pregnant. There also are women who cannot use the IUD because of adverse side effects. Others might prefer the diaphragm because they may expect to have intercourse infrequently and find it inconvenient to take an oral contraceptive every day just to be protected during an occasional sexual encounter.

A diaphragm provides only minimal protection against venereal disease if the man does not wear a condom. The cervical area and the uterus, Fallopian tubes, and ovaries are protected against immediate infection, but venereal disease organisms that enter the vagina could migrate through the cervix after the diaphragm has been removed.

Coitus Interruptus

Coitus interruptus, the birth control method performed by withdrawing the penis from the vagina before ejaculation, is one of the least effective of all serious efforts to prevent conception. The reason simply is that it works much better in theory than in actual practice. Some men are able to control ejaculation so that semen does not enter the unprotected vagina. But others, such as the many who experience premature ejaculation, might fail the test. Ejaculation is an autonomic nerve reflex which is at best difficult to control once it is triggered. Even a small amount of semen accidentally deposited in the vagina at the start of withdrawal may cause the woman to become pregnant. All men are not as quick on the draw as the biblical Onan.

The Rhythm Method

The rhythm method is not quite as risky as coitus interruptus, but it requires in most instances that a couple have the ability of Juda and his daughter-in-law to call their shots accurately. The rhythm method, the only birth control technique accepted officially by the Roman Catholic Church, is based on the concept that a pregnancy can be avoided if a couple is able to forego sexual intercourse during the days in which the woman is most likely to be fertile. The fertile period, of course, covers a few days before and during ovulation.

A woman with a classic 28-day menstrual cycle might be expected to ovulate on or about the 14th day after the start of her last menstrual period, or the half-way point in the cycle. However, only a small percentage of women—perhaps about ten percent—actually have a textbook-type

28-day menstrual cycle. All the rest have menstrual cycles that are longer or shorter than 28 days, and some are more regular than others. Many women never have the same length of menstrual cycle two times in a row.

There is some evidence that menstruation tends to begin about 14 or 15 days after ovulation, regardless of the length of the menstrual cycle. But for practical purposes the rule merely assures a woman that when she menstruates she probably ovulated two weeks earlier. In other words, by using the calendar for contraceptive guidance, a woman can be sure of only two things: if she doesn't menstruate, she's probably pregnant; or if she menstruates, she probably is not pregnant. And this much she probably could figure out without using the basic rhythm method.

There are a couple of variations to the rhythm method that can increase somewhat a woman's chances of avoiding pregnancy. One involves a change in the appearance of the cervical os, the tiny opening into the cervix, that occurs at the time of ovulation. For some women the cervical os dilates, increases a bit in size, at about the time of ovulation. Also, the amount of sugar present in the mucus on the cervix increases measurably. The changes in the opening of the cervical os can be observed by using a mirror and a speculum, an instrument for opening the vaginal orifice to inspect the cervical os. The sugar changes can be checked with a test kit available at drugstores. The kit contains small strips of yellow tape which will turn a dark green or blue at about the time of ovulation when a bit of mucus from the cervix is placed on the tape. The shades of color are darkest at the time of ovulation.

The second variation involves doing a daily temperature check, using a special thermometer called a basal body thermometer. It is designed to make it easier to read changes as small as one-tenth of a degree Fahrenheit. The basal body temperature, which should be recorded every morning before getting out of bed, can be used by some women to enhance the accuracy of the rhythm method, because the body temperature normally changes a fraction of a degree with ovulation.

The temperature can be measured rectally or vaginally, just so it is measured the same way each day. It may show a quick drop of perhaps four or five tenths of a degree at ovulation. Then the temperature jumps perhaps a full degree above the low point, or about half a degree above the preovulation average, and it remains near the higher level until menstruation begins. With the onset of the menstrual period, the temperature returns to a normal basal level. Because human body temperatures can fluctuate with the time of day, or because of infections and other factors, it probably will take several months of charting daily basal temperatures before a woman can tell what may be normal or abnormal in the daily readings.

The human ovum generally is fertile for about the first 24 hours after ovulation but is vulnerable to sperm deposited in the vagina as much as two or three days before ovulation. Therefore, some doctors recommend that a woman using the rhythm method should avoid intercourse for seven days before the ovulation and three days afterward, or a period of about 10 days spanning the usual midpoint of the menstrual cycle.

The rhythm method also can be used by couples trying to achieve conception. By estimating the approximate time of ovulation, they can engage in sexual intercourse on the appropriate days that provide the best chance for conception.

IUD's

The first IUD's, or intrauterine contraceptive devices, may have been stones inserted by their Arab owners into the uteri of female camels to prevent them from becoming pregnant on long caravan treks across the desert. But thousands of miles away, in the Dutch East Indies, women had been using a similar procedure for hundreds of years; they inserted molded balls of latex from native rubber trees into their wombs to prevent pregnancy. It's not known whether the Arab cameldrivers and the East Indian women arrived independently at the notion that by inserting a foreign object into the uterus the female reproductive system might be fooled into thinking that a pregnancy already had started. But apparently the technique was successful though quite risky. After all, the oral contraceptive is based on a similar principle of preventing pregnancy by making the female reproductive system mimic a pregnancy that already may have begun.

The question of exactly how an IUD prevents a pregnancy hasn't really been resolved, despite the popularity of the devices, which now are used by about 10 percent of American women during their fertile years. Some doctors believe the IUD does not prevent fertilization but merely irritates the lining of the uterus so that the ovum, fertilized or not, is simply expelled from the uterus. There is evidence that irritation of the lining causes a release of a substance that has a spermicidal effect and destroys spermatozoa that enter the uterus. Some experts suggest that a substance that kills the spermatozoa also probably would destroy the fertilized ovum.

Attempts to develop safe and effective human IUD's started in Europe at the beginning of the 20th century. The first commercial IUD's were made of animal membranes. Those used today generally are made of plastic, with or without a coating of copper, and are marked with an additional coating of barium so that they can be located on X-ray film.

Like a diaphragm, an IUD needs to be tailored somewhat to the individual woman. She must visit a physician who does a pelvic examination to determine the size and shape of the uterus and its position in the pelvis. The doctor usually recommends that the examination and IUD insertion be made during or immediately after a menstrual period when the cervical os is slightly dilated.

Modern doctors use the utmost caution in inserting an IUD because of individual sensitivities to the device and procedure. All the equipment is sterilized and the patient may be given a local anesthetic. The greatest discomfort from an IUD insertion is likely to be experienced by young women who have not been pregnant and have never before undergone dilation of the cervix. The cervix must be dilated in order to insert the IUD, which should fit snugly inside the uterus. There can be some discomfort associated with the installation since the inserter, or device used to install the IUD, is larger than the IUD.

Several different types of IUD's are used. Some are loops of plastic material that are T-shaped, Y-shaped, or coils; and one is shaped like a tiny shield. A plastic

IUD may be designed with a built-in molecular "memory" of the shape it is supposed to take after it is inserted into the uterus. It can be inserted in a smaller compact shape and then expand to fill the space in the uterus, somewhat like an outdoorsman's pop-up tent expands from a compact size for carrying into a larger, roomier size for practical use.

Each IUD has a plastic filament tail that extends through the cervical os. The IUD tail provides several clues for the doctor and patient. One clue is the length of the tail, which should extend a precise distance if the IUD is in its proper place. If the tail is too long or too short, it is a sign that the IUD has moved out of its proper position in the uterus. Another clue, which may be of some help to a doctor other than the one who installed the IUD in the first place, is the pattern of the IUD tail, or string. Each manufacturer uses a different color or width of string, or some other identification sign such as a tail with tiny knots in it. The tail's chief function is to serve as the means for removing the IUD.

Each doctor has his own reasons for prescribing a particular type or brand of IUD, depending upon his experience and current information about effects of the various kinds available. IUD's, like oral contraceptives, are basically similar, but changes in their design and effectiveness occur periodically, and the model that is "in" today may be outmoded by an improved version that could be introduced tomorrow. An IUD that causes adverse effects should be removed or replaced. Even if a device results in no serious problems, it should be checked periodically by the doctor.

Among problems encountered by women using the IUD method of birth control are automatic expulsion of the IUD, which some doctors attribute to failure to install the IUD properly. Other problems include a slightly increased risk of infection of the uterus, a risk of perforation of the uterus by the IUD, some discomfort experienced mainly by the man during intercourse, and a chance of pregnancy, particularly an ectopic pregnancy, or one that occurs outside the uterus, such as in a Fallopian tube.

The IUD usually is not recommended for women with a disorder or abnormality of the reproductive system, such as a tumor or cancer of the uterus or cervix, or inflammation of any part of the system.

Oral Contraceptives

Are oral contraceptives new? Medical historians probing the records of alchemists and practitioners of witchcraft over the centuries have identified more than 100 kinds of plant leaves, roots, and berries used in potions intended to prevent conception. Some botanicals used in ancient birth control potions in Asia and Europe actually contained chemicals associated with human fertility. Women in Sumatra believed they could avoid pregnancy by eating betel nuts each morning at sunrise for three consecutive days. Siberian women once believed they could prevent conception by drinking an herbal tea made with chickweed each day that they were not menstruating. In the Middle East and North Africa, there were women who believed that eating castor beans with their meals would reduce the risk of pregnancy.

The early stages of the development of modern oral contraceptives may seem equally outlandish. In the 1940's, for example, women with abnormal menstrual rhythms were given hypodermic injections of hormones obtained from farm animals. Five injections of natural estrogen, followed by five injections of natural progesterone each month for three months, helped 15 percent of the patients treated. Later, women were given estrogen therapy in the form of capsules containing a crystallized substance prepared from the urine of pregnant mares. It was described by the manufacturer as "practically odorless and without unpleasant taste." Thousands of animals were needed to obtain hormones that cost thousands of dollars per ounce.

Nature's way of controlling ovulation is approximately what happens when a woman uses oral contraceptive pills (see page 405). The hormones create the physiological illusion of a normal reproductive cycle except that an ovum is not released and follicle development is suppressed by the condition of pseudopregnancy. When the monthly supply of oral contraceptive pills has been used, the hormonal support of the endometrium ceases and the lining sloughs off in a typical menstruation. The pills not only mimic nature in suppressing the development of what normally would be the next ovum, they offer such additional protection as causing formation of a thick spermicidal mucus at the cervix to discourage any spermatozoon that might attempt to enter the uterus.

The oral contraceptive is regarded as the nearly perfect birth control device. A woman taking the proper formulation exactly as directed is virtually immune to pregnancy because no ovum is released and conception therefore cannot occur. However, the oral contraceptive falls a bit short of being an ideal medication, even

with some 40 different brands with varied formulations to choose from. There are as many adverse side effects from oral contraceptives as there are brands and formulations. The side effects range from increased blood pressure, stroke, and myocardial infarction down to simple problems like headaches, fluid retention, and nausea. Fortunately, from the experiences of literally tens of millions of women around the world who have used various oral contraceptive formulations since the pill was introduced in 1960, doctors have been able to sort out the side effects and risks according to formulations and contributing factors other than the hormones.

For example, if a woman develops fluid retention or nausea, her doctor might advise a different pill that contains less estrogen per dose. If she develops headaches or high blood pressure, the doctor might recommend either a lower dose of estrogen or an alternative method of birth control. The doctor may consider the involvement of contributing factors to the pill's effects, such as age and lifestyle. The risk of heart attacks among pill users is increased considerably if the patients smoke cigarettes. Older women seem to be at risk from the side effects of oral contraceptives. A woman smoker over the age of 40 might be advised to avoid oral contraceptives entirely.

Oral contraceptive hormones are potent chemicals that can cause dramatic changes in a woman's physiology. Each woman using or contemplating the use of the drugs should discuss frankly with her doctor the factors in her own health condition and lifestyle that might interact with the hormones. Also, there are points to be considered regarding the alternatives.

Those who favor use of the pill often point out, for example, that despite the risks of using oral contraceptives a woman may face greater dangers to her health if she becomes pregnant.

Abortion As a Last Resort

At least a few experienced physicians recommend that couples use condoms and/or diaphragms as birth control measures, and in the event of a failure resort to abortion. Since laws governing abortions have changed in recent years, the risk of complications has been reduced considerably and the main obstacles for many couples are of a moral or religious nature. In any event, an abortion is not a simple procedure, even when performed in the first trimester of the pregnancy.

An abortion performed by qualified medical personnel is equivalent to a minor surgical procedure. The clinic may require a complete medical history and physical examination, including blood and urine laboratory tests, Pap smear, chest X-ray, and test for gonorrhea. A local anesthetic usually is administered, but a general anesthetic may be available for a woman who wants to go to sleep while pregnant and wake up without a pregnancy; a general anesthetic also may be available on standby in case complications develop. Some clinics insert a cervical dilator a day before the abortion so entry to the uterus will be easier. The woman may be given instructions about pre-operative routines, such as consuming no food or beverage after dinner the night before the procedure. Certain medications may have to be curtailed or adjusted.

An abortion performed during the first three months of pregnancy may be done

with a suction device that is inserted into the uterus. If there are no complications, the procedure is over in a few minutes and the woman is allowed to get dressed and leave after a brief rest in a recovery room. She should be able to return to her daily routine after an additional day of rest. Sexual intercourse should be avoided for

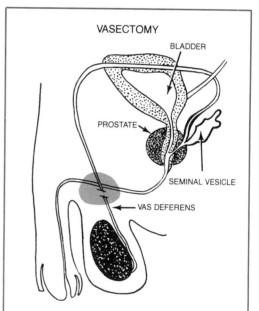

VASECTOMY

BLADDER

PROSTATE

SEMINAL VESICLE

VAS DEFERENS

A common method of "permanent" birth control for men is the comparatively safe and simple operation called a vasectomy. As the diagram shows, the two vas deferens, or tubes carrying sperm from the testes to the ejaculatory duct area of the prostate and seminal vesicles, is cut and a small piece of the ducts is removed. Although a woman still could become pregnant from spermatozoa still in the vas deferens pipeline, new sperm presumably would be unable to move across the break in the duct. Restoration of fertility sometimes is possible by means of a new operation to rejoin the severed ends of the vas deferens.

at least two weeks. There will often be postoperative bleeding that has been described as comparable to a very heavy menstrual flow.

Abortions after the first 12 weeks may involve a dilation and curettage (D & C) procedure, or the administration of prosta-glandins or a salt solution called hypertonic saline, which are injected into the sac of amniotic fluid surrounding the fetus. Abortions after the 12th week of pregnancy are much more complicated, expensive, and risky.

See also Chapter 6: *Sex Organs.*

QUESTIONS AND ANSWERS
BABIES BY CHOICE

Q: *I had a tubal ligation after giving birth to two children by my first husband. Now I have remarried and my new husband would like to have children. Can the tubal ligation be repaired?*

A: Frankly, there is a less than 50 percent success rate in performing a successful tubal ligation repair. During the original operation, a section of the Fallopian tube is removed. As a result, when the two remaining ends are rejoined they will be of different diameters. A further complication is a high incidence of tubal pregnancies in women who have been able to accomplish conception after a tubal ligation repair. So, while it's possible, the condition is not bright for a successful pregnancy.

Q: *Is it easier to restore fertility in a man who has undergone a vasectomy?*

A: As in tubal ligation repair, it is possible to surgically rejoin the ends of the vas deferens tubes that were cut in the original procedure. However, since a section is removed from each tube during a vasectomy, the remaining ends will never match exactly in diameter. When the procedure has been successful enough to allow spermatozoa to appear in the semen once more, the sperm often are not viable enough to fertilize an ovum. One explanation for the sperm failure is that the spermatozoa are treated as foreign tissue by the rejoined tube surfaces and are rejected much as bacteria or viruses would be treated by antibodies defending their home turf. See illustration, page 407.

Q: *I have read that a woman on the pill can become pregnant if she develops a stomach flu. Can this be true?*

A: There is pretty good evidence that stomach flu and several other kinds of gastrointestinal disorders can result in failure of the hormones in oral contraceptives to be absorbed adequately from the intestinal tract. A woman who develops diarrhea while using the pill might want to consider the use of alternate forms of contraception for the remainder of the menstrual cycle, because the effect of the GI disorder could be equivalent to skipping the pill for each day that the symptoms persist.

Q: *Since hormone therapy is used sometimes to stop a tall girl from growing taller, will oral contraceptives keep a short girl from reaching average height?*

A: While it is true that estrogens are used occasionally to hasten the end of long bone growth in young girls who appear to be growing too tall too soon, it's unlikely that the estrogen in oral contraceptives would stunt a girl's growth. An exception might be made for a girl who started using oral contraceptives at a very early age. But most young ladies already have reached their maximum height by the time they take the pill.

Q: *I was told that women on the pill should take vitamins also. Do you agree?*

A: There have been several published studies showing that the estrogen in oral contraceptives can cause a deficiency of vitamin C and a couple of B vitamins, mainly vitamin B-6. Most people who eat a well-balanced diet get enough vitamin B-6, which actually is a collective term for three nutrient chemicals present in a wide variety of animal and plant foods. But the vitamin is associated with female reproductive physiology, and deficiencies have been observed in pregnant women. It would be wise to mention the matter to your doctor on your next visit. Signs of a B-6 deficiency include changes in the skin and mucous membranes of the mouth area, as well as anemia, and these can be checked quite easily by the doctor.

Q: *Is a saline abortion a safe procedure?*
A: It is relatively safe if done very carefully. Unfortunately, the method has been associated with an assortment of complications that has resulted in the hypertonic saline abortion technique being discontinued in some clinics. The complications can result from accidental injection of the saline solution, which is a 20 percent salt solution, into the wall of the uterus or the fetal blood supply system. When such accidents occur, the misdirected salt solution can result in death of the patient or damage to the uterus that requires a hysterectomy.

Q: *How can you be sure an abortion clinic and its doctors are safe to use?*

A: You can start by finding a doctor who can give you some guidance in this area. All doctors are not enthusiastic about involvement in abortion matters, and you may not see eye-to-eye with your own doctor on this subject. Then check the credentials of the clinics and personnel you may be dealing with. Most authorized family planning agencies can provide information about abortion clinics in your own community. Of course, you can always visit one or more clinics to see it for yourself before the actual need for an abortion arises. Shopping for a proper abortion clinic might seem a bit unusual, but if you expect to use the services of one someday, why not plan ahead?

13

PREGNANCY AND CHILDBIRTH

Pregnancy should not be considered as an illness that afflicts the mother. Although some body functions are altered temporarily by the effects of approaching motherhood, pregnancy actually is a natural process that has been going on for perhaps millions of years. And the chances for a safe and successful delivery have never been better than they are today.

An expectant mother may hear many old wives' tales about the hazards of pregnancy from well-meaning friends. Although complications may develop in a few cases, most pregnancy problems can be prevented or corrected with proper medical care and the basic rules of good health and hygiene.

Hazards to the Unborn Child

For the developing child, the first nine months of life—from conception to delivery—can be the most dangerous period of existence. From the first days as a tiny cluster of multiplying cells inching through a Fallopian tube until the delivery when atmospheric oxygen fills the lungs, the individual is a helpless creature. A new baby may be subjected to a myriad hazards, ranging from contact with stray viruses or strange drugs that cross the placenta from the mother, to the ruthless Russian roulette of genetic defects that can snap the thread of life before the infant leaves the womb.

The embryo usually is most sensitive to the environmental hazards encountered by the mother at a very early stage of development. During the first few weeks after her last menstruation, a woman may not be certain that she is pregnant. During the first few weeks of embryonic life the new individual is most vulnerable to risk factors transmitted from the mother's exposure to her environment. These factors may be associated with infectious diseases, abuse of drugs—both the legal and socially acceptable drugs as well as the illicit kinds—and pollutants in the water, food, and air.

Until the 1950's many doctors assumed that the placenta formed a true protective barrier that isolated the embryo from dangerous substances that might enter the

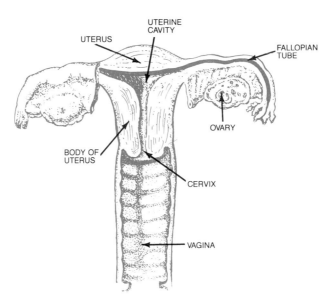

Conception generally occurs in a Fallopian tube after an ovum, or egg cell, is released from an ovary and is fertilized by a male's sperm while the ovum is moving toward the uterus. A fertilized ovum will become implanted in the endometrial lining of the uterus and develop into an embryo.

mother's body tissues. But the tragedy of the thalidomide babies in Europe demonstrated that a sedative designed to be safe and effective for mothers could cross the placental barrier and cause gross physical deformities in the embryo. Medical scientists have since found that many seemingly innocent substances used by the mother may be responsible for congenital defects in newborn infants. Because of the often unknown hazards of potential teratogens, the medical name for substances that cause birth defects, doctors now advise women expecting to become pregnant to avoid exposure to substances suspected of contributing to congenital defects. Changing a lifestyle after pregnancy begins may be too late to help the embryo.

Formation of the Zygote

Within ten days after ovulation, which is a few days before a woman would miss her usual menstrual period, the fertilized ovum, or zygote, usually will be implanted in the lining of the uterus and will begin to develop into a human. The zygote may reach the lining of the uterus as early as five days after ovulation, or approximately ten days before the woman's next menstrual period might normally begin. By the time many, if not most, women realize they are pregnant, the zygote already has established its base of operations in the endometrial lining of the uterus and has taken the first steps toward developing its true embryonic tissues.

The human child develops from the fertilized ovum, or zygote, by a series of cell divisions. The fertilized ovum divides into two cells, the two cells divide into four, then eight cells, and so on. By the time the zygote reaches the uterus it has taken on the appearance of a very tiny mulberry. Through a simple doubling of cells, the zygote will have multiplied into a million body cells after 20 such divisions. After perhaps fewer than 50 such generations of cell divisions, the original ovum may have produced all the body cells a human needs to begin life on its own.

The development of a human child actually is a more complex process than might be indicated by a multiple series of cell divisions. As the cells multiply, they differentiate into specialized cells of various shapes and sizes. Information built into the human genetic code tells the new cells that some are to become skin, others are to become blood cells, liver tissue, or part of the central nervous system. Some cells will eventually grow faster than others, and some, such as nerve cells, will lose their ability to divide and grow after reaching their mature size and function. Still others, like the epithelial cells lining the intestinal tract, will continue replenishing their kind for the rest of the individual's lifetime. All of the developmental steps follow in an orderly sequence which is repeated in each individual in every generation.

The zygote gets its initial food supply from the blood and sugar-enriched endometrial lining of the uterus. The tiny cluster of cells burrows deeply into the lining, which seems to dissolve into a small pool of nutrients surrounding the cells. At this stage the cells form a unit sometimes called a trophoblast. Fingerlike projections, known as villi, develop from the surface of the trophoblast and invade the endometrium to absorb more nutrients. The villi soon number in the hundreds and develop tiny blood vessels, then slowly evolve into a true placenta. The nutrients absorbed by the villi are passed along to a primitive umbilical cord which begins to appear in a watery environment inside a tiny cavity called the amnion. The true

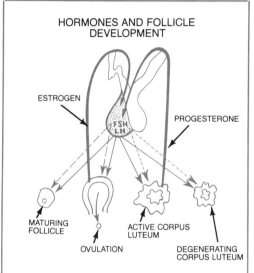

HORMONES AND FOLLICLE DEVELOPMENT

ESTROGEN
FSH LH
PROGESTERONE
MATURING FOLLICLE
OVULATION
ACTIVE CORPUS LUTEUM
DEGENERATING CORPUS LUTEUM

The female reproductive cycle involves a complex hormonal feedback system of the pituitary gland at the base of the brain and the ovaries. The follicle-stimulating hormone (FSH) of the anterior pituitary gland stimulates the ovary to cause a follicle containing an ovum to mature and release the ovum. This process is called ovulation. The same follicle-stimulating hormone causes the development of spermatozoa in the male testes. The ovary produces the hormone estrogen that feeds back to the anterior pituitary, which stimulates the production of a second ovarian hormone, progesterone, from the corpus luteum that develops from the ruptured follicle. If the ovum fails to become fertilized and implanted in the uterus, the feedback message to the pituitary carries the instruction to begin another menstrual cycle by releasing another round of FSH.

umbilical cord appears during the fifth week, and the amnion slowly increases in size until it eventually holds about two quarts of amniotic fluid.

When fully developed, the umbilical cord is about one-half inch in diameter and two feet long, sometimes much longer and sometimes much shorter. It encloses two arteries and one large vein which carry blood between the developing child and the surface of the placenta. There is no direct exchange of blood between the mother and the developing infant. The mother's blood circulates through cavities between the placenta and the uterus, literally bathing the villi extending into the lining of the uterus. Proteins, fats, carbohydrates, oxygen, and other nutrients are absorbed from the mother's blood through the villi. Waste products of the embryo's metabolism are released into the placental pool and are picked up by the mother's circulatory system and excreted.

Signs of Pregnancy

After the trophoblast becomes implanted in the uterus, it begins producing the chorionic gonadotrophic hormone, or HCG. When a woman becomes pregnant, traces of HCG begin to appear in her blood and urine. Discovery of the hormone led to the development of pregnancy tests. A small amount of urine from a woman who has missed her period is injected into a laboratory animal. If HCG is present in the urine, it will cause the ovaries of female animals to develop ruptured follicles. A few drops of the urine placed on a microscope slide with a drop of antiserum from a rabbit injected with HCG and a couple of drops of a latex preparation will result in clumping of the latex particles if the woman is not pregnant. If HCG is present in the urine, the particles will not clump, thus indicating pregnancy.

Other evidence of pregnancy can be

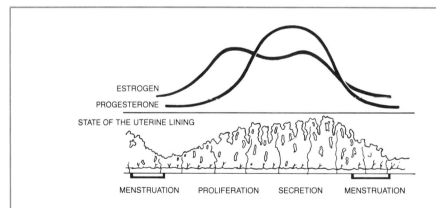

Drawing shows how the estrogen hormone level increases until ovulation and progesterone level peaks with corpus luteum formation in the ovary. Meanwhile, the uterine lining proliferates in preparation for the arrival of a fertilized ovum. If conception fails to occur, estrogen and progesterone production taper off, and the lining of uterus sloughs off as the menstrual flow. Menstrual cycle patterns are the basis of the rhythm method of birth control.

found in the traditional signs and symptoms used before the development of laboratory pregnancy tests. A woman who becomes pregnant may experience an increased frequency of urination because of growing pressure of the uterus on the bladder, breast enlargement, the nausea and vomiting of "morning sickness," a sustained increase of about one degree Fahrenheit in body temperature as measured in the morning, a bluish coloration called cyanosis in the vaginal area because of the congestion of blood veins there, and a softening of tissues around the cervix and vagina. These signs are not proof-positive of a pregnancy, but they are sufficiently good clues to warrant a visit to a doctor's office for an examination.

Development of the Embryo

During the early weeks of a pregnancy, the placenta is nearly as large as the embryo. But in the fifth month of gestation, the growth rate of the developing child increases sharply, and at the time of delivery a baby will weigh about six times as much as its placenta.

During the seventh or eighth week the embryo is less than an inch in length and weighs about $\frac{1}{28}$th of an ounce. Nevertheless, that tiny creature is nearly 50 times as large as it was at four weeks. In the third month an embryo will undergo a 14-fold gain in weight, although it will barely tip the scales at one-half ounce. At this stage the embryo will need only about two inches of space as it lies folded within the amniotic sac; if it could stretch to its full length, it would be about three inches tall.

By the end of the fourth week the embryo that was little more than a cluster of cells in its second week normally has acquired definite animal-like features, including a heart, brain, optic vesicles that will become eyes, and primitive jaws. During the second month, as the umbilical cord becomes more prominent, the face with eyes, ears, and nose becomes more human in appearance. The buds of the limbs appear with the fingers and toes outlined. A liver grows beneath the tiny heart and, along with other internal or-

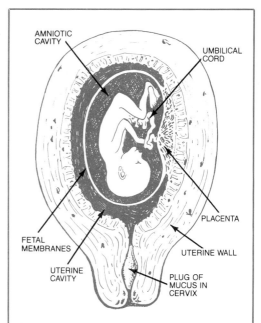

Illustration shows how a fetus develops within the uterus. The developing infant is cushioned by fluid that fills the amniotic cavity, and it receives oxygen and nutrients through the umbilical cord which draws its supplies of nourishment from the mother's blood supply. The placenta, which receives food and oxygen from the blood vessels in the mother's uterine wall, removes the waste products of the fetus into the mother's blood supply.

gans, moves deep into the embryonic body.

At the end of two months the human body pattern is pretty well established, and mostly minor changes will appear as growth continues. The embryo has acquired nerves and muscles, which it can contract so that independent movement is possible. From this point in its development, the individual is no longer considered an embryo and is promoted to the status of fetus.

Growth of the Fetus

Independent movement by the fetus is a milestone in its development, although several more weeks will pass before muscle activity will become strong enough to be felt by the mother. But as if rehearsing for life outside the womb, the fetus goes through an almost daily routine of muscle exercises. It can open its hand or make a fist, move the lips and make a swallowing action, nod the head or turn it, and move the arms and legs as if swimming in the amniotic fluid.

In the meantime, the fetus doubles in length and increases its weight six-fold. Weighing in at almost four ounces and measuring more than four inches in length, it is big enough and strong enough to make its presence felt by the mother. At first the mother feels only a flutter once or twice a day. But the intensity and frequency of movement gradually increase until the mother may feel the movements 100 times each day as the delivery date approaches. The first movements, or quickening, held special significance in the Middle Ages, when people believed the fetal activity marked the beginning of the soul and an independent life for the child.

Quickening varies with different women and even in different pregnancies of the same mother. The mother may become so familiar with the signals caused by jabbing elbows and kicking feet that she may become concerned if they stop for a day or two. Usually, an interruption in quickening is not a cause for alarm during the first six months, but the doctor should be consulted if fetal activity stops during the last three months. The amount of activity sometimes depends upon the amount of space for prenatal play, and as the end of the pregnancy approaches, the fetus may have little room for any activity except kicking. The amount of fatty tissue on a woman may affect her sensitivity to the fetal activity. A normally thin pregnant woman could be expected to feel more kicking and jabbing than a well-cushioned neighbor at the same stage of pregnancy.

At five months, the fetus begins to grow hair on the head and body. The heartbeat can be heard with a stethoscope. The eyelids are still fused but they can make blinking motions. The chest muscles can make respiration movements, even though the fetus will remain immersed in a half-gallon of fluid for several additional months. The child will be able to move the muscles involved in facial expressions. At this time he will be about 12 inches long and will weigh approximately two pounds. Quickening may become active to the point where a kick or jab by the fetus can be observed as a movement in the mother's abdominal wall. But vital organs are not mature enough at this stage to function normally if premature delivery should occur.

At seven months, the fetus will have about 70 percent of its normal length at birth. The rate of weight gain will be slowed somewhat, and the child may weigh about two pounds. If delivered prematurely, a fetus at seven months will have a good chance to survive. But it will look like a wrinkled old person because the subcutaneous fat needed to pad out the body is deposited later. Even when transferred to the womb-like security of an incubator, the premature infant will appear in a stupor, unable to detect the difference between day and night. Breathing usually is difficult, cries are almost inaudible, and although the sucking reflex has been present for several weeks it doesn't seem to be able to feed or even indicate if it is hungry. According to the built-in time clock of a 28-week-old fetus, it is still in its mother's womb; although dumped abruptly into the real world, it will assume the fetal position and appear to be floating in the warm, timeless environment of the amniotic fluid.

A premature infant generally gains nothing in the way of development as a result of entering the outside world ahead of schedule. A child delivered at seven months reaches the same stage of maturity at normal term as a child delivered at the usual nine months. At nine months plus one week, a full-term infant and a premature infant conceived at the same time can be expected to have the same degree of physical development and behavioral pattern. During its period in the incubator, a premature infant undergoes the same pattern of development it would experience if it remained in the uterus.

Pregnancy Timetable

The length of a human pregnancy is approximately 265 days from conception to delivery, or 280 days if figured by the LMP method, a bit of medical shorthand

sometimes used to figure from the Last Menstrual Period. Since conception occurs about halfway through an average menstrual cycle, both numbers are roughly correct. But there often are several unknown variables involved, including the precise date that fertilization actually occurred after the start of the LMP. Because of these variables, doctors seldom make bets on the dates that babies may choose as their birthdays.

During the 265 days—more or less—of prenatal life, the body weight of an individual increases about six billion times. From birth to adulthood, the gain in weight for an average human is only 20 to 30 times. In the last month of normal fetal life alone, an infant increases its weight by nearly 40 percent. A number of changes in body proportions also occur during development of an individual from prenatal life to adulthood. For example, a human in the early fetal stages is nearly 50 percent trunk and 43 percent head and neck, and the legs represent only about two percent of body volume. But by the time the individual reaches adulthood, the head and neck account for only about 10 percent of body volume, while the legs have increased in proportion to 29 percent. The trunk decreases from 50 percent of the body volume in the early fetal stages to 44 percent at birth, but it increases again to about 50 percent in the mature person.

Changes in the Pregnant Woman's Body

The nutritional needs of the mother vary somewhat from conception through nursing because each phase of pregnancy makes somewhat different demands on hormones, proteins, vitamins, and energy reserves of the mother's body. The endometrium, for example, requires larger than usual levels of glucose, a carbohydrate, while helping the trophoblast to feather its nest in the uterine lining. The glucose used to sustain the budding embryo during this period is drawn from the mother's own stores of glycogen, or body starch.

Since this activity usually begins before the mother knows for sure whether or not she is pregnant, what the mother eats before pregnancy can be almost as important as what she eats during the time she is carrying the child. Women who conceive when they are in an undernourished or malnourished state may find it difficult to catch up with the stresses of pregnancy after the fact of conception has been confirmed.

The placenta, the only source of essential nutrients for the developing fetus, becomes the equivalent of an extra body organ. The fetus has a frankly parasitic existence for nine months or more, depending upon whether the mother becomes the source of nursing nourishment after the birth of child.

The mother's body during pregnancy may store more nitrogen than is needed for protein by the developing fetus. But the nitrogen reserve is part of nature's insurance policy to protect the mother during the period of birth, when her body will lose more nitrogen than it normally would be able to accumulate. The mother's body also may accumulate more calcium than is needed for building teeth and bones in the fetus. The difference develops because the mother's tissues require added calcium for metabolic activities and to insure adequate calcium levels in the mother's blood at the time of delivery when there is a chance of hemorrhage.

Weight Gains During Pregnancy

The amount of weight gained by the mother during pregnancy is only an indirect measure of the state of nourishment of parent and child. It does not reveal the proportions of nitrogen, calcium, or other nutrient elements stored in the mother's body tissues, or the amounts consumed at any point in the development of the fetus. However, the rate of weight gain can be a guide to the general health of the mother and child.

A healthy mother-to-be can expect to gain from 25 to 35 pounds during the 40 weeks of gestation. A large woman with a heavy body build might gain more than a smaller woman, but there is no general agreement on this point. The rate of weight gain accelerates during the pregnancy period, amounting to little more than a pound per month at the beginning, but increasing to a gain of a pound per week during the final month.

The pattern of weight gain can be more important than the amount of weight gained. A sudden spurt in weight after the 20th week might be a sign of edema, or fluid retention. The amount of amniotic fluid, plus the added fluid in the mother's tissues at the time of delivery, can equal the weight of the fetus under normal circumstances, so a mother may be only vaguely aware of a greater than normal fluid gain.

Some women may gain too much weight during pregnancy, which can be as risky as not gaining enough weight at a proper rate of gain. They may rationalize that they must "eat for two," which might even be translated by the woman as eating enough for two adults. Actually, the calorie need for an average woman during pregnancy may amount to only 1,800 to 2,100 per day, or around ten percent more than would be needed to maintain a normal weight for a nonpregnant woman.

Proper Nutrition For the Mother-To-Be

A nonpregnant woman, according to the U.S. National Research Council, needs a daily protein intake of about one gram per kilogram, or about two pounds of body weight. Thus, a woman whose normal weight is 130 pounds would need approximately 65 grams of protein per day. During pregnancy the amount of protein consumed per day should be increased by about 25 grams. If the mother nurses the baby after its birth, her protein intake should be boosted by some 40 grams.

A three-ounce piece of roast beef or bluefish contains about 22 grams of protein, as does a half-cup of tuna fish salad, a hamburger patty, or one-fourth of a broiled chicken. A cup of milk provides around nine grams of protein, along with a number of essential minerals and vitamins. The main difference between whole milk, skim milk, and buttermilk is the amount of fat content; they all have the same minerals and vitamins in similar amounts. One ounce of cheese or a cooked egg, for variety, provides about six grams of protein.

There are a number of arguments in favor of high-protein diets for pregnant women. One is that the fetus, being a thriving parasite, may begin drawing upon the protein reserves in the mother's body tissues if the dietary intake of proteins is not sufficient. A source of protein in the mother's body that might be depleted is the mother's blood plasma. Studies of mothers in blockaded European countries during World War II, when protein foods were scarce, found that babies gen-erally were born smaller and three weeks prematurely as compared to prewar babies.

The parasitic fetus also may draw upon the mother's own calcium reserves if the amount of calcium in the mother's diet is not adequate. A fetus requires an average of about one-tenth of a gram of calcium per day during its life in the womb, although nearly 60 percent of the calcium is utilized by the fetus during its last month in the uterus. In order to maintain her own daily calcium needs and to accumulate the reserves the body may need to carry the mother safely through delivery, the mother should plan meals that provide at least one and a half grams of calcium each day. A quart of milk per day contains most of the mother's daily calcium needs, but in certain cases the doctor might advise against that much milk because it might contribute an overabundance of other nutrients. An excess of phosphorus, for example, can interfere with normal utilization of calcium. In such cases the doctor might recommend alternative calcium sources, such as canned salmon or sardines.

The mother's calcium intake, in any case, should be matched with vitamin D, which helps the body make effective use of calcium in the diet. Vitamin D usually is added to milk by commercial dairies because it isn't naturally available in cow's milk, so the mother-to-be should read the labels to make sure she gets the vitamin with the milk.

Among other vitamins of particular concern to a pregnant woman is the B-6 complex that is needed for protein metabolism, including both the breaking down of amino acids from dietary proteins and the building of new proteins from the amino acid units. Deficiencies of vitamin B-6 often occur in pregnant women, as well as in women using oral contraceptives. B-6 deficiency usually is manifested in the form of skin disorders, depression, irritability, and a general feeling of weakness. In pregnant women the signs of a B vitamin lack also may include anemia and a tendency to hemorrhage after delivery.

Identifying Potential Birth Defects

During the fourth month of pregnancy, the doctor may want to check on the condition of the developing fetus by analyzing amniotic fluid cells, a technique known as amniocentesis. This is a relatively low-risk method of diagnosing possible birth defects at an early stage of pregnancy. The fetus and placenta are located in the uterus by the use of ultrasound imaging, which produces a silhouette of the child and its surroundings. Locating these objects is important so that amniotic fluid can be extracted with a hollow needle while avoiding contact with the fetus and placenta. The needle insertion is virtually painless, although it must pass through the abdominal wall of the mother and the wall of the uterus.

About a half ounce of amniotic fluid is withdrawn in this procedure, sometimes described as prenatal diagnosis. The information gained from the study of fetal tissue cells and the fluid itself can be immensely valuable to the parents and doctors, although the test itself may cost several hundred dollars and results may not be available for several weeks.

By obtaining cell samples sloughed off by the skin, medical personnel can study the genetic material in the nuclei of the cells and determine months in advance of birth whether the child will be a boy or a girl. The girl baby will have an XX sex chromosome combination, and a boy will have an XY sex chromosome pairing. Also, by analyzing the cell chemistry of the fetus, a rather close estimate can be made of the precise age of the fetus.

Many chromosomal abnormalities, which would forecast probable birth defects, can be detected by studying the genetic material in the cell nuclei. With a few rare exceptions, every body cell of an individual should contain the same chromosome characteristics as the original body cell, the zygote formed by the union of the ovum and spermatozoon. The rare exceptions in which more than one chromosome pattern is represented will signal abnormalities.

More than 60 different genetic defects or congenital disorders can be found through prenatal diagnostic techniques. These include Down's syndrome (mongolism), Cooley's anemia, neural tube defects such as spina bifida, hemophilia, and a form of muscular dystrophy. Chemical analysis of amniotic fluid can tell the doctor whether the developing fetus is getting a sufficient amount of oxygen. Amniocentesis also can provide clues regarding possible problems of an Rh blood factor incompatibility that would require a blood transfusion for the child.

A substance called alpha-fetoprotein found in the amniotic fluid during the embryo stage of development is a more reliable indicator of the health of the developing infant than the X-rays and ultrasound techniques previously used to detect certain possible defects. Just the fact that alpha-fetoprotein is present in the amniotic fluid in abnormally high concentrations usually is a clue that something may be amiss in the uterus.

Fetal Development in the Later Stages

The ultrasound equipment used to locate the fetus and placenta for taking a sample of amniotic fluid without pricking the fetus or puncturing the placenta also is employed in the later stages of fetal development. For example, ultrasound may be used to determine the position of the fetus in the uterus and the size of the fetus as the delivery date approaches. Information of that sort can help the mother and doctor learn whether any delivery problems such as a breech presentation might be expected or if a caesarian delivery should be planned.

When the due date approaches, the mother usually receives a few signals that the baby is getting ready to move out of the womb and into the real world. One signal is the movement of the baby, usually head-first, into the lower part of the pelvis. The situation often is identified as lightening, although the doctor also may use the term "engagement" to describe the effect of the fetus becoming more or less locked into a delivery position. In some cases the baby might change its mind and float into a higher position in the uterus for another week or so before moving into another lightening position.

The lightening usually will be felt by the mother in one or more ways. She may have an increased urge to urinate because of added pressure on the bladder, and at the same time her breathing becomes easier because of reduced pressure of the baby against the chest area. The mother also may feel pressure in the area of the pubic bone, and may experience increased difficulty in walking because of pressure directed toward the hip joints. Women who have delivered previously may experi-

ence the lightening differently because of wear and tear on the pelvic tissues from the earlier pregnancies.

At this stage, if other signs of delivery are present, the doctor may be able to determine the position of the baby by palpation through the abdominal wall. The exact location of the baby in the mother's pelvis may be recorded according to the stations, or positions, of the fetal head with respect to the pelvic bones. The stations range from a +3 if the head of the fetus is well up in the pelvis to a –3 if the head is down about as far as it can go in the pelvis. The "0", or zero, station is marked by a pair of pelvic bone spurs along the birth canal.

Period of Labor

Labor occurs in several stages, not including false labor which is characterized by brief uterine contractions and a mild aching sensation in the abdomen. False labor has no real significance except that it often results in a trip to the hospital and a return trip home when the doctors and nurses determine that the signs of true labor are missing. What distinguishes true labor is dilatation of the cervix, regular forceful contractions of the uterus, and movement of the fetus toward the birth canal. The woman may notice the dilatation of the cervix by the discharge of a mucus plug that has been blocking the cervical os. The mucus plug, usually tinged with blood and sometimes called "show," is not a true labor signal; it may occur at any time from a day to a week before the start of true labor.

The pains of labor vary according to the emotional and physical condition of the mother, the strength of the uterine contractions, and the relationship between the fetus and the pelvic tissues as it moves through the birth canal. The pains, or contractions of the uterus, become increasingly frequent, powerful, and prolonged as labor progresses through the first stage. Labor pains are the usual effect; it is unusual for a woman to feel little or no discomfort while giving birth.

The fetal membranes break at the start of true labor. In about 90 percent of cases, delivery occurs within 24 hours of the rupture of the membranes, which serve as a protective barrier against infection. The membranes hold the amniotic fluid, some of which may be lost immediately; in many instances the descending baby blocks the flow of a part of the fluid, which later follows the fetus out of the birth canal.

The first stage of labor, which begins with the dilatation and other changes of the cervix, ends with the complete dilatation of the cervix to a diameter of about 10 centimeters, or four inches. The first stage usually averages around 15 hours for a first child and about eight hours for a mother who has delivered previously. But the normal range of time for the first stage might extend from one to 24 hours.

Childbirth

The second stage, which may last from a few minutes to a few hours, depending upon such factors as the position and presentation of the fetus, begins with the full dilatation of the cervix and ends when the baby has finally been delivered. In a classic vertex, or head-first, delivery, the baby moves in three phases: first the head, then the shoulders, and finally the body and legs.

The doctor and nurses do not try to speed up the delivery because of the risk of damage to the mother and child. Gentle, gradual delivery with help from the mother, who bears down with her abdominal muscles to expel the baby, generally is all that is necessary. A small surgical incision, an episiostomy, may be made to prevent tearing of tissues around the vaginal opening. After the head is free and the infant's airway is clear, it can breathe on its own if necessary while the rest of the body is moving through the birth canal. If the umbilical cord is wrapped around the infant's neck, it can be clamped and cut by the doctor at this point in delivery to prevent complications. Otherwise, the umbilical cord is cut and tied later.

The third stage of labor is the delivery of the placenta. The placenta usually is expelled several minutes after the baby is delivered, but there may be complications such as hemorrhage, infection, entrapment of a part of the placenta in the uterus, or inversion of the uterus. Thus, the childbirth adventure is not truly finished until, as the saying goes, "both the mother and baby are doing fine."

Emergency Child Delivery

In handling an emergency child delivery, the steps are essentially the same. The first stage of labor is hard work and lasts several hours. The mother needs rest, relaxation, and reassurance. If the baby's head appears with the bag of water over its face, the bag can be broken with the fingers. But otherwise, fingers should be kept away from the birth canal except to catch the baby. Any pulling or pushing can damage the baby or mother. Let nature handle the delivery at its own pace.

The baby's head and back should be supported to keep it out of fluid or other material at the birth site. The baby's skin

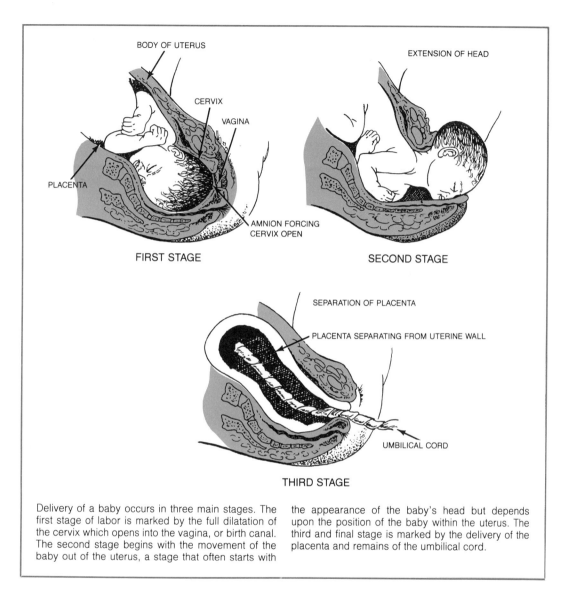

BODY OF UTERUS

CERVIX

VAGINA

PLACENTA

AMNION FORCING
CERVIX OPEN

FIRST STAGE

EXTENSION OF HEAD

SECOND STAGE

SEPARATION OF PLACENTA

PLACENTA SEPARATING FROM UTERINE WALL

UMBILICAL CORD

THIRD STAGE

Delivery of a baby occurs in three main stages. The first stage of labor is marked by the full dilatation of the cervix which opens into the vagina, or birth canal. The second stage begins with the movement of the baby out of the uterus, a stage that often starts with the appearance of the baby's head but depends upon the position of the baby within the uterus. The third and final stage is marked by the delivery of the placenta and remains of the umbilical cord.

is slippery, so it may be helpful to wrap clean towels around its legs and body to hold it. The baby should be held by its ankles, the head down but supported, so that any fluid accumulation in the chest and throat can drain. The baby should start crying at this point in the delivery. After crying has started, the baby should be wrapped to keep it warm, the head exposed so it can breathe. It should be placed on the mother's abdomen. The umbilical cord will still be attached.

It may help to "milk" the baby's throat by stroking the outside from the base of the throat toward the chin while the head is held slightly downward. This will help clear the air passages so the baby can breathe adequately. If the baby is not breathing properly, administer mouth-to-mouth resuscitation. But be gentle about it. Blowing too hard into the infant's lungs can cause serious damage.

The umbilical cord should be tied with strong cotton tape or cloth. Do not use string because it may cut through the cord, which contains arteries and veins. The umbilical cord should be tied in two places: first, tie a square knot about four inches from the baby's abdomen; next, tie a knot about three inches out from the first knot. Cut between the knots with a scissors, if one is available; sterilize the tape or cloth and the scissors before tying and cutting the cord if boiling water or other cleansing methods are available. This may be after the placenta has been expelled from the mother's uterus.

The abdomen over the uterus should be massaged gently to keep it firm. The mother should be encouraged to rest for about eight hours and to try urinating about eight hours after delivery.

Do not wash the white coating off the baby's skin until a doctor has had a chance to check the child. The white waxy coating is a natural protective surface. The baby should be kept warm, and feeding should begin at the first 12 hours of life.

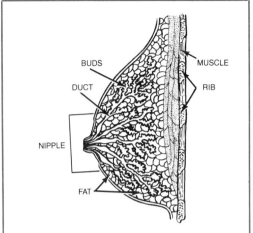

During pregnancy the hormones associated with maintaining the developing infant, estrogen and progesterone, contribute to the enlargement of the female breast in preparation for nursing the baby after it is born. Milk is formed in the buds and is excreted through the ducts leading to the nipple, which is composed of numerous milk duct outlets. Other hormones stimulate regular production of milk as a result of the baby's sucking action at the nipple. Much of the structure of the female breast, in addition to the milk-producing tissues, consists of fat deposits.

A record should be kept of all details of the birth, including the exact moment delivery was completed, the date, place, mother's name, father's name, their address, sex of the child, blood type of mother if known, and the name of the person attending the emergency delivery.

QUESTIONS AND ANSWERS
PREGNANCY AND CHILDBIRTH

Q: *When is a baby considered premature?*
A: If it is born before the usual 40 weeks following the last menstrual period. However, unless the exact date of conception is known, it is difficult to apply the term to any particular baby that may appear to be born a few days or more ahead of schedule. It has been estimated that 95 percent of all babies are born either earlier or later than expected.

Q: *What is meant by the "birth canal"?*
A: The birth canal is another term for vagina, which becomes the passage from the uterus to the outside through which a baby is delivered normally. It shortens in length while expanding in diameter to accommodate passage of the baby.

Q: *What is the purpose of massaging the uterus after delivery?*
A: Massaging the uterus helps it contract after the fetus and placenta have left the organ, and contraction helps reduce the risk of excessive blood loss.

Q: *Is amniocentesis ethical if the objective is to decide whether the mother should have an abortion?*
A: Whether amniocentesis should lead to abortion is a question beyond the main purpose of prenatal diagnosis. A couple who discover they may have a mongoloid child, for example, would be given a time advantage in making preparations for the changes in their lives and the special care of the child that would be required. Information obtained from amniocentesis is not limited to a search for future infants with birth defects. For example, it can inform the parents about the sex of the child. Doctors can provide the results of prenatal diagnosis to parents, but the parents make their own decision about use of the information.

Q: *There has been a trend in recent years toward having the baby delivered at home. Is homebirth safe?*
A: Homebirth is not new, of course, since it has been going on for generations in all parts of the world. Generally, having a baby at home can be safe as long as nothing goes wrong. Unfortunately, there can be complications such as hemorrhaging, an unusual presentation of the baby into the birth canal, a health disorder of the mother such as hypertension or diabetes, and so on. Also, the mother and her friends and relatives often require all sorts of standby measures such as having an ambulance service available, as well as a nearby hospital emergency room and doctors who are expected to be ready to rush to the mother's home if the delivery doesn't go according to plan. For most women, it is much easier to simply check into a good hospital with a well-equipped obstetrics department, so that the birth can be handled in a professional manner.

Q: *What ever happened to the old-fashioned midwife as a person who could help with delivering babies?*
A: The old-fashioned midwives in America are being replaced by highly trained nurse-midwives. The modern midwife is a registered nurse who receives two years of postgraduate training in obstetric nursing and receives a master's degree in nursing. As of this writing, there are nearly 2,000 certified nurse-midwives who work mainly in hospitals and public clinics in inner-city and rural areas. Generally, they manage the uncomplicated maternity cases with a qualified obstetrician as a backup professional for cases that develop difficulties.

Q: *Is it O.K. to use aspirin and other drugs after the first trimester?*

425

A: That's a question you should discuss with your doctor. Studies show that the average number of medications used by pregnant women is ten, and that some congenital defects may be due to drugs used by mothers during their pregnancies. Thus, a mother-to-be would be wise to avoid taking any drug while pregnant, unless the drug is necessary to preserve the life and health of the mother.

Q: *Could a childhood case of rickets cause a woman to have delivery problems in later life?*

A: Some women develop an abnormally flat pelvis because of rickets, and the shape of the pelvis can make delivery difficult. Some women have pelvises that are ideally shaped for motherhood, but others do not. For those not gifted with an ideal pelvis, doctors have ways of helping them achieve motherhood, anyway.

14

BASIC BABY AND CHILD CARE

The birth experience is a traumatic, abrupt change of life for most babies, regardless of the tender loving care given an infant. Until the moment of delivery the baby has spent its entire life floating in a warm, moist, cozy environment, and receiving all its bodily requirements by nature's intravenous feeding system, the umbilical cord.

At the moment before birth, the child did not even have to breathe to get oxygen; oxygen was supplied through the umbilical cord. In the next moment, the infant must quickly learn to inhale oxygen and exhale carbon dioxide and water vapor in order to survive. No longer can the child depend upon the mother to provide a constant warm temperature for its body; suddenly it must adjust its body to whatever sort of temperature and humidity it encounters in the delivery room. The infant must learn within hours to feed itself from the mother's breast, since its regular source of nutrients was stopped when the umbilical cord was cut and tied.

So, it's really not surprising that an infant enters the real world in a stupor, or that he appears tense and jittery, and

cries a lot. Usually, the child becomes rather well adjusted to his new lifestyle within a couple of weeks. He may appear to be deaf at first, but he will react to noises within a few days. He will show an ability to distinguish light from darkness at about the same time. During the first couple of weeks he will regain the small amount of weight lost on his day of birth because of temporary dehydration of body tissues and adjustment to a milk diet.

The Apgar Rating Scale

In the first moments after birth, a child today is examined for five factors that indicate its condition and ability to survive. The system was developed by Dr. Virginia Apgar, an expert on congenital problems, and is named for her. The five basic conditions are heart rate, respiration as indicated by crying, muscle tone, skin coloration, and reflex irritability or reaction to a stimulus such as touching the sole of the foot. The degree of response in each category is rated by the numbers 0, 1, and 2. The conditions are checked at least twice, and sometimes three times, immediately after birth, usually at one minute after delivery and again five minutes later. A third check sometimes is done at two minutes after birth.

If a newborn infant appears to be having trouble because of respiration or other problems, attention is devoted toward immediate treatment of the difficulty.

A typical Apgar rating chart looks something like this:

CONDITION	SCORE		
	0	1	2
A Appearance (Color)	Blue, pale	Body pink, extremities blue	Completely pink
P Pulse (Heart rate)	Absent	Below 100/min.	Over 100/min.
G Grimace reflex	No response	Grimaces	Cries
A Activity (Muscle tone)	Limp	Some limb motion	Active motion
R Respiration	Absent	Irregular, slow	Strong crying

A rating of ten points, representing a total of two points in each category, would be perfect, but few infants actually score this high, mainly because a newborn child rarely has a score of two on appearance. There usually is some cyanosis or bluish coloring in the extremities immediately after birth, even in infants who are delivered spontaneously or with very little need for assistance by doctors or nurses.

Any child that scores between seven and nine points on the Apgar scale is considered normal. About 90 percent of babies will score at least seven points, and those with at least six points seldom require any special treatment beyond routine delivery care. An infant scoring from four to six points is considered moderately depressed. A child in this range, for example, might have a strong heartbeat but show signs of breathing difficulty and poor circulation as evidenced by pale or bluish skin.

A severely depressed baby—that is, one scoring less than four points on the Apgar scale—should be given emergency treatment to insure adequate breathing, heartbeat, and other life functions. Oxygen therapy, external cardiac message, aspiration of fluid from the air passages, or even a blood transfusion may be ordered, depending upon the problem. Infants with low scores on the Apgar scale risk suffering temporary or permanent central nervous system damage because of oxygen deprivation if adequate circulation cannot be established immediately.

Infant Development

From a beginning as a virtually helpless organism when delivered into the outside world, a typical baby makes tremendous strides in his ability to cope with the external environment within a very short time. Although barely able to tell night from day at the start, his eyes develop rapidly so that he can distinguish objects in the room about him and his eye muscles enable him to track moving objects.

The rate of development in different average children is unlikely to be the same. A child that makes cooing sounds a week before other infants of the same age is not necessarily a genius, any more than a child might be regarded as retarded if he is a week behind schedule in learning to make the cooing sounds. As various children develop, mothers become aware that any child is likely to be slightly ahead of the average timetable in some areas of be-

HOW A CHILD USES HIS EYES AND EARS

Characteristic:	Appears usually between the ages of:
First follows object with eyes	Birth and 6 weeks
Pays attention to sounds nearby	Birth and 6 weeks
Makes sounds other than crying	Birth and 6 weeks
Eyes follow movement from one side of head to the other	2 months and 4 months
Laughs	6 weeks and 3½ months
Squeals	6 weeks and 4½ months
Brings hands together in front of face	6 weeks and 3½ months
Turns toward adult voice	4 months and 8 months
Passes object from one hand to other	5 months and 7½ months
Grasps very small object on flat surface	5 months and 8 months
Says "Dada" or "Mama"	6 months and 10 months
Imitates speech sounds of parents	6 months and 11 months
Brings together two toys held in hands	7 months and 12 months
Uses "Dada" to identify father or "Mama" to identify mother	10 months and 14 months
Scribbles with pencil or crayon	12 months and 24 months

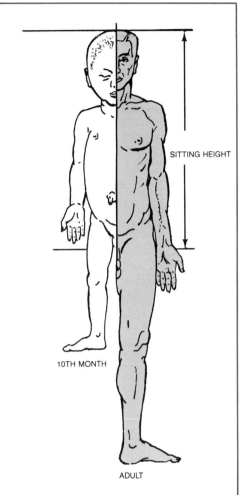

SITTING HEIGHT

10TH MONTH

ADULT

Between birth and adulthood, an individual undergoes many changes in body proportion in addition to gaining considerably in height and weight. The illustration (not to scale) shows some of the changes in features between a one-month old baby (at the 10th month after conception) and an adult male. Among other changes, the baby's head becomes much smaller and the legs much longer in proportion to the rest of the body as the person grows older.

havior development and behind schedule in other areas.

A "premature" baby may develop a characteristic later than one who was delivered at normal term. The difference in development will be approximately equal to the weeks or months ahead of term that the child was born. For example, a child born one month prematurely may not show a particular characteristic until one month longer after birth than a baby born after a full nine-month pregnancy. The trait or characteristic usually appears at an average time dating from the conception rather than the date of delivery.

HOW A CHILD HANDLES HIS BODY DURING FIRST YEAR OF LIFE

Characteristic:	Appears usually between the ages of:
Holds head up while lying on stomach	Birth and 4 weeks
Holds head upright lying on stomach	5 weeks and 3 months
Holds head steady when held in sitting position	6 weeks and 4 months
Rolls over on bed	2 months and 5 months
Sits without support when placed	5 months and 8 months
Gets himself into sitting position	6 months and 11 months
Supports weight on legs when held steady	3 months and 8 months
Stands while holding a support	5 months and 10 months
Stands alone for a moment	9 months and 13 months
Stands alone well	10 months and 14 months
Walking while holding onto furniture	7½ months and 13 months
Walks alone across a room	11 months and 15 months

HOW A CHILD REACTS WITH OTHER PEOPLE

Characteristic:	Appears usually between the ages of:
Looks at your face	Birth and 1 month
Smiles when you smile at him	Birth and 2 months
Smiles on his own	6 weeks and 5 months
Pulls back when you pull toy he holds	4 months and 10 months
Tries to get toy out of reach	5 months and 9 months
Feeds himself crackers	5 months and 8 months
Drinks from cup by himself	10 months and 16 months
Uses spoon, spills little	13 months and 24 months
Plays Peek-A-Boo	6 months and 10 months
Plays Pat-A-Cake	7 months and 13 months
Plays with ball on the floor	10 months and 16 months

Nursing the Baby

One of the early signs of eye development can be observed during feeding when the infant begins studying the mother's face while it is nursing. The true mother's milk does not begin flowing until two or three days after the baby has been delivered. The breasts begin to secrete a thin, yellowish milky fluid a few days before the baby is born, and the newborn infant can subsist on that until the true mother's milk begins to flow. Breast feeding can begin almost any time after birth. The baby's mouth contact with the nipples on the mother's breasts helps stimulate hormones that control the production and flow of milk, so breast feeding actually is an activity that requires cooperation between the baby and mother.

Normally, the average mother's production of breast milk is proportional to the baby's demand for food once a breast-feeding routine is established, so that nursing occurs about every three or four hours. The nursing act does not require actual sucking by the infant. The milk flow is started by a rhythmic biting action of the child. It is not uncommon for the mother's milk to flow out of the breasts spontaneously, thereby demonstrating that a sucking action is not needed. However, poor feeding habits by the baby or ineffective nursing procedures on the part of the mother can result in a gradually diminished milk flow.

Nursing at only one breast during a feeding can lead to breast engorgement. The nursing action at one breast stimulates the flow of milk in both breasts. As a result, one breast may become overfilled and cause engorgement distress. The pituitary hormonal system that monitors breast milk production and consumption may get a signal that breast filling is excessive, and milk output thereafter may be reduced. The mother, therefore, should nurse the child at both breasts during each feeding, rather than nurse the child at alternate breasts.

Normal milk production starts at a low level of perhaps four ounces a day at first and gradually increases over a period of ten days to two weeks to around ten ounces a day. Once regular milk flow is started and the effort is not diminished by illness or reduced production because of failure to empty the breasts, a mother can sustain a baby's needs for milk without serious difficulty. Some women with well-established milk flow, such as wet nurses, are able to supply breast milk to several infants.

Nursing a baby usually requires only a few minutes of the mother's time at each feeding. From 60 to 90 percent of the infant's milk is provided in the first four to five minutes of nursing. Allowing the baby to be at the breast more than seven minutes at a time can be a cause of complications such as maceration and cracking of the nipples, or mastitis, the inflammation of the breasts.

Some mothers find it helpful to let the nipples dry in the air for about five minutes after each nursing period, or to expose the nipples to the warmth of an electric light bulb held about six inches away from the breast. Otherwise, the nipples should be dried carefully with a clean cloth or half a sanitary napkin pad. A few experienced mothers begin toughening the nipples during the third trimester of pregnancy by washing the nipples daily with a mild soap and water, using a washcloth. After drying the nipples, the woman applies a thin film of liquid petrolatum. Alcohol or scented soaps or handcreams should not be used on or around the nipples because those materials may cause the skin to become dry and irritated, and perfumed soaps and creams often contain substances that can produce an allergic reaction.

If the nipples become cracked or sore, or if the breasts are so firm the infant has difficulty in grasping the nipples with his mouth, the mother can discharge milk from the breasts by milking the breasts by hand. The milk can be caught in a sterilized container, such as a baby bottle, and stored for feeding the baby at the next regular nursing period.

Women who prefer not to breast feed a child even though they are capable of doing so have several alternative ways of accomplishing the process of "drying up" the breasts. One method is by administering sex hormones daily for perhaps the first week after delivery. There are several hormone formulations available for this purpose. Another way is to simply not nurse or otherwise encourage milk production, and to wear a tight compression binder around the breasts. Aspirin or other analgesics and ice packs may be needed to relieve the discomfort that may persist for several days, but the breasts will cease functioning as a source of mother's milk within about 72 hours. A similar procedure is used if breast inflammation interferes with nursing, or when weaning becomes necessary.

Breast Feeding vs. Bottle Feeding

As for the controversy regarding breast feeding versus bottle feeding, most of the reasons for bottle feeding are based on factors involving the mother's health and lifestyle. Breast feeding has no disadvantages from the baby's point of view if the mother is healthy, willing, and adequately endowed with milk. Breast feeding is convenient and inexpensive. The milk is easily digestible, free of bacteria, served at the proper temperature, and without problems caused by mistakes in preparing the correct formulation. The child also receives passive antibodies from the mother for protection against a number of infections, and gains some emotional satisfaction. Breast feeding also is said by mothers to be emotionally satisfying for them, and it helps speed the return of the uterus to its prepregnancy size.

Women who object to breast feeding usually say they find the routine restrictive to their professional or social life. There also may be health reasons which may or may not include the use of drugs that could affect the health of the child. A woman who enjoys smoking or drinking alcoholic beverages may find it necessary to curtail those activities if she breast feeds her baby. A mother who is not sure about which food, beverage, or drug might affect the baby through breast feeding should check with her doctor.

Many new mothers find it convenient to have baby bottles and a formula available for days when illness or other conditions make it difficult to nurse the baby at the breast. The bottles also can be used for orange juice and water. Although milk is an adequate source of food and fluid at first, the baby soon develops a need for sources of water and vitamins beyond those provided by mother's milk. Vitamins C and D, particularly, may have to be added to the baby's diet in the early weeks after birth. They can be provided in the form of liquid drops administered with an eye dropper or through nursing bottles containing or-

ange juice or a vitamin D-enriched milk formula. Water can be provided in a separate nursing bottle; it should be boiled first and allowed to cool to room temperature.

The baby may spit up some of its milk, an event that varies in frequency with different babies. Usually, this is not a sign of illness but merely the result of air bubbles in the digestive tract or an overfilling of the stomach. Spitting up may be more frequent at first and diminishes as the baby's digestive tract develops with time. Burping or bubbling the baby after a meal helps remedy the situation. However, the parents should not confuse spitting up with vomiting, which usually is marked by spasmodic abdominal contractions as well as the loss of stomach contents. Vomiting in a newborn child can be a sign of a serious defect in the digestive system, requiring immediate medical attention. Vomiting in a baby after it has demonstrated the ability to manage milk meals without difficulty usually is a sign of illness and should be brought to the attention of the doctor. In some cases the vomiting may be accompanied by other signs of illness such as a rash or fever, which should be noted in discussing the problem with the doctor.

Infant Feeding and Diet

Most babies have their own timetables for feeding when they are first born, but they usually can be shifted into schedules that conform with the family routine without too much trouble. If the baby can adjust to feedings every four hours during the first few weeks or months, the day can be organized to begin with the first feeding at, say, 6 A.M. or 7 A.M., or whatever hour is most convenient for the family. Each successive feeding can be scheduled for four-hour intervals after that.

As the baby learns to spend more of the night sleeping, he often will be willing to go without one middle-of-the-night feeding after the first month. By the age of three months, he will begin to sleep through the night without interrupting the parents for a feeding. As the number of meals per 24-hour-period decreases, however, the amount of food per feeding should be increased so that the day's total intake remains about the same.

Graduating from liquid to solid foods can occur gradually during the second or third month. This transition often needs to be done with a bit of trickery because babies tend to be suspicious of any food substance that does not taste like milk and does not have a consistency like milk. The trick is to make solid food appear at first to be a different kind of milk. After orange juice or fortified formulas, some parents try to get the baby to eat yogurt, which is a natural step between milk and solid foods. Fruit-flavored yogurts can lead to strained fruits, followed by strained vegetables, which can be gradually worked into the baby's diet by offering, one kind at a time, naturally sweet vegetables such as carrots and squash.

Cereals can be introduced into the baby's diet in a similar manner, using finely milled grains such as farina or rice, and mixing the cereal with milk to give it a creamy consistency. It's not necessary to add sugar to the baby's cereal, or other foods for that matter, since most fruits and vegetables are sources of carbohydrates, and even milk is a source of carbohydrates in the form of milk sugar.

Parents should be cautious about adding either sugar or salt to baby food to make the natural food seem more palatable. Babies are not sensitive to flavors in the same way that adults are; what may be tasty to an adult may not be the baby's idea of a flavorful food. Commercial baby food manufacturers have been known to flavor their products to make them appetizing to parents who like to taste the baby foods before giving them to their offspring.

Babies often refuse to accept a new food the first time it is added to their diets. The youngest one in the family has a built-in reflex that enables him to reject anything that has a strange taste. A baby who spits out solid foods as fast as they are offered is demonstrating a natural reflex action, not a finicky attitude. Parents are advised simply to keep trying until the baby eventually accepts the food. If the food is not used within two or three days, however, it should be discarded to prevent spoilage.

It is during the transition to new and solid foods that allergies begin to appear. This is another reason why solid foods should be tried a little at a time and one at a time. If the child develops a rash, vomits, or otherwise displays a serious reaction to a food, it may be a sign of an allergy. Withdraw the food for a few days to see if the symptoms diminish, then try again with the food that appeared to cause the reaction. If the child repeats the symptoms, the parents can assume that the food was a factor. A record should be kept of any severe food reactions, and the matter can be discussed with the baby's doctor during the next visit. It is possible that a variation of the food, perhaps one that is prepared in a different manner or by a different manufacturer, would not cause the reaction.

Immunization Against Disease

There is some evidence to support the belief that babies who are breastfed get some extension of the immunity to disease that protects them through the first days after birth. The mother's own antibodies to diseases such as measles and diphtheria can be transmitted through the placental barrier. However, others cannot. Antibodies that are not transmitted through the placenta include those that resist infections of chicken pox and whooping cough.

Since the baby usually begins to become less dependent upon the mother's milk after the first few months of life, it is risky to delay immunization against diseases for which vaccines are easily available. The basic immunization plan recommended for infants provides for injections of killed or inactivated disease agents for whooping cough, diphtheria, tetanus, and poliomyelitis at the age of two months. Whether the antigens are administered in two or three primary injections as single or combined agents depends upon the age of the child and the immunization products used. A reinforcing dose is administered between seven months and one year later. The reinforcing dose actually is a third, or fourth, primary dose that is necessary to insure immunity; it is not the same as a booster shot.

The basic immunization shots for whooping cough, or pertussis, diphtheria, tetanus, and polio often are given in a series at the age of two months, four months, and six months. At the age of 15 months, injections of measles, mumps, and rubella, or German measles, should be given; by the age of 18 months, the reinforcing dose should be administered.

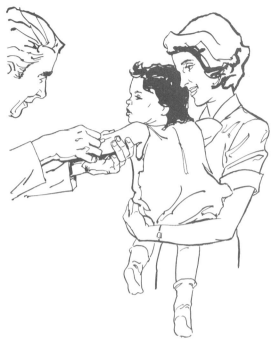

Many common diseases that resulted in death and disability for children of previous generations can now be prevented by proper immunization, starting as early as two months of age for most infants. During the first year the child should be immunized for diptheria, tetanus, pertussis (whooping cough), and poliomyelitis. At 15 months the child can be immunized for measles, rubella, and mumps.

Booster shots for whooping cough, diphtheria, tetanus, and polio should be scheduled between the ages of four and five years, or before the child enters school. In some communities proof of immunization may be required before a child will be admitted to a school. The booster shot schedule immediately before school days begin assumes that the basic immunization was carried out when the child was an infant. Otherwise, the primary and reinforcing injections simply have to start when the child is about four years of age and may have been exposed unnecessarily

IMMUNIZATION SCHEDULE FOR CHILDREN

At Age	Vaccine
2 months	DTP (Diphtheria, tetanus, and pertussis, or whooping cough). Oral Polio
4 months	DTP. Oral Polio
6 months	DTP (Some doctors also recommend an additional dose of oral polio.)
15 months	Measles, Rubella, Mumps
18 months	DTP. Oral Polio
4–6 years (before school)	DTP Booster, Polio Booster
14–16 years	TD (Tetanus-diphtheria toxoids, adult type)
Thereafter	Tetanus-diphtheria (TD) booster should be given every 10 years or following a dirty wound if a booster has not been given in the preceding 5 years.

to a variety of dangerous disease organisms for a good share of his early childhood.

Vaccinations for smallpox, once a routine procedure, are no longer required unless the child has been exposed to the disease or an epidemic threatens. Because the disease has been virtually wiped out in all parts of the world and the only known smallpox viruses are in medical laboratories, exposure or an epidemic are unlikely.

Immunization to a number of other diseases, such as influenza, can be obtained if and when needed. Hepatitis and scarlet fever shots offer some protection to a child who has been exposed to either of the diseases, but the immunization is not given routinely. Rabies shots also are available, but they are only administered to youngsters who may have been bitten or scratched by an animal known to be rabid, or by an animal that cannot be located to check for rabies infection.

Immunization for plague, yellow fever, typhus, cholera, typhoid, or Rocky Mountain spotted fever might be recommended for children likely to accompany their parents to geographic areas where exposure to the diseases might be expected.

With the exception of the Sabin polio vaccine, all immunizations are by injection; the Sabin polio vaccine is administered orally by a few drops of weakened live viruses on a sugar cube. German measles vaccine, like the Sabin polio vaccine, is prepared from weakened live viruses. The Salk polio vaccine and other vaccines, such as those for influenza and whooping cough, are prepared from killed antigens. The agents used for immunization against tetanus and diphtheria are prepared from toxoids, which are nonpoisonous substances made from toxins, or poisons, of the disease organisms.

Childhood Diseases

A record of all immunizations, including dates of injections and the type of vaccine, should become a part of the child's permanent health record. Copies should be made for use when requested by school officials, camp physicians, and other doctors who take over the health care of the child when the family moves to a new neighborhood.

Whooping cough (pertussis) is caused by a contagious bacteria that usually is inhaled by the patient getting the disease. It gets into the air by being sprayed from the mouths of people already infected. The disease symptoms begin with watery eyes, sneezing, loss of appetite, and a hacking cough. The cough progresses into a pattern of five to 15 coughs followed by a whooping noise (from which the disorder gets its name) when the child takes a deep breath. After a few breaths, the pattern may begin again. The coughing spells may continue around the clock, day after day, until recovery begins about a month after the disease starts.

Whooping cough can be quite serious in small children. A small percentage of whooping cough cases involving infants become fatal. But hospitalization often is necessary. Medications usually are administered only for complications such as pneumonia, or as sedatives to help the child get some sleep. The only truly effective treatment is immunity provided by vaccination or by experiencing the disease. However, one whooping cough attack does not provide lifelong protection; it merely results in milder symptoms if the disease is caught again.

Diphtheria also is a bacterial disease involving the respiratory system. It is spread mainly by contact with infected persons. The infected person need not be seriously ill with the disease but simply a carrier of the disease organism. The bacteria become trapped in the throat area, especially in the tonsils, where they multiply and produce a toxin that is poisonous to the surrounding tissues. The toxin can be carried by the bloodstream to the heart, kidney, lungs, or other body organs where further tissue damage results.

The disease symptoms usually begin with a low-grade fever, sore throat, and difficulty in swallowing. Fever and chills, nausea, and headache are among symptoms often felt by children. A tell-tale sign of diphtheria is the appearance of a dirty gray membrane that forms in the lining of the throat and becomes so firmly attached that removal of the film causes bleeding. Small children may not complain of the symptoms of diphtheria until the membrane has appeared in the throat.

Patients generally are hospitalized in isolation wards and given antitoxin made from horse serum. Because of the possibility of a serum reaction, a horse serum sensitivity test is made first to see if the child shows signs of allergy. The patient also is administered antibiotics and is watched for signs of complications such as effects on the heart and central nervous system. Bed rest is important and recovery is slow. If the heart muscle has been affected by the diphtheria toxin, even normal physical exertion can prove fatal. Patients who recover may experience irregular heartbeats, and their electrocardiograms may show mildly abnormal patterns.

Tetanus is a bacterial disease marked by spasms of the voluntary muscles and convulsions; it is often identified by the common name of lockjaw. The term is appropriate because facial muscles generally are affected with the result that an infected patient has difficulty opening his jaws. The infection can develop from seemingly small wounds, as well as burns, and from the use of hypodermic needles that have become contaminated by the bacterium. The disease organism can be carried in animal feces or in soil that has been contaminated by animal feces; the bacterial spores of tetanus can remain dormant in the soil for years. A housing development on land that formerly was a farm could bring young children into contact with tetanus organisms.

Restlessness, irritability, headache, fever, chilliness, sore throat, or headache that may be associated with muscle stiffness about a week after a wound, even a slight wound, may have been contaminated could suggest a tetanus infection. Stiffness of the jaw is an important clue. As the disease progresses, the child may develop convulsions but be unable to speak or cry because of the lockjaw effect.

Treatment usually requires administration of antitoxins, sedation, and control of symptoms. Because of difficulties in eating and breathing, the patient may be fed intravenously and have artificial breathing equipment attached to maintain normal respiration. Since a common effect of tetanus is constipation, enemas often are required. A catheter also may be needed to assist in emptying the bladder.

Because a tetanus infection does not make a person immune to future attacks, the patient is given a series of tetanus immunization shots after being discharged from the hospital. A person who has not received a booster shot within the past five years may be given a booster injection at the time of an injury that could result in tetanus infection.

Diphtheria, tetanus, and pertussis vaccines are combined in a DTP shot recommended for infants beginning at two months of age, with a reinforcing dose about one year later. The DTP booster is given about the time the child enters school. Tetanus-diphtheria toxoid boosters should be given when the child is 12 years old and repeated every five to ten years after that. The oral polio vaccine is repeated when the child is less than 18 months old, and again before starting school.

A baby may show some discomfort after receiving vaccine injections. If the child displays signs of a swelling around the injection site, a fever, or irritability, the doctor may recommend giving one baby aspirin tablet, which is equivalent to about one-fourth of an adult aspirin tablet, and perhaps repeating the dose once after four hours.

Babies may show reactions to other immunization vaccines. Some infants may develop a fever and/or rash after a measles vaccine injection, for example. This is generally not a serious situation, and the doctor may reduce the effect by giving a dose of gamma globulin with the vaccine. The gamma globulin also may be administered as temporary protection in case the infant is exposed to measles before being immunized. But the gamma globulin is not a substitute for the measles vaccine which should be given as soon as the doctor advises.

Colic and Other Digestive Disorders

Baby health problems for which there are no protective vaccines often relate to the digestive tract, food allergies, vomiting, and colic. Colic is a term commonly used to describe the situation in which the baby, after being fed, develops cramps that are intense enough to make him scream. The cries of pain usually are accompanied by tense abdominal muscles and a drawing up of the arms and legs. The child's face becomes red. In many cases, the problem is a digestive system that has not matured properly for that stage of life, and the child eventually gets over the problem.

In the meantime, the parents may simply have to learn to live with the situation for three or four months. The colic spells will tend to occur only after certain feedings, such as in the evening, and will gradually diminish as the infant grows older. The parents should make the child as comfortable as possible during periods of colic. The child can be rocked, held, patted gently, and a pacifier may help. In severe cases a doctor may prescribe a sedative that can be given in liquid form.

However, all signs of discomfort in a child too young to talk and explain its problems to the parents may not simply be caused by colic. An ear infection or some other disorder could be the source of pain. The parents would be wise to check for other possible causes of discomfort before assuming that it is colic.

Some babies may cry when having a difficult bowel movement after feeding. Various individual babies cry while passing a soft stool, but show no discomfort in passing a relatively hard or large stool. A baby's bowel movement tinged with bright red blood may be a sign of a disorder in the anal canal. Loose bowel movements accompanied by signs of blood can be a sign of infection. Breastfed babies are more likely to have frequent loose stools until they begin eating solid foods along with the mother's milk. But otherwise, an infant's bowel movements can vary so much in frequency and content that one or two examples may have little or no significance as far as the child's general health is concerned.

Doctor's Examinations

Good baby care routines usually include regular visits to a doctor for examination of the baby, beginning two to four weeks after the mother and child have been discharged from the hospital. The visits should be repeated every two months for the first year, even if the child appears to be in good health, and every four to six months during the second year. The visits will include measurement of body height and weight, sensory screening for adequate hearing and vision, immunizations, and medical history information. The doctor may request further laboratory studies of blood and urine during the visits for babies who may be susceptible to genetic diseases. The doctor may check for signs of tumors that may begin to appear as an infant grows.

Rates of Normal Growth

During the first year the infant continues to grow at a rapid pace. Its weight nearly doubles in the first five months and triples by the end of the 12th month. The child also grows in length during the first year. The growth rates gradually taper off through early childhood and spurt upward again as the period of adolescence begins.

The most remarkable area of growth in the first year is in the brain. The brain increases from about 25 percent of its adult size at birth to 75 percent during the first 12 months, then slows in the rate of growth over the following years until adolescence. Because of the tremendous growth in brain tissue during the period of infancy, it is important that adequate nutrition be provided to assure optimum development. It also is essential that the infant be protected from disorders that could affect brain development and result in mental retardation.

QUESTIONS AND ANSWERS
BASIC BABY AND CHILD CARE

Q: *One baby book recommends suspending toys over the baby's crib so it can develop arm and leg muscles by reaching or kicking at the toys. Is this a safe thing to do?*
A: The American Academy of Pediatrics recommends that hanging toys be suspended well beyond the reach of the baby in its crib. The academy also advises that parents remove large toys from the crib when the baby is unattended. When the baby is able to move about in the crib it may use large toys as objects to climb or step on in order to get over the railing of the crib.

Q: *Our baby has colic but it continues to gain weight. Is it possible that he cries about something other than the food?*
A: Anything may be a mysterious cause of crying for a child unable to explain his feelings. In regard to the colic symptoms, it is quite normal for a child to gain weight during his colicky period.

Q: *What are nipple shields and what are they used for?*
A: Nipple shields are rubber devices that a nursing mother can place on her breasts when her nipples are sore or retracted. The baby can continue to be breastfed by using the rubber nipple on the nipple shield which draws milk from the breast by creating a partial vacuum when mouthed by the infant.

Q: *Most of the information about breast feeding versus bottle feeding is loaded in favor of breast feeding. What are some of the good arguments in favor of bottle feeding an infant?*
A: One argument often used is that a mother is better able to control the amount of milk consumed in a single feeding because she can measure the amount of formula put in a bottle and the amount consumed by the baby. As a result, the baby would be less likely to become overweight by overfeeding.

Another reason given is that bottle feeding gives the father and other family members an opportunity to participate in feeding the baby, while at the same time giving the mother more free time for other activities.

Q: *When is a baby ready to sleep in a regular bed rather than a crib?*
A: Probably when it has developed to the point where it can easily climb out of a crib. Then, having the baby sleep in a regular bed is safer because falling out of a crib can be more dangerous than falling off a regular bed mattress, which is lower in height. The child's ability to sleep in a regular bed can be tested by letting him take a few naps in a regular bed while spending his nights in the crib.

Q: *When is it safe to take a baby outdoors for fresh air and sunshine?*
A: A baby can be allowed some fresh air and sunshine at a very early age, provided it has protection from wind, sun, and cold. A properly wrapped baby in a carriage usually will benefit from the experience. But protection from the sun is important because infants cannot tolerate much direct sunlight; they have sensitive skin that burns easily.

Q: *What should be done about thumbsucking by a baby?*
A: Thumbsucking seems to be an instinctive pleasure for babies and should not be a problem unless it continues after the teeth erupt, when the habit could result in a misalignment of the teeth. However, very few youngsters continue thumbsucking into the period of life when their teeth may be threatened. One approach that may be helpful is to encourage the baby to use a pacifier instead of a thumb because it usually is easier to get the child to quit

using a pacifier substitute as he grows older. Try not to make a big issue of the problem when dealing with the child. Don't put mittens on his hands or restraining devices on his arms.

Q: *Is there any special trick in getting a baby to shift from breast milk to cow's milk?*
A: Yes. Do it gradually so the baby has a chance to get used to the taste of cow's milk. The same rule applies in switching a baby from a bottled formula to regular milk. Start the child off by allowing him one bottle a day of fresh, whole, pasturized milk that has been boiled and allowed to cool. Like other new foods, he may not accept the cow's milk at first, but he will get used to it with time.

Q: *My baby spits out food offered by spoon, even if it is a liquid. Does this reaction indicate he isn't ready for solid food?*

A: Teaching a baby to eat from a spoon is a major obstacle for most parents in switching a child from a bottle to solid foods. He probably resents the spoon more than the food because it requires learning a new way to eat just when he has become familiar with feeding from a bottle and/or breast. So make the transition gradual. Interrupt the bottle or breast feeding about halfway through a meal and offer some food in a spoon. Then finish up the meal with breast or bottle feeding. The child probably will treat the food in the spoon as some kind of poison at first, but he gradually will learn to like being spoonfed as the spoon phase of feeding gradually expands to fill the mealtime periods and the bottle or breast phase declines.

Very thin cereal mixed with milk and blended into a smooth fluid could be the first spoon food offered to a baby.

15

THE UNSEEN AGENTS OF INFECTION

We humans live in an ocean of invisible organisms, some friendly and others not so friendly. The organisms are invisible in terms of our ability to see them without the aid of microscopes. But for the unfriendly organisms, those that cause disease, relative size is not important. A virus, which is approximately the size of a DNA molecule, can kill an elephant. Enough bacteria to start an epidemic could hide under the period at the end of this sentence. The tiny creatures reproduce so rapidly that a single bacterium on your breakfast toast could increase the population of its own species more than 30,000 in your body by lunchtime.

Viruses, bacteria, protozoa, fungi, mycoplasmas, rickettsias, and the very tiny worms known as nematodes still cause most of the diseases that affect people and other animals, despite the emphasis by the news media and fund-raising organizations on disorders caused by other factors. The diseases caused by the microscopic organisms are of special concern because they are contagious. While cancer, heart disease, arthritis, and genet-

ic diseases are very serious disorders that account for a major share of human deaths and disabilities, they are not contagious. You can't "catch" cancer or heart disease by direct or indirect contact with a patient suffering from the disease.

The infectious disease organisms, often called microorganisms because of their small size, or microbes for short, probably are not truly malicious creatures. They might be viewed simply as parasites that find people and animals a fertile source of food for their own survival. The fact that each organism may produce somewhat different disease effects is due to the great variety in the living habits of the microbial parasites. Some of the microbes produce toxins, or poisonous substances, which cause the signs and symptoms of disease in terms of tissue damage. Some toxins are excreted by the microbe; others may be released when the microbe is attacked by antibodies that are a part of the host body's defense system.

A virus generally does its damage by capturing and enslaving the reproductive machinery in the nucleus of a tissue cell. The virus breaks or slips through the protective membranes of the living cell and forces the cell to use its own energy and nutrient resources to produce more viruses which can invade other cells.

How Microbes Cause Disease

The microorganisms that cause disease in humans often work in ways that can be misleading to people who expect that they are safe from harm if the microbes are not in the host body, or that the body has not been invaded if there are no signs and symptoms of disease. An example of a very dangerous disease that can be caused by microbes without their direct contact with human body tissues is botulism. A frequently fatal disorder, botulism results from eating food that contains a toxin excreted by a bacterium that may have lived in the food before it was prepared for consumption.

Regarding the second misleading aspect, pathogenic, or disease-causing, microbes quite frequently live in the bodies of humans and other animals at a low-level state of activity. Doctors may refer to this situation as a subclinical infection. The microbe can be shown to be present in the tissues of the patient, although he does not exhibit any clinical signs and symptoms of the disease. The subclinical type of infection may be more common for a particular disease than cases of actual illness caused by the pathogen. People who have subclinical infections may develop a kind of steady-state relationship between the microbe and their bodies. The microbe thrives peacefully in the human tissues without causing serious problems, and the human tissues adapt to the presence of the parasite without producing a symptom-generating reaction.

People with steady-state subclinical in-

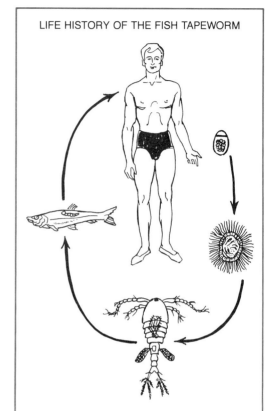

LIFE HISTORY OF THE FISH TAPEWORM

Fish and other animals often are intermediate hosts in the spread of disease. The fish tapeworm lays its eggs in the intestinal tract of an animal and the fertilized eggs are excreted in feces. If the eggs are washed into a lake or stream, the egg becomes a tiny hairy creature that is swallowed by a small crustacean, which in turn is catch by a freshwater fish. A human who eats the fish, raw or poorly cooked, becomes infected with the tapeworm.

fections may become carriers of a disease and unwittingly transmit pathogenic microbes to other persons who are more sensitive to the disease effects. A classic example of a disease carrier was the American woman known as Typhoid Mary who was responsible for an epidemic of typhoid cases through her contacts with the public, although she was not herself a victim of the disease organisms that she carried in her body.

For reasons not clearly understood even by doctors, some microbes select only certain organs or body tissues as their targets. The respiratory system, for example, is usually the infection site picked by influenza viruses and pneumonia bacteria. Although the respiratory tract is a logical target for microbes that may enter the body through the nose, they also have access to other body tissues such as the gastrointestinal tract. Or they can invade the bloodstream and attack almost any organ, including the heart, liver, and kidneys, which handle large amounts of circulating blood every hour.

Also not entirely understood are the reasons why some disease organisms are more likely to produce symptoms in children or in elderly persons, but not both, when factors such as possible malnutrition, genetic influences, and immune system conditions are eliminated. Some diseases can be explained in terms of hereditary or ethnic factors. Blacks with sickle-shaped red blood cells, for example, appear resistant to malaria because their hemoglobin-deficient red blood cells are less likely to attract the malarial disease organism. However, blacks, as well as Eskimo and American Indian populations, are more sensitive to tuberculosis infections than persons of Caucasian or Oriental ancestry, presumably because Europeans and Asians have acquired some tolerance for the tuberculosis bacterium from exposure spanning many centuries.

A person who is abnormally sensitive to infectious diseases sometimes is described as a compromised host. An otherwise normal individual can become a compromised host because of some change in his immune defense system, unless he happens to be one of those rare individuals who is born with a deficient immune system. An immune defense system can be altered by the administration of drugs employed in chemotherapy or organ transplants; the drugs are called immunosuppressive because they work by suppressing the body's natural antibody reaction system. The use of antibiotics can lower the body's natural defenses by wiping out some friendly bacteria that ordinarily would eliminate pathogenic invaders. Diseases such as leukemia can make a patient more susceptible to infections by robbing him of his natural immune defenses.

Most infectious disease organisms enter the human body through an opening, which could be the nose, mouth, urethra, or a break in the skin. Once inside the body, the pathogens frequently establish a local base of operations which the patient observes as a lesion near the point of entry. An early sign of a venereal infection, for example, is a sore or lesion in the genital area, or possibly a discharge from a nearby infection site.

From the base of operations near the body surface, the disease organism can travel through a passageway such as the urethra, esophagus, or trachea, or along tissue layers, to areas deeper inside the body. Eventually, the pathogen can enter the bloodstream through the lymph system or blood vessels, and travel to distant parts of the body where new sites of parasitic activity can be established. Poliomyelitis is an example of a disease that may enter the body at one point and eventually migrate to a distant area where the most serious damage occurs. The polio virus enters through the mouth and causes an initial minor illness similar to influenza, with symptoms that include nausea, vomiting, diarrhea, and/or constipation, and then moves on to attack the central nervous system.

Signs of Infection

Because of the rather consistent pattern of infectious diseases, doctors often try to jog the memory of patients or family members about events that may have preceded the symptoms. Often, it will be recalled that an insect bite, a small red pimple, or some other unusual feature appeared on the skin or at a body orifice a few days before the serious symptoms started.

Fever and chills are common symptoms of an infection. The fever may be the result of several different kinds of disease influences. The fever may be an expression of increased metabolism by the body tissues, resulting in the production of excess body heat. Another cause could be a protein substance released by the interaction of antibodies and microbes; the protein substance, called a pyrogen, has an effect of turning up the body's thermostat, a temperature-regulating center in the hypothalamus portion of the brain. The chills actually are associated with the disease's effect on the body's thermostat. The autonomic nervous system causes rapid muscle contractions, felt as shivering, in order to generate the body heat needed to match the new thermostat setting in the hypothalamus.

An infection may be accompanied by an inflammation of the soft tissues of the body. The condition sometimes is called cellulitis, but is has nothing to do with the fatty deposits involved in spot-reducing body exercises. The cellulitis of inflammation may be marked by painfully tender and swollen areas of skin and subcutaneous tissues. One or more lymph nodes often can be involved as a sign of an infection. Like soft tissues, they may be tender, painful, and inflamed.

Depending upon the individual case, the signs and symptoms that accompany an infection may require treatment of palliation in addition to the therapy administered for the disease itself. Cellulitis, for example, may cause complications requiring surgery if mucous membranes of the throat become involved. Chills and fever often need treatment with aspirin, and in some cases application of cold compresses or alcohol baths, while antibiotics or other medications are directed toward controlling the pathogen causing the symptoms.

Viruses: Properties and Effects

The smallest bacterium is about one-tenth of a micron in diameter, a micron being about 1/250,000th of an inch. But that bacterium is about five times the size of the smallest virus that could be involved in human disease. There are hundreds of different viruses that can produce infections in humans, and they may differ in size and shape as much as do the vast array of bacteria. Some, including viruses that cause influenza, may suddenly produce a new breed of its own kind of pathogen. This sends the vaccine makers back to the drawing board to develop a new form of medication to combat its effects.

Viruses as a group include representatives with several unique properties. For example, viruses can produce cancers in some animals, even though evidence that human cancers can be caused by viruses has been challenged by medical scientists. Another unique characteristic of some viruses is that they can exist only in certain parts of the world where there are species of animal life that live in close proximity to humans. The animals and humans form a continuing cycle of infection that may be broken if the animal species isn't available to sustain the infection in humans.

Still another unique property is the remarkably slow incubation period of some viral diseases. It has been demonstrated in animal studies that signs and symptoms of certain viral diseases may not appear for more than a year following exposure. It is assumed by many doctors that similar slow incubation periods may occur in human viral infections. The virus, no more than a crystalline core of nucleic acid, might even wait for several or many years before being triggered to come out of its cellular closet and begin attacking a host.

Some of the more common human viral diseases begin with a feverish rash, and for that reason may be identified by doctors as exanthematous viral diseases. The group includes regular measles, also known as rubeola or nine-day measles; rubella, which also may be called German measles or three-day measles; roseola infantum, or pseudorubella; chicken pox, or varicella; herpes zoster, or shingles; herpes simplex, which goes by the common names of fever blister or cold sore; and smallpox, which sometimes is identified by the medical name of variola.

Exanthematous viral diseases occur chiefly in humans, although monkeys can be infected with regular measles. Human viruses are transmitted from person to person and occur throughout the world. The same virus is the cause of both chicken pox and shingles, although children are usually the victims of chicken pox and adults are almost exclusively the targets of attacks of shingles. Herpes simplex can be transmitted by two different strains of the virus. One, sometimes identified as HVH (for Herpes Virus Hominis) Type 1, usually affects the lips, mouth, and sometimes the eyes. HVH Type 2 affects the genitalia and usually is transmitted as a venereal disease. This type of herpes virus and rubella, or German measles, are of particular concern to pregnant women because the infections can damage their offspring.

Respiratory Viral Diseases

A group of respiratory viral diseases sometimes is subdivided by doctors into upper and lower respiratory tract viral infections. The common cold is an example of an upper respiratory viral disease. There may be as many as 100 different strains of viruses that can produce common cold symptoms, which can include a scratchy throat, sneezing, runny nose, and, mainly in children, a fever. The variety of symptoms can mimic many other disorders ranging from hay fever to whooping cough. The ailment may be complicated by bacterial infections in the middle ear and sinuses. Because of the myriad strains of viruses that can cause common cold symptoms, it has not been practical to design a vaccine that could be used as a preventive measure for the problem.

A doctor might recommend bed rest, steam inhalation to relieve chest tightness, antihistamines, aspirin, and cough syrup as needed for appropriate symptoms. Antibiotics are not prescribed except to control secondary infections involving bacteria.

Viral infections of the lower respiratory tract can be quite serious and occasionally fatal. The viruses involved in lower respiratory tract infections usually are of different types from those causing the common cold. Influenza, or flu, viruses are of a specific size, composition, and pattern of activity despite the recurrent shifts in prevalent types since the microbe was first identified nearly 50 years ago. Symptoms may vary according to the type of influenza virus—A, B, or C—but the onset of a flu infection may be marked by chills and fever, general aches and pains, headache, sensitivity to light, and possibly a sore throat and coughing. Like the common cold, there is no agent that can be administered to cure the infection. The only relief is for symptoms and includes bed rest, analgesics, throat gargles, cough medicines, steam inhalation, and antibiotics if needed to control secondary infections of bacteria.

Symptoms similar to either or both the common cold and influenza can be produced by four types of parainfluenza viruses, each of which usually is relatively mild, self-limiting, and of short-lived duration. They differ somewhat from other respiratory viruses in attacking during the summer or autumn, rather than in the winter.

Still another kind of viral respiratory infection can be caused by a group of microorganisms called adenoviruses. The virus itself is rather distinctive, appearing under the lens of an electron microscope as a 20-faced geometric figure. One might think that a disease organism shaped like an alien from a science-fiction movie would be easy to identify and control. However, there are more than 30 subtle variations of this virus with different protein-coating components, tiny fibers that extend from corners of the surface, and in some instances an adenovirus may be accompanied by a still smaller incomplete virus. Each variation may account for different symptoms or groups of symp-

toms that may include fever, sore throat, cough, and even viral pneumonia. Adenoviruses also can cause a form of conjunctivitis that can accompany or not accompany respiratory symptoms.

Enteroviruses

A large family of viruses that attacks through the gastrointestinal tract is given the name of enteroviruses. This group includes the poliomyelitis virus, the coxsackie viruses that cause symptoms similar to those of polio but without paralysis, and the echo viruses that are responsible for many human diseases, ranging from respiratory complaints to diarrhea and including aseptic meningitis. Echo is an acronym formed from enteric cytopathogenic human orphan; when first isolated from the human gut the viruses were considered orphans because the medical researchers did not know what diseases they caused, but now they know.

Coxsackie viruses are responsible for a number of sore throats, headaches, fevers, aches and pains, vomiting, and loss of appetite in infants and small children. These symptoms result from a disorder known as herpangina, which also causes sores or lesions in the mouth anywhere from the tongue to the tonsils. A similar disorder caused by a coxsackie virus causes lesions on the hands and feet as well as in the mouth, and occasionally in the anal-genital area. The infection is known by the appropriate common name of hand, foot, and mouth disease.

A more severe version of a coxsackie infection causing the common childhood complaints of headache, fever, sore throat, and general feeling of ill health is known as epidemic pleurodynia. In addition, the youngster may have severe pains in the lower chest or abdomen and pains in the limbs. The onset of symptoms may resemble those of appendicitis or a heart attack, and there may be complications such as inflammation of the membranes in the chest area. Except for complications, most acute symptoms subside within a few days, and the patient usually recovers within a week or two. There is no known therapy for the infection, and treatment is limited to relieving the symptoms.

Aseptic meningitis is marked by headache, fever, vomiting, loss of appetite, and pain and stiffness in the neck and back. When the illness begins it may be difficult to tell whether the symptoms are those of aspetic meningitis or a form of poliomyelitis. Laboratory tests often are needed to identify the virus responsible, and in a case of aseptic meningitis almost any of the enteroviruses may be involved. In some cases of aseptic meningitis, the patient may have a skin rash resembling measles. The disease usually is treated as if it were a case of nonparalytic polio. Recovery from the acute symptoms occurs within a week in most patients.

Poliomyelitis

Poliomyelitis is a preventable enterovirus disease. In areas of the world where children are immunized with polio vaccines, the disease has virtually disappeared. It occurs in North America almost exclusively in persons who have failed to be immunized. But the disease still is prevalent in underdeveloped regions of the world and occurs in all seasons in tropical areas.

Polio as a health threat in the industrialized countries of the western world developed inadvertently because of improved sanitation practices beginning in the 19th century. Previous to that time, polio virus-

es apparently affected everyone as a subclinical infection, and any person who survived childhood probably had become immune to the disease. After the use of flush toilets, the practice of hand washing, and other hygiene measures were popularized, the natural immunity acquired from daily contact with polio viruses was lost. Sanitized people thus ironically became the victims of polio epidemics by contact with carriers of the virus. An unimmunized person could become infected today by contact with polio carriers in a country with poor sanitary conditions.

A polio infection may become a disease condition as a so-called minor illness, with fever, headache, sore throat, and vomiting. In some mild cases, the symptoms subside and there is complete recovery. In severe cases, there is a second phase of more severe symptoms which follow the minor illness by several days. The patient experiences fever with severe headaches, deep muscle pains, and stiff neck and back. As the disease progresses, the patient experiences weakness, loss of sensation, and/or paralysis of various muscles. The area of the body that becomes paralyzed depends upon what part of the central nervous system is damaged by the polio lesion.

About half of all polio patients suffer some disability, which may range from mild to severe and permanent. A small percentage of polio patients, mainly cases involving viral damage to brain tissues, die.

Other Viral Diseases

Mumps, infectious mononucleosis, scarlet fever, and rabies are among other viral diseases affecting humans. Rabies, along with yellow fever, encephalitis, tick fever, and a number of exotic diseases with names like O'nyong-nyong and machupo, are viral diseases that generally involve contact between humans and animals or insects. The animals may be of the domestic type, like cats and dogs, or wild, like rats and birds. The insects usually are ticks, mosquitoes, or sandflies. Virus diseases that man can get from rodents, including mice and hamsters as well as rats, can also be transmitted from human to human.

Rickettsial Infections

Somewhere in between viruses and bacteria is a group of disease organisms called rickettsias which carry disorders such as typhus and Rocky Mountain spotted fever from animals to humans. Like viruses, the rickettsial organisms require the living cells of the host, but like bacteria they have cell walls and their own metabolic apparatus. They usually enter the human body through an insect bite and invade the cells that line small blood vessels. Typical symptoms include a lesion at the bite site, where the creatures originally set up housekeeping, plus a rash and headache. The headache and certain other effects, such as interruption of blood flow to body tissues, are complications of the damage to blood vessels by the rickettsias.

Typhus is an example of a widespread rickettsial infection. The disease organism is carried by the human body louse, a tiny vampire-like insect that feeds on human blood and is found especially in tropical regions. The louse has a reflex habit of defecating when it eats and tends to deposit feces on the human skin while feeding on human blood. The louse feces contains the rickettsia, which is rubbed into the bug bite when the victim scratches the bite.

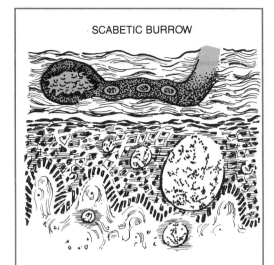

SCABETIC BURROW

Scabies is an example of a disease caused by a tiny insect that burrows under the skin and lays its eggs in the tunnels, causing an intense itching sensation in the infected person. The disease can be spread by contact with the skin or clothing of an infected person.

After an incubation period of less than two weeks, the infection begins to produce symptoms of a high fever and a severe headache that defies treatment. Dark, sometimes bleeding sores may appear on the skin.

Because rickettsias are part bacteria, they usually can be controlled by antibiotics. Symptoms are treated with aspirin for headaches and application of sponge baths to reduce fever. Cardiovascular failure, pneumonia, and gangrene are possible complications. The risk of death increases with the age of the patient. However, persons venturing into areas where typhus is a health threat can obtain protection by innoculation of typhus vaccines.

A milder form of the disease, known as endemic typhus or murine typhus, is transmitted by a rat flea. Symptoms of the infection are similar to typhus, and treatment is with antibiotics. A vaccine to protect against murine typhus also is available. The rat flea, which is carried by mice, inhabits the warm areas of the North American Gulf and South Atlantic coasts.

Rocky Mountain spotted fever is a rickettsial disease transmitted to people through the bite of the hard-shelled wood or dog tick. At one time it was believed the disease was limited to the Rocky Mountains area of the U.S., but it is now known to be prevalent in many other parts of the western hemisphere. Attacks are most likely to occur between May and September, when the ticks are most active and people are most likely to be exposed to brush and weeds infested by the insects.

Symptoms include headache, fever, chills, muscular pains and weakness, and a skin rash that begins on the hands and feet and spreads to other body areas. Like the typhus rickettsia, the spotted fever rickettsia tends to attack and damage the blood vessels, increasing the risk of thrombosis and gangrene in affected tissues. Treatment involves the use of antibiotics, and a vaccine is available for outdoor workers and others likely to encounter the ticks.

Bacterial Infections

Bacteria are seemingly innocent one-celled plants, except that some are pathogenic and capable of killing a human. Most bacteria that cause human disease are toxin producers. An invasion of the body tissues by pathogenic bacteria results not only in the effects of toxins excreted by the organisms, but in the effects of battles between the invading plant cells and the body's defending forces which may result in the release of additional unpleasant substances into the patient's tissues. A significant share of the body's blood supply and energy resources may be commandeered to fight a bacterial infection, which is the reason a sick person may experience pain and fatigue. The doctor will advise the patient to get plenty of rest, instead of competing with the anti-infection apparatus for the body's natural resources, during an illness.

Bacteria are classified in several ways by the medical profession. Little, round bacteria are likely to be identified as cocci. The singular form of cocci is coccus, but a pair of cocci is called diplococci. If the cocci occur in clusters they are called staphylocci; if they occur in strips they are known as streptococci. A coccus may be associated with a disease it causes, such as the gonococcus that is responsible for gonorrhea. An example of a diplococcus germ is the pneumococcus that causes bacterial pneumonia.

There are also rod-shaped bacteria that are called bacilli—or bacillus in the singular—and spiral-shaped bacteria known as spirilla, or spirillum. Tuberculosis is caused by a tubercle baccilus, and syphilis is an example of a spirillum infection.

Bacteria also may be identified by doctors as gram-positive or gram-negative, which refers only to the way the bacteria react when stained with a dye called Gram's stain. Some strains of bacteria retain the dye and are called gram-positive; those that do not are called gram-negative bacteria. The Gram's stain helps doctors identify a strain of bacteria that might resemble another type in some ways.

A diplococcus that causes pneumonia, for example, retains the purple color of the stain, but a diplococcus that causes

FORMS OF THE TRUE BACTERIA

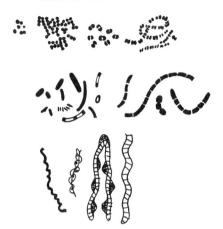

Bacteria often are given names according to their basic shapes. A spherical or round bacterium, for example, is known as a coccus. A cylindrical or rod-shaped bacterium is called a bacillus. Spiral-shaped bacteria usually are called spirochetes. Pairs of cocci are called diplococci, strings of cocci are streptococci, and cocci that live in clusters are known as staphylococci. Staphylococci often are associated with pus-forming skin infections. Streptococci are responsible for infections like rheumatic fever and scarlet fever. Baccili are involved in tuberculosis, leprosy, and diptheria. Spirochetes include the germs that cause syphilis and cholera. Bacteria names also may indicate the disease; for example, gonococci are diplococci that cause gonorrhea.

meningitis would not retain the Gram's stain. Thus, when viewed under a microscope after staining, pneumococcus is identified as a gram-positive bacteria, and meningitis as a gram-negative bacteria.

Staphylococcal and streptococcal bacteria generally are gram-positive. Staphylococcal infections often involve wounds because the bacteria are present normally on the skin surfaces of perhaps one-fourth of all people and in the nostrils of about half of all humans. Furuncles, carbuncles, and abcesses are likely to involve staphylococcal germs. However, staphylococcal infections also can be a cause of pneumonia, osteomyelitis, and enterocolitis.

Staphylococcus germs can be transmitted from person to person by skin contact, as in shaking hands, and can infect as a complication of surgery, a skin disorder, or a burn, as well as through a wound or break in the skin. A patient receiving immunosuppressive therapy for cancer or an organ transplant may be particularly vulnerable.

The same general treatment procedure is followed for most cases of staphylococcal infections, regardless of the source of infection or the site. The therapy is based on removal of the pus produced by the disease organisms, usually by draining an abscess, and the application of an effective antibiotic. Since some strains of staphylococcus germs are resistant to antibiotics, doctors try to identify the strain of the germ before prescribing a specific antibiotic.

Streptococcus infections usually are more virulent and complex than those caused by staphylococcus bacteria. There are many groups and subgroups of streptococci. One group, called pyogenic streptococci, causes such diseases as acute glomerulonephritis, scarlet fever, rheumatic fever, and septic sore throat. A strain known as streptococcus pneumoniae is the most common cause of lobar pneumonia. Some strains of streptococci are called hemolytic because they produce a substance that destroys red blood cells.

Many individuals are innocent carriers of streptococcus germs. The germs can be recovered from the throat, intestinal tract, or lungs of seemingly normal, healthy people. When a carrier of streptococci becomes sick, medical personnel may be confused by the discovery of the germs which often have nothing to do with the illness at hand, although they might cause an acute disease in another person.

Among common gram-negative bacteria that may cause infections are salmonella diseases, which include typhoid fever, acute gastro-enteritis, shigellosis or bacillary dysentery, cholera, whooping cough, tularemia, and the bubonic plague.

Diphtheria, botulism, tetanus, and certain types of food poisoning other than botulism but including one form of staphylococcal food poisoning, are caused by bacteria that produce toxins. In a case of staphylococcal food poisoning as well as botulism, the bacteria does not have to be present in the food since the toxic effect is caused by the substances left by the bacteria.

Tuberculosis and leprosy are caused by a type of bacteria sometimes called mycobacteria. Tuberculosis germs generally are associated with lung infections, but they often invade the blood and lymph vessels to involve the heart, central nervous system, bones, gastrointestinal tract, and other organs such as cancer cells and certain viruses that spread to distant body tissues after becoming established at an original disease site.

Examples of bacterial diseases caused by spiralla are syphilis, relapsing fever, and leptospirosis, each of which may be transmitted in a different manner. Syphilis, a venereal disease, and three nonvenereal diseases with similar symptoms—yaws, pinta, and bejel—are spread by direct contact with infected persons. Relapsing fever is transmitted by ticks or body lice. Leptospirosis is carried by wild animals and transmitted to humans by direct contact with an infected animal, or by contact with water or soil contaminated by the diseased animal.

Protozoal Diseases

Protozoal diseases, caused by one-celled animals, include amebic dysentery, African sleeping sickness, toxoplasmosis, and malaria. Malaria usually is transmitted by the bite of an infected anopheles mosquito that usually lives in tropical areas. The disease also has been transmitted in North America by blood transfusions from infected humans, by contaminated hypodermic needles, and by carriers from malaria-infested area, such as military personnel returning from duty in tropical countries.

Toxoplasmosis is a not uncommon protozoal disease that can be acquired from eating meat that has not been properly cooked. It is somewhat unique as a human protozoal disease in that the disease organism can be transmitted through the placenta of a pregnant woman to her unborn child. The pregnancy may end in miscarriage or stillbirth, or the child may be born with a toxoplasmosis infection.

Sulfa drugs and other medications are used to treat cases of toxoplasmosis infections in humans. Special antimalarial drugs are available for treating effects of malarial parasites.

QUESTIONS AND ANSWERS

THE UNSEEN AGENTS
OF INFECTION

Q: *Why is malaria a health problem today? Aren't the drugs developed during World War II effective anymore?*

A: Two antimalarial drugs developed during World War II were chloroquine and primaquine. Chloroquine ordinarily destroys the disease organism during one stage of its life cycle, while it is in the blood. Primaquine attacks the form that invades the liver, where the sporozoites, or malarial parasites, divide into numerous new cells. However, since the 1960's malarial protozoa have displayed increasing resistance against the drugs, first in Asia and now in South America.

New antimalarial drugs are still being introduced, but they also may lose their effectiveness after a few years. The *Plasmodium*, as the infectious malarial protozoon is called, seems quite adaptable to new drugs. Also, since an invasion of human body tissues by a malarial parasite does not evoke the kind of antibody reaction produced by most bacteria and viruses, there is little hope of developing a vaccine or of people developing permanent immunity to the disease.

Q: *Is hepatitis always caused by a virus infection?*

A: There are two viruses, Types A and B, which along with alcohol, account for most of the cases of hepatitis that occur worldwide. However, hepatitis occasionally can be caused by bacteria that are associated with tuberculosis, leprosy, and salmonella. Several kinds of fungus and helminths (worms), syphilis, leptospirosis, ameba, and malarial protozoa also can produce hepatitis symptoms.

Q: *Has the cause of Legionnaire's disease ever been identified?*

A: The disease organism was identified through laboratory studies of tissue samples taken from Legionnaire's disease patients as a rod-shaped bacterium, a bacillus. Doctors now believe the disease that produces pneumonia-like symptoms has been around for decades and probably was the cause of many previously unexplained deaths. But the Pennsylvania epidemic of 1976 helped bring the problem into focus so that people stricken by the disease in the future can have their cases diagnosed and treated quickly and properly.

Q: *Why are flu epidemics so hard to control?*

A: One reason is that Type A influenza, the virus that causes most of the trouble, mutates periodically into a new strain. Millions of people may have been immunized against the previous strain, but the mutation creates a whole new ballgame for public health doctors who must develop a new form of influenza vaccine. Meanwhile, the influenza virus needs only a short incubation period to produce symptoms and spread from one population group to another.

Q: *Would it be possible for a new kind of virus to start an epidemic in North America?*

A: One hopes it would not be probable, but it certainly could be possible. Doctors know of several highly infectious and deadly disease viruses, such as green monkey fever and Ebola hemorrhagic fever, for which there are no known medications to prevent or treat their effects. These diseases thus far have been confined to remote regions of the world like the jungles of Africa. But as recreational and business travel to those areas increases, there is a constantly increasing risk that a traveler could become infected with one of these exotic viruses in Sudan, Zaire, or another African country today, and could return home via jet airplane to spread the disease through a large population center like New York City or Los Angeles tomorrow. As evidence that such an event could occur, a man returning to Washington, D.C., from West Africa recently was stricken with Lassa fever, a disease so virulent that even medical personnel avoid direct contact with the patient. Fortunately, the disease did not spread.

Q: *I read in a newspaper story recently about a man in New Mexico developing bubonic plague. Didn't that disease disappear with the Middle Ages?*

A: Plague, which occurs in bubonic (enlarged lymph nodes) or pneumonic (respiratory) forms, is considered to be endemic in the western United States. The disease is harbored by rodents, including prairie dogs and squirrels as well as rats and mice, and is transmitted to humans by the bite of a flea that acquires the disease organism from the animals. As an example of how a dangerous disease like the plague can be acquired, rabbit hunters in western states can get bubonic plague by handling the carcasses of rabbits that live in burrows contaminated by diseased rats.

People who are likely to be exposed to plague germs, such as travelers to Southeast Asia, can receive inoculations of a vaccine made with killed plague bacilli. Antibiotics are used in the treatment of plague cases. Thus the disease is still with us, but doctors now have weapons to control outbreaks.

Q: *What is extrapulmonary tuberculosis and how does one get it?*

A: Extrapulmonary tuberculosis usually is a complication of tuberculosis of the lung. Extrapulmonary means that it has spread from the lungs to other tissues. The infection can travel through the lymph system or the digestive tract from contaminated secretions coughed up from the lungs.

16

CANCER
THE UNCONQUERED
KILLER

It has been said that cancer is caused by everything and cured by nothing. This is, of course, a simplistic description of the enigma of the disease that accounts for more deaths in the industrialized world than any other medical problem with the exception of heart disease. There have been numerous surveys and studies that have "discovered" an association between myriad factors in the environment and cancer of one sort or another. And cancer is one of the few diseases that has continued to increase in mortality rates during the past few decades despite progress in finding effective therapies.

Actually, the outlook for control of this insidious killer disease is not as hopeless as might appear from statistical reports of increased numbers of cases. These studies often indicate that better diagnostic techniques and improved public awareness of signs and symptoms can lead to detection of cancers that might previously have been overlooked. More also is being learned about which factors in the environment are likely causes of human cancers and how to cope with those factors.

And there are medical and surgical treatments for certain types of cancers that can be effective when started in early stages of the disease.

It's quite important to put the matter into a proper perspective, to understand that there are many types of cancer. Although the various types can be described as abnormal tissue growths of cells that have "gone wild," spreading throughout the body to invade other tissues and disrupt normal body functions, there are more than 150 different kinds of cancers which involve different types of body tissues and may be caused by different agents. Some cancers, for example, are sarcomas, which affect mainly bones and muscles. Others are carcinomas, which are involved in tissues of glands as well as of the breast, uterus, stomach, and skin. The rate of growth and other effects of a cancer may be determined by the type of cell tissue in which it first appears.

Not all tumors are cancerous. Tumors that are noncancerous are identified as benign tumors. Tumors that are cancerous often are called malignant tumors. A benign tumor can be destructive in that it may grow so large that it interferes with the normal functions of an organ. Or a benign tumor may ulcerate and bleed. But, in general, a benign tumor does not spread beyond its original tissue site; it does not invade other tissues directly or indirectly by metastasis—the process by which cancer cells migrate from the original tumor to other sites in the body by riding in the bloodstream. However, it is possible for a benign tumor to change into a malignant tumor. A mole on the skin, for example, may develop as a benign tumor but suddenly turn malignant and expand its growth rapidly through the skin tissues.

Possible Causes of Cancer

Cancers can be caused by viruses, although this relationship has been demonstrated more clearly in other animals than in humans. Hormones, particularly synthetic hormones that have been used in animal feeds and as human medications, have been shown to stimulate the growth of cancers in people. Radiant energy, from sunlight, X-rays, and other sources, has been linked to cancers of the skin, bone marrow, and thyroid gland. At least half, and perhaps as many as three-fourths of all cancers, are believed to be caused by exposure to chemicals in the environment, including chemicals produced by the burning of tobacco. Most human lung cancers have been attributed either to the combustion products of cigarettes or exposure to asbestos fibers used in modern building construction.

Modern civilization itself is sometimes blamed for the incidence of cancer in the western world. However, there are references in the Old Testament to diseases identified as cancer. Physicians at the beginning of the Christian era reported performing amputations, hysterectomies, and mastectomies in an effort to control cancers considered then to be incurable. Doctors have known for more than 200 years that cancer can be caused by certain chemicals and radiation. The effect of modern civilization has been to introduce new chemical agents and sources of radiation, and to make the potential causes of cancer available to everybody.

Of the many thousands of chemical agents that might be a direct cause of cancer, only about a dozen actually have been proven to be true human carcinogens. But the dozen agents include substances that are virtually impossible to avoid in most parts of the world, such as the benzpyrene produced by the burning of gasoline, diesel fuels, and many organic molecules; and aflatoxin, which is produced by molds that grow on a wide variety of plant products and finds its way into milk ingested by a cow eating contaminated feed. It is even more difficult to avoid a carcinogenic substance known as nitrosamine which, like cholesterol, can be produced by the human body's own tissues.

In addition to cancer-causing agents that seem to be everywhere in the environment, there are cancer-causing factors that seem to be associated with geographic and lifestyle influences. Among Seventh Day Adventists in the Los Angeles area, for example, the incidence of lung cancer for this religious group that abstains from smoking and drinking of alcoholic beverages was found to be about ten percent of the level observed in their neighbors. Their lifestyle, however, apparently offered no special protection from cancers of the uterus, prostate, and other organs. The incidence of lung cancer has been found to be higher in Finland than in neighboring Sweden, and higher in American blacks than in American whites. Cancers of the digestive tract vary as much as 20-fold from one country to another, perhaps because of differences in diet or substances in drinking water. Some studies have found that the risk of cancer increases for smokers who also consume alcoholic beverages. Other studies that have investigated possible factors such as eating vegetarian meals, as opposed to meals rich in animal fats and proteins, have produced conflicting results. Not too surprising, therefore, is the growing notion that anything and everything can be a cause of cancer.

How Cancer Cells Develop

Most information about how a cancer cell develops is based on retrospective data. In other words, a cancer is found and medical scientists work backwards to try to trace the origin of the tumor. The trail generally leads to the concept that some event occurred to change the genetic material in the tissue cell where the cancer started. Ordinarily, it is assumed, a cell's genetic material, which is composed of DNA molecules, directs the cell's activities, including reproduction. A normal tissue cell reproduces by dividing into two daughter cells that are in effect the clones of an original cell. The cell or tissue composed of a group of cells presumably contains in its genetic material the orders to form an organ or part of an organ, or to produce new cells to replace old, worn-out cells, and to stop when that task is completed. But when a virus, which usually is nothing

more than a wild DNA molecule, or a chemical molecule or jolt of ionizing radiation, enters a normal cell, it may be able to change the entire template or set of instructions for normal cell functioning. Instead of stopping its growth activity when the altered cell's membrane bumps into the membrane of a neighboring cell, the neoplastic or malignant cell invades the neighboring cell and converts its protoplasm and chromosomal material to its own use. Depending upon the type of cancer and tissue, the new cell will spread its own kind slowly or rapidly. But if not stopped, the new growth will eventually spread throughout the body, robbing all normal cells of their blood and other components, until the host body is destroyed.

Ironically, a cancer cell strain once established is virtually immortal. It doesn't die but simply continues to grow as long as there is host material available to provide nourishment. Cancer cell strains removed from cancer victims continue to thrive in test tube cultures of research laboratories long after the cancer patients have died.

Some oncologists, medical scientists who specialize in cancer, believe that a cancer can start from a single cell altered by a single virus or chemical molecule. Others think there is a threshold level requiring a large dose of cancer-causing agent to start a tumor, and that normally healthy tissue cells can withstand a small exposure to a carcinogen. Still others suggest that perhaps more than one agent may be involved in starting a cancer at the cellular level. For example, an interaction between an invading virus and a chemical within a cell might be the triggering force. The various theories are offered to explain why a cancer may not appear until 10, 15, or 20 years after exposure to a known cancer agent, or why only a minority of individuals may develop cancer after an entire population group has been exposed to a cancer-causing substance.

How Big a Risk?

As a rule of thumb, the risk of cancer for any individual increases as he grows older. The risk rate for some types of cancer has been estimated to increase by one percent for each year of a person's age, so that at the age of 50 the chances of developing a cancer are 50 percent, 75 percent at age 75, and so on. While this data is something of a statistical game that could never be applied to any particular person, there is evidence that more people than is generally realized have a cancer somewhere in their bodies. During autopsies of persons who have died in accidents or as a result of a cerebrovascular disease, pathologists often find cancerous growths that had not yet reached the stage of producing typical signs or symptoms of the disease.

Warning Signs

Cancer usually does not cause pain in the early stages, but there are other signs and symptoms that can be cancer clues for both the patient and the examining doctor. They include the typical seven early warning signs.

1. Any lump or thickening, especially in the breast, lip, or tongue.

2. Any irregular or unexplained bleeding from a nipple or any body opening, including signs of blood in urine or stools, and any unexpected bleeding or discharge from the vagina such as vaginal bleeding after menopause.

3. A sore on the skin, lips, mouth, tongue, or elsewhere that fails to heal.

4. Any significant change in the size or color of a wart, mole, or birthmark.

5. Indigestion or loss of appetite that persists in the absence of factors such as food allergies, influenza, etc.

6. Persistent hoarseness, coughing, or difficulty in swallowing.

7. Any change in normal bowel habits that is more than temporary.

Cancer of the rectum may be signaled by a change in bowel habits to a pattern, perhaps, of periods of constipation followed by periods of diarrhea. There also could be rectal bleeding and/or a feeling of a mass in the rectum, or a sensation that the bowel movement was not complete. Some patients may experience abdominal cramps.

Persistent indigestion with a lack of appetite and loss of weight could be signs of stomach cancer. There also could be stomach pains after eating and/or vomiting. Anemia can be another sign of stomach cancer. Any bleeding from the upper portion of the digestive tract will not have the red coloration of bleeding from the lower bowel because of the effect of digestive juices on the blood. Blood loss at the stomach level results in a black, tarry coloration in the stool.

Blood in the urine, difficulting in urinating, or an increasing urge to urinate during the night can be signs of cancer in the bladder or kidney. These also could be signs of prostate cancer in a man.

Skin sores that do not heal easily, or changes in the size or coloration of moles, warts, birthmarks, and even scars, could be signs of skin cancer.

Headaches, changes in vision, dizzy spells, paralysis, or nausea and vomiting not explainable in terms of dietary difficulties, could be signs of a stroke, brain tumor, or cancer.

Chest pains and a cough that persists for two weeks or more could indicate the presence of lung cancer. Other signs might include blood in the sputum or coughing up blood, strange respiratory noises in the chest, or a feeling of breathlessness when there has been no particular exertion to account for the shortness of breath.

Persistent hoarseness can be a sign of cancer of the larynx.

Cancer of the uterus often is marked by unexpected, unusual, or irregular vaginal bleeding that may occur between menstrual periods, after menopause, or following sexual intercourse. Unusually heavy bleeding during a menstrual period also could signal a disorder.

Cancer of the breast may reveal itself through bleeding or other discharge from a nipple, or the appearance of any lump or nodule in the breast which may be painless or painful.

Cancers of the mouth area, including the tongue and lips, may begin as a sore or ulceration that does not heal, or as a path of white tissue that replaces the normal pink coloration. The thickened white patches, called leukoplakia, can be either precancerous tissue changes or benign growths.

A biopsy, or laboratory microscope examination of a sample of tissue suspected of being cancerous, usually is made before a definite diagnosis of cancer can be rendered. For certain types of cancers, such as leukemias, or blood cancers, other kinds of laboratory tests may be helpful. However, cytologic examinations—studying suspicious biopsy cell samples under a microscope—provide the final diagnostic clues for most cancer cases.

Metastasis of Cancer Cells

Because of the tendency of cancers to metastasize, or spread to other organs, early detection and treatment are important. Once a malignant tumor has started to spread to other organs in other parts of the body, the chances for a cure or control of the cancer decline rapidly.

With a few exceptions, cancer cells that metastasize usually migrate to the lungs and liver, as well as the bones. The lungs and liver are among common secondary cancer sites because any foreign body that enters the bloodstream is likely to be carried through the lungs or liver at least once. The kidneys and heart also are major routes of the circulatory system, but they are not metastasis targets. Because

ORIGIN AND GROWTH OF MALIGNANT CELLS IN THE SKIN

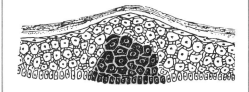

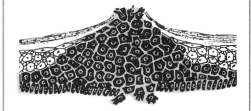

One type of skin cancer, a papilloma, may begin developing beneath the surface of the skin (dark-colored cells). Its presence may be noticed at first as a lump beneath the skin. As the cancer continues to grow and spread, it eventually breaks through the surface of the skin.

CARCINOMA OF SKIN

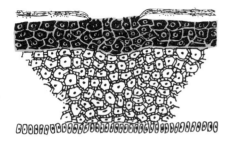

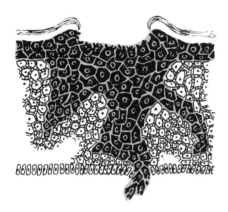

A type of skin cancer that may begin on the surface and gradually erode downward into deeper tissues is a squamous cell carcinoma. It may appear at first as a small skin ulceration, but it works progressively deeper into vital tissues as it grows. Cancer cells that eventually invade lymph or blood vessels can spread quickly to other body areas.

cers associated with moles that have changed from benign to malignant tumors, can spread rapidly to the lungs, lymph nodes, or other organs. Cancers that develop from exposure of epidermal cells to ultraviolet rays of the sun tend to migrate to the lymph nodes. Most skin cancers involve cells at the bottom layer of the epidermis—the melanomas that start from melanocytes, the pigment-forming cells, and the basal and squamous cells that form the living cells of the epidermis.

Skin cancers are less likely to become life-threatening than other malignant tumors for several reasons, including the fact that they are more easily detected and treated. When basal and squamous cell skin cancers and melanomas are treated in the early stages, the prognosis for complete recovery is close to 100 percent. Therapies can include surgery to remove the skin cancer, chemotherapy, and/or radiation. The treatment chosen may depend in part upon the cosmetic effect; a chemotherapy lotion may be tried first on a facial area that might be disfigured by a surgical scar. The amount of surgery would depend upon how far the tumor had spread. A melanoma that goes untreated in the early stages may burrow beneath the epidermis and require a deep excision.

Leukemia

Blood cancer is a bit of a misnomer in that the disease actually involves the blood-forming part of the bone, the marrow. But the signs of the disease, known as leukemia, appear in the white blood cells, or leukocytes, which become numerous and fail to mature. As the leukocytes proliferate, the red blood cells and blood platelets are reduced in number, so that anemia devel-

of the peculiarities of various types of cancers, it is not uncommon for cancer symptoms to appear first at a secondary site that has been invaded by cells carried from the original tumor. The first symptom of a soft tissue cancer, for example, may be bone pain of a secondary cancer site.

Contrary to popular belief, skin cancers can metastasize and invade tissues deep in the body. Melanomas, the kind of skin can-

ops along with increased susceptibility to infections and hemorrhages.

Leukemia can develop in one of several different forms. It may be classified as acute or chronic, depending upon the progress of the disease and condition of the white blood cells. In chronic leukemia, the white blood cells are more mature and may have some ability to function as mature cells. White blood cells in acute leukemia are likely to be immature and ineffective in combating infection.

There also are classifications of leukemia according to the specific type of white blood cells involved—lymphocytes, monocytes, or myelocytes. In addition, the different forms of leukemia generally affect different age groups. Acute lymphoid leukemia occurs in small children, and the chronic form of lymphoid leukemia affects adults who are past middle age. Acute myelocytic leukemia affects mainly young adults, and the chronic form occurs in adults between 30 and 50 years of age.

Leukemia is one of the forms of cancer that is increasing in incidence because of improved methods of detecting the disease. It is a leading cause of death among children. The cause in most cases remains unknown, but suggested causes include exposure to ionizing radiation, benzene that is present in gasoline, viruses, and hereditary or familial factors. When the disease occurs in one of a pair of identical twins, there is a strong possibility that the other twin will show symptoms also.

Symptoms of leukemias include fever, pains in the bones and joints, and swollen lymph nodes, liver, or spleen. Treatments vary somewhat according to the type of leukemia, but the therapies generally include blood transfusions, chemotherapy, and radiation. Bone marrow grafts have been used for some acute leukemia patients. Patients often need to rest because they tire easily, and require protection against injuries that can start bleeding. They should have warm clothing and bedding because they are more sensitive to cool temperatures than normal individuals.

Cancers of the Bone

Bone cancers usually are secondary cancers caused by cells that have metastasized soft tissue organs elsewhere in the body. They often are discovered because of pain and swelling that resembles the signs and symptoms of arthritis or bursitis. Diagnosis often is made during X-ray studies of the bones and joints, or sometimes during treatment of a fracture.

Multiple myeloma is a type of bone cancer involving destruction of bone tissue by cells that originate in the marrow. The patient experiences bone pain and may show signs of anemia. X-ray photos of the affected bone often show punched-out areas of destruction. Sarcomas, or cancers of the cartilage and bone-forming cells, are among other kinds of primary bone tumors. A sarcoma can turn bone to mush, which is approximately what happens after the cancer gets started in a long bone of the body. The sarcoma also can spread into neighboring muscle and other soft tissue. It often is necessary to amputate a limb invaded by sarcoma to prevent the cancer from spreading to other parts of the body. Radiation and chemotherapy may be administered.

Breast Cancer

Breast cancers may develop painlessly or painfully as tumors within the ducts that carry milk to the nipple. The nipple may produce a discharge or it may retract as the cancer grows. The skin of the breast sometimes turns red and forms a dimple or an ulcer. But a lump in the breast is the usual sign, even though all breast lumps are not cancers. A lump in the breast may be a benign tumor—in most cases, only a doctor can tell for sure.

Most women learn to conduct a monthly self-examination for lumps in the breasts. The procedure involves several simple steps, such as standing before a mirror and holding the back erect with the elbows and hands held behind so the breasts protrude. She looks for dimpling or puckering of the skin or any changes in the nipples. The nipples should be squeezed to see if blood or any other fluid is discharged. In the second stage of the procedure, the woman lies on her back with a pillow beneath the shoulders. In this position, she carefully feels all areas of each breast with the fingers, pressing the breasts gently against the rib cage, to see if any lumps can be felt. The examination should be extended into the armpits, where the lymph nodes are located.

A woman who is not sure of how to handle self-examination for lumps in the breast should get instructions from her doctor. Some doctors supplement the breast examination by palpation and by X-ray mammography or thermography, which sometimes may detect a tissue abnormality that could be missed by palpating the breasts with the fingers. As in other forms of cancer, however, the use of a biopsy often is needed to determine if a growth is benign or malignant.

Surgery is the standard method of treating breast cancer in the United States. The surgical procedure usually follows one of four possible approaches, de-

pending upon the size of the tumor and other individual case factors. The surgeon may remove only the lump, the breast, or the breast plus the adjacent lymph nodes in the armpit; or he may perform a radical mastectomy, which consists of removing the breast, the lymph nodes, and the muscle tissue beneath the breast.

If it appears likely that the cancer may have spread by metastasis from the breast, doctors may administer chemotherapy and/or radiation treatments. In some cases additional surgery may be required to remove the adrenal or thyroid glands, the ovaries, or other glands.

A number of risk factors have been associated with cancer of the breast, such as a failure to bear children before a certain age, having a mother or aunt who had breast cancer, etc. However, as with other forms of cancer, the relationships are mainly statistical, and for every patient who fits the pattern a doctor can find a woman who developed breast cancer even though her medical history runs contrary to all the reported genetic and lifestyle links.

Cancer of the Uterus

Cancer of the uterus usually develops in cells of the endometrium, the layer that lines the organ. The most common sign of the disease among women in their fertile years is abnormal bleeding—bleeding that occurs after intercourse, bleeding that occurs between menstrual periods, or bleeding that is unusually heavy during a regular menstrual period. For women beyond their fertile years, a sign is bleeding that occurs at any time after the menstrual periods have ceased.

Diagnosis of uterine cancer usually is based on examination of biopsy material removed in a D & C procedure—the commonly used abbreviation for dilatation and curettage. The uterus is dilated and the lining is scraped, a procedure similar to that used in treatment of benign growths such as fibroids or as an abortion technique. The D & C may be performed in a hospital under a general anesthetic or with a local anesthetic.

If the presence of cancer is confirmed by the biopsy examination, the uterus is removed along with the ovaries and Fallopian tubes. Depending upon the individual case, a uterus may be removed through the vagina or through an opening made by an incision in the abdomen. The cervix may or may not be removed along with the uterus. But the vagina usually remains intact.

If the woman is postmenopausal, removal of the uterus and ovaries will have little effect on her hormonal activity. If she is still in her fertile years, some therapy may be needed to help the patient through the sudden menopause.

Cervical Cancer

Cervical cancer causes symptoms similar to those of cancer of the uterus, such as abnormal bleeding in the vaginal area. Diagnosis is much simpler, however, because of the availability of the Pap smear test. The Pap test allows the doctor to scrape a few cells from the surface of the cervix for the biopsy sample to be examined under a microscope. The Pap test is so remarkably accurate that it can be used to predict possible cervical cancer in a patient's future by detecting the presence of tissue cells that are of a type that eventually become malignant. Nevertheless, a biopsy is performed even if the Pap test

indicates a positive cancer case. The biopsy may be supplemented with direct observation of the cervix and surrounding tissue.

Treatment of cervical cancer may be limited to radiation, but in many cases the cervix and uterus are removed surgically. If the cancer has been diagnosed at a late stage of development, the ovaries and Fallopian tubes, plus other tissues, may be removed along with the entire uterus.

Cancers of the Prostate and Testes

Men are not excluded from the threat of cancers that affect the reproductive system. The most common forms of the disease involving the male sex organs are cancer of the prostate, which afflicts mainly men who are beyond middle age, and cancer of the testes, commonly called testicles, that generally occurs in younger men.

The prostate surrounds the male urethra, just below the urinary bladder. Because of its location, the prostate can interfere with the flow of urine from the bladder. Difficulty in urination, with or without the appearance of blood in the urine, can be an early sign of a prostate disorder, including cancer of the prostate. Symptoms of pain or pressure in the lower pelvic region may occur in a more advanced stage of prostatic cancer.

Despite its location in the pelvic region, the prostate is somewhat accessible for palpation or needle biopsy when a problem with the organ is suspected. An examining physician can palpate the prostate through the wall of the rectum. A biopsy needle can retrieve tissue samples through the rectum or through the skin between the anus and the scrotum.

Treatment for cancer of the prostate may require surgical removal of the gland, which seems to have no particular function except that of contributing to the seminal fluid which helps transport spermatozoa from the male to the female reproductive system. Therapy may include the use of radiation to control growth of the tumor. For some patients, such as those who may be too feeble to tolerate surgery, doctors may administer female sex hormones, which have the effect of slowing growth of cancer of the prostate. Male sex hormones, on the other hand, may have the effect of increasing the rate of growth of prostatic cancer.

Cancer of the testes may begin as painless or painful lumps in the scrotum. The scrotum may become enlarged and an examining doctor often can tell by shining a light through it whether the swelling is due to an accumulation of fluid or to a tumor. Testicular tumors often are treated by surgical excision, regardless of whether the growth is due to cancer. When that procedure is followed, a biopsy sample can be taken from the excised testicle to determine the presence of cancer so that further steps can be taken if needed. These steps might include a search for secondary cancers in and beyond nearby lymph nodes and radiation treatment of the tissues.

Some doctors use a more conservative approach to obtaining biopsy material in cases of suspected testicular cancer. They simply remove a sample tissue of the testis through the wall of the scrotum, leaving the testicle in place until the biopsy results show for certain that cancer is present.

Cancer of the testes occasionally may occur in a boy whose testicles have not descended normally from the abdomen where they form during the fetal stage. A male baby should be examined at birth or shortly after to determine if the testicles have descended into the scrotum to reduce the risk of testicular cancer developing some years later.

Cancers of the Kidneys and Bladder

The presence of blood in the urine, a sign of cancer of the prostate, might also signal the development of a tumor in one of two other major organs that are associated with the urinary tract, the kidneys, and the bladder. Kidney cancer can begin without pain, or pain and fever can be among the early symptoms of the disease. An advanced case of kidney cancer may be detected because of a persistent pain in the side or back—in the usual kidney area—and palpation of the area by a doctor might reveal a lump or abnormal surface.

Biopsy samples may be removed during surgical exploration while the patient is under a general anesthetic, or by a hollow needle inserted through the skin while the patient is under a local anesthetic. When exploratory surgery is not a part of the diagnosis, the doctor may use instead a technique called pyelography, in which a radio-opaque dye is injected into the circulatory system of the kidney before it is X-rayed. The X-ray picture usually will show sufficient detail of the kidney tissue structure to enable the doctor to tell where a tumor is located, its size, the possible extent of damage, etc.

When the presence of cancer has been confirmed, the usual method of treating the condition is to remove the diseased kidney. The surgeon also may excise neighboring tissues, such as the ureter, which is no longer needed after its kidney has been removed. Most otherwise healthy individuals can live a rather normal life with only one kidney.

Bladder cancer can produce urine that is colored with blood to a degree that may indicate the severity of the bleeding; the redder the coloration, the heavier the bleeding. However, the severity of bleeding may or may not be a clue as to the extent of cancer invasion; a small cancer can produce heavy bleeding, while a large advanced tumor may cause no bleeding at all. In the absence of bloody urine, symptoms of bladder cancer can include discomfort during urination and an increased urge to urinate more frequently.

Malignant tumors of the bladder occur in two different forms, solid and papillary. The papillary tumors, which are nipple-shaped projections, often are benign growths, although they can eventually become malignant and invade the walls of the bladder if not removed. Solid lesions may appear like ulcers and most often are the type that account for blood in the urine or urinary frequency and discomfort.

Papillary tumors can be removed by use of instruments that are inserted into the bladder to scrape them from the lining much like a D & C operation is used to remove tumors from the lining of the uterus. Examination of the interior of the bladder and removal of the polyp-like growths is made possible with a cystoscope, a pencil-shaped instrument that is inserted through the urethra and is equipped with a light and a knife for cutting away papillary tumors. The procedure is carried out while the patient is under an anesthetic.

Solid lesions are not as easily treated, and when biopsy has determined that the lesions are cancerous, the only way to extend the life of the patient is by surgical removal of bladder tissue. The procedure may involve removal of only the part of the bladder that has been damaged by the cancer, or of the entire organ; it all depends upon the individual patient and the extent of cancer invasion. Radiation therapy may be administered when the patient is not regarded as a good surgical risk.

Brain Cancer

Brain cancers sometimes are identified as gliomas, although technically the term applies only to certain structures within the brain tissue. Symptoms and signs of brain cancer are similar to the effects of strokes in that changes in function and behavior usually are related to the specific area of the brain that is damaged by the disorder. As a result, one patient may experience headaches or dizziness, another may lose the ability to coordinate his legs in walking, and a third might show only a tendency toward nausea and vomiting that can not be accounted for by a gastrointestinal disease.

Often, a diagnosis of brain cancer depends upon X-rays, brain scans utilizing radioactive materials injected into an artery, or computerized axial tomography, a technique that scans an organ and produces a series of images that represent slices of the organ.

When the exact cause of the problem has been diagnosed, treatment depends in part upon accessibility of the tumor. One that can be removed surgically without destroying vital nerve fibers controlling breathing or heart contractions might be excised. A tumor that could not be removed without probably causing increased damage to the brain probably would be treated with radiation or chemotherapy.

Cancers of the Digestive Tract

Cancers of the digestive tract vary with the part of the body that is the site of the tumor. Mouth cancers, including those of the lips, often appear at first as hard sores that seem slow to heal and usually have more red coloration or less than the surrounding tissue, and may even be white. Mouth cancers often occur in areas that are in contact with natural teeth or dentures. A mouth cancer may or may not be painful, but usually it is detected at an early stage as a result of self-examination or a periodic dental checkup.

Cancers that develop farther back in the mouth, around the base of the tongue, in the tonsils, or at the top of the throat, may escape early detection unless the vocal cords are involved. Because of difficulties in swallowing or persistent hoarseness, a patient may seek medical care before the cancer becomes well advanced. Otherwise, symptoms of cancer in throat tissue may be a feeling of soreness or of a "lump in the throat," after the tumor has become large enough to become an obstacle to breathing or swallowing.

Biopsy followed by surgery or radiation therapy are the usual methods of dealing with cancers in the upper part of the digestive tract. The exact procedure chosen depends on the cancer site and the extent of cancer growth. If the cancer has invaded the larynx, it may be possible to correct the problem by removing the vocal cord on one side; the patient would be able to continue using the voice box, although his voice would not sound the same as before surgery. If the entire larynx must be re-

moved, the patient learns to speak with the help of electronic aids or by swallowing air into the esophagus and forcing it out again while the lips and teeth help to form understandable sounds. But the speech pattern of a person who has undergone a laryngectomy is somewhat limited by the amount of words or syllables that can be produced with each gulp of air.

Difficulty in swallowing can be a symptom of esophageal cancer as well as cancer of the mouth or throat. The patient may experience pain or choking sensations when swallowing food or liquid, and a loss of appetite because of the swallowing problem. But this effect may not be noticed until the cancer has advanced beyond its early stages. Surgery to remove the diseased portion of the esophagus is the usual corrective treatment, although radiation may be administered if the tumor is discovered at a very early stage. When a portion of the esophagus is removed, the stomach portion may be attached to the remainder of the upper portion of the food tube, or a plastic tube prosthesis may be attached to span the gap left by excision of the cancerous length of esophagus.

Stomach cancer generally signals its presence by symptoms of pain and indigestion which, in turn, lead to loss of appetite and loss of weight. Vomiting may become a frequent complaint. Eventually, there may be traces of blood in the feces, although the feces coloration will be black rather than red because of chemical changes produced in the blood as it passes through the digestive tract. Peptic ulcers can cause similar symptoms, so a careful diagnosis is needed to determine the cause of stomach distress.

The examination procedure includes "barium X-rays," or X-ray pictures taken after the patient has swallowed a milk-shake-like fluid containing barium that produces a rather clear outline of the inner surfaces of the digestive tract. Other tests include a gastroscope examination using a lighted tube that is inserted into the stomach to permit the doctor to inspect the lining; the gastroscope also is equipped with a knife blade to enable the doctor to remove biopsy samples.

Treatment for stomach cancer is generally like that for cancer of the esophagus. The diseased portion of the stomach is excised, and the remaining portions are sewed together to produce a somewhat smaller digestive tract. If it is found necessary to remove the entire stomach, portions of neighboring tissues also may be excised, and the esophagus is attached directly to the small intestine. A similar surgical procedure is followed when needed for treatment of peptic ulcer cases, although peptic ulcers are considered benign lesions and neighboring tissues do not have to be removed along with the diseased area.

Below the stomach, the most common cancer sites are in the large intestine, or the colon and rectum, and in the pancreas. Bleeding, cramps, and diarrhea are the most likely symptoms of a malignant tumor in the large intestine; the bleeding may be heavy and the blood is likely to be red. Signs of cancer can be confirmed, and early cancers detected before they produce discomforting symptoms, by an examination of the lower bowel that often is included as part of a periodic medical checkup. Most of the length of the large intestine in which cancers are most likely to occur can be observed with a proctosigmoidoscope, another lighted tube device that can be inserted into a body cavity to enable the doctor to inspect the inside of

an organ. In this case, the device is inserted through the anus. The examination may be supplemented with barium enema X-rays and exploratory surgery, which is performed under a general anesthetic so that the doctor can obtain biopsy samples from the portion of the large intestine that is beyond the reach of the proctosigmoidoscope. Most cancers of the bowel develop at the rectal end of the large intestine.

If the presence of cancer is confirmed, the diseased portion of the colon and/or rectum is removed by a surgeon. When possible, only the diseased section is removed, along with neighboring lymph nodes. If it is necessary to remove a large cancerous portion of the rectum, the surgeon produces a colostomy, which is an opening in the abdomen through which feces can be removed. A patient with a colostomy learns to irrigate the remaining portion of the colon each day to remove any fecal matter, after which the opening is covered with a plastic cap, so the patient can work or engage in most normal activities in the outside world without the handicap being noticeable.

Cancer of the Pancreas

Cancer of the pancreas causes abdominal pain and digestive problems that eventually may involve the liver and gallbladder, since the bile produced by the liver and the digestive enzymes produced by the pancreas share a common exit duct into the small intestine. Jaundice, the yellow coloring of the skin due to the bile disorder, thus can be a sign of pancreatic cancer as well as of liver or gallbladder problems.

There is no true cure for cancer of the pancreas. The only kind of treatment that

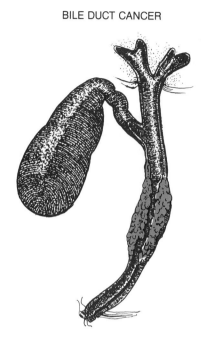

BILE DUCT CANCER

Drawing shows how a cancer can gradually destroy an internal organ, in this case the bile duct leading from the gall bladder. Cancer cells may run wild and accumulate so that they restrict or block the lumen of an organ, thereby interrupting normal physiological processes. Some cancers may cause pain; others are painless and when they cannot be observed from outside the body the first signs of an internal cancer may be the appearance of blood in urine, feces, vomit, or sputum after cancer cells erode the walls of blood vessels supplying the affected organ.

offers the patient a chance to extend his life is surgical removal of the organ. After the pancreas is removed, the patient must receive insulin and pancreatic enzymes as medications in order to survive.

Lung Cancer

Lung cancer is one of the most common of the neoplastic diseases among humans. The symptoms are a chronic cough, short-ness of breath, chest pains, and bloody sputum. Diagnosis is made on the basis of X-rays and biopsy examinations from samples obtained by several possible methods, including needle aspiration of tissue, exploratory surgery, and use of a bronchoscope that is inserted through the patient's throat. Radiation and chemotherapy are of some help in relieving symptoms and extending the life of the patient, but surgical removal of the affected lung tissue is the only effective treatment.

Thyroid Cancers and Lymphomas

Thyroid cancers usually develop slowly and cause the gland in the neck to enlarge, causing a condition like that of goiter which results in a swollen neck because of lack of iodine in the diet. Hoarseness and difficulty in swallowing and breathing are other symptoms. Most thyroid cancers can be controlled by surgical removal of most of the gland and the neighboring lymph nodes. Additional therapy may be provided by radiation exposure to radioactive material swallowed as a "cocktail" and absorbed by the thyroid tissues.

Although the lymph system is a favored target for migrating cancer cells looking for a secondary target, the lymph organs also are capable of causing their own type of cancer. The tumors, called lymphomas, occur in several forms, one of which is known by its common name of Hodgkin's disease. Symptoms include a swollen lymph node that remains swollen for several weeks, fatigue, itching, and a fever that seems to occur daily. Diagnosis is made from microscopic examination of the tissue of an involved lymph node. Radiation and chemotherapy are the usual types of treatment for lymphomas.

GLOSSARY

A FEW MORE WORDS ABOUT CANCER

Ames test A simple inexpensive test, named for Dr. Bruce Ames, for identifying substances that might be a cause of cancer. Bacteria are exposed to a sample of the substance, which might be a chemical in cigarette smoke, for example, to see if the chemical causes a change in the chromosomes of the bacteria. A substance that alters the genetic material of the bacteria may or may not be a cancer-causing substance, but in most cases it is later found to be a carcinogen.

anemia A disease condition characterized by an abnormally low proportion of red blood cells or hemoglobin in the bloodstream. The cause of anemia can be a loss of blood due to an ulcer or cancer that slowly drains the red blood cells faster than they can be replaced.

angioma A tumor, usually benign, involving the blood or lymph vessels.

anorexia A loss of appetite; a common sign of a cancer of the digestive tract.

arsenic A chemical element that has been identified as a cause of certain types of cancer. Ironically, arsenic at one time was used as a medication to treat cancer.

asbestos A chemical commonly used as insulating material in building construction and recently identified as a cause of lung cancer and other respiratory disorders in persons who inhale the asbestos fibers. There also is some evidence that asbestos fibers can enter the body through drinking water taken from lakes or other sources contaminated by refuse from mines or factories processing asbestos.

basal cell cancer A type of skin cancer involving cells from the lower, living tissue area of the epidermis. Basal cell cancers usually are slow growing tumors and often can be treated by radiation therapy.

benign A medical term that is used to identify tumors that are not cancerous. Although the word suggests a friendly or benevolent tumor, the description is true only by comparison with the malignant variety. Benign tumors of certain types, such as moles, can turn into cancers, and a large benign tumor can interfere with normal functioning of neighboring tissues or organs.

benzene A chemical commonly associated with gasoline and the production of gasoline at petroleum refineries. It is believed to be a causative factor in cases of leukemia.

benzpyrene A chemical produced by the combusion of a wide variety of organic materials, ranging from tobacco to barbecued hamburgers, and a substance believed to cause cancer.

biopsy The removal of a small sample of diseased tissue from a patient for examination under a microscope. The biopsy study is used to determine whether the tissue cells may be normal or cancerous. Most abnormal tissue growths are subjected to a biopsy examination before surgery or other treatments for cancer are undertaken.

blocking factor A substance believed by some medical scientists to be produced by cancer cells to enable the cancer to block the body's natural immune system, which otherwise might resist the spread of cancer.

bone marrow The soft, spongy material in certain bones of the body, mainly the long bones of the limbs, in which red blood cells, white blood cells, and blood platelets are manufactured.

bone marrow test A diagnostic technique used in cases of suspected bone cancer or leukemia. A bit of bone marrow is extracted for study by the doctors for evidence of cancer.

bronchoscope An instrument used by doctors to examine the bronchi, or tubes leading to the air sacs of the lungs from the end of the trachea. The light-equipped device is lowered into the trachea after the patient has been given a sedative and a local anesthetic. The bronchoscope can be used to retrieve foreign objects inhaled into the bronchi or to remove biopsy samples of tissues.

buccal Pertaining to the cheeks, particularly the mucous membrane surfaces on the inside which can be the site of mouth cancers.

Burkitt's lymphoma A cancer of the lymph tissue. It is believed to be caused by a viral infection.

butter yellow The name of a yellow dye once used as food coloring material. After its use was discontinued as a food additive, butter yellow was identified as a carcinogen.

carcinoma A type of cancer that develops in the skin and in the membrane linings of organs.

chemotherapy The administration of drugs designed to control the growth and/or spread of cancer cells. Generally, any drug that kills cancer cells also kills normal cells, but chemotherapy drugs destroy more cancer than normal cells because they take advantage of unique characteristics of cancer tissues, such as the way cancer cells reproduce. In many cases, doctors use combinations of several chemotherapy agents, each designed to attack a different phase of cancer cell life.

chondrosarcoma A type of bone cancer affecting the cartilage portion of the bone at first, but spreading into other tissues if uncontrolled.

chromosomes Chains of genetic material that form in the nucleus of a cell at the time it divides into two daughter cells. It is at this point in cell life that a carcinogen is believed to disrupt the normal genetic package of the cell so that it goes "haywire" and becomes the start of a strain of abnormal cancerous tissue cells.

circumcision Surgical removal of the prepuce, or foreskin, from the penis. Statistical studies associate a higher incidence of cancer of the penis and cancer of the cervix with male sexual partners who have not been circumcised.

cordotomy A surgical technique for relieving the pain of cancer by inserting an electric needle into the spinal cord of the patient. The needle disrupts the flow of sensory nerve impulses from the cancerous area of the body to the brain so that the pain is no longer experienced.

cryosurgery The application of supercold liquid nitrogen, or a similar material, to a tumor to kill the cells by literally freezing them to death.

cytology A method of studying the condition of tissue cells that are generally obtained from body fluids or surfaces rather than from solid or soft tissues. The cell samples may be obtained from urine, sputum, stomach washings, or mouth or nose smears.

deoxyribonucleic acid Also conveniently known as DNA, a complex molecular configuration that is the basic chemical component of all genetic material. The arrangement of units in a DNA molecule determines the physical and certain behavioral characteristics of all individuals. Chromosomes are composed of DNA molecules.

DES An abbreviation for diethylstilbesterol, a synthetic sex hormone that has been used as a livestock feed additive to increase the growth rate of the animals, and as a medication to prevent miscarriages in pregnant women. DES later was found to be an agent that could result in tumors in certain strains of mice and in uterine cancer in the daughters of mothers who received DES therapy.

D & C Abbreviation for dilatation and curettage, a therapeutic and diagnostic technique employed in connection with problems involving the endometrium, or lining, of the uterus. The uterus is dilated and the inside membrane scraped; the tissue scrapings are used as biopsy material. Fibroid tumors are removed in this manner, and the technique is used for abortion.

dyes Chemicals used as artificial colorings may be cancer-causing agents. Potential human carcinogens generally are dyes made from aromatic amino or aromatic azo compounds.

dysphagia Difficulty in swallowing; a symptom of possible cancer of the mouth, throat, or esophagus.

dysplasia A type of abnormal cell that often is found to be precancerous. When evidence of dysplasia is found in a sample of Pap smear cells, a cervical biopsy is recommended.

dyspnea A shortness of breath that is associated with a variety of health problems, including lung cancer.

epidural block A type of nerve block sometimes used to relieve the pain of cancer by injecting a drug into an area near the spinal cord where nerves from the affected tissue area enter the cord.

Ewing's sarcoma A type of bone cancer that tends to occur most frequently in cylindrical bones such as the long limb bones. Symptoms include pain, fever, and a blood disorder, leukocytosis.

exfoliative cytology A medical term sometimes used to indicate studies of cells shed by tissues and retrieved from body fluids or surfaces, as in the example of Pap smear test cells.

familial polypsis An inherited intestinal disorder characterized by the development in the bowel of polyps that can be precancerous.

fever therapy A method applied occasionally to control temporarily the growth of cancer cells by inducing a fever in the patient. The technique is somewhat controversial but is believed to help in some cases by destroying cancer cells or activating the body's immune system to resist the cancer. Fever also has been suggested as a cause for some of the rare cases of spontaneous regression, in which a usually fatal cancer suddenly stopped growing for no apparent reason.

gamma rays A type of radiation sometimes used in diagnosing and treating cancers. The gamma rays are emitted by radioactive chemicals and are capable of destroying body cells, including cancer cells.

genital herpes An infectious disease transmitted by a virus similar to but different than the common cold-sore virus. The genital herpes virus is a venereal disease agent that is suspected to be a possible cause of cervical cancer.

HeLa cells A strain of cancer cells removed from the uterus of a patient in 1952 and used in experimental cell cultures to study substances that may stimulate or control the growth of new cells of the strain. The name of the strain is derived from the first letters of the name of the patient who died after the cancer was removed.

Hodgkin's disease Also known as Hodgkin's lymphoma, a type of cancer that develops in the lymph system. It is characterized by painless but progressive enlargement of the lymph nodes and spleen, weakness, sweating, and fever. Treatment is by radiation and chemotherapy. It affects mainly persons below the age of 30, particularly men.

hospice An extended care facility for cancer patients whose disease has progressed to a terminal stage. The hospice usually provides comfort and guidance for members of the patient's family as well as medical care for the patient.

hyperthermia A type of treatment that is a sort of variation of fever therapy. Patients are subjected to temperatures around 110 degrees Fahrenheit after being anesthetized, and the heat kills many of the cancer cells without destroying normal body cells.

hysterectomy A surgical procedure in which the uterus is removed from the woman's abdomen. The technique usually is employed as part of the treatment for cancer of the uterus and/or cervix.

ileal bladder A urinary bladder fashioned by surgeons from intestinal tissue to replace a normal bladder that has been removed surgically because of cancer.

immune mechanism Also known as the immune system, it is the means by which the body defends its own tissues against strange or foreign tissue cells, whether they be bacteria, viruses, or transplanted organs. The mechanism is important in cancer care because of evidence that cancer tends to develop in persons whose immune system is unable to resist the invasion of the strange growth of cancer cells. Some studies suggest that persons whose bodies readily accept transplants of tissues from the bodies of other individuals are particularly vulnerable to cancers.

isotope scanning A diagnostic technique sometimes used in examining a suspected cancer case. A radioactive substance is injected into the bloodstream and is followed by radiation detection devices to see if an affected organ has undergone apparent changes. Because cancer cells can be more active than normal tissue cells, some cancers may tend to accumulate the radioactive material in their tissues, thereby producing a "hot spot" area of radioactivity.

keratosis A type of skin disorder marked by scaly, thickening areas of epidermis which may be precancerous.

Laetrile A substance derived from apricot pits and other fruits for use in controlling the growth or spread of cancer. One argument used by proponents of Laetrile treatment for cancer is that the disease is caused by a vitamin deficiency, a lack of vitamin "B_{17}," and the material in apricot pits cures the deficiency.

Laetrile backers also have claimed that cancer is the result of embryonic tissue cells that remain at large in the body after formation of the fetus and develop into wild growths that can be controlled only by the administration of Laetrile. Use of Laetrile is permitted in some countries, but it has been banned by the U.S. Food and Drug Administration as treatment for cancer.

laryngectomy Surgical removal of the larynx when the voice box has been damaged by cancer. The larynx usually is replaced by an electronic device or an artificial opening in the windpipe that permits the patient to speak by swallowing air into the esophagus and "belching" the air through the mouth; the tongue, teeth, and cheeks form the proper shapes for converting the moving air into spoken words.

leukemia A cancer of the bone marrow or lymph nodes that results in abnormal white blood cells which crowd out the red blood cells and blood platelets so that patients suffer from oxygen deficiency and increased susceptibility to hemorrhages and infection. There are several different variations of leukemia. Treatment approaches include chemotherapy, antibiotics, blood transfusions, and bone marrow transplants.

leukoplakia White patches that appear on the lips and inside the mouth. They often precede cancer of the tongue.

lumpectomy A term sometimes used in referring to a surgical procedure in which a lump is removed from a woman's breast, rather than removing the entire breast as in a mastectomy.

lymphogram A diagnostic method sometimes used by doctors for locating cancerous tissues in the lymphatic system. A radio-opaque dye is injected into the lymphatic system before the suspected body areas are X-rayed.

lymphoma A cancer of the lymph tissues. Hodgkin's disease is an example of a lymphoma form of cancer. There also are types of lymphomas with symptoms similar to Hodgkin's disease that have different patterns of development and require different kinds of treatment.

malignant tumor Another term for cancer.

mammography A method of examining the breast for the presence of abnormal tissue growth by using X-ray equipment. The use of mammography has been a source of controversy because of the possibility that exposure of the breast to X-rays might induce cancer as well as diagnose the disease.

mastectomy Surgical removal of the breast because of the presence of cancer in its tissues. There are several kinds of mastectomy procedures, ranging from removal of the lump of tissue containing the cancer to excision of the entire breast, the surrounding lymph nodes, and the chest muscles beneath the breast.

melanoma A type of skin cancer that develops from melanocyte tissue of the epidermis. Melanocytes are the pigment-forming cells of the skin.

multiple myeloma A type of bone cancer that is marked by muscle and bone pains, weakness, weight loss, and pallor. X-rays often reveal holes in the bone caused by destruction of bone tissue by the cancer. It is one type of bone cancer that may affect the skull.

myelocytic leukemia A form of leukemia that develops from myeloid, or red bone marrow, tissue. It affects a different kind of white blood cell than lymphocytic leukemia, the other major form of the disease.

oat cell cancer Sometimes called oat cell carcinoma, a type of lung cancer in which the clusters of cancer cells resemble grains of oats. Oat cell cancers generally are treated with chemotherapy because the disease cannot be controlled effectively with lung surgery.

orchiectomy Surgical removal of a testis, or testicle.

osteosarcoma A type of cancer that involves bone tissues.

palliative treatment Medical care that is directed toward relieving the symptoms rather than curing the cause of the symptoms. Palliative treatment of cancer may consist of pain-killing drugs, surgery to block a nerve route or to excise a tumor causing pressure on a neighboring organ, etc.

Pap test A diagnostic technique developed by the American physician George Papanicolaou for early detection of cancer of the cervix by removing exfoliative cells from the surface of the tissue and examining the cells on a microscope slide.

polyps A mass of cells that protrudes from a mucous membrane, usually as an overgrowth of normal tissue. However, polyps also may become malignant tumors. Cervical polyps, for example, occasionally develop into cancers. Polyps often are identified as pedunculated if they are attached by a thin stalk, or as sessile if they have a broad base.

proctosigmoidoscopy Examination of the rectum and sigmoid colon areas of the large intestine with the aid of a lighted tube.

radiation therapy The use of radiation, ranging from X-ray machines to radioactive isotopes, to kill cancer cells. Radiotherapy usually requires precise targeting of the radiation so that cancerous tissue is destroyed without damaging normal tissue cells surrounding the cancer. Radiation can cause cancer in normal cells. It is used in diagnosing cancer as well as in treating the disease.

retinoblastoma A rare type of eye cancer.

sarcoma A type of cancer that occurs in the muscle or bone. A bone cancer may be identified as an osteosarcoma, and a muscle cancer as a myosarcoma; but more likely, a bone or muscle cancer is identified more precisely according to the specific type of osteosarcoma or myosarcoma involved.

seminoma A type of cancer of the testis that develops from gonadal cells.

squamous cell cancer A skin cancer of the squamous cells which lie at the base of the epidermis. See illustration, page 459.

symptomatic treatment Another term for palliative treatment in which medical care is directed toward the relief of pain and discomfort rather than the cure of the disease itself. Symptomatic treatment is instituted when doctors decide that further attempts to cure the disease would be futile and wastefully expensive for the patient's family.

terminal care Medical and other care given a cancer patient who is terminally ill. Curative treatment usually is ended and *symptomatic treatment* is started. The patient may be moved from the hospital to a hospice or to his home when doctors decide that they can do nothing further to help the patient survive.

thermography A diagnostic technique sometimes used to detect cancers which may produce more metabolic heat than normal tissue cells. By checking for thermal hot spots, a cancer may be found.

ultrasound A diagnostic method that uses high-frequency sound waves that are transmitted into the patient's body. Abnormal tissue surfaces, such as those produced by cancers, are expected to cause echo patterns that differ from those of normal tissue surfaces that reflect the ultrasound waves.

urostomy An artificial opening in the abdominal wall made to release urine after a cancerous bladder has been removed by surgeons.

vinblastine An anticancer drug that is produced from the vinca, or periwinkle, herb. Vinblastine often is used in the chemotherapy of Hodgkin's disease. Vincristine is another cancer chemotherapy medication manufactured from the periwinkle plant.

Wilm's tumor A specific type of kidney cancer that affects children. It also may be called nephroblastoma or embryonal carcinosarcoma; the latter term indicates that the tumor contains embryonic tissue.

xeroderma pigmentosum A type of precancerous disease in which the skin and eyes are extremely sensitive to light, beginning in childhood and becoming progressively severe with continued exposure to sunlight. Freckles develop into keratoses which in turn become malignant tumors. The disease is hereditary, due to lack of a gene that normally enables skin cells to repair damage caused by energy of ultraviolet rays.

QUESTIONS AND ANSWERS
CANCER

Q: *Since cancer of the uterus develops from the endometrium, is it possible to have cancer in a placenta attached to the lining of the uterus?*

A: Yes. Placental cancers do occur occasionally, and it usually is possible to determine whether the cancer is placental or uterine by means of laboratory tests. Placental cancers produce a substance that can be detected in a sample of blood taken from a mother's vein. These cancers usually are treated with chemotherapy.

Q: *Can a fetus develop cancer as a result of exposure by the mother to a cancer-causing agent?*

A: Yes. There are cases of children developing leukemia after the mother's pelvic area was X-rayed while she was pregnant. Certain drugs taken by the mother during pregnancy also are capable of causing cancer in the offspring. This was discovered after uterine cancer developed in daughters of mothers who took DES medications to prevent miscarriages right after World War II.

Q: *Do men get the same kinds of cancers as women?*

A: In general, yes. But there is a difference in the distribution of the most common types. Nearly one-third of the cancer cases involving women are tumors of the breast and reproductive organs. Some men develop breast cancer but this is a relatively rare form of cancer for males. About ten percent of cancer cases among men involve the reproductive organs, mainly the prostate.

Men have a greater incidence of lung cancer than women, by a ratio of 33 to 19 percent, but women may catch up as more of their sex continue smoking cigarettes—the apparent cause of most lung cancer cases. Beyond the statistics for lung cancer and cancers of the male-female reproductive organs, the cancer incidence rates are fairly equal. Both sexes, for example, get skin cancer, leukemias and lymphomas, and pancreas cancers at the same rate. And cancer of the colon and rectum is the second leading cause of cancer in both men and women, after lung cancer in men and breast cancer in women.

Q: *If a boy is not circumcised at birth but is circumcised later, will his chances of developing cancer of the penis, or cervical cancer in his wife, be reduced?*

A: The information about the role of circumcision in controlling some sex organ cancers is mostly circumstantial; in other words, it is based mainly on statistical surveys. But the evidence shows that penile and cervical cancer is lower in Jewish populations, which practice circumcision at birth, than in non-Jewish populations that do not have their boy babies circumcised. However, in Moslem populations which practice circumcision at puberty rather than at birth, the incidence of penile and cervical cancer is higher than in Jewish communities, but lower than in populations that do not practice circumcision.

Q: *Is there any proof that breathing cigarette smoke from other people will cause cancer?*

A: One long-term study of the effects of exposure to "second-hand" tobacco smoke found that wives of husbands who did not smoke lived four years longer on the average than wives of cigarette-smoking husbands. But the study did not show the cause of death for wives who breathed the cigarette smoke of their spouses.

Q: *Why is there concern about diet as a factor in cancer?*

A: One reason for increasing interest in dietary factors is evidence that fatty foods cause an overproduction of bile acids by the liver; the bile acids help digest fats. But bile acids also may be carcinogens, or co-carcinogens, which means that they may react with other substances eaten or inhaled by the patient to cause cancers. That aspect of diet and cancer was revealed by data showing that patients with cancer of the large intestine had abnormally high levels of bile acids in their stools.

Another dietary factor suspected of being a cause of cancer is the nitrates used as a preservative in some processed meats, such as hot dogs and bologna. Sodium nitrate and potassium nitrite have been used as food preservatives for many years to prevent the development of botulism, a rare but deadly form of food poisoning. They may be used to preserve fish and poultry in addition to processed meats. The cancer angle is that nitrites may combine with amino acids in the digestive tract to form substances called nitrosamines, and nitrosamines have been identified as carcinogens in animals. The inference is that nitrosamines could cause cancer in humans as well.

Q: *Is it true that certain hair dyes can cause cancer? If the reports are true, how do the dyes get from the hair to tissues inside the body?*

A: Like many possible causes of human cancer, the association is based on experiments with laboratory animals and statistical surveys of the humans who develop cancers; humans obviously cannot be used as test animals in cancer experiments. The evidence shows that certain ingredients of human hair dyes cause cancers in the liver and other tissues of laboratory rats. Some epidemiological studies have found a higher incidence of cancer in women who dye their hair. Thus it is assumed that hair dyes containing the same ingredients can be the culprits.

As for the second part of your question, chemicals in hair dyes can be absorbed into the body through the skin, particularly in areas such as the scalp where there are a lot of hair follicles. Very few ordinary chemicals are absorbed directly through the unbroken skin. But hair follicles provide tiny shafts that penetrate beneath the epidermis, the top barrier level of the skin. And once a chemical, or a disease organism, reaches the deeper tissue layers of the skin, it can spread to other body areas.

Q: *Does cigarette smoking increase the chances of lung cancer for people who work with asbestos, or vice versa?*

A: Studies of men who worked in World War II shipyards, where asbestos was present in large amounts, have found a higher than expected incidence of respiratory disorders, including lung cancer. The incidence of lung cancer was found to be even higher for men exposed to asbestos who also smoked cigarettes. The two factors, asbestos and cigarettes, were determined to be synergistic, which means that they worked together to produce a total relative risk that was higher than either of the factors alone. Whether the asbestos increased the risk for cigarette smokers, or vice versa, really doesn't matter.

Q: *Why are bone cancers harder to cure than some other kinds of cancer?*

A: One reason is that bone cancers are more difficult to detect in the early stages. They usually are deep inside the body, and the symptoms they produce tend to mimic other diseases, such as arthritis or bursitis. If a patient thinks he has arthritis, he may delay a trip to the doctor's office for examination much longer than he would if he had any idea that the condition actually was a bone cancer. In some cases of bone cancer it can be difficult to find the proper clues even during a careful physical examination. Unfortunately, by the time definite signs and symptoms of bone cancer have developed, the cancer has progressed beyond the early stages and may have spread to other tissues.

But bone cancer is something of an exception to the general rule that early diagnosis and adequate treatment can improve the outlook for a person with cancer. Nearly half of all cancers develop in parts of the body that can be examined easily by a doctor during an ordinary office visit. And many of the other types of cancers can be diagnosed and treated in the early stages, when patients are aware of the symptoms and seek professional help before the situation gets out of hand.

17

HEART DISEASE
NUMBER ONE HEALTH THREAT

Heart disease is still the leading cause of premature deaths in America and most of the western world despite progress since the 1950's in finding causes and cures for the various forms of heart failure. Your chances of dying of heart disease are more than twice as great, and for some women nearly three times as great, as the risk of death from cancer. If other diseases of the circulatory system, such as cerebrovascular accidents and arteriosclerosis, were combined with heart disease, you would be four times as likely to die of a cardiovascular disorder as of cancer, which still is the number two killer.

Among the various forms of heart disease, the most common cause of death is ischemic heart disease involving the coronary arteries. Ischemia is a deficiency of oxygenated blood in some part of the body, often caused by an obstruction or constriction in a blood vessel supplying that part. The coronary arteries are the blood vessels supplying the heart tissues.

Heart disease resulting from obstructed or constricted coronary arteries is a disorder that appears to be associated with the diets and/or lifestyles of the industrialized world. This disease is virtually unknown among the blacks living in tropical Africa, but black persons living in North America are just as likely to be afflicted as their white neighbors.

Ischemic heart disease is just one of a number of disorders affecting the heart, although it may be the most likely form encountered by a doctor treating an adult patient. It also may be associated with cardiovascular complaints affecting other parts of the body. An interruption in the flow of freshly oxygenated blood to the leg muscles, even though a temporary interruption, can cause a painful condition called intermittent claudication; walking can produce the symptoms and rest can alleviate the pain. An ischemic effect in a blood vessel of the brain will produce signs and symptoms of a stroke. It is not unusual for a patient to suffer from more than one kind of ischemic effect, such as heart and brain disease, at the same time, since a common cause of artery narrowing, atherosclerosis, can occur throughout the body.

How the Heart and Circulatory System Work

The problem of ischemia also illustrates the main function of the heart, which is to move blood rich in fresh oxygen and nutrients to every living cell in the body. The matter is even more complex because the circulatory system, through feedback controls, tries to distribute oxygen and nutrients, and remove waste products, from various body tissues according to their immediate needs. A tennis player or football player requires oxygen and nutrients for various muscle cells in a rather sporadic pattern. He may be standing still, almost resting in a standing position, one second, and burning energy at an exhausting pace of arm and leg motion the next second. This requires a bit of quick shifting of gears by the circulatory system to move oxygen and nutrients at different speeds to different organs or muscle groups as the immediate need changes.

The normal cardiovascular system is rather elastic and resilient, and it can handle quick shifts in demand for blood without difficulty. It is essentially a self-contained, closed-circuit system for moving blood by the pressures of muscle contractions and partial vacuums produced by other muscle actions. Blood moves from the left ventricle of the heart into the aorta, the major artery of the body, and by branches from the aorta into other arteries. Beyond the arteries are smaller muscular vessels called arterioles that divide into capillaries, which may be very thin and fragile. The body contains many miles of capillaries, some so fine that red blood cells must pass through them in single file. But the capillary beds are so vast they could drain the body's entire blood supply, except that the control of blood released into the capillaries is exercised by the arterioles.

The capillary beds are so extensive that every living cell in the body is in contact with a capillary wall membrane. Oxygen and nutrients pass from the capillaries to the cells, and carbon dioxide, water, and other waste products of cell metabolism are collected by the passing flow of blood. The bloodstream continues on into small vessels called venules, which drain into veins. The veins empty into the vena cava, the major vein of the body, which delivers the used blood into the right atrium of the heart.

After the blood leaves the capillaries, it has a darker, bluish coloration because of having given up the oxygen molecules that account for the typical red coloration of blood. Blood is under less pressure in the veins, which therefore have thinner

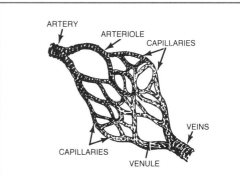

General pattern for the circulation of blood through the hundreds of billions of individual cells throughout the human body. Arteries which branch off from the aorta have smaller branches called arterioles which in turn form numerous capillary branches. Used blood returning to the heart flows into venules linked to the capillaries. The venules in turn flow into veins that empty into the vena cava, which is connected to the right atrium of the heart.

walls. But many of the veins have valves to prevent a backflow of blood, and muscle groups in the limbs help to move venous blood back toward the heart by squeezing the veins as the muscles contract.

The four-chambered human heart—some animals have hearts with fewer than four chambers—is a relatively small organ considering the amount of work it performs over a lifetime. An adult heart is only about five inches long and weighs between eight and ten ounces. It is mostly muscle, called the myocardium, that is different in cell structure from the skeletal muscles of the body and from the smooth muscles of other internal organs. The heart muscle is covered on the inner surface with a membrane, the endocardium, and on the outside by another membrane, the pericardium.

Blood that returns through the vena cavae—actually there are two, a superior and an inferior vena cava, one collecting blood from above the heart and one from below—enters the right atrium, one of the four heart chambers. Most of the blood drains passively from the right atrium into the right ventricle immediately below it, but the atrium walls give a little squeeze at the end of this phase of the heart, or cardiac, cycle to force the rest of the blood into the ventricle.

The right ventricle pumps the used blood into the lungs where carbon dioxide and water vapor are released, to be exhaled during respiration, and fresh oxygen is acquired. The refreshed blood is returned by the pulmonary veins to the left atrium, which drops the blood into the left ventricle to be pumped into the aorta on the next ventricular contraction.

The heart normally beats at a pace of about 70 per minute, or at an average rate

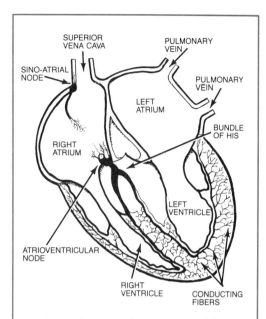

Heart muscle contractions are started by an electrical signal from the sino-atrial node, the natural pacemaker situated between the right atrium and the vena cava, the main vein of the body. The signal passes to the atrioventricular node and is conducted by the bundle of His, which divides to carry the impulse message to muscle fibers throughout the heart.

of once every eight-tenths of a second. Each contraction, called a systole, pumps about two and a half ounces of blood into the arteries. At 70 contractions a minute, this amounts to a movement of roughly five quarts of blood per minute. When a person engages in strenuous work or exercise, the heart pumps considerably more blood per minute. The amount of blood pumped by a heart during each contraction is called the stroke volume, and the amount pumped per minute is the cardiac output. These amounts will vary from time to time in the same person and from one individual to another.

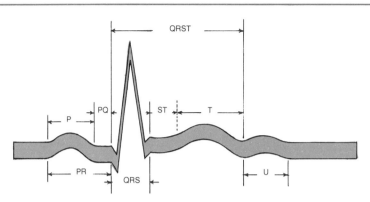

The illustration shows the pattern of a typical tracing made by an electrocardiograph of a patient's heart beat. Since the contraction of the heart muscle at each beat involves a small discharge of electricity, doctors can translate the patterns made by normal and abnormal heart tissue and determine the prob- able cause of an abnormal tracing. In this pattern, the "P" portion of the tracing represents the contraction of the atria; "Q", "R", and "S" portions are pro- duced by contraction of the ventricles; the "T" seg- ment represents the relaxation of the ventricles; and "U" indicates the atria's refilling for the next beat.

The contractions of the heart are controlled by a group of specialized nerve cells of the autonomic nervous system. This is the same part of the body's nervous system that controls the caliber of the blood vessels with impulses that order the muscle fibers of an artery to constrict or dilate the vessels. The nerve cells that initiate the rhythm of the heart are a part of the sino-atrial node, sometimes referred to as the body's own heart pacemaker. Located between the right atrium and the superior vena cava, it generates an electrical signal that spreads through the rest of the heart.

The impulse that begins at the sino-atrial node travels across the right atrium to a second part of the heart's conduction system, the atrioventricular node, located at a point in the lower right atrium where a septum, or interior wall, separates the four chambers of the heart. Fibers from the atrioventricular node travel down through the septum, separating into branches that loop up again through the outside walls of the ventricles. The pattern of the electrical impulse within the heart muscle becomes important when the normal rhythm is disrupted by a type of disorder known as heart block.

Kinds of Heart Failure

A failure of any of several links in the cardiovascular system can result in a condition in which the heart is unable to supply the amount of blood required to maintain normal distribution of oxygen and nutrients to the body's cells. Any disorder that causes this effect may be identified with heart failure. Heart failure can be due to a myocardial infarction or heart attack, to hypertension, an infection such as rheumatic heart disease, or a birth defect.

Heart failure can occur suddenly or develop gradually, as in certain cases of congestive heart failure in which fluid accumulates in the abdomen, legs, or lungs because it is forced out of the circulation system.

When fluid is forced out of circulation and into the alveoli of the lungs, the situation becomes complicated because the fluid in the tiny air sacs prevents oxygen from crossing the membrane to reach the red blood cells in the capillaries extending from the pulmonary arteries. Breathing is impaired and the patient experiences a shortness of breath, or dyspnea, which is quite similar to the effect of drowning.

Left ventricular failure Dyspnea and congestive heart disease sometimes are associated with a condition known as left ventricular failure. Failure of the left ventricle can result from ischemia, a myocardial infarction, or hypertension. The strain on the left ventricle that eventually results in failure also can be due to a defective heart valve or a stenosis or narrowing of the aorta. This causes regurgitation of blood and difficulty for the ventricle to expel blood into the arteries of the body as fast as it accumulates in the heart chamber. The muscle of the left ventricle can hypertrophy, or increase in size, to cope with the condition for a while, but eventually it loses the battle, and heart failure of the left ventricle occurs.

When pulmonary edema develops as a result of left ventricular failure, the patient may notice a dry cough and/or breathlessness from physical exertion. Depending upon the severity of the case, the patient may develop difficult breathing symptoms even from such a simple task as walking for any distance on level ground. He may not be able to get out of bed or, occasionally, he may not be able to rest while lying in bed because of the fluid accumulation in his lungs—that is, the pulmonary edema. In order to breathe adequately, he may have to sit up in bed.

Symptoms of this form of heart disease often can be treated with drugs or surgery. In some instances, fluid accumulation in body cavities as a result of heart failure can simply be siphoned out of the body. Diuretics often are prescribed to help the body get rid of edema. A diuretic may work by inhibiting the natural tendency of the kidneys to reabsorb fluids from the blood while it is being "cleaned" of waste products. The diuretic also can inhibit the kidney tendency to reabsorb sodium, which is a vital substance in normal body chemistry, although too much sodium will make the body retain water. The doctor usually prescribes a diet that eliminates any unnecessary sodium-rich foods. A similar procedure for reducing excess body fluids generally is followed in the treatment of hypertension.

Other drugs may include one of the various forms of digitalis, such as digoxin. Digitalis drugs, prepared from the leaves of the foxglove plant, cause the heart to pump more forcefully, thereby improving the circulation of blood and promoting the normal elimination of excess fluid. The amount of digitalis needed to maintain proper heart function in a heart disease patient may vary greatly depending upon the patient. There is only a narrow margin between the size of a dose that is too little to be effective and the dose size that may be toxic. Thus, the drug treatment for heart failure literally has to be tailored by the doctor to fit each individual case.

Right ventricular failure The right ventricle ordinarily is not as strong as the left ventricle because normally less effort is required by the heart muscle to push blood through the lungs than through the rest of the body, and it may fail more easily. Failure of the right ventricle often is a result of failure of the left ventricle. This is because ineffective functioning of the left ventricle may put more demand on the right ventricle to move the blood forward through the lungs and the other organs of the body. Since the primary function of the right ventricle is to move blood forward through the lungs, pressure in the pulmonary arteries is increased. That in turn causes the right ventricle to hypertrophy, or enlarge. An enlarged right ventricle, like an enlarged ventricle on the left side of the heart, can continue pumping blood for quite a while, but eventually it will fail.

Right ventricular heart failure can produce symptoms similar to those of left ventricular failure, such as edema and breathlessness. Right ventricular failure may make the patient feel fatigue quite easily and spend a lot of time in bed. Bed rest, in fact, is a part of the therapy often recommended for victims of right ventricular failure. Digitalis drugs and diuretics may be prescribed, also.

Because of increased pressure in the veins associated with right ventricular failure, the patient's veins are likely to become distended. In some cases, distention of veins in the stomach can cause symptoms of nausea and vomiting, and distended veins in the liver may result in signs of jaundice.

Coronary Heart Disease

As with many other medical problems, signs and symptoms of heart disease often appear in the guise of other conditions. This situation can be misleading to the ordinary person, although a doctor who is a good diagnostic detective is quite likely to check out the clues of heart disease that appear to have nothing to do with the heart. Many laypersons might ignore a dry cough, fluid accumulation in the legs, distended veins, fatigue, or

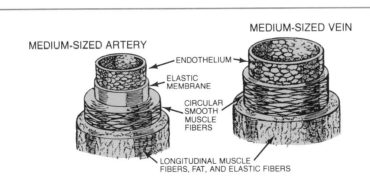

Arteries and veins are similar in construction except that arteries generally have thicker walls. A typical artery has one layer of muscle cells with circular fibers and another layer with muscle cells that run length- wise. An artery also has a layer of elastic membrane, a feature absent in veins. Larger blood vessels may be supplied with blood capillaries and nerve fibers that supply the muscle tissue.

breathlessness after mild exertion as signs and symptoms of heart disease, because they have been led to believe that heart troubles give their warning with a sharp pain in the chest.

Most cases of heart disease that involve chest pains are the result of ischemia that disrupts the normal flow of blood in the coronary arteries. The two coronary arteries, which begin near the base of the aorta, move in generally opposite directions around the surface of the heart. One goes to the left and the other to the right with branches that supply the myocardium, or muscle tissue of the heart, the nodes and conduction systems, and other structures. The arteries provide blood to a dense web of smaller vessels throughout the heart muscle fibers. The used blood from the heart tissues is returned through coronary veins that run parallel to the coronary arteries.

The coronary artery blood flow differs somewhat from the forward movement of blood in other arteries in that there is very little blood movement when the heart contracts. That is because the pressure of contractions inhibits the blood flow, so blood movement occurs mainly during the diastole, or relaxation, phase of the cardiac cycle. Also, the myocardium is more sensitive to oxygen deprivation than the skeletal muscles; it doesn't provide the several minutes of oxygen debt that is offered by the skeletal muscles. Although it weighs only a bit more than a half-pound, the human heart consumes about 10 percent of all the oxygen received by the entire body. At the same time, the heart is a much more efficient organ than most man-made machines; it utilizes 80 percent of all the oxygen it receives and converts approximately 50 percent of all the fuel it receives into work energy. A fossil-fuel-burning engine as efficient as the human heart would be considered a remarkable energy-saving device.

Unfortunately, the major obstacle to maximum efficiency of the human heart is the disease that narrows the bore or caliber of the coronary arteries, reducing and eventually blocking normal blood flow to create the condition of ischemic heart disease. The condition, sometimes called arteriosclerosis, is characterized by a buildup of fatty deposits, fibrous tissues, and/or

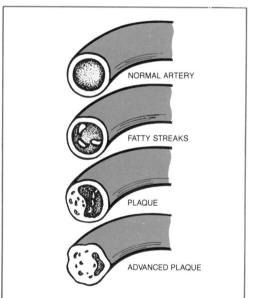

NORMAL ARTERY

FATTY STREAKS

PLAQUE

ADVANCED PLAQUE

Many cases of circulatory disorders, including strokes and heart attacks, are due to the accumulation of fatty deposits and minerals that gradually fill the inside of an artery so that normal blood flow is restricted and finally obstructed. When blood is unable to deliver fresh oxygen and nutrients to an area of body tissue, the body cells in that area die and the organ involved loses some of its capacity to function at an optimum level. A tissue deprived of freshly oxygenated blood often expresses its problem to the patient as a severe pain.

minerals on the intima, or innermost layer of an artery wall, that gradually reduces the opening. As the artery wall thickens it also tends to lose its elasticity. The accumulation of fatty substances, fibrous tissues, and minerals has the net effect of constricting the blood flow through the artery.

The fatty deposits, known as atheromata, were once thought to be a normal result of the aging process. But during the Vietnam and Korean wars, it was discovered during medical studies of soldiers that most American teenagers had fatty deposits in their arteries. More recently, it has been found that virtually every child by the age of ten has such fatty streaks or plaques in his arteries. The mineral deposits are mainly of calcium, and the fibrous tissue apparently is generated by smooth muscle cells of the media, or middle layer, of the arteries. Cellular debris and other materials also may become trapped in a sort of trash heap that gradually lines the arteries.

Because it may take several decades for arteriosclerosis to make its effects felt, ischemic heart disease usually does not begin to produce symptoms until after the age of 40. As time goes on, an increasing percentage of individuals begin to develop complaints associated with atherosclerotic or arteriosclerotic effects, which can include intermittent claudication of the legs and cerebrovascular accidents of the brain as well as heart problems.

There are three major types of ischemic heart disease: angina pectoris, coronary insufficiency, and myocardial infarction.

Angina pectoris Angina pectoris is marked by a pain in the chest that results from an inadequate supply of oxygen to the heart. The condition is relieved by rest and exacerbated by physical effort. The pain usually is described as vise-like crushing felt in the center of the chest, beneath the sternum or breastbone. It usually lasts only a few moments, probably because the symptoms are such that the patient stops whatever he is doing at the time and that has a resting influence.

The pain sometimes may radiate beyond the breastbone and/or down the left arm. It may be confused by the patient with myocardial infarction or with heartburn or other conditions. A careful examination by the doctor, who may perform a variety of special tests such as administering a drug such as nitroglycerin which relieves only angina pains, may be needed to establish the exact cause of the symptoms.

Because the ischemia involves an imbalance between the demand and supply of oxygen, there can be causes for angina pectoris other than narrowing of the coronary arteries. Tobacco smoking, for example, can result in a diminished flow of oxygen to the heart muscle; so can a respiratory disease. Cold weather, a large meal, anger, or anxiety can be factors responsible for an attack, as can the postural position of the body. Some men who do strenuous work or exercise may find that the particular type of muscle activity they perform does not cause the chest pains, but that some other kind of effort may trigger an attack.

Treatment for angina pectoris may require some minor changes in lifestyle, such as reducing the number of calories consumed each day in order to control weight, curtailing the use of cigarettes, avoiding sudden exertion but exercising the body in ways that build endurance, and controlling other possible medical problems such as high blood pressure. Medications include drugs of the nitroglycerin type, vasodilators, and beta-blockers. Nitroglycerin drugs tend to reduce heart muscle effort while widening the bore of the blood vessels, as vasodilators also do. Beta-blocking drugs block receptors of a part of the autonomic nervous system so that the heart rate is reduced along with the work load of the heart.

When other forms of therapy fail to relieve the ischemia effects, surgery may be recommended. The surgical approach might provide a bypass or other kind of artery transplant to assure an adequate flow of freshly oxygenated blood to the heart muscle.

Coronary insufficiency Acute coronary insufficiency is a variation of angina pectoris except that the pain may develop quite suddenly and with little or no exertion. Some patients develop the symptoms while resting. Since acute coronary insufficiency sometimes is regarded as an intermediate step between angina pectoris and myocardial infarction, or a heart attack, the patient often is administered anticoagulants. These drugs are designed to prevent the formation of blood clots in the arteries. Other medications may include beta-blocking agents.

Complete bed rest may be prescribed for an acute coronary insufficiency patient. The bed rest and medicines often are sufficient to control insufficiency.

Myocardial infarction Myocardial infarction is the result of an obstruction of a part of the coronary artery system, resulting in the death of an area of heart muscle tissue. Exactly what happens to the patient when a myocardial infarction occurs depends in part upon what part of the heart muscle is involved and the extent of

the damage. The patient may feel severe pain that begins suddenly and continues until a potent pain-killing drug is administered. Another patient, however, may have no serious pain but will experience instead an abnormal heart rhythm or the symptoms of failure of a ventricle. The patient usually has a fever and may show signs of shock, although he may also appear to be well. The pain, when it occurs, may be similar to that of angina—starting under the breastbone and possibly radiating throughout the chest and/or down the left arm.

In severe cases, the patient may fall unconscious and death can occur almost immediately.

Although there are wide individual variations in the way a myocardial infarction makes itself known, these are the common symptoms of a heart attack:

1. A heavy, squeezing pain or discomfort in the center of the chest.
2. Pain which may radiate to the shoulder, arm, neck, or jaw.
3. Feelings of anxiety.
4. Sweating.
5. Nausea and/or vomiting.
6. Shortness of breath.
7. Dizziness or fainting.

A heart attack victim may have one, several, or all of the above symptoms, but he also may have none of these symptoms and experience an effect that may be mistaken for indigestion. A detailed medical examination that includes the use of electrocardiograms and special laboratory tests of substances in the blood usually is needed to determine the severity of a myocardial infarction.

When a person experiences signs or symptoms of a myocardial infarction, a doctor should be notified immediately—every minute counts, literally. In many

ANEURYSM OF
THE DESCENDING PORTION
OF THE AORTA   MYOCARDIAL INFARCT   COARCTATION OF THE AORTA

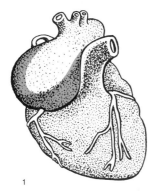
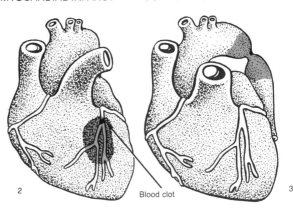

1   2   3
                                          Blood clot

1. One type of heart dysfunction is caused by an aneurysm of the aorta, in which the main artery supplying the body becomes abnormally enlarged, usually due to a weakening of the wall of the blood vessel. The disorder often is associated with hypertension and may be repaired with a Dacron plastic blood vessel graft if detected in an early stage.

2. A myocardial infarct is a common cause of a fatal heart attack. A blood vessel supplying the heart muscle becomes blocked by a blood clot so that oxy-gen and nutrients cannot reach the area of heart muscle normally served by the obstructed blood vessel. As a result, the heart is unable to function normally.

3. Coarctation of the aorta is a condition marked by a narrowing of the main artery leading from the heart. Because of the restricted blood flow beyond the coarctation, circulation to the lower part of the body depends upon enlargement of vessels that normally would be small arteries. The disorder often is associated with heart valve disease or hypertension.

communities, about half the heart attack victims die before they can be given professional medical care. In many of these cases the death can be attributed to a delay in alerting a doctor or in getting the victim to a hospital emergency room. In some instances, death could be prevented by administering mouth-to-mouth resuscitation to the patient.

Once in a hospital, the patient is admitted directly to a CCU, or Coronary Care Unit. An intravenous tube is attached to the patient's arm for feeding and administration of certain medicines. An electrocardiograph is connected for continuous monitoring of the heart during the crisis period. Oxygen may be administered by mask, respirator, or a catheter. The patient's stay in the CCU generally is determined by the amount of time required for his condition to stabilize so that recovery procedures can be accelerated. Usually, the minimum length of time for a patient to remain in the unit is three days, but a week or more may be necessary. After release from the Coronary Care Unit, the myocardial infarction patient may spend an additional week or two of gradually increasing ambulation, progressing from sitting up in a chair to walking a short distance and perhaps climbing stairs.

Abnormal Heart Rhythms

Normally, the atria and ventricles contract in a more or less regular pattern that produces a normal electrocardiogram pattern. A number of pattern variations may appear after a patient has undergone a myocardial infarction. Some abnormal heart rhythms also are observed in persons who have never experienced any form of heart disease.

Tachycardia One kind of abnormal heart rhythm is a tachycardia, which means simply a rapid heartbeat. There are several variations of tachycardia, which generally can be traced to specific areas of the heart. A tachycardia may occur as a regular rhythm of 100 beats per minute. In one variation, the ventricles may contract only once for every two contractions of the atria. In another variation, sometimes called atrial flutter, the atria contract three or four times as fast as the ventricles, which continue to contract at a regular pace. Atrial fibrillation is marked by rapid, irregular contractions. The abnormal atrial rhythms often can be controlled by the use of drugs, the administration of a small energy electric shock, or by manual manipulation of the carotid sinus which contains nerve endings that influence the circulatory system.

More urgently serious are abnormal rhythms of the ventricles. In ventricular tachycardia, the ventricles may contract at a rate of 140 or more beats per minute, and the patient can die quickly unless a normal rhythm can be re-established quickly with drugs or electric shock. Ventricular fibrillation is characterized by irregular contractions that may exceed a rate of 300 per minute. Although the ventricles contract, they do not pump blood, so the net effect is one of heart failure; death occurs if the condition is not treated quickly with electric shock.

Premature ventricular contractions produce what are known as ectopic heartbeats. An occasional ectopic beat is not considered dangerous, but when several premature ventricular contractions occur in succession, or when a regular heart rhythm is disrupted regularly by premature ventricular beats, the abnormality may signal the threat of ventricular fibrillation or tachycardia. Efforts are made by medical personnel who observe the irregular heartbeats to control the condition with medications.

Heart block Since all of the heart normally contracts in an orderly regular rhythm as the electrical impulse spreads from the sino-atrial node, any disruption in the transmission of the impulse can alter the rhythm of the contractions of the atria and ventricles. A failure in the transmission of the impulse is called a heart block. An interruption in the flow of the impulse along the right wall of the heart is known as a right bundle branch block; a failure of the impulse to flow from the bottom of the septum through the left side of the heart is a left bundle branch block. Occasionally, an impulse fails to leave the sino-atrial node and the result is a dropped beat, or a complete heartbeat skipped.

A complete heart block can occur, with all transmission from the atria blocked, but the result is not necessarily fatal. The heart has more than one built-in "pacemaker," so the ventricles may contract to the rhythm of a conduction node below the level of the atrial block. Pacemakers below the sino-atrial node, however, transmit impulses at a slower rate. Thus the heart rate may drop from 70 per minute to from 30 to 60 per minute, depending upon the pacemaker that continues functioning.

A heart that continues to function at a slower pace will have a lower cardiac output. The patient will experience fatigue more easily and may feel breathless more of the time. If the patient already suffers from a cardiovascular problem, the heart block could be a serious and life-threatening complication.

One complication of heart block is a condition known as Stokes-Adams attacks, in which the victim may feel dizzy and faint because of missed heartbeats. But after a brief period of unconsciousness, during which he may have no pulse and the skin will become cyanotic, he may suddenly recover consciousness and color will return to the skin. The recovery is due to an automatic restarting of the heart and circulation. Unfortunately, all Stokes-Adams attacks do not have happy endings, so it should never be assumed that a patient who faints because of this condition will recover automatically. Each attack should be treated as a medical emergency, which it is in fact.

Patients with heart block or other malfunctions of heart rhythm usually can be restored to normal life activities with the help of an artificial pacemaker. The pacemaker is an electrical device that can control the beating of the heart with battery-powered rhythmic electrical discharges. The electrodes that deliver the discharges can be placed on the outside of the chest wall or implanted inside the chest as an internal pacemaker. The electrode usually is implanted at the base of the right ventricle of the heart, and the battery-powered generator is located under the skin near the right armpit.

The artificial pacemaker may be designed so that it takes over only when the

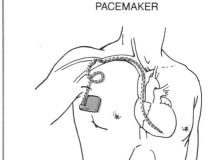

PACEMAKER

Many thousands of patients with heartbeat disorders are able to lead normal lives with the help of an artificial pacemaker. An electrode is snaked into the right ventricle of the patient's heart through blood vessels such as the jugular vein. A battery to power the pacemaker is sewed beneath the skin near the armpit. A minor operation is required every few years to replace the batteries. An artificial pacemaker usually generates an electrical impulse to trigger heart contractions only when the natural pacemaker fails.

patient's natural pacemaker fails to generate an impulse needed to produce a heart contraction.

Heart Valve Abnormalities

Heart failure sometimes is associated with failure of a heart valve. The valves actually are flaps of tissue that prevent a backflow of blood and help to keep it moving forward through the cardiovascular system. There are four valves at the entrances and exits of the heart ventricles. The valves are controlled by sets of small, cone-shaped papillary muscles attached to the walls of the ventricles that contract or relax as needed to open or close the valve flaps.

The two valves opening from the left ventricle are the mitral valve, a two-cusp, or flap, valve that separates the left atrium from its ventricle, and the aortic valve, which separates the left ventricle from the aorta.

On the right side of the heart are the tricuspid valve, between the atrium and ventricle, and the pulmonary valve that separates the right ventricle from the pulmonary artery.

The heart valves can be affected by several kinds of insults over a lifetime so that normal function is impaired. Rheumatic fever, for example, can result in an inflammation of the valve cusps so that they tend to stick to each other along the edges where they meet when closed. The valve flaps also can become fibrous and rigid from mineral deposits in later years. The

papillary muscles and their cords can become fibrous and shortened over the years.

Mitral stenosis is a condition involving a narrowing of the mitral valve as a result of one or more of the effects of aging and disease. Because of the narrowed opening between the left atrium and left ventricle, blood cannot be moved in adequate amounts from the left ventricle to the general body circulation. At the same time, blood can accumulate in the left atrium after it returns from the lungs, causing a buildup of pulmonary vein pressure and a loss of fluid into the air sacs of the lungs. The result is reduced cardiac output complicated by pulmonary edema. Responsibility for moving the blood forward shifts to the right ventricle, which then would become enlarged and eventually fail.

If the mitral valve fails to close properly, blood is forced back into the atrium with each contraction of the ventricle. The left atrium may enlarge in an effort to accommodate the regurgitated blood volume.

Stenosis of the aortic valve, from similar causes, will reduce the amount of blood that can be pumped to tissues throughout the body, although the left ventricle may enlarge in an effort to push the same amount of blood through a smaller opening. The extra effort, meanwhile, can create a greater demand on the coronary artery supplying oxygen to the left ventricle, and the patient may experience the pain of angina pectoris. Unless the condition is corrected, the left ventricle will fail.

Patients with diseases of the heart valves sometimes can be aided by medications that tend to restore normal heart action, such as digitalis drugs. A more permanent solution, however, is the re-

---

HOW A ONE-WAY VALVE WORKS

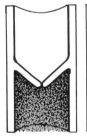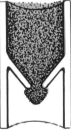

The flow of blood in the human body depends in part upon a series of valves designed by nature to keep the flow going in one continuous circuit. Heart valves prevent blood from flowing back into the atria when the ventricles contract, or returning to the left ventricle from the aorta. Smaller valves in the veins prevent blood from pooling in the lower part of the body while being returned from the feet to the heart.

placement of a diseased valve with an artificial valve or surgical repair of the valve cusps. When stenosis is due to edges of the valve flaps becoming fused, special instruments can be inserted into the heart to pry the cusps apart, thus enlarging the opening into or from the ventricle.

Diseases, including stenosis, of the valves of the right side of the heart are similar to those of the mitral and aortic valves. Right-sided valve disorders, however, may be reflected in abnormal conditions of the veins and liver. Tricuspid regurgitation, for example, can result in surges of the blood in the jugular veins, and pulsations may be observed in an enlarged liver. Treatment of problems of the valves on the right side of the heart also is similar to those on the left side, although defects of the pulmonary valve generally are less threatening than those involving the aortic valve.

Congenital Heart Defects

Pulmonary valve disorders often are congenital defects. Pulmonary stenosis at birth can result in the onset of congestive heart failure in a child, but the condition is easily corrected by surgically enlarging the valve opening.

Coarctation of the aorta is another congenital defect of the cardiovascular system. The aorta develops a severe constriction that virtually blocks the normal flow of blood, but the defect may not be detected until related symptoms such as hypertension occur in later life. Other arteries usually enlarge and bypass the coarctation, so the defect may escape notice unless a careful medical examination of the infant is made.

Defects in the ventricular or atrial septa are among the more common congenital heart abnormalities. An opening in the wall between the two atria results in a condition in which the heart functions as if it had three chambers, rather than four, with a common atrium. The defect often is not detected until later in life when abnormal heart functioning leads to an examination. A ventricular septal defect is likely to be more serious because contractions of the ventricles will push blood from the left side to the right side of the heart. Unless corrected surgically, the child will suffer from fatigue and breathlessness, and eventually will experience heart failure.

An opening between the aorta and pulmonary artery that serves the fetal circulation sometimes fails to close after birth, requiring surgery to prevent infant heart failure if the opening is large. In many cases the opening remains small and presents few problems, but doctors often recommend that congenital defects such as this, called persistent ductus arteriosus, be corrected when the child is small, in order to reduce the risk of serious heart problems in later life.

Still another congenital heart disease which may require surgical treatment in early childhood is the tetralogy of Fallot. Tetralogy of Fallot is so called because it involves a combination of four heart defects and was first described by a French physician named Fallot. The four defects are: (1) a ventricular septal defect, (2) a pulmonary stenosis, (3) a misplaced aorta that receives blood from both the left and right ventricles, and (4) an enlarged right ventricle.

Children with this disorder usually have a bluish, or cyanotic, skin coloration because used blood that lacks oxygen is shunted from the right side of the heart to the left and out of the aorta without going through the lungs. The young patient may suffer such a lack of oxygenated blood that he may become unconscious after mild exertion. The child often learns instinctively to rest in a squatting position after playing a while, because this posture helps the cardiovascular system recover from the strain of physical activity.

Surgery to correct the four defects may be carried out in stages or in a single operation that closes the opening between the ventricles, opens the obstructed pulmonary valve, and reroutes the aortic blood flow through another artery near the heart.

GLOSSARY

HEART DISEASE

Medical names and terms relating to heart disease are the subjects of this Glossary, which includes words in italic type that refer to separate entries in this list.

adrenergic blocking agent A drug that blocks the normal response of an organ or tissue to nerve impulses transmitted by the adrenergic, or sympathetic, nervous system. Blocking sympathetic nerve impulses to the heart and blood vessels tends to decrease the rate and intensity of heart contractions and to reduce constriction of the blood vessels.

There are two classes of adrenergic blocking agents, alpha and beta blockers. Both can be used in cardiovascular disorders, although beta blockers are employed more often. Some are used to control high blood pressure, especially when the condition is associated with a hyperactive heart, and to treat *angina pectoris* by reducing the work load of the heart. See also *beta blocking agents*.

aneurysm A ballooning of the wall of a vein or artery due to the weakening of the vessel wall by disease, injury, or birth defect.

angina pectoris A disorder of the heart marked by chest pain that is due to a greater demand for oxygen by the heart muscle than can be delivered by the coronary arteries supplying oxygenated blood to the heart.

angiocardiography A diagnostic technique involving injection of a radio-opaque dye into the bloodstream. X-rays taken after injection of the dye show the inside dimensions of the heart and blood vessels carrying the fluid.

anoxia A lack of oxygen. When living tissue of the human body is deprived of oxygen it dies, an effect of a blocked artery to the heart or any other organ resulting in an infarction.

antiarrhythmic drugs Medicines prescribed for certain heart disease patients to correct abnormal heart rates or rhythms.

anticoagulant drugs Medicines prescribed to control the threat of blood coagulation. The substances do not dissolve existing blood clots that may block arteries, but they can prevent new clots from forming and existing clots from becoming larger.

aorta The main artery trunk that receives blood from the left ventricle of the heart and distributes blood to smaller arteries that carry it to tissues throughout the body.

aortic stenosis A narrowing of the opening in the valve between the left ventricle and the *aorta*. The stenosis disrupts normal blood flow from the heart to the arteries of the body.

arrhythmia Any variation from the normal rhythm of the heartbeat.

arterioles The smallest vessels that are still considered arteries. Abnormal constriction of the arterioles can result in high blood pressure since the same amount of blood must pass through a smaller caliber of blood vessel.

arteriosclerosis A term used to identify several kinds of arterial diseases, characterized by a thickening and hardening of the walls of the blood vessels. The disorder can be caused by an accumulation of fibrous tissue, fatty deposits, and/or minerals such as calcium. Arteriosclerosis is due mainly to fatty deposits and sometimes is called atherosclerosis.

arteritis The term used to identify any inflammation of the arteries. Modifying terms help to describe specific kinds of artery inflammation, such as temporal arteritis for inflammation of the arteries about the temples.

asymmetric septal hypertrophy A medical mouthful sometimes abbreviated as ASH, the term is used by doctors to identify a rather common type of heart problem marked by an enlargement of the walls of the left ventricle, with the septal wall becoming thicker than the outer wall. The abnormality results in obstructed blood flow and less effective heart contractions. The patient may experience symptoms of dizziness and chest discomfort.

atheroma A fatty deposit on the inner wall of an artery. The accumulation of atheromas results in the disease condition called atherosclerosis. See illustration, page 483.

athlete's heart A supposed form of heart damage resulting from prolonged strenuous physical exercise.

atrioventricular valves Another name for the valves that separate the atria from the ventricles of the heart. The one on the right side is the tricuspid valve; the one on the left side is the mitral valve.

atropine A drug sometimes administered to treat *arrhythmia* or an abnormally slow heart rate.

auricle Another name for atrium, an upper chamber of the heart.

autonomic nervous system Another name for the involuntary nervous system that maintains automatic control of heartbeat, *blood pressure*, and other body functions.

bacterial endocarditis A bacterial infection of the membrane lining the heart. The lining of the heart valves often is affected and may suffer permanent damage from the infection.

Barlow's syndrome A medical name for a disorder involving the mitral valve between the left atrium and left ventricle of the heart. The condition, also called "floppy mitral valve," may permit blood to be pushed back into the atrium, instead of into the *aorta*, when the left ventricle contracts. Patients with this problem may experience chest discomfort and abnormal heart rhythm.

baroreceptors Sensory nerve cells that detect changes in blood pressure and in the diameter of blood vessels. The information they transmit to the brain results normally in adjustment of artery calibers and blood pressure to meet the needs of the moment.

beta blocking agents Drugs that stop nerve impulses which normally trigger increased heart activity. Sometimes called beta blockers, the substances are administered to reduce effects of *angina pectoris* and/or *hypertension*. See also *adrenergic blocking agent*.

bicuspid valve Another name for the mitral valve. It may be called bicuspid because it is composed of two cusps, or flaps, that move to open or close the opening between the heart's atrium and ventricle.

biofeedback A technique used for training patients to exercise control over certain autonomic nervous system functions by conscious effort reinforced with lights or sounds. In controlling heart rate, for example, electronic devices connected to the body trigger the lights or sounds whenever the heart rate exceeds a normal limit. The same kind of control can be produced without electronic biofeedback devices through consciously controlled relaxation.

blood pressure The force exerted against the walls of arteries by the flow of blood.

blue baby A common name for a condition, such as a defect in the septum separating the two sides of the heart, that results in a lack of oxygenated blood flowing to the tissues of the infant. The bluish coloration, or *cyanosis*, is due to a mixing of blood from the right and left ventricles through the defect. Other disorders, such as premature birth or respiratory difficulties, also may account for the blue baby effect.

bradycardia An abnormally slow heart rate, which usually is anything slower than 60 beats per minute.

Buerger's disease A blood vessel disease that results in such poor circulation that gangrene, or tissue death, is caused in the affected body area. The condition is related to the use of nicotine, a substance that can constrict the bore of blood vessels.

bundle of His Also called the A-V, or atrioventricular, bundle, this is a group of fibers that helps to conduct impulses for heart contractions along the muscular septum that separates the left and right sides of the heart. The bundle of fibers, named for a German doctor, transmits impulses from the atrioventricular node, or *pacemaker*, located near the base of the right atrium. The bundle divides into left and right branches, one going to the left ventricle and the other to the right ventricle.

capillary The smallest of the blood vessels of the body. Capillaries link the *arterioles* of the circulatory system to the venules, which merge to form veins for returning blood to the heart and lungs.

carbon dioxide A waste product of metabolism, or "calorie burning," in which carbon atoms from glucose molecules in tissue cells combine with oxygen atoms carried in the bloodstream to release life-sustaining energy.

cardiac arrest What happens when the heart stops beating and blood stops flowing.

cardiac cycle The series of events involved in one complete heart contraction from the end of one *systole* to the beginning of the next systole.

cardiac output The amount of blood that can be pumped by a patient's heart during a period of one minute—normally, about five quarts.

cardiac reserve The difference between the amount of blood pumped by a patient's heart when resting and the amount that can be pumped during maximum physical effort. The figure usually is the difference between about five quarts per minute and twenty-five quarts per minute.

cardiomyopathy A medical term used to identify diseases that involve only the myocar-

dium, or muscle tissues, of the heart, such as *myocardial infarction*.

carditis A word sometimes used to suggest any inflammation of the heart tissues.

carotid arteries Arteries that run on either side of the neck and branch around the middle into an internal and an external carotid artery.

carotid body An oval mass of cells located near the point where the internal and external branches of the *carotid arteries* leave the common carotid artery. The carotid bodies, on either side of the neck, contain nerve endings that monitor the acidity of the blood as well as the oxygen and carbon dioxide content. The receptors help adjust the heart and lung activity automatically to maintain normal levels of blood chemistry. When the oxygen level drops, for example, the carotid bodies send the appropriate signal for increasing the respiration rate in order to enlarge the oxygen supply.

carotid sinus A wide point on the common carotid artery, where branches of the internal and external *carotid arteries* begin. The carotid sinus contains the *carotid body*.

chlorthiazide A type of diuretic drug used to promote the flow of urine in patients with high blood pressure and *edema* associated with heart dysfunction.

chordae tendinae Fibrous cords that hold the valves between the upper and lower chambers of the heart. They are connected at one end to the papillary muscles in the ventricles, and at the other end to the cusps of the *atrioventricular valves*.

cineangiography X-ray motion pictures of the heart made by injecting into the bloodstream a radio-opaque substance that produces a shadow on the X-ray film. The technique permits moviemaking of the patient's heart while it actually is pumping blood.

claudication Pain or lameness that can be caused by defective blood circulation in the limbs.

clofibrate A drug generally used to reduce the triglyceride component of fats in the blood.

clubbed fingers Fingers with short broad tips and overhanging nails that develop in children born with certain kinds of heart defects, as well as in adults with certain heart, lung, or other disorders. The fingers sometimes are described as resembling "drumsticks."

coagulation The changing of fluid blood into a thickened or solid form that becomes blood clots.

coarctation of the aorta A pinching or narrowing of a section of the *aorta*; a condition that may occur as a *congenital heart defect*.

collateral circulation Blood circulation that develops in neighboring vessels when a main vessel becomes blocked.

commissurotomy A surgical procedure for widening a heart valve that has become narrowed by scar tissue. The valve flaps are spread apart along their natural lines of closure with a blunt tool.

congenital heart defect One that was present at birth. It may be either an inherited defect or one that developed during the fetal stage of life.

congestive heart failure A heart disorder, which is not necessarily a true failure, in which the heart is unable to pump as much blood as is needed to maintain normal body functions. Congestion results when, as a result of ineffective pumping action, fluid accumulates in the lungs, abdomen, or legs, or in more than one body area.

coronary arteries Two arteries that arise near the base of the *aorta* and spread to the left and to the right sides of the heart, distributing fresh blood to the heart muscle fibers.

coronary bypass surgery A surgical method of relieving restricted blood flow in *coronary arteries* by providing alternate routes. Pieces of arteries or veins are removed from other parts of the body and are grafted into the *coronary arteries.*

coronary heart disease A heart ailment caused by the narrowing of a coronary artery that restricts blood flow to the heart muscle.

coronary insufficiency A condition in which the *coronary arteries* are unable to deliver enough freshly oxygenated blood to the heart muscle to meet the heart's needs. The result can be *angina pectoris* or a *myocardial infarction*, although the condition also may cause no particular discomfort in certain patients.

coronary occlusion Another name for heart attack. A clot or other obstruction in a coronary artery hinders the flow of blood to some part of the heart muscle, causing that part of the heart to die.

coronary thrombosis A *coronary occlusion* in which the obstruction in the coronary artery is a blood clot.

cor pulmonale A form of heart disease in which the lungs are a cause of the problem. High blood pressure in the vessels of the lungs, for example, causes the heart's right ventricle to enlarge so that blood can be circulated through the pulmonary artery network.

coumarin The name of a type of *anticoagulant drug* that delays the clotting of blood.

cyanosis A medical term for the bluish coloration of the skin when there is not enough oxygen in the blood to give it the typical red coloring.

decompensation Inability of the heart to maintain adequate circulation, a condition that causes tissues to become waterlogged.

defibrillation The technique for controlling *fibrillation* of the atrium or ventricle by applying an electric shock to the chest area.

depressant A term used to identify any drug that reduces the activity of any function of the body.

dextrocardia A medical term used to describe a congenital abnormality, which is not necessarily a defect, in which the heart and its blood vessels are reversed.

diastole The period of relaxation during the *cardiac cycle* of heartbeats. The term is usually applied to the part of the cycle in which the ventricles relax while blood fills the chambers from the atria above. But the term also can refer to a period of atrial diastole.

digitalis A drug prepared from leaves of the foxglove plant. It is used to treat some types of heart failure because the drug causes the heart muscle to pump more forcefully and effectively.

dilation A stretching or widening of blood vessels.

ductus arteriosus A big medical term for a shunt between the *aorta* and pulmonary artery that is a normal part of circulation during the fetal stage of life. Normally, it closes around the time of birth. But the ductus arteriosus may remain open, requiring surgical correction to maintain normal blood circulation for the infant.

dyspnea A medical term for shortness of breath.

echocardiography A diagnostic method by which ultrasound pulses are transmitted into the body and the echoes returning from the surfaces of the heart are converted into a recorded image of the movements of a patient's heart.

edema A swelling of body tissues or body cavities due to accumulation of fluids. The fluids usually originate in the circulatory system but are forced out of the blood vessels because of a disorder such as congestive heart failure.

effort syndrome A term sometimes used to identify a functional heart disease marked by rapid heartbeat, fatigue, dizziness, and dyspnea as a result of exertion, even though no disorder of the heart or other organs can be found to account for the symptoms.

Eisenmenger's syndrome A type of high blood pressure disorder resulting from a congenital defect in heart anatomy. The condition causes oxygen-rich blood to be pumped back into the lungs, and oxygen-poor blood to be returned to the general body circulation.

electrocardiogram Abbreviated as either EKG or ECC. A record of electrical activity associated with contractions of the heart.

embolism The blocking of a blood vessel by an embolus, which most often is a blood clot.

endocarditis An inflammation of the endocardium, the smooth membrane forming the lining of the heart.

endothelium The thin, smooth lining of blood vessels and the heart.

enlarged heart A condition in which the heart is larger than normal. The cause may be hereditary, physical activity, or a disorder that causes the heart to work harder so that the muscle tissue develops *hypertrophy*.

epicardium Another term for pericardium, the membrane that provides a protective outer covering for the heart muscle.

epinephrine Also called adrenalin, a hormone secreted by the adrenal glands. It can raise the blood pressure, constrict the *arterioles*, and increase the rate of heartbeat.

erythrocyte Another term for red blood cell.

essential hypertension Also called primary hypertension, it is a euphemism for high blood pressure for which no organic disorder can be found.

extracorporeal circulation Circulation of blood outside the patient's body; for example, by means of a heart-lung machine during heart surgery.

extrasystole A heart contraction that occurs prematurely and interrupts the normal rhythm of the heart.

fibrillation A kind of cardiac arrythmia, usually occurring as rapid uncoordinated contractions of the heart muscle. The haphazard systoles usually result in an inability of the heart to pump blood effectively. Heart failure may occur if the condition is not quickly corrected with drugs or electric shock. See also *defibrillation.*

fibrin An elastic, threadlike protein that is dissolved in the blood as fibrinogen and converted by enzymes to the basic fabric of blood clots. The clots sometimes can be converted back to the liquid state by an enzyme called fibrinolysin.

fluoroscope A piece of equipment that permits the doctor to view the heart and other organs in action through X-ray images projected onto a screen similar to that of a TV tube.

foramen ovale The medical name for the congenital defect of a hole in the heart between the two atria.

gallop rhythm A heart sound that sometimes resembles that of the hoofbeats of a galloping horse.

heart block An abnormal condition in which the electrical impulse needed to trigger contraction of the heart muscle is slowed or stopped along the route of the heart's conduction system.

hemoglobin The oxygen-carrying red pigment of red blood cells.

heparin A naturally occurring anticoagulant used to treat or prevent blood clots.

hypercholesteremia A condition marked by an excess of cholesterol in the patient's blood.

hyperlipoproteinemia A disorder caused by an excess of lipoproteins in the blood. Lipoproteins are complexes of fatty substances, such as cholesterol or triglycerides, and certain kinds of proteins. Persons afflicted with this disorder are more likely to experience strokes or heart attacks.

hypertrophy Enlargement of a tissue or an organ such as the heart due to an abnormal growth of its tissue cells.

hypoxia A less than normal supply of oxygen in the blood.

iatrogenic A disease condition that has been caused by a doctor or his assistants. An iatrogenic heart disease, for example, could be a heart ailment resulting from something said by an examining physician that was interpreted by the patient as evidence of a heart disorder.

infarct An area of tissue that has died or been seriously damaged by an interruption in the supply of oxygen-rich blood to the area.

intermittent claudication A pain that occurs, usually in a leg muscle, because of inadequate blood supply to the area during periods of exercise or exertion.

interventricular septum The muscular wall that divides the ventricles, or lower chambers, of the heart.

intima The innermost layer of a blood vessel. It includes the endothelial lining.

ischemia A local, usually temporary, lack of oxygen in an area of living tissue. Ischemic heart disease is marked by a deficiency of oxygen delivery to the heart muscle because of a decreased blood supply resulting from a blocked or constricted artery.

jugular veins Veins that return blood from the head and neck to the heart.

leukocytes White blood cells.

lipid A fatty substance, such as cholesterol or triglycerides.

lumen The bore or passageway inside a tubular organ such as a blood vessel.

mitral stenosis A narrowing of the opening in the mitral valve between the upper and lower chambers of the left side of the heart.

murmur An abnormal sound produced by blood flowing through the heart. The cause often is an obstruction that diverts the fluid flow.

myocardial infarction Death or damage to an area of heart muscle because of an interruption of arterial blood to the area.

myocarditis An inflammation of the myocardium, or heart muscle, which may be due to disease organisms, injury, or drugs.

neurocirculatory asthenia A functional disease, sometimes called soldier's heart as well as effort syndrome. It identifies a group of symptoms that resemble those of heart disease although examination of the patient fails to reveal any evidence of organic heart damage.

nitroglycerin A vasodilator drug prescribed to relax the muscles of the blood vessels in *angina pectoris* and other disorders.

norepinephrine Also known as noradrenalin, a hormone substance that can increase *blood pressure* by constricting the small blood vessels.

normotensive A medical term meaning simply normal *blood pressure*.

occlusive A closing or shutting off, as when a *coronary occlusion* closes off a *coronary artery*.

organic heart disease A disorder that is characterized by evidence of a structural defect in the heart or surrounding blood vessels. It may be compared to functional heart disease in which no damage or abnormality of the heart and circulatory tissues can be found to account for the symptoms.

pacemaker A small group of specialized cells that produces the rhythmic electrical impulses which cause the heart muscle fibers to contract. An artificial pacemaker is an electronic device implanted in the chest to produce the electrical impulses when the natural pacemaker fails.

palpitation A sensation of an abnormal heartbeat, sometimes described as a "fluttering" of the heart.

papillary muscles Tiny cone-shaped muscles anchored in the walls of the heart ventricles that open and close the heart valves.

paroxysmal tachycardia A period of abnormally rapid heartbeats that begins suddenly and ends just as suddenly.

percussion A diagnostic technique used by doctors in studying the heart and lungs by tapping the chest and listening for abnormal sounds that might indicate, for example, fluid accumulation.

pericardial tamponade An accumulation of fluid between the layers of the pericardium, the membrane covering the outside of the heart.

pericarditis An inflammation of the pericardial membrane.

peripheral resistance The resistance of the walls of the *arterioles* to the flow of blood. When the resistance increases, the *blood pressure* rises.

peripheral vascular disease Any disease of the blood and lymph vessels that are outside the immediate area of the heart.

pheochromocytoma An adrenal gland tumor which can increase the production of the hormones *epinephrine* and *norepinephrine*. The hormones can increase the heart rate and cause a rise in *blood pressure*, plus other symptoms such as headaches and sweating.

phlebitis An inflammation of a vein, usually in the leg, often leading to the formation of a blood clot in the vein.

plasma The liquid portion of the blood after all cells have been removed.

platelets Small disk-shaped bodies in the blood which are involved in the formation of blood clots.

polyarteritis nodosa A medical name for a disease marked by inflammation and destruction of small- and medium-sized arteries. The cause is unknown. Tissues supplied by the diseased vessels become impaired.

polycythemia An abnormal blood condition marked by an excess of red blood cells; the excess cells can thicken the blood and interfere with its normal forward movement through the circulatory system.

pressor A substance that tends to increase blood pressure.

primary hypertension Another name for *essential hypertension*, or high blood pressure of unknown cause.

propranolol A beta blocking drug used to control *angina pectoris*, hypertension, and other cardiovascular disorders.

prosthesis An artificial device that substitutes for a body part. An artificial heart valve would be an example of a prosthesis.

pulmonary Pertaining to the lungs, as in pulmonary artery or pulmonary edema.

pulse pressure The difference in blood pressures in an artery between systolic and diastolic readings.

pulsus alternans A pulse beat that alternates between weak and strong pulsations.

Purkinje fibers Specialized muscle fibers in the ventricles that are associated with electrical impulses that cause heart contractions.

quinidine A drug sometimes used to control abnormal heart rhythms.

rauwolfia A drug obtained from the root of the Indian snakeroot plant that can be used to lower high blood pressure and slow the heart rate. A related substance from the same plant is reserpine.

Raynaud's disease A circulatory disorder characterized by pallor and numbness in the fingers, toes, and occasionally other exposed skin surfaces, due to a transient constriction of *arterioles*. The effect is associated with cold temperatures, use of nicotine, and emotional stress.

regurgitation The backward flow of blood through a defective valve.

revascularization Restoration of blood flow in arteries that have been blocked or constricted by disease or injury.

risk factor The chance of developing a disease, such as hypertension, because of exposure to an influence that may be associated with the disease. Family history, obesity, and cigarette smoking are examples of factors that can increase one's chances of developing hypertension.

sclerosis Hardening; *arteriosclerosis* means hardening of the arteries.

secondary hypertension High blood pressure produced by, or secondary to, a known cause such as kidney disease.

shunt A passage between two blood vessels or two sides of the heart.

sinus rhythm Normal heart rhythm controlled by the heart's natural pacemaker, the sino-atrial node.

syncope A fainting spell, sometimes caused by insufficient blood supply to the brain.

systemic circulation The blood circulation through all parts of the body except the lungs. This represents the blood flow from the left ventricle via the *aorta*.

systole The period of contraction of a heartbeat.

tachycardia Abnormally fast heartbeat, usually any rate that exceeds 100 beats per minute.

thrombus A blood clot that forms inside a blood vessel or the cavity of the heart.

vagus nerve A nerve that extends from the brain to the abdomen, via the neck and chest. It is able to slow the heart rate when stimulated.

varix A varicosity or abnormally swollen blood vessel. A varicose vein of the leg is an example of a varix.

QUESTIONS AND ANSWERS
HEART DISEASE

Q: *My father is 60 years old and has pulmonary artery disease. Would it help him to get a heart transplant?*

A: Probably not. Most heart transplants today are restricted to persons less than 50 years of age who do not have additional cardiovascular problems. The pulmonary artery disease you mention probably involves hypertension of the pulmonary arteries, which would be a condition that usually increases the risk of heart transplant failure.

Q: *What kind of heart disease patients are accepted for transplants?*

A: Nearly half of all heart transplant recipients today suffer from a disorder called myocardiopathy, a heart muscle damage condition that may be caused by an infectious agent.

Some other types of heart disease for which transplants were considered a decade or more ago can now be treated with drugs and surgical techniques that have been developed in recent years. The drugs include the adrenergic beta blocking agents. A surgical method that has solved a previously difficult problem for advanced heart disease patients is the coronary bypass technique, in which veins or arteries from other parts of the body can be grafted into the coronary artery network.

Q: *I have heard there is a new surgical technique for treating coronary artery stenosis while the patient is under just a local anesthetic. How does it work?*

A: The surgical technique to which you refer is one that had been used in previous years to correct stenosis of blood vessels in other parts of the body and, more recently, was adapted to treatment of constrictions in the more vulnerable coronary arteries. The way it works, briefly, is this: a catheter is inserted into an artery in the leg or arm after the patient has been given a local anesthetic. The catheter is maneuvered into the aorta and then into the opening of the coronary artery with the help of a fluoroscope, which permits the doctors to view the heart and other internal organs with an X-ray image while they actually are working. From the position at the opening of the coronary artery, a second catheter carried inside the first one is maneuvered into the artery toward the stenotic portion. Then a balloon at the end of the smaller catheter is filled with a liquid that causes it to expand. The balloon may be inflated, then deflated, several times to push the artery walls farther apart at the stenosis. The balloon is inflated for only a few seconds at a time so that the artery is never completely obstructed long enough to interfere with blood flow to the heart muscle.

Q: *There have been news stories reporting that people who take aspirin every day will not get heart attacks. Are the reports true?*

A: This is a matter that you should discuss with your own physician. While there have been experimental animal studies and statistical surveys of human subjects indicating that aspirin may reduce the risk of heart attacks and strokes, scientists are not really sure about how aspirin affects the cardiovascular system to possibly prevent blood clot formation in people. Also, aspirin can have certain adverse effects such as stimulating the signs and symptoms of peptic ulcers. Thus, a person who is ulcer-prone but shows no evidence of developing a stroke or heart attack could create a real health problem by taking aspirin to avoid a disorder that is merely a possibility.

Q: *Can jogging or marathon running prevent heart attacks?*

A: This subject is still controversial despite numerous studies reported in medical journals.

As more marathon runners are autopsied after death from accidents or other causes, the evidence seems to be accumulating to support the contention that marathon running will not insure protection against myocardial infarction or other forms of coronary heart disease. Some runners have died of heart attacks, one during a marathon race; some who died in automobile or other accidents were found to have coronary arteries with signs of atherosclerosis. But this evidence should not be interpreted as some sort of proof that running and jogging are not worthwhile exercises. Such information would require data from studies of many thousands of joggers and runners over a period of several decades, so the answer may not be available until the twenty-first century.

Q: *Will heart surgery for angina pectoris affect a patient's sexual performance?*
A: There is some evidence to indicate that sexual function may suffer if angina treatment by coronary bypass surgery is delayed too long. More than 90 percent of a group of patients who received early treatment for angina through coronary bypass treatment found their sexual performance "satisfactory," whereas in a similar group of patients, who had delayed treatment for angina, most claimed sexual dysfunction as an aftereffect of the surgery. However, it also has been found that patients who delay treatment for angina generally tend to be more depressed than those who seek early corrective treatment. So it's possible that attitudes toward sexual activity among heart patients may be only a part of a larger complex of psychological factors associated with a potentially life-threatening disease.

Q: *I have a yellowish wart on my face and my doctor told me it might be a sign of heart or blood vessel disease. I think he's kidding. What do you think?*
A: I think your doctor probably found a xanthoma on your skin. A xanthoma is not a wart, although it might resemble one. It is a small, slightly raised patch or nodule that is caused by abnormally high levels of cholesterol or other lipids in the bloodstream. Since people who have xanthomas usually have blood lipid disorders of the type associated with cardiovascular disease, I think you should believe your doctor.

Q: *My internist recommended that I take a "stress test" because of the results of my last electrocardiogram. Does this have something to do with mental stress?*
A: A stress test is a diagnostic technique used to determine the body's ability to handle physical exertion, or physical stress. A stress test usually is taken in a medical laboratory equipped with a treadmill or a stationary bicycle, and electrocardiograph equipment that can be connected to the patient while he is exercising on the treadmill or stationary bicycle. Instruments also may be used to measure blood pressure and respiratory function while one exercises. Since an electrocardiogram usually is recorded while the patient is in a resting position, it may not give a true picture of how the heart and lungs perform in a work or play situation. Thus, the stress test.

Q: *What is meant by a "silent" heart disorder?*
A: The term "silent" refers to the insidious early stages of heart disease, before the symptoms of pain or shortness of breath, fainting, dizziness, or other effects suddenly make themselves felt. Periodic medical examinations, including electrocardiograms, often can detect the "silent" symptoms of cardiovascular degeneration so that treatment can begin before the condition becomes deadly serious.

Q: *Is there a time of day when a heart attack is most likely to happen?*
A: For most people, a heart attack is most likely to occur around three or four o'clock in the morning. The reason is that for most people—those who follow a typical workday schedule—this is the hour when the heart rate reaches its slowest pace, oxygen distribution to body tissues is at the lowest point of the day, and the chances of the body coping with a cardiovascular accident are the least. Exceptions to this

rule of thumb would be persons whose biological clocks are not set for typical workday schedules, such as workers on night shifts.

Q: *Why are men more likely to have heart attacks than women?*
A: Until recently, it was believed that all women were immune from heart attacks during their fertile, or child-bearing, years because of their female sex hormones. Some doctors now suspect that other factors may have been involved in the earlier statistics. Recent studies have found that cigarette smoking among premenopausal women can alter the risk considerably. Women under the age of 50 who smoke from one to 14 cigarettes a day are four times as likely to have a heart attack as women who do not smoke. But women under the age of 50 who smoke 35 or more cigarettes a day are 21 times as likely to experience a myocardial infarction.

Men generally are expected to have a heart attack rate four times higher than women, in the under-45 age groups. But with more girls and young women smoking cigarettes, the difference is expected to narrow in future years.

Q: *If the human body produces its own cholesterol, is there any point in worrying about cholesterol in the diet?*
A: While it's true that human body tissues can produce their own cholesterol, which in limited amounts has a number of important functions including the formation of certain sex hormones, the amount of cholesterol contributed by an average American's body amounts to somewhat less than half the total amount circulating in the blood vessels. In other words, the cholesterol a person gets from foods generally more than doubles the amount in his arteries. It is the excess cholesterol, not cholesterol per se, that increases the risk of atherosclerosis and heart disease.

Q: *Is cholesterol the only fat substance that is involved with atherosclerosis and heart disease?*
A: Actually, there are other lipid, or fat, molecules in the diet that are more closely related to cardiovascular problems. But cholesterol is a sort of barometer that can be used to measure the amount of fats in a person's diet and blood. A high cholesterol level in a patient's blood indicates a higher than normal intake of fatty foods in general.

Q: *What are good sources of protein that would also contain little or no cholesterol?*
A: Egg whites, fat-free milk, and fish—but not shellfish. Veal and poultry are relatively good sources of low-cholesterol protein if care is taken to remove any fatty tissues. Egg yolks and organ meats should be avoided as among the richest sources of cholesterol in foods.

18

STROKES AND HIGH BLOOD PRESSURE

High blood pressure does not always result in a stroke, and strokes are not always caused by high blood pressure. But strokes occur from two to four times more often in persons with hypertension, or high blood pressure, than in people with normal blood pressure. And high blood pressure is the most easily treated cause of strokes.

Unfortunately, only about half the people suffering from abnormally high blood pressure are aware of their condition. Blood pressure can increase to potentially dangerous high levels without warning signs or symptoms that most patients would detect. The first warning that something may be wrong might come during a medical examination for a seemingly unrelated problem. Untreated hypertension can cause damage that is marked by heart problems, such as angina pectoris, or by kidney disease. High blood pressure on a weakened artery in the brain tissue can result in a cerebral hemorrhage, or as it sometimes is called, a CVA, for cerebrovascular accident.

A cerebrovascular accident is medical terminology for stroke. It is the third lead-ing cause of death, after heart disease and cancer, in that order. Until the 1960's, when the risk of death from stroke began to drop, cerebrovascular disorders ranked ahead of cancer as the second most common fatal disease category. For American women, the risk of death from a stroke trails cancer by a very small statistical margin.

Strokes and hypertension can affect anybody, although there are some variations in risk according to age, sex, and geographic area. Except for women living in the Deep South, strokes are relatively rare among Americans under the age of 35. After the age of 45, the incidence of strokes increases markedly, and strokes become rather common occurrences for persons over the age of 65.

What Causes a Stroke?

Exactly what is a stroke? A stroke usually means a sudden attack of clotting or bleeding within the brain that may result in damage to brain tissues. Paralysis is a common effect of a stroke. The stroke can be caused by a ruptured blood vessel, resulting in a cerebral hemorrhage type of CVA, or it can be due to a blockage or obstruction of a blood vessel similar to the type of thrombosis that would lead to a heart attack. It's also possible that several kinds of alterations in normal blood circulation, other than a ruptured or obstructed artery, could produce stroke symptoms. It's not at all unusual for a cerebrovascular accident to have a transient, or temporary, effect and for the victim to recover almost immediately. In other cases, a patient may suffer a stroke that results in paralysis on one side of the body, but the symptoms disappear after a week or two; or the condition may become stable and be followed by gradual recovery over a period of months. In other words, not all strokes are alike.

Of course, some CVA's can be fatal or produce permanent disabilities. A cerebral hemorrhage that does not cause early death or become progressively worse in its effects within the first few days or weeks, however, may be reversible, offering hope that some degree of recovery can be expected. A hemorrhage that involves the brain stem is much more likely to become a fatal stroke than a CVA that affects the frontal lobes; the brain stem is responsible for normal functioning of vital body processes such as breathing and heart rate, while the frontal lobes are associated with activities of an emotional or moral nature. An injury to the frontal lobes might result only in diminished initiative or increased carelessness by the patient. The brain stem, in addition to con-

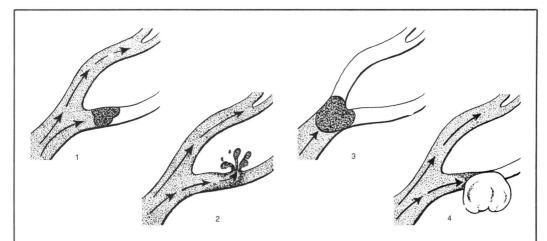

Drawings show four ways in which disrupted blood flow to the brain can result in a stroke: (1) illustrates a small blood clot blocking a small blood vessel, resulting in the death or damage of an area of brain tissue which is supplied by the blocked vessel; (2) shows a rupture of a blood vessel in the brain, a condition often resulting from high blood pressure in a weakened artery; (3) blood flow to more than one branch of an artery may be blocked by a large blood clot that becomes lodged at the very point where the artery branches; and (4) a tumor growing in the brain tissue may press against an artery and thereby interrupt or stop completely the normal flow of blood to a section of the brain.

trolling nerve pathways for the heart and lungs, plays an important role in the ability to swallow. A generation ago, doctors often checked the ability of a new stroke victim to swallow adequately because this provided a clue as to the possible location and extent of damage caused by a CVA.

Because of the close association between blood pressure and stroke, an early therapeutic procedure used in helping a patient to survive a cerebral hemorrhage is to lower the blood pressure with medications. This not only reduces the risk of further damage to surrounding brain tissues, but it cuts the chances of additional hemorrhages.

How the Body Maintains Blood Pressure

Normally, a certain amount of blood pressure is required in order to circulate oxygen and nutrients in the blood to tissues throughout the body and to remove waste products such as carbon dioxide produced by cellular metabolism. The blood pressure is maintained by the heart's pumping action. Blood is pumped from the left ventricle into the aorta which supplies the arteries. The arteries are connected with the capillaries, the ultimate part of the blood distribution system, by vessels called arterioles, which are muscular tubes that regulate the blood pressure in the circulatory system. When an arteriole bore is narrowed, the force of the blood, or the blood pressure, builds up against the walls of the blood vessel. The effect is similar to that of a garden hose that delivers water from a faucet at a higher pressure than a hose of wider diameter or a hose of more flexible tubing material. When the arterioles fail to function normally, the blood pressure will be altered.

The muscles in the arteriole walls de-

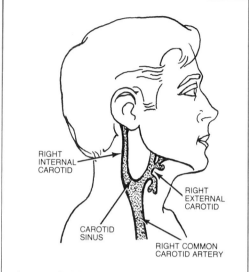

RIGHT INTERNAL CAROTID

RIGHT EXTERNAL CAROTID

CAROTID SINUS

RIGHT COMMON CAROTID ARTERY

A person's blood pressure is monitored automatically by nerve receptors in the carotid artery which carries blood from the heart to the head. The receptors are located in the carotid sinus, where the neck artery divides into internal and external branches.

pend upon signals from the nervous system to control the size of the bore in the vessels. The size of the opening in the arterioles normally varies according to the immediate needs of the tissues being supplied with freshly oxygenated blood. After a big meal, for example, the arterioles may need to supply extra blood to the capillaries spread through the digestive system. On a hot day, the body's control system may find it necessary to enlarge the arterioles carrying blood to the skin surfaces in order to reduce excess body heat. Or, if a person is running, the muscles involved in moving the body would need an extra blood supply. If two or more events that demand extra blood flow occur at the same time, the circulatory system could be in big trouble—a good

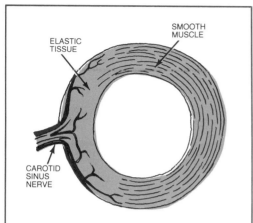

Close-up view shows how carotid sinus nerve detects changes in blood pressure. Changes in the volume and pressure of blood flowing through the vessel cause the elastic tissue in the carotid sinus wall to stretch or contract, changes that are detected by the endings of nerve fibers in the carotid wall.

could range from simple discomfort to circulatory collapse, depending upon the general health of the individual and other factors.

Theoretically, if all the arteriolcs and capillaries happened to relax at the same time, they could swallow the body's entire blood supply within a few seconds. One reason this is unlikely to happen is that ar-

reason not to enter a track meet on a hot summer day immediately after eating a big lunch!

A normal, healthy arteriole is a major controller of the flow of blood being pumped continuously by the heart. By contraction and relaxation of the smooth muscle fibers in the walls of an arteriole, the size of the bore of an arteriole when fully relaxed may be as much as five times the diameter of the same arteriole when fully contracted. Ordinarily, arterioles dilate to meet the needs of surrounding tissues for oxygen and nutrients in the blood; they contract when the tissue cells have an abundance of oxygen and nutrients. In the hypothetical case of a person running a race in the hot sun after a huge meal, three competing organ systems would place an abnormal demand on the body's circulatory function. The effects

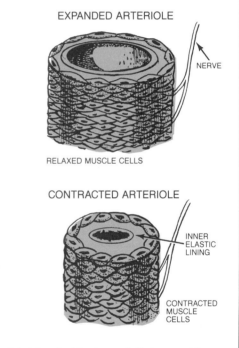

Arterioles, the blood vessels that connect the arteries to the capillaries of the body's blood distribution system, affect blood pressure by expanding or contracting. Arterioles have relatively thick muscular walls and nerve endings from the autonomic nervous system. The link between the nervous system and the arteriole muscle tissue explains how emotions such as fear or anger can result in changes in the bore, or opening, of the arterioles and, in turn, blood pressure. Contraction of the arteriole walls increases blood pressure.

terioles normally are under a moderate degree of constriction at all times. The effect is quite similar to muscle tone in the skeletal muscles. An increase in the tone of the arteriole muscles, resulting from an increase in impulses from the sympathetic nervous system, can cause a measurable rise in a person's blood pressure. A similar effect can be produced with a small amount of a hormone called epinephrine, a natural chemical secreted by sympathetic nerve endings. An injection of epinephrine into the bloodstream of a human will cause the arteriole muscles to constrict and will raise the blood pressure to hypertensive levels.

A tumor of the adrenal glands, located atop the kidneys, can produce an overabundance of norepinephrine, a hormone related to epinephrine. The tumor, called a pheochromocytoma, may secrete only normal amounts of norepinephrine when the patient is not agitated or nervous. But if he becomes angry or excited, the adrenal tumor can result in an outpouring of the hormone that sends the blood pressure skyrocketing to levels of 200 millimeters of mercury or more. A variety of disorders of the kidney also can result in abnormally high blood pressure readings. If arteries to both kidneys should become obstructed or restricted, the patient's blood pressure can gradually increase to levels that are nearly double normal or average readings.

Still another cause of hypertension can be a disorder affecting the part of the brain that controls the muscle tone in the arterioles. A lesion in the hypothalamus, for example, can result in an increase in sympathetic nerve impulses transmitted to the arterioles, making them constrict more than necessary and thereby raising the pressure of blood flow.

Ironically, one of the body's many marvelous control systems can increase the blood pressure during a cerebral hemorrhage, which was a result of high blood pressure in the first place. This system consists of baroreceptors, or pressoreceptors, that are nerve endings in the walls of arteries that detect changes in the diameter of the blood vessels. During hemorrhage, blood pressure normally would drop, but the baroreceptors detect the change and signal the nervous system to constrict the arterioles, so that blood pressure is elevated back toward the level before the start of bleeding.

Causes of Hypertension

Disorders involving the kidneys, the adrenal glands atop the kidneys, and the brain and central nervous system are among the known causes of hypertension. Other known causes include the narrowing of major arteries, such as the aorta, which places an abnormal demand on the circulatory system to squeeze blood in normal quantities through the narrowed opening. Such cases of hypertension sometimes are classed as secondary hypertension, which in many instances can be controlled or corrected to restore blood pressure to normal levels. Surgical removal of a diseased kidney or adrenal gland, or repair of a restricted or obstructed artery, usually ends the patient's blood pressure problem. However, the known and correctable causes of hypertension account for only five to ten percent of all cases of high blood pressure.

Essential hypertension is the term used to identify the type of high blood pressure that has no identifiable cause and accounts for 90 to 95 percent of all cases of hypertension. Essential hypertension is a disorder that has challenged medical scientists for many years. Although it affects more than 10 percent of the population and accounts for 20 percent of all deaths in some areas, the cause of essential hypertension has generated many theories but few facts. Various studies have suggested it might be the result of a kidney abnormality or a glandular disorder, since both factors can be shown to be causes of secondary hypertension. It also has been suggested that essential hypertension may be the result of abnormal activity in the brain center that controls the size of arterioles.

Strong evidence indicates that essential hypertension may be inherited. Some studies have shown that a person has a 50 percent chance of developing essential hypertension if one parent had the disease, but the odds increase to 90 percent if both parents had it. The exact factor that may be inherited is unknown. It has been speculated that victims of essential hypertension may inherit genes that cause a production of overly active arterioles, defective arterioles, or possibly a deficiency of arterioles which restricts normal blood flow.

Certain environmental factors are associated with essential hypertension. They include obesity, cigarette smoking, emotional stress, and the excessive use of table salt or other forms of sodium in the diet.

Doctors who treat patients with hypertension often ask a number of questions about the family history of the patient to determine if either or both parents, or any brothers or sisters, had high blood pressure. Other questions might relate to causes of death of family members, such as stroke, heart failure, heart attack, or kidney disease. The doctor may try to de-termine how long the patient has had high blood pressure; untreated hypertension generally progresses toward damage to vital organs. Once organ damage begins, the average survival time for the untreated patient is about six years.

The heart is the organ most commonly damaged by hypertension because it must respond to the elevated blood pressure problem by pumping harder. In responding, the heart increases gradually in size until it becomes unable to cope with the problem. Congestive heart failure often is a result of hypertension. Atherosclerosis, a disorder marked by the accumulation of fatty deposits on the inner surfaces of artery walls, is complicated by hypertension. When the coronary arteries supplying blood to the heart muscle are affected by atherosclerosis, hypertension can lead indirectly to angina pectoris, the type of chest pains exacerbated by physical effort, or to serious heart muscle damage such as myocardial infarction. Hypertension can reduce kidney function by restricting blood flow to that organ, which handles more than a quart of blood every ten minutes; any interference with normal kidney function results in a failure of that organ to rid the body of toxic waste products.

The statisticians who estimated that death from hypertension could be expected about six years after the start of organ damage also have calculated that an average hypertension patient could expect to live about 20 years from the onset of the disease if it went untreated. But not all doctors agree on what blood pressure levels mark the boundary between normal blood pressure and high blood pressure, although most agree that the risk of death and damage to organs increases more or less directly with the severity of the hypertension, or the increased levels of blood pressure readings.

Measuring Blood Pressure

Blood pressures vary from person to person and from day to day in the same person, so the level at which blood pressure is considered abnormally high may not always be the same set of numbers. Further complicating the situation is the fact that blood pressure readings vary according to circumstances under which they are measured. Unless a patient has a blood pressure reading that is critically high, most doctors prefer to take a series of measurements over a period of weeks or months before determining whether a serious problem exists and the best method for treating the individual case.

To obtain careful blood pressure readings, the patient usually is checked at least once in each arm and in both a sitting and standing position. The blood pressure also may be checked while the patient is recumbent, or lying down. Some doctors prefer what is called a casual blood pressure measurement; that is, blood pressure is measured while the patient is seated quietly in the doctor's office with the arm resting on the desk and at the level of the patient's heart.

Many doctors and most insurance companies diagnose high blood pressure as one that measures 140/90, or 140 millimeters of mercury on the systolic reading, over 90 millimeters on the diastolic. The systolic reading measures pressure resulting from contraction of the heart ventricles; the diastolic pressure represents the blood pressure during the resting phase of the heart, or the brief period between contractions of the ventricles.

Some physicians classify a patient as hypertensive if his blood pressure measured 140/90 or higher on three successive visits to the doctor's office. They apply that rule to younger patients but allow an older person to have a slightly higher systolic blood pressure measurement before treating him for hypertension. A person over 60 years of age, for example, might be considered normal with a blood pressure reading of 160/90. But a patient of any age with a blood pressure measurement of perhaps 200/120 would be considered hypertensive, and there would be no delay of two or more return visits to determine whether or not the blood pressure was still at that critically high level.

While hypertension generally is considered to develop without signs or symptoms other than the indications revealed by a doctor's diagnostic tests, many patients associate hypertension with headaches, nosebleeds, and dizzy spells. However, some careful studies have indicated that the only symptom that seems to have a definite cause-and-effect relationship with high blood pressure is dizziness, which reportedly occurs only in some patients with very high blood pressure.

Controlling High Blood Pressure

When high blood pressure has been established, the doctor may prescribe weight reduction if the patient is overweight, curtailed smoking if the patient smokes cigarettes, and a reduced use of sodium products such as table salt and processed foods with high sodium content. Processed foods that might have to be curtailed include cheeses, sausages, lunch meats, etc.

Obesity tends to be directly related to high blood pressure; the greater the weight gain, regardless of the patient's original weight, the greater is the tendency to hypertension. Scientific studies show that when overweight people reduce their body weight, their blood pressure falls to or near normal levels. Thus, a doctor who advises weight reduction as part of the treatment for high blood pressure has adequate evidence to support his recommendation.

Salt-free Diet and Nondrug Therapy
The role of salt in the diet in relation to hypertension is like the association between obesity and high blood pressure—it is a matter of experience rather than a direct cause-and-effect link. People with hypertension simply do not seem to be able to tolerate excess sodium in their diets as well as people with normal blood pressure. When people with high blood pressure followed their doctor's orders and curtailed sodium intake, their blood pressure dropped. In studies of large populations around the world, similar results have been found: Eskimos who have a virtually saltless diet seldom are found to be hypertensive, whereas a very high incidence of hypertension has been found among Oriental populations who use sodium products freely in their diets.

Surveys of hypertensive persons who smoke cigarettes and those who do not smoke show a higher risk of premature death among people with high blood pressure who continue to smoke.

Compliance with the advice of doctors is a factor in controlling hypertension, as is true of most other disorders. Only about one-third of cigarette-smoking hypertensive patients who are told by their doctors to quit smoking actually do so. About half of all hypertensive patients follow the doctors' orders to curtail the use of sodium products in their diets. A greater propor-

tion of high blood pressure patients try to control their body weight, but many overweight hypertensive people refuse to accept the possibility that they might be at least a bit on the obese side of the scale for their height and build; in fact, about one-half of those surveyed in one study considered their weight to be "about right." Hypertensive patients who fail to accept medical advice probably will be victims of strokes and other types of organ damage in future years.

Rest, relaxation, and endurance types of physical exercise are among the other nondrug methods of treating high blood pressure. In many cases of noncritical hypertension, the nondrug methods of therapy are sufficient to control high blood pressure. When the nondrug approaches fail to reduce blood pressure significantly, there are several forms of medication that can be effective.

Diuretics and Drug Therapy One is the use of diuretics, which is often a first step in drug therapy for hypertension. The purpose of using diuretics is to decrease blood volume and the work load of the heart. The drugs used for this purpose reduce the water content of tissues by restricting the ability of the kidneys to retain salt; as more sodium is excreted, water is lost under normal conditions. Blood volume and heart output eventually return to pretreatment levels, but the drugs continue to interfere with retention of sodium by the kidneys.

Another type of antihypertension drug, called an adrenergic blocker, has several effects, including decreased cardiac output and reduction of sympathetic nerve impulses that cause arterioles to constrict. A third group of antihypertension drugs, called vasodilators, have the opposite effect of norepinephrine in that they relax the arterioles and thereby increase the flow of blood at a lower pressure.

Nearly all antihypertension drugs have adverse side effects for some individuals that cause a varying percentage of patients to drop out of blood pressure control programs. The adverse effects often include a dry mouth, an urge to get out of bed at night to urinate, and sexual dysfunctions ranging from impotence to the growth of mammary glands in males. Headaches, diarrhea, and nasal congestion are among other complaints. Several drugs administered for hypertension interfere with medications that may be needed by a patient. One type of adrenergic blocker can cause a diabetic coma in patients using insulin, or it can produce heart failure in certain heart disease patients. Another type of adrenergic blocker may produce adverse effects if the patient using the drug consumes an alcoholic beverage.

In summary, a patient often must choose between two possible evils: the effects of high blood pressure or the effects of medicines used to control hypertension. However, doctors usually take a conservative route and use the smallest dose of a drug least likely to produce adverse effects for starters. If a mild diuretic will bring the patient's blood pressure down to a persistently normal level with a minimum of side effects, there is no need to try anything stronger.

Treating Stroke Patients

When a stroke occurs despite efforts to prevent one, the doctor usually tries to obtain as much information as possible about signs and symptoms, and events that might have preceded the problem. If the patient becomes unconscious or unable to communicate effectively, a spouse or other family member or friend may be called upon to contribute information that will help diagnose the precise problem, so that treatment will be applied to the correct cause. A stroke caused by a cerebral hemorrhage, for example, may follow complaints by the patient of headaches, dizziness, and confusion.

Signs or symptoms that can help the doctor pinpoint the area of tissue affected and the cause, such as a blocked artery rather than a ruptured artery, may include memory loss, changes in personal habits, headaches, changes in vision or the ability to hear distinctly, hallucinations, feelings of weakness or loss of sensation in a particular part of the body, or loss of coordination or equilibrium. A brain hemorrhage associated with hypertension may be accompanied by fever, slow heartbeat, and fluctuations in levels of consciousness.

If the patient is able to communicate, even though he might have lost the ability to speak because of a stroke, the doctor can obtain additional clues. The doctor may ask the patient to perform certain simple tasks, such as lifting the right arm in the air, reading a newspaper item, or identifying objects in a magazine illustration. His responses can help locate the site of damage to brain tissue since a good number of brain areas have been "mapped" with respect to the function of sensory and motor nerve cells located in them. For example, if the stroke patient has developed a stutter that did not exist before, doctors will have a pretty good idea of where the brain tissue has been damaged and may even be able to locate the branch of the artery in the brain that was involved.

Visual tests may be given to determine whether there has been any significant change in the acuity of either eye within a short period of time. In other words, a person with 20/20 or 20/30 vision who suddenly experiences a great change from that range of vision may have suffered a lesion in a portion of the brain affecting that visual factor. He also could suffer a loss of visual fields, which would affect peripheral vision; that is, he may fail to blink when a threatening gesture is made from a direction other than straight ahead. Or one pupil may be larger than the other, regardless of exposure to varying intensities of light.

Swallowing ability, control of the tongue in normal movements of eating, tendon reflexes such as the Babinski reflex, and reactions to touching the skin or cornea of the eye may be part of the list of neurological tests that would be performed in diagnosing the effects of a stroke. Electroencephalography (EEG), lumbar puncture, and laboratory tests of spinal fluid, brain scanning, and computerized axial tomography (CAT), as well as X-rays of the skull with radiopaque dye injected into the arteries of the brain, may be used if needed for further studies of stroke effects.

All stroke patients do not receive all of the possible diagnostic tests that are available. The use of X-rays and radiopaque dyes, a technique called angiography, may be recommended in a case in which a patient may have some symptoms or signs of a stroke, but further evidence is needed to verify the diagnosis, or in a case of stroke in which the patient has taken a turn for the worse after apparent improvement. Use of the dye enables the doctor to visualize on the X-ray film the condition of various arteries in the brain.

Stroke patients usually are placed in an intensive care unit (ICU) of a hospital for at least the first few days. Some hospitals have special groups, called Stroke Teams, that are trained to handle stroke cases. A hospital also may have a neurological unit that is specially equipped to care for stroke patients.

Until the condition of the patient has been stabilized and a final diagnosis has been made, a stroke victim may receive nutrients through feedings of intravenous (IV) fluids dripping from a bottle or bag through a tube into a vein. Some patients may be fed by a tube inserted through the nose into the esophagus. The calories and nutrients fed a stroke patient during the first few days are carefully controlled, and so is the amount of fluid permitted. Catheters or other devices for urine collection usually are needed both to keep the bed dry and to enable the hospital staff to measure the fluid output and analyze the urine in the laboratory at regular intervals.

Medications generally are administered to prevent restlessness, to control blood pressure, and to relieve headaches and fever. Because some medications can produce a rapid drop in blood pressure, there may be a risk of hypotension, or inadequate blood pressure. To prevent such an occurrence, the stroke patient may be placed in a postural position like that used in first aid treatment for shock—that is, with the head lower than the feet while blood pressure is being stabilized at a normal level. Although high blood pressure can be life threatening, blood pressure that drops too rapidly or reaches an abnormally low level can deprive the brain of essential nutrients and oxygen. The doctor and his assistants therefore try to achieve a delicate balance of blood pressure that will supply an adequate amount of fresh blood to the brain tissues, but not enough pressure to exacerbate the bleeding problem.

Hematoma of the Brain

Blood accumulated in the brain from a ruptured artery forms a large hematoma, which is similar to the "blood blister" on a finger that has been smashed accidentally with a hammer. A hematoma can be located in the brain with the help of angiography or CAT scanning, which produces a series of X-ray type images that resemble slices of a body area. By studying the angiograms or CAT pictures, and the signs and symptoms of the stabilized stroke victim, doctors may decide whether or not it would be worthwhile to operate in order to remove the hematoma. The size and location of the hematoma, plus the age and condition of the patient, are among the factors considered.

If a hematoma is small and not a life-threatening problem, the doctors probably will decide not to attempt removal. A large hematoma in the frontal lobe of the brain or a hematoma in the cerebellum might be considered worth removing to save the life or improve the condition of the patient. Certain other types of hematomas, such as those involving vital brain-stem tissues, could present great risk to the patient by efforts to remove them.

The surgical technique in treating a hematoma of the brain may vary according to whether an aneurysm is involved. Strokes that result from a brain hemorrhage often can be traced to aneurysms, which are areas of arteries in which the walls have become weakened so that blood leaks between layers of the vessel wall or

the walls become dilated and thin, like an expanded rubber balloon If an aneurysm is found, surgeons may repair it while draining the hematoma. In other cases the hematoma will simply be drained so it will no longer cause unnecessary pressure on neighboring brain tissue.

Rehabilitation of Stroke Victims

After hospitalization and nursing care have helped a stroke patient to survive the CVA, efforts are started to rehabilitate the individual. The rehabilitation process may require a wide array of medical specialists, including occupational and physical therapists, psychologists, speech therapists, and social workers and counselors. The patient may have to spend time in a nursing home or rehabilitation center, or both. The patient's home environment often must be altered to accommodate the recovered patient, who may be permanently disabled in one or more functions.

Persons who work with stroke patients during the rehabilitation process may have some difficulty in communicating with the victim, especially if he has suffered some loss of normal language usage. The patient may not be able to follow complex ideas and should be presented with single concept messages. The language used in speaking to a stroke patient should be precise, and the voice should be slow and quiet. It is not necessary to use baby talk, and in most cases there is no need to shout at a stroke patient simply because he appears to be slow at grasping the meaning of words.

Stroke patients who have suffered some paralysis may have to wear braces and/or supporting devices. But some exercise in-

GETTING UP FROM CHAIR

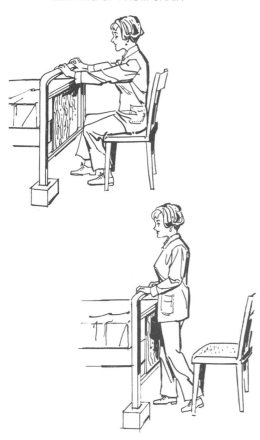

A victim of a stroke often has to gradually relearn such simple tasks as rising from a sitting to a standing position because of interruption of motor nerve functions resulting in various degrees of paralysis. Placing a chair near a headboard or footboard of a bed allows the patient to practice changing his or her body posture positions.

volving all the limbs, including those not affected by the stroke, should be performed daily. The arms and legs should be moved through their full range of motion several times to prevent muscle atrophy or loss of function. Because the patient is

likely to spend a considerable amount of time in bed, it is important that strength and mobility be maintained in all usable muscles.

Even while the patient may be bedfast, efforts should be made to train him to turn from side to side and raise himself to a sitting position without help, although assistance may be required at first. The bed should have a firm mattress with a bed board under the mattress. In some cases a short mattress may be more comfortable if it permits the heels to be free of pressure. A footboard usually is necessary to help prevent tightening of the heel cords. Pillows or rolled towels can be placed under the knees.

As the patient's recovery progresses, he should learn to sit on the edge of the bed and maintain his balance. Then he should learn how to move his body from the bed to a chair or wheelchair, and vice versa, in-

GRAB CHAIR FOR SUPPORT

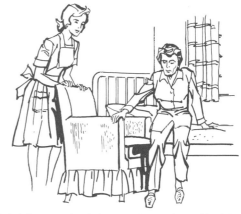

In helping a stroke victim to get into and out of bed during the rehabilitation process, it can be helpful to have a large solid chair next to the bed to provide support for the patient's body.

and to stand and pivot on a leg if the leg was not affected by the stroke. The stroke patient may have to relearn to bathe himself, feed himself, brush his teeth, and so on.

MOVING FROM WHEELCHAIR TO EDGE OF TUB

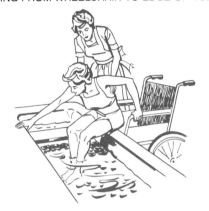

During rehabilitation a stroke victim can learn to take tub baths with the help of a wheelchair and a bench in the tub. In moving from the wheelchair to the bench in the bathtub, and back, the patient should be accompanied by a person who can give assistance as needed to prevent accidents.

The physical therapist may participate in the rehabilitation program by determining the range of motion or limitations of the patient's bones and muscles. With information collected while evaluating the patient's abilities, the physical therapist will advise the patient and his family regarding exercises and activities that will help to restore the strength and functioning of the victim's bones and muscles.

The role of the occupational therapist supplements that of the physical therapist by helping the victim to adapt to normal life routines with whatever abilities have not been lost. The occupational therapist

may train a stroke victim to perform tasks with one hand if the other side has become paralyzed, to use special devices and equipment designed to help handicapped individuals in self-care, and to counsel the patient's family about the special self-care techniques. This part of the rehabilitation program also may include training of the patient to follow simple instructions, since many stroke victims experience some loss of ability to concentrate or to maintain a long attention span.

Strokes in Young Children

Although most information about strokes and their effects relates to older adults with fragile blood vessels, doctors have recently become aware that children also can be the victims of strokes. In fact, it is possible for a newborn baby to have a stroke. However, strokes that afflict children are most likely to be of the type that results from obstruction of an artery in the brain, rather than from a ruptured aneurysm associated with high blood pressure.

There is a great range of signs and symptoms of strokes in infants and children. Some doctors believe that some children who were classified in the past as victims of brain damage or cerebral palsy actually were young stroke patients. Aphasia, marked by a difficulty in identifying objects properly, has been found in some cases to be the result of a stroke affecting the brain center associated with speech.

Young victims of strokes may experience the same kind of effects observed in older patients, such as headaches, fever, altered states of consciousness, and/or a feeling of weakness. Hemiplegia, the type of paralysis that affects the side of the body opposite that of the affected brain area, or hemiparesis, a slight or mild form of paralysis of one side, may occur in children as signs of a stroke. Also, as in older patients, some children may experience transient stroke effects and recover completely within a short period of time. Children below school age who develop stroke aphasia are more likely to overcome the speech problem than older children.

Medications, surgical options, and rehabilitation programs also can help children to recover from strokes.

GLOSSARY

STROKES AND HIGH BLOOD PRESSURE

Following are terms often used by doctors and other medical personnel when discussing the diagnosis and treatment of patients suffering from stroke or high blood pressure. Words in italics refer to separate entries in the list that provide further information on the subject.

airway The breathing passages that extend all the way from the nostrils to the alveoli, or tiny air sacs, at the end of the bronchioles in the lungs. One of the most important first aid measures in assisting a stroke victim is to keep the airways open. Any flexion of the head or neck by a stroke victim who tends to lose consciousness can restrict the airway, and reduce or obstruct the flow of oxygen into the lungs and of carbon dioxide from the lungs.

akinetic mutism A condition that may occur when a stroke victim loses the ability to speak but can demonstrate awareness with eye movements. Some patients suffering this form of mutism may be able to communicate by whispering simple words.

amaurosis fugax A medical term meaning temporary blindness in one eye. This effect can occur as a result of a transient circulatory problem, or mild stroke, that interferes with the normal flow of blood in an artery supplying the eye.

ambu bag A piece of equipment carried by ambulance crews to provide resuscitation to victims of strokes and similar disorders. It delivers a standard amount of respiratory gases to the lungs of the patient at a normal breathing pace, functioning somewhat as a mechanical version of mouth-to-mouth resuscitation.

ambulation The ability of a patient to move about with or without the aid of crutches, walkers, or other devices.

aneurysm A defect in the walls of a blood vessel. Blood may leak through layers of the artery walls or a weakened wall may balloon outward and eventually rupture to cause a brain hemorrhage.

anger An emotional effect of a stroke may be aggressive feelings by the victim who feels frustrated in his efforts to resume normal physical functioning while recovering gradually. Anger and anxiety are not unusual expressions of a stroke victim's reactions to disability and to being dependent upon others.

angiography A diagnostic technique employed by doctors in tracing the flow of blood through arteries in the brain.

anticoagulant A type of medication that interferes with normal blood coagulation processes. It may be used in treating certain kinds of strokes involving an obstructed artery. However, anticoagulants are not recommended for many patients who tend to bleed easily or who are hypertensive and might experience a cerebral hemorrhage.

antihypertensive therapy The use of medications and other techniques usually known to be effective in reducing the blood pressure of a patient suffering from *hypertension*.

aorta The major artery feeding blood from the left ventricle of the heart into smaller arteries that distribute the blood to tissues throughout the body.

aphasia A loss of the ability to communicate effectively with language. A stroke victim may suffer varying degrees of inability to speak in a manner that is easily understood. An aphasia victim might recognize common objects, for example, but be unable to identify the objects by their common names.

atherosclerosis A degenerative disorder of the arteries which may become narrowed and lose their resilience so that normal blood flow is restricted and/or obstructed. Atherosclerosis is commonly associated with aging and may affect several body areas at about the same time. The condition accounts for the high incidence of strokes among heart disease patients.

auscultation A technique used by doctors to check for evidence of blood vessel disorders. The doctor listens with a stethoscope for a *bruit*, or murmur, in arteries of the head and neck areas.

bilateral Affecting both sides of the body. A stroke involving both cerebral hemispheres of the brain could result in paralysis or other disabilities on both sides of the body.

bladder care Stroke patients often need special help in maintaining bladder emptying or control. If nerve cells involved in bladder control are affected by a stroke, the patient may become incontinent. If the patient is unconscious, a catheter is usually inserted into the bladder to insure emptying and to provide a means of measuring daily urine output.

body image Stroke patients often develop a distorted perspective of their bodies and physical abilities. A patient may have difficulty, for example, in realizing that his legs will no longer support his body and may fall to the floor while attempting to walk across the room.

bowel care Like *bladder care*, bowel care is often needed by stroke patients, especially during the early stages of recovery, to maintain normal functioning of the bowels. Special diets and medications may be given to prevent constipation and fecal impaction.

brain scan A technique for producing an indirect picture of the blood vessels in the brain by injecting a radioactive substance into an artery. The radioactive material does not enter the brain tissue but remains in the blood vessels to produce an X-ray-like image of normal and abnormal arteries.

bruit An abnormal sound produced by blood flowing through an artery that is restricted or obstructed. The artery distortion can produce eddy currents similar to those caused by obstacles in a stream bed. Instead of flowing quietly, as in a normal artery, the bloodstream is distorted and produces sounds heard as murmurs.

Burr hole A hole that sometimes is drilled into the skull of a patient who has suffered a cerebral hemorrhage. The pool of blood from the hemorrhage, which has nowhere to go because it is confined by the bones around the brain, may be drained through a hole in the head. The procedure is used only when draining the *hematoma* is likely to improve the health of the patient.

carotid artery One of the main arteries supplying blood to the head. Disorders involving the carotid artery can produce a variety of symptoms, including the effects of stroke, migraine-like headaches, and altered vision. See illustration, page 506.

cerebral hemorrhage Bleeding into brain tissues from a ruptured *aneurysm* or another type of blood vessel defect, usually associated with *hypertension*. Symptoms may range from a temporary mental disturbance to loss of consciousness and vital functions, depending upon the area of the brain affected and the volume of blood lost.

cerebrospinal fluid A fluid that flows in parts of the brain and the central canal of the spinal cord. Cerebrospinal fluid serves as a watery protective cushion for the delicate nerve tissues of the brain and spinal cord.

cerebrovascular A word that means the blood supply of the brain. A cerebrovascular accident is known as a CVA.

cerebrum A term that may be used to refer to the entire brain, although technically it should be applied only to the two cerebral hemispheres occupying the upper part of the skull.

cigarette smoking A factor that has been associated directly and indirectly with stroke by various studies. One major epidemiological survey, the Framingham Study, found that cigarette smoking increased the chance of stroke by 300 percent. Although other studies have not confirmed these results, they have found a link between cigarettes and heart disease that is related to the incidence of strokes.

collateral circulation Blood vessels that duplicate somewhat the distribution of blood to various tissues. If blood flow in one of the vessels becomes obstructed, a neighboring blood vessel provides compensating circulation. Recovery from a stroke often depends upon the establishment of collateral circulation in the brain.

comprehensive stroke center A hospital or extended care facility staffed and equipped for the care and rehabilitation of stroke victims.

computerized axial tomography An X-ray type of device that scans successive sections of a body or organ and produces a series of pictures showing the condition of tissues as they would appear in biopsy or autopsy "slices." The device is also called a CAT scanner.

condom drainage Instead of inserting a catheter into the urinary bladder of a male stroke patient, doctors may attach a condom to the penis to collect urine. In addition to controlling problems of urinary incontinence, urine collected in the condom can be measured to monitor fluid output.

confusion One of the common signs, along with headaches and dizziness, associated with the onset of a stroke. A patient may complain of feelings of confusion before other signs and symptoms of a *cerebral hemorrhage* appear.

contraceptives Oral contraceptives are associated with an increased incidence of cerebral infarction, resulting from a blocked artery in the brain, in young women. Although a direct cause-and-effect link has not been established, a higher proportion of strokes of this type has been found in women using oral contraceptives when compared with other women of the same age who do not use the pill.

decubitus The plural is decubiti and the term simply means bedsores. Because a stroke patient usually spends a great amount of time in bed during the early stages of recovery, he is likely to develop decubiti unless care is taken to prevent this problem.

dementia A mental condition related to arteriosclerotic degeneration of the arteries of the brain. Patients with this condition, which often is associated with a completed stroke, may show lack of judgment and insight, poor memory, and failure to recognize people and places.

diplopia A type of visual disturbance marked by "seeing double," which can be a symptom of a transient or mild stroke.

diuretic A substance, usually administered in the form of a medicine, that reduces the amount of fluid in the body tissues by increasing the patient's flow of urine. Diuretics commonly are prescribed as the first stage of treatment for *hypertension.*

Doppler flowmeter A diagnostic device that uses sound waves to study the flow of blood in an artery. The equipment can be used to measure the direction of flow in a blood vessel and then to estimate the size of blood flow.

drop attack A manifestation of restricted or obstructed blood flow in the brain that is marked by the sudden failure of the legs to support the body's weight. The patient may be unable to stand and may or may not lose consciousness.

dysphagia Difficulty in swallowing, which is a frequent effect of strokes. The condition results in problems of eating as well as difficulty in controlling salivation. Stroke victims may require help in eating without choking on the food.

echoencephalography A diagnostic technique for studying soft tissues inside the skull by use of an ultrasonic device that works in a manner similar to that of sonar. The sound waves aimed at the brain produce silent echoes that are translated into pictures on a cathode-ray tube. Tumors and other structures, normal and abnormal, can be detected in this way.

edema An abnormal accumulation of fluid. Cerebral edema can be dangerous because the fluid has nowhere to drain and its increasing pressure may damage delicate brain tissues.

EEG An abbreviation for electroencephalography, a method of studying brain function by recording "brain waves" in a manner similar to that used in producing electrocardiograms. Nerve cells in the brain tissue generate a variety of different electrical wave patterns which can be recorded with tracing pens and interpreted by experts. One type of EEG pattern, for example, is the alpha wave which is generated when the mind of the patient is in a state of normal relaxation.

embolism The blocking of an artery by a clot or other foreign object, which may be of natural origin. Embolism is one of the causes of a stroke.

facial muscles Lesions in different nerve centers of the brain resulting from strokes can be responsible for changes in facial expressions. Muscles on one side of the face may become weakened, or the upper and lower face areas can become altered in ways that produce a loss of normal symmetry of facial surfaces.

focal signs Stroke effects that involve a specific area or organ of the body. For example, a stroke can result in blurred vision in one eye, a loss of the ability to use the tongue in forming spoken words, or weakness on one side of the body, while the rest of the body is unaffected.

hematoma A collection of blood from an internal injury, which in the case of a stroke could be a *cerebral hemorrhage*. A hematoma outside the skull would appear as a bruise or "blood blister." Inside the skull, the bleeding can damage vital nerve centers and cause death. Small hematomas that are not life-threatening usually are not treated, nor are large hematomas requiring surgery that could

have fatal results. Certain hematomas that can be removed with a fair degree of safety to improve the condition of the patient may be drained or otherwise removed surgically.

hemiparesis Slight or mild paralysis, which may be characterized by weakness and numbness, that affects only one side of the body.

hemiplegia Paralysis that affects one side of the body. Generally, the side paralyzed is on the side of the body opposite the CVA or other type of brain lesion responsible for the disorder.

hemorrhage Another word for bleeding, although the term usually is used to describe loss of blood that may be massive or life-threatening because of a vital area involved, such as a *cerebral hemorrhage*.

hypertension High blood pressure.

hypotension Low blood pressure, or the opposite of *hypertension*. Blood pressure that is lower than average generally is not a cause for concern, but a sudden drop in blood pressure as a result of treating *hypertension* can result in shock.

incontinence An inability to control the bladder or bowels, a not unusual result of some types of strokes.

infarction An area of body tissue that dies because of an interruption of blood flow to the cells. A cerebral infarction will result in a loss of normal function in some other part of the body that normally is controlled by nerve cells in the infarct area.

ischemia An interruption of normal blood flow to a tissue area. The cause may be an obstruction or a constriction in the artery. An ischemia can lead to an *infarction*.

ligation A surgical technique for controlling the flow of blood to an area where a hemorrhage is occurring or may occur. The artery is tied off at a point ahead of the trouble spot, which could be an *aneurysm*.

motor system The nervous system network involved in body functions that require skeletal muscle movements. A stroke can cause motor defects that alter a patient's gait in walking, or his ability to button a sweater, if a motor nerve cell in the brain controlling that function is damaged.

numbness A loss of normal feeling, perhaps accompanied by a mild tingling sensation, that may result from a mild or transient stroke.

nystagmus Eye movements that may be associated with feelings of faintness or dizziness. There are several different patterns of eye movements in nystagmus; a typical one is a rotary movement of the eyeballs around a visual axis or a hypothetical fixed point in front of the eyes.

ocular Referring to the eyes. Abnormal ocular movements, such as those of *nystagmus,* are not uncommon signs of a stroke that can occur before, during, or after the CVA is diagnosed.

oral secretions A polite reference to salivation, or drooling, which a stroke patient may be unable to control and which can cause choking if it is accompanied by *dysphagia.*

physiatrist A medical doctor who specializes in the diagnosis and treatment of physically handicapped patients. The medical specialty sometimes is called physical medicine.

prognosis The doctor's prediction of how a patient is likely to recover, based on the doctor's experience in such matters and the information obtained from diagnosing the patient's condition.

progressive stroke A term sometimes used to describe a stroke case that is still developing or worsening, although it may eventually stabilize.

quadriparesis A mild or transient paralysis or weakness that affects arms and legs on both sides of the body.

resuscitube A plastic tube that can be used for mouth-to-mouth resuscitation without actually touching the lips of the rescuer to those of the victim.

retinal emboli A diagnostic test for persons who have or are likely to develop a CVA frequently reveals tiny emboli in the small arteries of the patients' retinas. Doctors often study the blood vessels on the back inner surface of the eyeballs for signs of circulatory disorders; it is one of a very few places where blood flow can be observed without the use of surgery.

Roentgenogram Another word for X-ray picture.

saccular aneurysm A sac-like swelling in a weakened artery wall.

singultus A mysterious medical term for hiccoughs, another effect along with *dysphagia* and salivation that can result from a stroke that damages brain tissue involved in controlling the oral cavity.

stenosis Another word for restricted or obstructed blood flow in an artery.

subarachnoid An area of the membranes that form a protective covering for the brain. One membrane layer is the arachnoid and another is the pia mater. A subarachnoid hemorrhage is one in which the bleeding occurs between the arachnoid and the pia mater membranes.

subdural The area between the arachnoid and the dura mater, which is the outermost and toughest of the three membranes covering the brain.

thrombosis The occurrence of a blood clot inside a blood vessel. A cerebral thrombosis is a clot that obstructs an artery in the brain, causing an ischemic infarct, or stroke.

TIA An abbreviation for transient ischemic attack, a mild or temporary stroke. The stroke may be mild or temporary because the constriction or obstruction of an artery is not severe enough to cause the death of brain tissue, and/or the area might receive *collateral circulation* resulting in eventual recovery.

vasodepressor A drug that can lower the blood pressure by depressing the control over blood flow exerted by the arterioles, or by reducing the resistance to blood flow offered by the small blood vessels of the body.

vasodilator A drug that causes the blood vessels to dilate and, in effect, lowers blood pressure.

vasopressor A drug or other substance that contracts the muscle layers of blood vessels.

ventilation In medical terminology, this refers to the process of ventilating the lungs or aiding in the exchange of gases between the alveoli, or terminal air sacs of the bronchial tubes, and the air in the environment outside the body.

ventricle A small cavity. The heart has ventricles and the brain has a half-dozen ventricles in various parts of the organ. A cerebral ventricle normally might be filled with *cerebrospinal fluid*, but after a hemorrhage the space may become filled with a *hematoma*.

Venturi mask A type of oxygen mask that administers oxygen at a measured rate of gas per minute. The device may be used to aid the breathing of a stroke victim while he is recovering in the hospital.

vertigo A form of dizziness or light-headedness experienced by some patients with cerebrovascular disorders. *Nystagmus* often is a sign of vertigo.

visual fields The peripheral vision of a patient as measured by an ophthalmologist or other doctor. An occasional effect of a stroke is a reduced field of vision. The patient may have normal or near normal vision for looking straight ahead, but may lose the ability to detect objects or motions on either side of his body. In testing a stroke patient for visual fields, the examining physician might make a threatening gesture at the side of the patient; if the patient should blink, it would be a sign that the visual fields were not impaired. The blink test for visual fields can be administered to a stroke patient who may have lost his ability to speak, as well as to a patient who has not developed *aphasia* as a result of a CVA, or cerebrovascular accident.

QUESTIONS AND ANSWERS
STROKES AND HIGH BLOOD PRESSURE

Q: *I have read in the newspapers that death from hypertension is declining. Is it true and what is the reason?*
A: It is true that death rates from hypertension have been falling over the past decade. The risk has been reduced by more than one-third. There are several reasons, one of which is the development of drugs that control blood pressure for most patients. Other factors include better screening of the population to identify persons with high blood pressure and the changes in lifestyles made by those who are found to be hypertensive.

Q: *What changes in lifestyles change blood pressure levels in people with hypertension?*
A: By lifestyle changes, we mean using less salt in foods, reducing body weight, eliminating cigarette smoking, and doing whatever else may be helpful to improve the general health picture.

Q: *Will exercising prevent the risk of a stroke?*
A: To be honest, we know of no documented evidence showing that lack of exercise contributes to strokes. But there is some indirect circumstantial evidence that exercise may be beneficial, since sedentary people are more likely to develop heart disease and heart disease seems to be associated with an increased chance of stroke. Also, if exercise helps a person lose weight, the blood pressure probably will fall. And anybody willing to exercise vigorously enough to lose weight probably will be motivated to follow other lifestyle changes to reduce the risk of stroke.

Q: *What can an ordinary person do in the way of first aid to help a stroke victim?*
A: The first thing you should do is summon professional medical help: call a physician, a hospital emergency ward, a police or fire department ambulance service, or whatever emergency medical services may be available in your neighborhood. In some areas, a toll-free telephone number is available for advice in such matters, and a local operator may be able to help.

If emergency medical help for some reason is not immediately available, a physician may give instructions by telephone for helping the victim survive until help can arrive. An important factor is to maintain an open airway to the lungs, which means the victim should not be placed on his back or have a pillow under his head, since flexing the neck and head will tend to restrict the upper airway. Mouth-to-mouth resuscitation may be needed if the normal respiration rate drops below eight per minute.

The doctor may advise taking the victim to a hospital emergency ward as quickly as possible. If an ambulance is not available, the patient should be transported in a station wagon, truck, or similar vehicle that has a flat area where the patient can be placed in a proper postural position. The most dangerous way to transport a stroke victim is in the front seat of a two-door passenger car.

Q: *Is it always necessary to move a stroke victim to a hospital emergency ward? What if it is just a "mild" stroke?*
A: If a doctor determines that a stroke is a mild one by examining the patient at home, and if the patient does not appear to be seriously ill, the doctor might agree that hospitalization is not necessary. However, it's generally safer to admit a stroke patient to a hospital for further diagnosis and observation, particularly if the cause appears to be a cerebral hemorrhage. A stroke patient usually is not considered safely recovered from even a mild stroke until the

condition is stabilized, and that may require several days.

Q: *Is primary hypertension the same as essential hypertension?*
A: Both terms are used to identify a case of abnormally high blood pressure for which no specific cause, such as an adrenal gland tumor or kidney disease, can be found.

Q: *What is a sympatholytic drug?*
A: That is a type of drug that helps blood pressure to decrease by dilating or expanding the bore of the blood vessels.

Q: *I have heard that transcendental meditation will control blood pressure. Why isn't TM used for hypertension patients instead of drugs?*
A: Because it doesn't help most patients, according to studies made of experiments using meditation and biofeedback. The techniques can be shown to lower blood pressure under laboratory conditions, but the effects don't seem to carry over into everyday life situations. One reason may be that a hypertensive person would have to spend most of his time meditating in order to make the technique a continuing success.

Q: *How does hypertension contribute to heart disease?*
A: The higher the blood pressure, the harder the heart must work to pump blood through constricted arteries. The heart eventually becomes enlarged from the added work load, and congestive heart failure results.

Q: *Why do blacks suffer more from hypertension than white people?*
A: The reason for this difference isn't known for sure. Statistical studies show that non-whites are more likely to develop hypertension and are more likely to die of hypertensive effects than whites. There may be a genetic reason since the risk of developing hypertension seems to increase with the number of family members who are high blood pressure patients. And studies among twins show that one of a pair of identical twins, who have developed from the same egg cell, is more likely to develop hypertension if the other twin has the disease than if the twins are fraternal, meaning that they developed from two separate ova, or egg cells.

Q: *Will the use of oral contraceptives increase the chances of a woman having a stroke?*
A: There have been published reports indicating that young women using oral contraceptives have a significantly higher incidence of strokes than women of the same age who do not use the drugs. The type of stroke found in these patients is one that results from a blocked artery in the brain rather than a cerebral hemorrhage. The relationship is something of a controversy and mystery, particularly in view of the fact that the brain lesions have been found during autopsies and the victims showed no previous symptoms of stroke effects.

Q: *What do bruits have to do with hypertension and strokes?*
A: Bruits are abnormal sounds produced by blood flowing through an artery. The sound is usually that of a soft murmur caused by a constriction or other defect in a blood vessel, and is an important clue in diagnosing a potential stroke case. Blood flow in normal arteries is silent by comparison.

19

ARTHRITIS
THE GREAT HANDICAPPER

Heart disease ranks as the greatest threat to chances for a North American to live out his normal lifespan. It also is the leading cause of restricted activity for persons afflicted with most of the various forms of heart disease. A recent survey by the U.S. National Center for Health Statistics found that approximately 15 percent of the American population is unable to lead normal lives because of physical handicaps that limit their abilities to work or participate in other activities that most people take for granted. The most common reason given for limited activity was heart disease. But running a very close second was arthritis and rheumatism.

A close examination of the data shows that heart disease holds a slight edge as the overall handicapper only because of the fact that men seem to be heart-disease prone. When the figures for the male population are taken out of the picture, the data shows that arthritis and rheumatism actually account for a greater proportion of disability than heart disease for all age groups of the female sex.

Osteoarthritis, also known as degener-ative joint disease, is such a common affliction that many doctors assume that everyone will develop the disorder if they live long enough. The doctors have some good evidence that a good many patients will eventually have symptoms of degenerative joint disease because signs of the disorder appear on X-rays of 20 percent of all Americans. The X-ray evidence usually precedes the start of symptoms.

As with many other health problems, the incidence of degenerative joint disease increases with age; by the age of 70 the odds are about eight to one that any North American will begin to feel the effects of this form of arthritis.

Degenerative joint disease is only one of about 100 different kinds of arthritis and rheumatism. The medical definition of arthritis limits the condition to diseases involving an inflammation of the joints. Rheumatism has a broader application and may be applied to any disorder of the muscles, tendons, connective tissues, and bursae, as well as the joints. However, the terms often are used interchangeably by the public.

The American Rheumatic Association

and the American Arthritis Foundation have classified the various kinds of arthritis under 13 main categories, with a dozen or more disorders in some of the categories. A category of infectious agents associated as causes of arthritis and rheumatism includes ten species of bacteria, in addition to parasites, fungi, viruses, and rickettsial agents that may be disease factors. The list actually could be virtually endless if such factors as an occupational hazard of piano playing, carpal tunnel syndrome, were added.

The two main types are osteoarthritis, or degenerative joint disease, and rheumatoid arthritis, which is one of the most disabling of all diseases.

Osteoarthritis

Osteoarthritis is characterized by the degeneration or wearing away of the cartilage cushions between the bones of a joint. Particularly affected are the weight-bearing joints of the body, such as the hip and knee joints. Normally, the cartilage helps dissipate the force of the person's body weight by serving as a kind of modified water bed. The cartilage contains water molecules that are dispersed when pressure is placed on the surface of the cartilage, and when the compression effect of the weight is released, the water molecules return to their normal position. As one grows older this function declines, and the chemical composition of the cartilage changes so that it contains more fibrous material of the kind that occurs in tendons and less of the watery cushion type. At about the same time, the ends of the bones begin to hypertrophy, developing deposits called bone spurs.

A similar phenomenon occurs in the spinal column where the cartilage cushions

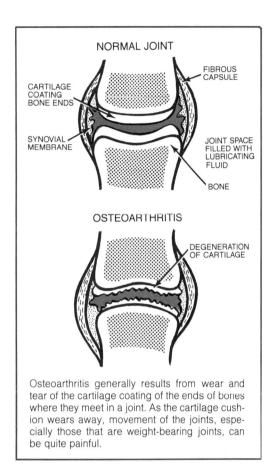

Osteoarthritis generally results from wear and tear of the cartilage coating of the ends of bones where they meet in a joint. As the cartilage cushion wears away, movement of the joints, especially those that are weight-bearing joints, can be quite painful.

separating the vertebrae gradually lose their fluid-cushioning capacity and undergo chemical changes as a person grows older. The effect of osteoarthritis in the spinal column is an increasing problem of backaches.

The exact cause of the changes is not clear. Some medical scientists believe that at least part of the cause is tiny fractures of the cells at the ends of the bones. Cartilage itself lacks nerves and blood vessels, so it must depend upon fluid that is released from circulation in the bone where the bone and cartilage meet. The tiny fractures result in the formation of a kind of scar tissue that prevents the nutrient fluids from reaching the cartilage, which as a result gradually degenerates. This explanation often is expressed in a more direct and simple manner as a "wear-and-tear" effect.

Evidence that tiny fractures of the bone tissues may account for the development of osteoarthritis is found in patients who develop osteoarthritis in joints other than those involved in bearing the body's weight. Construction workers tend to develop osteoarthritis in their elbows and shoulders when the job requires repeated pressure on the joints of the arm. On the other hand, medical investigators have found that patients who are unable to use a particular joint because of a disability do not develop the disease in the disabled body area.

Osteoarthritis that develops with no particular cause is called primary degenerative joint disease. When the signs and symptoms are associated with a specific injury or abnormality, the condition is classified as secondary degenerative joint disease; the disorder is secondary to the cause. The symptoms and treatments for both primary and secondary forms of osteoarthritis are essentially the same.

The symptoms of primary osteoarthritis usually begin later in life than those caused by injury or an abnormality, beginning after the age of 50 for most people and becoming quite common by the age of 65. The first symptom is an aching pain that is confined mainly to the affected joint and usually occurs when the joint is moved or when weight is placed on it. There usually is a period of stiffness after resting; the stiffness occurs when the victim arises after a period of sleep or after sitting for a while. The stiffness generally lasts only a few minutes. There may be joint tenderness, bony enlargement of the joint, and a restricted range of motion.

Osteoarthritis of the hips and knees can become gradually disabling unless medical care is administered in the early stages. The symptoms in the early stages tend to diminish after a brief period of exercise after resting. But exercise in the advanced stages of the disease tends to aggravate the condition, and the pain eventually may become continuous, except when controlled by medications. When the hip is involved, the disorder can be seriously disabling and affect other body systems as the loss of joint function and limitation of physical activity increase.

Sports injuries often precede an early onset of osteoarthritis. Damage to a meniscus, or cartilage within a joint, or to a ligament of the knee can alter the stability of the joint and cause osteoarthritis. The popularity of outdoor exercises, such as jogging and tennis, can be expected to result in an increase of degenerative joint disease in future years, particularly among individuals who engage in strenuous sports without adequate preparation. It could be ironic, as some doctors have observed, if people who extend their lives by improving their cardiovascular systems through outdoor exercise find that they also have gained more time to experience the symptoms of degenerative joint disease.

While osteoarthritis was once thought to be just a part of the normal aging process, we now know that aging itself is not responsible for the disease. The extra years merely give the osteoarthritis more time to develop. Improved diagnostic techniques and better knowledge of the disease process have revealed evidence that degenerative joint disease has started in young persons, even though the more obvious signs and symptoms will not surface for some years yet.

Other studies, reaching back into history, show that osteoarthritis probably is as old as the earliest animals with skeletons. Dinosaur bones display evidence of osteoarthritis, which some scientists suggest could have contributed to the extinction of the species. Today, some animals, ranging from pet dogs to racehorses, suffer from the disease. Neanderthal man was a victim of the disease, and so was the ancient Egyptian pharaoh Ramses II, who was so crippled by the ailment that he was unable to walk.

The ordinary patient today, of course, will receive better medical care for osteoarthritis than the richest and most powerful rulers of ancient days. Some of the remedies are new and some are not so new. They include hot packs, ultrasound therapy, and infrared heat, plus drugs such as aspirin that relieve pain and inflammation, and orthopedic treatments to relieve pressure on nerve roots. Isometric and other exercises designed to strengthen individual muscles are recommended, while vigorous exercises that could aggravate a diseased joint are restricted. Weight-reduction programs are prescribed when body weight may be a contributing factor. When necessary, artificial joints made of plastic or metal can be installed surgically to replace the natural joints that have been damaged by the disease.

Some patients of osteoarthritis, mainly women, develop bony knobs on the end and middle joints of the fingers. The knobs, called Heberden's nodes, may develop rather suddenly, with or without pain, and may affect the thumb as well as the other fingers. The nodes may begin as soft, tender swellings at the finger joints and gradually change into hard, painless knobs. Heberden's nodes usually do not affect the use of the fingers. It is believed that this form of degenerative joint disease is hereditary or familial, since patients often have mothers or sisters with the same condition.

Rheumatoid Arthritis

Women also are more likely to develop the second of the main types of arthritis, rheumatoid arthritis. This is a systemic disease; that is, it involves the entire body even though the most obvious signs and symptoms may appear in the joints. While rheumatoid arthritis can occur at any age from infancy to the Social Security years, the majority of cases begin between the ages of 20 and 40, the most productive years for many individuals.

Young women are about three times as likely to develop rheumatoid arthritis as young men, but the difference declines in later life. Only a small percentage of the total population is affected by rheumatoid arthritis, but the figure is somewhat deceptive because in America alone that proportion can amount to more than six million patients.

Why some people develop the disease and others do not remains something of a mystery. Those who become victims of rheumatoid arthritis have a substance in their blood called rheumatoid factors, although there is no evidence that the rheumatoid factors lead to development of the disease. Another factor seemingly unique to rheumatoid arthritis patients is the presence of a substance in the synovial membranes of their joints.

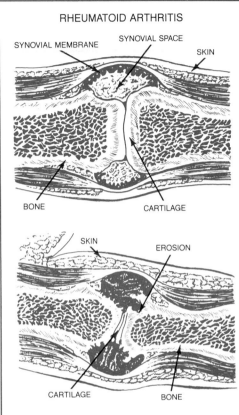

RHEUMATOID ARTHRITIS

SYNOVIAL MEMBRANE

SYNOVIAL SPACE

SKIN

BONE

CARTILAGE

SKIN

EROSION

CARTILAGE

BONE

Rheumatoid arthritis usually begins with inflammation of the synovial membrane around a joint. As the disease progresses, there is erosion of the cartilage edges of the bones, and eventually the patient may not be able to move the joint.

The synovial membrane is a lining of the joint cavity. When the disease begins, the synovium develops numerous folds and spreads over the cartilage cushion in the joint. The cartilage and adjoining bone surfaces degenerate, and the ends of the opposing bones of the joint may fuse. Ligaments, muscles, and other tissues surrounding the joint can become involved in the disease process and degenerate or atrophy. Knobs of tissue, some of it debris

from destruction of the joint, may form as rheumatoid nodules. Much of the treatment effort is directed toward controlling the deformity that develops in the joint.

Rheumatoid arthritis often begins with symptoms that are misleading to the patient, who may delay seeking professional medical help in the early stages. The symptoms can include a general feeling of fatigue and weakness, with some slight stiffness that continues for several weeks before the more serious effects appear. Then there can be swelling of one or more joints, usually in the hands and/or feet. Raynaud's phenomenon, a circulatory disorder in the extremities that causes numbness or coldness in the fingers or toes, may accompany the onset of swellings.

Because rheumatoid arthritis has the signs and symptoms of other possible diseases, such as systemic lupus erythematosus, doctors depend upon a certain combination of effects in making a firm diagnosis of rheumatoid arthritis. They include morning stiffness which usually lasts much longer than the morning stiffness of osteoarthritis, pain on motion or tenderness in at least one joint, swelling in one or more joints that is not merely a bony overgrowth like a Heberden's node, X-ray evidence of changes typical of rheumatoid arthritis, and laboratory test results showing certain data such as the presence of the rheumatoid factor.

The prognosis for recovery from rheumatoid arthritis varies as much from patient to patient as the signs and symptoms of the disease. Only about 10 percent of afflicted persons become seriously crippled or disabled. Others experience virtually no effects serious enough to warrant more than minimum medical treatment. Approximately three-fourths of all patients show improvement during the first year of treatment, and many are able to function somewhat normally at work or at home. However, most victims of rheumatoid arthritis can expect some degree of progressive joint damage and will require medical care for the rest of their lives, even though the medical care need only be supervisory and conservative.

Complete bed rest is required during the early stages of the disease. Anti-inflammatory drugs usually are prescribed. Splints or braces are employed to provide some rest and support for affected limbs. Rest may include immobilization of a joint through splinting and may be required to reduce inflammation. But some mild exercises are permitted to prevent loss of joint function where it might otherwise be threatened. Rest for the patient, in general, may be planned to include a longer than usual nighttime period of perhaps nine hours, plus a daytime nap or rest period of a couple of hours.

Drug therapy often begins with salicylates, which means aspirin in some form. The aspirin or aspirin-like drug used by a patient with rheumatoid arthritis may not be taken in the typical do-it-yourself manner, but is taken according to a doctor's written orders. Daily dosage may range from about 10 to 30 tablets, depending upon the effects the medicine has on an individual patient. The aspirin may be prescribed to be consumed at mealtime, and the meals are divided so that the patient has four somewhat smaller than usual meals each day, rather than three regular meals.

No particular diet is prescribed for rheumatoid arthritis patients, except that some advice may be offered regarding foods that might interact with the medication. Some patients may be sensitive to the gastrointestinal effects of aspirin or to other anti-inflammatory analgesic drugs which can contribute to peptic ulcers or stomach upsets. Overdoses of aspirin may have other effects on individual patients, such as a ringing in the ears or partial deafness.

During the period of active joint inflammation, the patient may be administered injections of gold salts. The gold salts help control the progress of the disease in early stages, but they usually are not beneficial in cases where joint destruction already has occurred. Gold salts can have adverse effects on some individuals who may require special blood and urine tests to determine their sensitivity to the therapy. After the treatments have started, these patients usually are examined at least once a week for signs of adverse effects, which often begin with skin disorders including itching and a rash. When such signs appear, the therapy usually is discontinued.

Other medications that may be used in addition to or instead of aspirin include penicillamine, indomethacin, phenylbutazone, corticosteroids, and hydroxychloroquine. One of the drugs was designed originally to treat disorders of copper metabolism, and another was developed for the care of patients with malaria. Certain immuno-suppressive drugs also may be tried. Because every patient with rheumatoid arthritis does not respond in the same manner to each available medication, a doctor may try several previously tested remedies before finding one, or a combination of drugs, that offers remission from the disease or relief from the symptoms.

Rheumatoid arthritis and osteoarthritis are generally nonfatal diseases in themselves, although under certain circumstances they might contribute to a shortened lifespan by hampering normal bodily activities. At the same time, the diseases are not truly curable. Thus, a doctor's choice of remedies often is directed toward finding drugs potent enough to control the symptoms but not so powerful that they might be more dangerous than the disease. Immuno-suppressive drugs, for example, have been used experimentally as a substitute for corticosteroids, but long-term use of the substances carries a risk of causing cancer.

Beyond rest and medications, treatment for rheumatoid arthritis patients includes exercises designed to prevent atrophy of muscle tissue and to preserve range of motion without increasing inflammation of the affected limbs. Other therapies are surgery to preserve joint function or to replace joints that have been destroyed, physical therapy, and patient training in the use of orthopedic and self-help devices to increase the range of normal activity that is possible. Braces, crutches, special shoes, and equipment that can assist crippled hands to function at work or home are some of the orthopedic and self-help devices that may be available.

The recovered patient also can benefit from such simple items as clothing that can be put on or taken off with a minimum need for normal finger manipulation, chairs and even toilet seats that are adjusted to a comfortable height for the patient who may have difficulty in lowering or raising his body, and cabinet or counter surfaces that are easily accessible in the kitchen or working area for a person who may be confined to a wheelchair or who is no longer able to work in a standing position.

Juvenile rheumatoid arthritis can afflict children of any age, but it most often begins when the youngster is about two or three years old. Girls are affected more often than boys. The disease usually has more symptoms that involve the entire body than the adult form of rheumatoid arthritis. About a quarter of a million children suffer from the disease in America alone.

The juvenile rheumatoid arthritis patient may have a high fever that peaks late each day for several weeks before the onset of the arthritis symptoms. The fever often is accompanied by a rash. Heart and lung involvement may occur with signs and symptoms of pneumonia, pleurisy, pericarditis, or myocarditis.

The body joint affected by juvenile rheumatoid arthritis usually is a large joint such as the ankle or knee. Although the joint inflammation of the juvenile version of the disease is the same as that of adult rheumatoid arthritis, nodules are less likely to occur at the affected joints. In relatively mild cases, the child—and the parents—may not recognize the seriousness of the condition. The child may seem to favor one leg or appear to be lame as a result of effects of the joint inflammation.

In addition to inflammation involving joints of the limbs, juvenile rheumatoid arthritis may affect the spinal column and/or the temporo-mandibular joint of the jaw. Complications can involve tendons, such as the Achilles tendon, and the eyes. Careful eye examinations are recommended for all juvenile rheumatoid arthritis patients during and after the active phase of the disease because of the possibility of eye damage.

Treatment for juvenile rheumatoid arthritis is about the same as for adult cases: aspirin and gold salt medications for most patients, rest and splints balanced with passive and active exercises, physical therapy, and surgery when necessary to modify any disabling effect.

Still's disease is another name often used to identify juvenile rheumatoid arthritis, although the term originally referred to only one of several forms of the disease.

Ankylosing Spondylitis

Another arthritic disease that sometimes is associated with the name of a doctor who first described the ailment is Marie-Strumpell disease, or ankylosing spondylitis. Ankylosing means a locking of a joint, usually as a result of damage to tissues that help form the joint. Spondylitis means an inflammation of the vertebrae. Ankylosing spondylitis, therefore, might be translated as a type of arthritis in which the spinal column tissues become inflamed and the joints between the bones become immobilized.

Ankylosing spondylitis affects mainly men below the age of 30. It may be genetic or familial since most of the victims have a certain blood factor present in the tissues of only a small percentage of the general population, and because those afflicted often have male relatives with the disease.

It begins insidiously like other types of arthritis. The patient may notice periods of low back pain which may seem to involve the sciatic nerve area. He also may experience some feeling of a stiff back upon awakening after sleep. But the symptoms gradually and progressively worsen as the aching and stiffness spread up the back to eventually include the neck. In many cases, the disease spreads into the shoulder and hip joints and sometimes involves the knee joints.

Muscle spasms may accompany the spinal ankylosing so that the patient finds it difficult to bend his back forward. In advanced cases, the spinal column may become fused in a forward curve that gives the patient a humpbacked appearance. The change in posture may involve the respiratory and cardiovascular systems.

There is no real cure for ankylosing spondylitis. The patient usually is given analgesics to relieve pain. Exercises designed to improve the posture are recommended. Hot packs may be applied to the muscles in the areas involved. In severe cases, surgery may be required to straighten a deformed spine. If untreated, the disease often runs its course in ten or more years, and a period of remission follows.

Gout

Gout is considered one of the forms of arthritis, although the cause is somewhat different and treatment permits most patients to pursue active and productive lives. The symptoms are caused by crystals of uric acid salts deposited in and around the joints and tendons. The disease is controlled in most cases by drugs and diet.

Like ankylosing spondylitis, most gout patients are men, and most of the small proportion of female gout sufferers are older, postmenopausal women. One reason is that premenopausal women generally have a lower level of uric acid salts in their blood than men; it is the uric acid content of the blood that is the source of the crystals deposited in the joints and tendons. Nearly all gout patients have an excess of uric acid in their system and are called hyperuricemic.

The deposits of uric acid crystals are called tophi—tophus is the singular form of the word. Tophi have been associated with gout for about 1,800 years; they were described by Galen, a physician to the Roman Emperor Marcus Aurelius. But the disease is much older than that; a drug used in treating gout was described in an ancient Egyptian papyrus about 3,500 years ago.

Technically, there are more than a dozen forms of gout. All are associated with various metabolic disorders, and many—if not most—cases are believed to be inherited forms of the disease. Generally, gout involves an abnormal production or accumulation in the body of uric acid. The uric acid is formed by the metabolism of purines, which are substances that occur in certain foods but also are produced by the body's own tissues. A patient could acquire an excess of uric acid, therefore, by eating more purine-rich foods than his body could handle, by producing too much purine from his own tissues, or by being unable to excrete uric acid as fast as it formed from purine metabolism.

Purines are found in meats, fish, and poultry, particularly in very high amounts in animal organ meats, such as liver, kidney, and sweetbreads, as well as in anchovies and sardines.

A typical attack of gout begins without warning, often during the night, with pain in a peripheral joint such as a toe. The pain may become progressively more intense as the skin surrounding the affected joint becomes hot, shiny, and a dark red or purple in coloration. The joint is very tender and may appear to be infected. The patient often has additional symptoms of chills and fever, and an abnormally rapid heartbeat.

The first attack may involve one joint, perhaps the big toe. But subsequent attacks of gout often involve several different joints and can spread to the elbow or knee from the toes or fingers. After an attack, the joint usually returns to its normal condition. The early attacks may last a few days, but later attacks, if the condition is not treated, may persist for weeks. If the gout becomes chronic, the intervals between attacks become shorter and the affected joints begin to lose their function. Tophi deposits may begin to appear in areas other than peripheral joints, affecting the shoulders and spine.

If untreated in the early stages, gout often can lead to complications involving the kidneys. The risk of kidney stones is much higher in gout patients than in the general population. Many gout patients develop other forms of kidney disease such as uremia.

Treatment of gout usually involves the use of drugs designed to control inflammation and to prevent the production of uric acid crystals. The medications also aid in dissolving pre-existing tophi, which melt into body fluids when the level of uric acid saturation is reduced. The available drugs are so effective that most doctors no longer advise patients to restrict their consumption of purine-rich foods. However, the medicines often have to be taken daily to prevent additional attacks. Diets to control the weight of gout patients still remain a part of the therapeutic regimen.

Pseudogout

An arthritic disease with symptoms similar to those of gout is marked by deposits of crystals of a substance sometimes identified as CPPD, for calcium pyrophosphate dihydrate, in the synovial membrane fluid of the joints. The disorder is called pseudogout, or chondrocalcinosis.

Pseudogout affects men and women about equally. Symptoms of pain and discomfort occur in the peripheral joints, with periods of remission between attacks. The patient may have other symptoms that vaguely resemble those of rheumatoid arthritis. One difference is that the crystal deposits usually are a result of joint degeneration, whereas in true gout the crystal deposits are the cause of joint discomfort. Also, the crystals can be observed as different under a microscope during laboratory tests.

Another difference is that colchicine, a traditional drug that has almost dramatic effects in controlling attacks of true gout, has no effect in reducing symptoms of pseudogout. However, there are drugs such as phenylbutazone and corticosteroids that are effective in treating most cases of pseudogout.

Lupus Diseases

Lupus is a group of rheumatoid arthritis diseases that affect mainly women of childbearing age. Lupus diseases are characterized by a disfiguring red rash that appears on the face and other body areas. The patients often are photosensitive, and attacks may follow exposure to strong sunlight.

Cutaneous lupus erythematosus, or chronic discoid lupus erythematosus (DLE), is a chronic and recurring version of the disease that lacks the systemic, or general body symptoms, characteristics of systemic lupus erythematosus (SLE). However, the skin lesions of both forms of the disease are similar.

Discoid LE, so-called because the red skin lesions are disklike, is further divided into two types of the disease depending upon the distribution of the skin lesions. One type of discoid lupus lesions occur only on the face of the patient; the other type of discoid LE may cause the lesions to occur elsewhere on the body, with or without the characteristic red rash on the face. The hair follicles may be involved and alopecia, a form of baldness, can be a result.

The lesions may continue or recur over a period of years, and a small percentage of the patients eventually develop the SLE form of the disease. The systemic LE often begins with a fever that erupts suddenly or develops gradually, accompanied by a general feeling of ill health and suggesting a smoldering infection of some kind. About 90 percent of the patients display symptoms of joint problems that closely resemble those of rheumatoid arthritis. The red skin lesions characteristic of lupus erythematosus appear on the body, including the face. Some lesions may be of the discoid variety, or they may take the form of the red butterfly pattern across the bridge of the nose that has become something of a trademark for SLE.

The disease frequently is complicated by disorders of the lungs, heart, and/or kidneys. Pleurisy is a frequent complaint; pericarditis is not uncommon. Kidney problems occur in a majority of cases. In some patients, complications involve central nervous or gastrointestinal symptoms.

Lupus forms of arthritis, although relatively rare, can be more dangerous than osteoarthritis, rheumatoid arthritis, or gout. The disease seldom occurs in an acute form, but the effects, particularly the complications, can be life-shortening. There are many types of treatment; because of the many variations of the disease and the individual patient's condition and complications, the treatment must be tailored for the specific case. Even the clinical condition of an individual case may change from time to time, making lupus a very unpredictable disorder for a doctor to treat.

In general, however, the outlook for many patients is good after their condition has stabilized. They can lead reasonably normal lives, although they usually must restrict physical activity and need more rest than other people. They also need regular medications and medical examinations to check their progress. They should avoid undue exposure to sunlight.

Other Arthritic Diseases

Another type of arthritis involving the skin is psoriatic arthritis. The patient experiences a rheumatoid-like arthritis along with a psoriasis of the skin and nails. The signs and symptoms of attacks and remissions may coincide. The typical subcutaneous nodules of rheumatoid arthritis are not present, but this form of the disease often progresses to a severe crippling condition.

Acute bacterial arthritis can result when almost any kind of bacteria invades a joint via the bloodstream and produces an inflammatory condition. Patients with joints weakened by rheumatoid arthritis or other disorders are particularly susceptible, but a person of any age can become infected in this manner. If the disease organism is not identified and destroyed immediately by the proper antibiotic, the joint may be permanently damaged.

GLOSSARY

ARTHRITIS

analgesia A loss of pain sensation. Analgesic medications are designed to relieve pain.

ankylosing spondylitis A disease that usually is characterized by inflammation and fusion of the bones of the spinal column. The disorder affects mainly young men. In severe cases it can result in a humpback posture because the spine tends to become locked into a forward flexion position.

arthritis A broad term meaning literally "disease of a joint." In modern medical application, the word generally is used to denote any disorder that involves both inflammation and degeneration of a joint.

arthrosis An alternative term sometimes used to identify a degenerative lesion of a joint. Osteoarthrosis may be used, for example, to denote a degenerative joint disease in which inflammation may be absent.

Baker's cyst A complication of osteoarthritis in which the synovial capsule of the knee joint herniates so that the fluid drains backward and downward.

baseball finger A swelling at the first joint of the finger which may be due to an injury, such as catching a baseball on the fingertip. The term also is applied occasionally to describe the Heberden's nodes that occur on the first joints of fingers of some patients with osteoarthritis.

Bryant's triangle A hypothetical triangle formed by bones at the hip joint. It is used occasionally by doctors to estimate whether the bones are out of alignment as a result of degeneration of the hip joint.

bursa A small fluid-filled sac that is located at joints in the body where friction might occur because of the movement of bones, muscles, and tendons.

bursitis An inflammation of a *bursa*.

carpal tunnel syndrome A painful disorder involving the wrist and finger joints resulting from pressure on a nerve that passes between the carpal bone of the wrist and a band of connective tissue. Repeated shock to the fingers and arms as a result of certain types of work can produce rheumatoid-like symptoms in the joints of the wrist.

cartilage A type of fibrous connective tissue.

causalgia A type of disorder caused by an injury to a nerve trunk of the body and marked by a severe burning pain in the area served by the nerve. A disabling pain involving the leg can be due to causalgia affecting the sciatic nerve, rather than a symptom of arthritis.

Charcot's joints Another term for neurogenic arthropathy; a kind of arthritis in which there is destruction of tissues in the joint but the patient is not aware of the pain that would accompany the damage under normal circumstances. The cause is a nerve disorder that interferes with the transmission of deep pain impulses. The knee, ankle, and elbow are among joints most commonly affected by this disorder.

chondromatosis A congenital disorder in which the *cartilage* at the ends of long bones fails to evolve into bone tissue. This results in an imbalance of an involved joint and, in some cases, a bone that is shorter than normal and is distorted.

cup arthroplasty A surgical technique, most often applied to the hip joint, in which a new ball-and-socket arrangement is fashioned with a smooth metal cup surface installed as a lining for the head of the femur, the long bone of the upper leg. An alternative technique is that of replacement arthroplasty in which a new femur head, usually made of metal, is installed in the upper end of the femur so that it will fit snugly in the hip socket.

degenerative joint disease A term that has generally replaced the word osteoarthritis in identifying the common disorder that is marked by the degenerative loss of cartilage in the joint and by a hardening of bone and cartilage surfaces with new bone growths in the joint that produce pain or discomfort. The disorder may or may not be accompanied by inflammation of the *synovial membrane* lining the joint cavity.

Dupuytren's contracture A disorder that results in a deformity of the fingers or toes because of a shortening and thickening of connective tissue beneath the palm or sole of the hand or foot. The effect often begins as a thickened nodule in the palm below the base of the ring finger, and gradually results in a contracture, or permanently flexed, finger. The deformity resembles an effect of rheumatoid arthritis, but Dupuytren's contracture is not a true form of arthritis.

electromyograph A device that measures muscular contractions; used in some cases to train patients to reduce tension and the related muscular pain.

extra-articular Outside a joint; an extra-articular disorder could be housemaid's knee, a painful inflammation of a *bursa* located between the patella of the knee joint and the skin.

facet joint A joint formed by small plane surfaces of neighboring bones. Facet joints are found in the spinal column's stack of vertebrae.

fascia A type of connective tissue that may appear as envelope-like sheaths to enclose other tissues. Muscles are enclosed in fascia sheaths. The fascia often produces its own lubricating fluid to reduce the friction of one muscle group rubbing against another.

fibromyositis Inflammation of fibromuscular tissue which may involve ligaments, joints, or other limb structures.

fibrositis An inflammation of the muscle sheaths of the limbs, accompanied by pain and stiffness. The term sometimes is used to identify a disorder known as muscular rheumatism.

frozen shoulder A common name occasionally applied to a disorder of the shoulder joint that is characterized by pain and restricted movement of the arm. In some cases the arm is carried in a sling to relieve pain, but the sling is removed for short periods to permit shoulder exercises designed to correct the problem. The condition also may be known by the term *periarthritis*.

gout Also called gouty arthritis; a disease characterized by inflammation of joints, mainly of the peripheral areas of the limbs such as toes and fingers, ankles and wrists. Cause of the inflammation is an accumulation of uric acid crystals in the joints as a result of abnormal uric acid metabolism. Treatment is directed toward relieving the symptoms and reducing the level of uric acid salts in the body fluids.

hemophilic arthritis A rare disorder that is a complication of hemophilia, a disease marked by hemorrhages because of a deficiency of a blood clotting factor. A patient with hemophilic arthritis may accumulate blood in the joint cavities, producing symptoms similar to those of arthritis, with joint degeneration after repeated episodes of blood loss into the joints.

hinge joints Joints that fold and open like a hinge. The flexion of the elbow sometimes is cited as an example of a hinge action.

humeroulnar joint One of the three joints forming the bones that articulate at the elbow.

manipulation A method of restoring function to a limb by carefully moving it through at least a part of the normal range of motion permitted by the joint.

meniscus A crescent-shaped cartilage in the knee joint. Damage to a meniscus, or the menisci, of a knee joint can contribute to early onset of symptoms of *degenerative joint disease*. Causes of damage most frequently are actions that place rotary stress on the knee joint, such as can occur during sports activities that require quick body turns while the body weight is on a single knee joint.

neuropathic arthritis A medical term for *Charcot's joints*.

osteoarthropathy Another medical term for *Charcot's joints*.

osteochondritis A joint disorder that is characterized by a part of the cartilage surface breaking loose from its attachment to a bone and becoming a loose body in the joint. The elbows and knees are the most common sites for this condition. The cause is believed to be an interruption in the blood supply to the joint, resulting in tissue infarction.

osteotomy An operation in which a damaged or diseased bone is cut and usually shaped to correct the deformity, such as a hip joint damaged by arthritis.

paratendinitis Also known as peritendinitis, a term applied to a disorder marked by tenderness and swelling which often is due to tendon friction resulting from repeated movements of a limb such as the arm. The treatment may consist simply of immobilizing the limb and allowing it to heal while resting.

periarthritis A medical term for *frozen shoulder*.

polymyalgia rheumatica A common disorder of persons beyond middle age, mainly women, who experience muscular pain and stiffness, symptoms that mimic arthritis.

pyogenic arthritis Another name for bacterial or septic arthritis, a disorder in which the causative agent is a disease organism that invades a joint.

Quervain's disease A joint disorder of the thumb and wrist, which become tender and swollen because of muscle and tendon friction.

synovial membrane A membrane lining the cavity of a joint. The membrane secretes a fluid, called synovia, which helps lubricate the joint. The synovial membrane often is involved in early stages of joint disease; it is easily inflamed and thickens, so that pain and congestion follow.

tenosynovitis An inflammation of a synovial lining of a tendon sheath. The cause may be an infection or frictional irritation. The symptoms are similar to those of *bursitis*.

trigger point An area of the body which triggers pain or discomfort in another part of the body when the trigger point is subjected to a stimulus such as excessive cold or heat, pressure, or skin puncture. Trigger points often are associated with rheumatic and arthritic disorders.

ulnar neuritis A disorder of the hand involving mainly the little finger side which develops numbness or tingling and loss of coordination of the fingers. It is a complication of osteoarthritis of the arm.

QUESTIONS AND ANSWERS
ARTHRITIS

Q: *Since some kinds of arthritis seem to run in families, is it possible that the diseases can be genetic?*

A: So far about a dozen of the various rheumatic diseases have been found to have "genetic markers," which are detectable in blood tests. The first of the arthritic diseases found to have a genetic marker was ankylosing spondylitis, and that breakthrough touched off a great deal of new research to find genetic clues in the other disorders. The people who develop ankylosing spondylitis generally have the genetic marker for that disease in their blood, but it is not found very often in the general healthy population. Those who appear to be healthy but have the marker in their blood might be at greater risk for developing the disease at some time in the future than those who lack that particular blood factor.

Q: *What decides whether somebody is likely to get, say, rheumatoid arthritis if he or she has the blood substance that is a genetic marker for the disease?*

A: The genetic markers are associated with the cells of the body's immune system, the part of the body that normally is equipped to resist disease of almost any kind, including cancer. The circumstantial evidence suggests that an infection from a virus or a bacterium causes the patient's immune system to fail and release the damage that is associated with the genetic marker for a particular kind of arthritis.

Q: *If you think you have arthritis should you take aspirin?*

A: First, you should make sure you have arthritis. A lot of aches, pains, and swellings that people experience are not arthritis at all. Arthritis is a serious matter that should be diagnosed by a physician; the diagnosis can involve from six weeks to two months or more of ob-

servation of signs and symptoms. In other words, diagnosing arthritis is not a do-it-yourself matter; any delay in accurate diagnosis and treatment can result in permanently disabling complications.

Second, if it is determined that you actually do have some form of arthritis—or another health problem with symptoms similar to those of arthritis—the doctor will recommend a specific treatment program which may include the use of aspirin. But, again, the use of aspirin in the treatment of arthritis is not a do-it-yourself type of therapy. The doctor may spend some time trying different daily doses and kinds of aspirin in order to find the most effective dosage level that does not cause adverse side effects. Some patients cannot tolerate aspirin because of other health conditions, or they may need to take an antacid medication with the aspirin to avoid heartburn or similar discomfort resulting from the required daily dose of aspirin.

Q: *Will acupuncture cure arthritis?*

A: Acupuncture is not recommended for patients with diagnosed arthritis. It may relieve the pain of arthritis temporarily, but there is a lack of scientific evidence that the therapy does anything for the swelling and inflammation that accompany the pain in rheumatoid arthritis.

Q: *Should people with arthritis move to the Sunbelt?*

A: Some patients claim their symptoms improve after moving from a cold, damp region to one that is relatively warm and dry. But there is no evidence that arthritis is caused or treated by climate alone. The change may improve the mental outlook for arthritis patients, which can be somewhat beneficial, but it has no long-term curative effects on the course of most forms of arthritis.

Q: *If you develop arthritis can you still hold a regular job?*
A: The answer to that question depends upon what kind of job the patient can handle and the extent of any disabling effects of the disease. Like the question of climate, a certain amount of limitation on a patient's ability to adapt to the outside world after an attack of arthritis depends upon his attitude toward his condition. The patient's job status and job environment can have more to do with his ability to hold a regular job than how bad the arthritis may be.

One study of the rehabilitation of patients with rheumatoid arthritis found that some persons with severe arthritis were still working 40-hour-weeks ten years after they developed the disease. But others whose arthritis disability was rated as mild to moderate claimed they were unable to continue working. Further investigation of the cases showed that the severely disabled patients who continued working were managers or supervisors, while those with mild to moderate disability who were unable to continue working had jobs with less status.

Q: *I have read about operations for artificial hip joints in people with arthritis. Is this a common operation?*
A: According to the Arthritis Foundation, about 100,000 adult arthritis patients undergo this kind of surgery each year.

Q: *What about children who are disabled by arthritis. Do they ever get artificial joints installed in their hips?*
A: Artificial hip joints for victims of juvenile rheumatoid arthritis have been tried successfully since about 1974. At one time doctors shied away from attempts to install synthetic joints in children because they could outgrow or wear out the artificial joints and have to undergo a second operation. Kids who have had the artificial joints installed are not running marathons, but they are able to walk and climb stairs without crutches, and some who previously were confined to a wheelchair now get around without it.

Q: *There is supposed to be a new kind of childhood arthritis going around. What's different about it?*
A: You probably are referring to Kawasaki disease, which was named for a Japanese pediatrician who discovered the disorder in the 1960's. Doctors are not really sure it is a "new" disease. Perhaps it's a condition that has been around for some time and was treated as something else because the signs and symptoms resemble scarlet fever as well as several other childhood illnesses. In addition to arthritis, symptoms of Kawasaki disease include a rash, fever, inflammation of the eyes and other tissues, and heart problems. Except for heart complications, Kawasaki disease does not appear to be life-threatening. Arthritis symptoms include red and swollen hands and feet, and some recurrent arthralgia pain in the knee and ankle joints. Treatment of Kawasaki disease usually involves administration of large doses of aspirin plus other therapies.

Q: *What happens to the sex life of arthritis victims?*
A: Arthritis victims usually do not lose their sex drive, although their sex life may be altered somewhat if joint deformities interfere with their previous approaches to sexual performance. If the arthritis victim has an understanding sex partner, they will experiment with new and different positions for intercourse and perhaps other methods of sexual stimulation. Many persons with chronic diseases are easily fatigued and take longer to become sexually aroused than before they were stricken.

Based on the experience of arthritis patients who have overcome the problem of pain and stiffness, aspirin or other analgesics can be taken in advance of planned sexual activities. A warm bath to relax muscles before starting sexual activities also is recommended. The fact that victims of rheumatoid arthritis severe enough to warrant artificial hip surgery were able to get married and become parents of normal, healthy children should be adequate evidence that an attack of arthritis need not interfere with a pleasurable sex life.

Q: *Are there any special diets that can cure arthritis?*
A: There are no known foods that cause arthritis and none that will cure it. Doctors may recommend weight-reduction diets for some arthritis patients who are overweight for the simple reason that excess body weight puts added pressure on the weight-bearing joints which are common targets of arthritis inflammation. And the doctor in charge of an arthritis case may advise a patient about certain foods that may or may not be compatible with medicines that have been prescribed. When aspirin is taken, for example, some foods may be preferred because of their buffering effect to reduce heartburn or other adverse reactions in sensitive patients.

Q: *My own doctor claims there is a new way of treating rheumatoid arthritis by filtering the blood. Could this be true?*
A: A technique called pheresis has been used to remove blood factors that are believed to be responsible for the inflammation and joint damage of arthritis. It has been used to provide temporary relief for patients with arthritis so severe that powerful drugs usually employed for treatment fail to work. The blood-filtering procedure also seems to make the drugs more effective. But the pheresis technique is not generally available to patients who can be treated by other methods.

20

GENETIC AND METABOLIC DISEASES

How often have you heard the expression "It runs in the family"? As medical scientists probe deeper into the structure and function of the molecules of inheritance, they are finding that many of the common and uncommon health threats we face have been transmitted through the generations directly or indirectly—much as eye color and balding patterns are predestined—from parents, grandparents, and great-grandparents. Only 20 years ago, the number of diseases identified as being inherited numbered in the hundreds. Today, medical researchers are counting genetic diseases in the thousands.

Many genetic diseases have rather obscure names, like striatonigral degeneration—a term you may never see again unless the symptoms of that motor function disorder show up in a member of your family or in the family of a friend. Other genetic diseases, such as Down's syndrome, cystic fibrosis, and sickle-cell anemia are better known to the general public because of fund-raising campaigns or publicity about the condition.

Some diseases are believed to involve a genetic factor simply because they tend to "run in families." There is evidence, for example, that lung cancer may be associated with a genetic defect since male relatives of individuals with lung cancer seem to run a greater risk of developing the same disease, and the risk increases if the male relatives are cigarette smokers. Breast cancer in women tends to occur more frequently in daughters of women with breast cancer. Down's syndrome, commonly known as mongolism, is rather well established as a genetic disease. Investigators also have found that Down's syndrome appears to have a genetic complication of leukemia. Down's syndrome patients are 15 times as likely to develop leukemia as persons who do not have mongolism.

Because of the myriad genetic diseases and many generations of intermarriage of genetic disease carriers over the centuries, it's unlikely that anybody in our modern mobile society could be called "normal"—if normal can be defined as completely free of one or more genetic diseases.

Family Medical History

Few people today are able to provide an accurate family medical history beyond one or two past generations. Often, it has been found that a diagnosis made by a doctor more than 75 years ago was not accurate enough to be reliable by today's standards. Hospital records of the 19th century may show, for example, that a 45-year-old woman died of "old age." But doctors today do not recognize old age as a cause of death, especially of a patient in her 40's.

Despite the problems of providing a long and accurate family medical history, this information is often the key to diagnosis of a patient's health condition. Doctors are taught that each patient is the current episode of his family's medical history. To better understand the signs and symptoms of the present, it is necessary to ask the patient pertinent questions about his family's past. For that reason, doctors spend a good deal of time during the first examinations of patients asking, "Are your mother and father still alive?" or "At what age did they die and what was the cause of death?" The doctor also may ask about diseases the parents and other family members have or have had, suggesting some possible diseases. There may be questions about the health of brothers, sisters, and distant relatives. This information, plus the patient's own medical history of diseases and injuries as far back into his childhood as he can recall, may add other clues to possible genetic diseases. Many disorders of adult life, including those associated with genet-

ic diseases, show a link with a childhood illness. Today's babies with juvenile eczema, for example, are likely to be the adults of tomorrow with hay fever or asthma, and the adult patient with heart valve disease was quite likely a rheumatic fever patient as a child.

Genetic Makeup of an Individual

The combination of inherited factors that makes each person the individual he or she is, was established at the moment of conception. Half of the genes that determine the form and function of all the tissue cells with which the individual starts life are contributed by the mother, and half by the father. The genetic package of an individual is called a genome. A gene, and there are countless thousands in a genome, are molecules of DNA, which is shorthand for deoxyribonucleic acid.

A normal complement of genes is contained in the genome, along with the 46 chromosomes normally present in each of the individual's body cells. Two of the human chromosomes are sex chromosomes; they determine the sex and sexual characteristics of the individual. The chromosome determining male sexual characteristics is called a Y chromosome. It is smaller than the X chromosome, which contains genes for many hereditary traits in addition to genes that determine the female sexual characteristics. If the genome contains two X chromosomes, the individual will be female. An X + Y chromosome combination becomes a factor that determines the male of the species. Occasionally, a trait associated with the X chromosome is identified with an X-linked gene.

With the exception of the X and Y chromosomes, the rest of the human genes are distributed on 22 more or less identical

MECHANISM OF SEX DETERMINATION

FEMALE   MALE

OVA   SPERMATOZOA

ZYGOTE   ZYGOTE

FEMALE   MALE

The many thousands of genes that determine a person's physical characteristics and other factors, such as susceptibility to certain diseases, are carried on chromosomes. Humans normally have 46 chromosomes, of which half are acquired from the mother and the remaining 23 from the father. The illustration shows how sex is determined by chromosomes. The mother's ova, or egg cells, contain two "X" chromosomes, which are necessary for a fertile female; the father contributes one "X" chromosome and a "Y" chromosome. The child of the parents will be a girl if it acquires an "X" chromosome from both the mother and the father, but a boy if it acquires a "Y" chromosome from the father. Many of the genetic disorders are associated with the sex chromosomes and are more likely to occur in boys.

TWO BROWN-EYED PARENTS—HIDDEN BLUE GENE

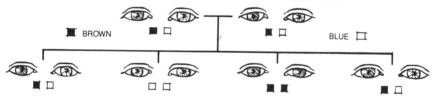

BROWN

BLUE

A recessive trait can be carried for one or more generations as a hidden gene and suddenly appear in a baby whose parents and other blood relatives do not show the hidden characteristic. An example is the occurrence of a blue-eyed child in a family of brown-eyed adults. Both the mother and father could have brown eyes, but each would carry in his and her chromosomes a recessive gene for blue eyes. At conception the offspring would receive a gene for blue eyes from both parents, while the brothers and sisters might receive one or both genes for brown eyes and have that eye coloration.

pairs of chromosomes. The genes on each of the pairs are lined up in precisely the same order for that particular set of chromosomes. For example, a gene for eye color on one of the chromosomes contributed by the mother will be in the same position on the same chromosome contributed by the father. The two genes may or may not be identical; one may produce blue eye color, and the other brown eye color. If both genes agree on the same eye color, the individual inheriting that set of chromosomes will have that eye color.

If one gene controls blue eye color and the other brown, however, one color—brown—will be the dominant gene, and the individual usually will have brown eyes. Blue eye color is a recessive trait and is most likely to occur only if both parents are blue-eyed. Usually, but not always. Because of the complex pattern of gene distribution it is possible for two brown-eyed parents to have a blue-eyed child. Thus, if both parents have one gene for brown eyes and one gene for blue eyes, the brown-eye gene will be dominant and will be responsible for their own brown eyes. But each can contribute the recessive blue-eye gene to their offspring, and the two matched recessive genes will result in brown-eyed parents with a blue-eyed child. The statistical odds show that two parents, each with one brown eye and one blue eye gene, could have one or more children with two brown, two blue, or one brown and one blue eye gene. But only the combination of two genes for blue eyes would result in a blue-eyed child.

Transmission of Genetic Diseases

Eye color is not a disease, of course, but the example shows how a gene that might result directly in a disease or contribute to a disease by making a person more susceptible can be transmitted from one generation to the next without making an appearance. A genetic trait can easily skip a generation, as happens with male baldness, which may be transmitted from grandfather to grandson through a daughter without affecting either the son or daughter of the grandfather.

Hemophilia is an example of a genetic disease that is transmitted from one generation to another and skips an intermediate generation, just as a male baldness pattern may appear in alternate generations. Hemophilia is a term applied to about a dozen inherited bleeding disorders caused by a defect in the body's ability to cause blood to clot normally. Because of the failure of the blood to clot adequately when the patient suffers a wound, a trivial injury can be life-threatening. The trait for this genetic disease is carried by a recessive gene in the mother and affects only her sons.

All genetic diseases are not entirely hereditary disorders carried by humans for countless generations. Some diseases can originate in gene mutations or chromosomal aberrations due to several possible influences, including environmental damage. Some gene mutations or chromosomal aberrations are lethal and disrupt the reproductive process so that the altered trait goes no further. But some gene mutations result only in a minor change in the family tree, adding more variety to the already existing infinite possibilities of gene juggling for future generations.

Types of Genetic Defects

Some genetic diseases are classed as single-gene defects. A defective gene can be X-linked, carried by both sets of a pair of chromosomes, and it can be a dominant or recessive gene. It may or may not occur in a person who may have one or more other genetic defects. An example of a single-gene defect is a disease called osteogenesis imperfecta, which involves various disorders of the bones and connective tissues. Another example of a single-gene defect is achondroplastic dwarfism, a cartilage disorder that leads to abnormally short limbs. Achondroplastic dwarfism also may be an example of a mutation since it usually occurs in families with no previous history of the disorder.

Another general class of genetic defects is called multifactorial inheritance, which means simply the result of an interaction of many different genes. Multifactorial inheritance also takes into account the effect of environmental influences, such as a virus infection of the mother during her pregnancy. The term is used to help explain a number of diseases that tend to run in families, although the distribution of cases from one generation to the next does not fit the typical pattern followed by inheritance of eye color, stubby fingers, curly hair, and other dominant-recessive traits.

Multifactorial inheritance can be used to explain why some members of a family seem more susceptible to a genetic disease than to others. The close members of a family—parents, children, brothers, and sisters—will have genomes that are more nearly identical than those of distant relatives. Therefore, a genetic defect that runs in the family is more likely to affect the immediate family than their cousins. The more distant the cousins, the less chance that they might have inherited the defect.

An example of the distribution of a genetic defect in the general population is that of cystic fibrosis, which is marked by digestive problems and respiratory difficulties associated with thick glandular secretions that block vital ducts of the body. The random chance of a baby being born with cystic fibrosis is about one in 2,500. However, the gene for cystic fibrosis is a recessive trait that is rather common; it is estimated that one out of 25 persons may be carriers of this recessive gene.

If a brother or sister of a cystic fibrosis patient is normal but inherits the gene and marries an unrelated person, who would have one in 25 chances of carrying the same recessive gene, the chance of having a child with the genetic disease would be one in 150. But if the normal brother or sister married a first cousin, the chance

that both marriage partners carry the gene would increase to one in eight, and the risk of their having a child with cystic fibrosis would be one in 48.

Genetic Counseling

The example of cystic fibrosis also points up the importance of genetic counseling in family planning programs. Men and women who are close members of the same family, such as first cousins, can expect an increased risk of having a child with a genetic defect if such a genetic disease exists in their family. Also, men and women who are unrelated but are members of families which include close relatives with a genetic disease, probably should seek family counseling regarding the possibility that both may be carrying a gene for the defect. The counseling may lead to the discovery that the two families do not have the same genetic disease. Of the several thousand possible genetic diseases, it's quite possible that disorders with similar symptoms may involve different causes. It has been calculated, for example, that some 60 different congenital problems can result in hearing loss. The risk of marrying an unrelated person with the same set of recessive gene defects has been compared to the chances of two card players drawing 13 cards of the same suits from a well-shuffled deck.

However, the risk of a normal sibling of a person with a serious genetic disease carrying the same gene defect is 25 percent. Where there is an apparent chance that the normal sibling might become the parent of a child with the same genetic disease, genetic counseling should be sought. Genetic counselors usually begin by helping the marriage partners trace their family trees and list the names, ages, and health conditions of first, second, and third-degree relatives. If there are any gaps, the counselors give advice about how to obtain the missing information for relatives who are no longer in contact with the immediate family. The family tree history also should include information about ethnic and religious backgrounds, since some genetic diseases are more likely to be associated with people of a particular cultural group, and young men and women traditionally have tended to marry people of similar backgrounds.

Tay-Sachs disease, which is characterized by central nervous system degeneration, blindness and seizures, and death in childhood, is an example of a genetic disease that often can be detected through genetic counseling and testing techniques. The disease is carried by a recessive gene in persons descended from Eastern European Jewish families. The chances that any man or woman with Eastern European Jewish ancestors will be a carrier of the Tay-Sachs disease gene are one in 30. The risk of a child with the disease being born to a carrier obviously becomes more likely if the marriage partner also has the same cultural background and carries the gene.

Genetic Defect Tests

There are genetic test centers throughout the country where blood samples can be tested to determine the presence of cer-

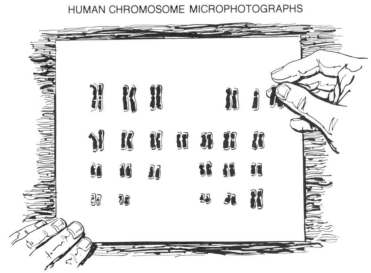

HUMAN CHROMOSOME MICROPHOTOGRAPHS

Genetic experts often can predict characteristics of a child before it is born by examining its chromosomes. A set of the chromosomes of the fetus can be obtained by amniocentesis, or the withdrawal of a small sample of aminotic fluid surrounding the fetus while it is in the mother's womb. The fluid will contain body cells, such as skin cells, that have been shed by the fetus. By finding a set of chromosomes in the nucleus of one of the cells through a microscope and photographing the chromosomes, the sex of the unborn child, possible genetic defects, and other information can be obtained. The illustration shows how a doctor can examine individual chromosomes that have been cut out of a photographic enlargement made from the original microphotographs.

tain genetic defects. They are called carrier tests, and they can indicate the presence of a potentially defective gene by measuring the level of a chemical that ordinarily is not present if the particular gene was normal.

A second kind of test that may be performed is called amniocentesis. It is done after pregnancy has started by analyzing cells extracted through a hollow needle inserted into the amniotic fluid in which the fetus floats. If the amniocentesis test indicates the baby may be diseased or malformed, the parents can decide whether to have the fetus aborted or to continue the pregnancy and provide care for a child that may be abnormal. Couples who feel they are at high risk of producing a child with a genetic defect also have the option of adopting children or providing a surrogate parent through artificial insemination.

Not all genetic diseases can be predicted by carrier tests or amniocentesis. Huntington's chorea, or Huntington's disease, for example, can affect 50 percent of the offspring of a carrier, but there is no way to detect the presence of the gene defect before the symptoms appear. The symptoms, which include involuntary jerky movements and personality changes marked by moodiness, obstinacy, and paranoia, usually do not occur until the victim is about 35 years of age. At that period of life, many victims already have married and become parents of children who will eventually be Huntington's chorea patients.

Chromosomal Aberrations

Down's syndrome, which appears in about one of every 700 live births and occurs most frequently when the mother is over the age of 35, is a genetic disease that is associated with a chromosome aberration rather than an inherited recessive or dominant gene. The characteristics of the disorder include general physical and mental retardation. The babies are placid and rarely cry. The muscles lack normal tone, the eyes appear to be slanted—hence the common term, mongolism—and the head may be misshapen. Many Down's syndrome children die at an early age of leukemia or heart defects, but others may live to old age.

Doctors who specialize in genetics describe Down's syndrome as Trisomy 21, meaning that the cause is related to the presence of three copies, instead of the normal two, of chromosome number 21 in the genome. In some instances one of the chromosomes is translocated; for example, the extra chromosome 21 has become attached to some other chromosome.

There are other genetic diseases associated with additional chromosome numbers 8, 9, 13, 18, and 22. Each chromosomal aberration is accompanied by similar physical abnormalities. A child with an extra chromosome 13, for example, is likely to be small at birth, have breathing difficulties, be mentally retarded, and appear deaf. The child also may have the condition known as dextrocardia, in which the heart is positioned in the chest toward the right side, rather than the left.

Anomalies also can result when pieces of chromosomes are missing or only a portion of a third chromosome is present. A condition known as the cat-cry syndrome, marked by an infant's crying sounds like the mewing of a kitten, plus other abnormalities, is caused by the absence of a part of chromosome 5. The presence of a piece of an extra chromosome 22 accounts for a condition called the cat-eye syndrome because of cat-like irises in the eyes of the child.

Various chromosomal aberrations are associated with a very wide range of variations from the normal human physical traits, although they are not necessarily responsible for every unusual physical feature in an individual human. Physical traits that have been traced in some patients to altered chromosomes include clubfeet, short neck, low-set ears, undescended testicles, long flexed fingers, stubby fingers, beaked nose, prominent nose, broad nasal bridge, cleft or high-arched palate, highly convex fingernails, maloccluded teeth, and a small mouth.

Tests for chromosomal aberrations are relatively simple for most doctors. The physician takes a small blood sample and mails it to a laboratory specializing in genetic studies. The laboratory produces a cell culture from the blood, stimulating the cells in the blood to reproduce. A drug often used in treating gout, colchicine, is added to the cell culture because it has the effect of freezing the action, so to speak, at a point in cell division when the chromosomes appear most distinctly. The chromosomes are then placed on a microscope slide and photographed. An enlarged photograph of the patient's chromosomes allows a genetics specialist and the family doctor to see what's normal and what's not about an individual patient's genetic material.

Diabetes Metabolic Diseases

A significant number of metabolic disorders, those that involve abnormal handling of nutrients by the body, are associated with genetic defects. Some of the disorders are genetically determined directly; others probably result from a combination of a gene or chromosome defect and an environmental influence that triggers the symptoms of the disorder.

At least one type of diabetes mellitus and one form of diabetes insipidus have hereditary links. The type of diabetes mellitus that is of a hereditary nature sometimes is designated as genetic diabetes to distinguish the disorder from other causes. The genetic basis for diabetes mellitus consists mainly of the evidence that a person who has close relatives with diabetes has a higher risk of developing the disease himself, that it is more likely to occur in both members of a set of identical twins than in both of a pair of fraternal twins, and that the disease can occur in the offspring when either the mother or father is a diabetic.

Because diabetes mellitus can develop either as juvenile onset or adult onset diabetes, meaning it can begin either in childhood or adulthood, some medical scientists have suggested that there might be two different genetic factors involved, one for each type. However, there is no typical genetic pattern of inheritance when both the father and mother are diabetic; the children may or may not develop diabetes. This fact supports the argument that what may be inherited is a susceptibility which is triggered into the actual disease symptoms by an environmental influence such as obesity, drugs, or a disease. Some studies show patterns of diabetes appearing in children after they recover from a viral infection.

Since the function of the genes is to control the formation of structural units of the body and the production of enzymes that control the metabolic activity of the tissue cells, defects in genes or chromosomes can result in abnormal metabolic activity as well as in abnormal physical traits. Diabetes mellitus is just one of hundreds of metabolic disorders with a genetic disease link.

Diabetes insipidus is a different kind of diabetes, although like diabetes mellitus it is marked by abnormal urine excretion. Diabetes insipidus occurs in two forms, both related to the influence or lack of influence of a pituitary hormone on the ability of the kidney tissues to form urine. Nephrogenic diabetes insipidus is a genetic disease caused by a defect in the X chromosome. It affects mainly males whose kidneys are unable to concentrate urine and allow the excess water to be reabsorbed into the bloodstream. As a result, the patient develops a tremendous thirst, excretes a very diluted urine, and suffers from severe water depletion. In a baby the disorder can lead to convulsions and permanent brain damage if it is not corrected by providing adequate fluid intake.

Amino Acid Metabolic Diseases

Amino acid metabolic diseases are among the most common of genetic disorders. One of the amino acid disorders, phenylketonuria, or PKU, is caused by an inherited recessive trait that results in an accumulation of phenylalanine in the body. Phenylalanine is an essential amino acid, but in a normal person the amino acid is converted to another substance, tyrosine. The enzyme needed to convert the phenylalanine to tyrosine, however, is virtually absent in PKU because of the defective gene that does not produce the enzyme.

PKU may produce no symptoms in the newborn child, but the infant may have skin, hair, and eye color that is lighter than other members of the family, a rash similar to that of infantile eczema, and lethargic body movements. If untreated, the accumulation of phenylalanine leads to severe mental retardation. However, screening programs are available to test infants before the disease progresses to a serious stage.

Ironically, the source of phenylalanine is milk and milk is used in testing the child. After the baby has consumed milk for several days, a few drops of ferric chloride solution are placed on a wet diaper. If the child has PKU, the urine spot on the diaper will turn a deep bluish-green. Since phenylalanine is an essential amino acid, it cannot be eliminated entirely from the diet without impairing the growth of the child. But special food supplements are available to provide—but not to exceed—the child's daily requirement of the nutrient.

PKU patients may or may not require lifetime treatment to control the symptoms. If a female PKU patient marries and has children, the offspring may show signs of brain damage because of the mother's inability to metabolize the phenylalanine in protein foods.

Another amino acid disorder is known popularly as maple syrup urine disease, although doctors may refer to the genetic defect as branched-chain ketoaciduria. The common name, maple syrup urine disease, is derived from the odor of the urine and sweat of the patient, which sometimes is a diagnostic clue—just as the urine and sweat of the PKU child has a distinctive "mousey" odor. Like PKU, delayed treatment can result in mental retardation and neurological damage. If untreated, maple syrup urine disease can be fatal, whereas PKU really is not a life-threatening problem.

The disease is caused by a genetic defect in the production of an enzyme involved in the metabolism of three amino acids, leucine, isoleucine, and valine. The amino acids accumulate in the blood, and eventually this condition leads to convulsions, coma, and, if untreated, death. Infants with maple syrup urine disease appear normal at birth but quickly show signs of deterioration. They become lethargic, flaccid, show diminished awareness, and refuse to feed. Death may occur within a few weeks if the condition is not corrected.

Diagnosis and treatment are similar to PKU. Chemical tests of the urine will confirm the disease if it is the cause of the symptoms. Treatment is based on restricting the amounts of the amino acids in the child's diet to no more than what is required to assure normal physical development.

Still another of the amino acid metabolism disorders based on genetic defects is homocystinuria, caused by a deficiency of an enzyme needed to convert the amino acid methionine to cysteine. Homocystinuria is second to PKU in frequency of occurrence. Symptoms of the disorder include a juvenile form of osteoporosis, a bone atrophy effect; displaced lenses of the eyes; a tendency to develop thromboses; and mental retardation. The symptoms are believed to be caused by abnormal development of the circulatory and connective tissue systems as a result of the amino acid metabolism deficiency.

Treatment of homocystinuria involves dietary control of amino acid intake after confirmation of the cause of the symptoms through laboratory tests of the patient's urine and blood.

Storage Diseases

A group of genetic-based metabolic disorders are called storage diseases because they involve excessive storage in the body of metabolites, or the products of metabolism.

Tay-Sachs disease is an example of a storage disease that involves a storage of excess lipid metabolites in the central nervous system.

Glycogen storage disease can result from lack of an enzyme, producing symptoms of hypoglycemia when the stored glycogen cannot be mobilized quickly into glucose to provide fuel for the brain and muscles.

Alkaptonuria is an amino acid metabolite storage disease in which a deficiency of an enzyme involved in the metabolism of tyrosine results in an accumulation of a substance called homogentisic acid. Unlike some of the other metabolic disorders that first appear at infancy, alkaptonuria does not begin producing significant signs and symptoms until the patient is middle aged. The homogentisic acid is associated with a dark pigment that gradually turns the urine equally dark. The acid also becomes deposited in the connective tissues, an effect that causes inflammation of a joint that is similar to rheumatoid arthritis or ankylosing spondylitis.

Galactosemia

Galactosemia is a relatively common genetic disorder marked by a deficiency of the enzyme needed to convert galactose, a sugar molecule in milk, into glucose. An infant who inherits this disease tends to show a lack of interest in either mother's milk or milk formulas and may vomit any milk that is swallowed. The child fails to progress in development and eventually develops liver disorders, cataracts of the eyes, and mental retardation. The cataracts often are a clue to the diagnosis, which can be confirmed with laboratory tests.

Treatment of galactosemia is based on elimination of milk and other foods containing galactose and substituting infant food preparations that contain maltose or other sugar molecules.

Genetic Disorders Affecting Ethnic Groups

For reasons that baffle even genetics experts, some diseases occur in clusters within different ethnic or regional populations, although the symptoms are quite similar. A genetic disorder called Niemann-Pick disease, which is characterized by cholesterol storage among other symptoms, occurs mainly among Eastern European Jewish populations, but it also has been discovered in unrelated populations in Nova Scotia. Another cholesterol metabolism disease, cholesterol acetyltransferase deficiency, seems to affect only Scandinavians.

Thalassemia, a type of anemia characterized by defective hemoglobin, occurs mainly among people of Greek or Italian ancestry.

Sickle-cell anemia, caused by a different form of hemoglobin anomaly, affects mainly blacks; about ten percent of American blacks carry the gene for sickle-cell anemia. American blacks also may be affected by another type of anemia known as hemoglobin C disease, which has symptoms similar to but different from those of sickle-cell anemia.

GLOSSARY

GENETIC AND METABOLIC DISEASES

allele Two or more alternative forms of a gene that may occur at a particular site on a *chromosome*. Each person normally has two alleles for each gene, one contributed by the mother and one from the father. The two alleles may be similar or different.

autosome A chromosome that is not a sex chromosome. Humans normally have 22 pairs of autosomes plus two sex chromosomes.

carrier A person who carries a recessive gene but does not show a trait or disease that may be associated with the gene. A mother may be the carrier of a gene for blue eye color although her own eyes may be brown.

chromatin A substance in chromosomes which can be stained with dyes in order to make the genetic material visible on a microscope slide.

chromosomal aberration An abnormal chromosome which could be caused by an environmental influence about the time of conception. Heavy consumption of alcoholic beverages by a mother, for example, or a virus infection could cause aberrations in previously normal chromosomes.

chromosome A microscopically small chain of genes which are composed of DNA molecules. Each gene normally has an assigned location on a particular chromosome.

congenital Refers to a condition present at birth, the cause of which may be either genetic or environmental.

cytogenetics The study of the activity of genes and chromosomes within tissue cells.

diploid A matched set of 22 pairs of autosomes plus the two sex chromosomes.

dominant gene The gene that determines a trait when the matching gene is recessive or is also the same dominant *allele*.

genetic code The pattern of chemical components in a gene that determines the function of the particular gene.

genome The complete set of genes in a pair of chromosomes.

haploid Literally, half of a *diploid*. Each male spermatozoon or female ovum normally contains one set of 23 chromosomes, or haploid. Upon conception, the 23 male and 23 female chromosomes form a diploid of 46 chromosomes.

heterozygous Possessing different alleles or genes at a location on two otherwise matching chromosomes.

homozygous Possessing identical alleles or genes at a given location on two matching chromosomes.

inborn error of metabolism A genetic defect resulting in a failure of an enzyme to be made available for a vital metabolic function.

locus Another term for location of a gene on a chromosome.

metaphase A stage of cell division in which the chromosomes line up in the nucleus and are most visible for study by cytogenetecists.

mitosis The process of cell division during which each *chromosome* duplicates itself by splitting lengthwise. Each of the two new cells receives 46 chromosomes that are identical with the original set. Normally, all of the trillions of body cells in a mature human contain a set of chromosomes identical with the set formed at the time of conception.

monozygotic twins Identical twins developed from the same original fertilized ovum.

multifactorial inheritance Inherited traits that are influenced by a great number of genetic factors accumulated over many generations.

mutation A spontaneous change in a gene. The new gene may be inherited.

proband A patient who is the basis for a genetic or heredity study.

recessive Referring to a trait that usually determines a genetic characteristic in a child only when it is carried by both the mother and father.

sex-linked gene A gene carried on a sex chromosome, usually the X chromosome.

translocation A relocation of genes from one chromosome to another or to a different place on the same chromosome.

trisomy Three chromosomes instead of the usual two. Trisomy errors often are involved in genetic defects. The extra chromosome may be found with its matching autosome or attached to an entirely different chromosome.

X and Y chromosomes The two sex chromosomes. A male normally has one X chromosome, and a female has two X chromosomes. The male receives a Y chromosome, which is smaller than the X chromosome. The female combination of sex chromosomes usually is indicated as XX, and the male as XY.

QUESTIONS AND ANSWERS
GENETIC AND METABOLIC DISEASES

Q: *What happens if a child on a special PKU diet is taken off the formula after he starts school?*

A: Generally, the experience has been that children who have been on the phenylalanine-free protein formula for a period of four or five years tend to suffer some degree of mental deterioration after the diet is discontinued. One European study found the average I.Q. of PKU children fell 11 points after the special diet was discontinued, and in an extreme case the I.Q. of a child fell from 106, which is in the normal range, to 75 over a period of four years.

About two-thirds of the children studied also developed abnormal EEG's (electroencephalograms), learning difficulties, and hyperactivity after they were allowed to drop the generally unpalatable PKU diet.

Q: *Has anybody actually seen a human gene or do genes exist only in theory?*

A: A decade or more ago, human genes were believed to exist because of evidence obtained from studies of genes in plants and animals and the circumstantial evidence of human heredity patterns. But in 1978 single genes were first observed through an electron microscope during research into factors associated with the development of Down's syndrome, or mongolism. The genes were photographed and scientists are now able to see what makes a normal gene different from a defective gene.

Q: *Is it possible to tell from the appearance of a black person whether he might be a carrier of the sickle-cell anemia gene?*

A: No. In fact, that subject has been studied rather thoroughly because of an unfounded notion that sickle-cell anemia carriers were physically smaller or intellectually slower than normal black children. The medical research found no difference between black youngsters within the ages of three and five who were sickle-cell anemia gene carriers and those with normal genes when they were matched for such factors as age, sex, weight, and intelligence.

Q: *How can doctors tell if a newborn baby is deaf, since that is one sign of a genetic defect?*

A: A newborn baby often appears to be deaf for the first few days outside the womb, but later he will appear startled if an unexpected noise occurs nearby. Actually, hearing in an infant can be detected earlier than normal vision. A baby may be unable to distinguish objects for several months, although he presumably can tell the difference between light and darkness during the first few days of life.

Q: *Are all genetic traits determined by either dominant or recessive genes?*

A: Not all traits work out into such simple patterns. Some characteristics such as body stature and skin color may appear as an intermediate balance between the extremes represented by the parents. Environmental factors also can influence the outward appearance of an individual. Good childhood nutrition, for example, can result in youngsters who are much taller and heavier than either parent, rather than offspring who represent some kind of average between parents or ancestors.

Q: *Could hair dye used by a mother account for a genetic defect in her child?*

A: There is some evidence that hair dyes can be absorbed through the skin to cause chromosomal damage. But whether the damage to chromosomes that has been observed in women who use hair dyes results in offspring with birth defects is a subject of controversy. Some medical investigators believe there is a greater risk of chromosome damage from virus infections such as rubella or from exposure to radiation—factors that have been documented. Whether women with dyed hair become more susceptible to chromosomal damage during a virus infection or a chest or dental X-ray is another unresolved question of genetic disease causes.

Q: *Just how common are genetic diseases, compared to another type of disease?*
A: A survey of more than 40,000 American infants found an average frequency of only 5.6 chromosomal abnormalities per 1,000 births. The worldwide incidence of diabetes mellitus, for comparison purposes, is about five percent, or almost ten times that of genetic diseases, and peptic ulcers affect about ten percent of the population. But such comparisons can be misleading since at least part of the diabetes and peptic ulcer causes probably involve genetic disease factors. In addition to children born with some genetic defects, estimated to total around 20,000 a year in America alone, as many as half of all spontaneous abortions in which a pregnancy is lost during the first three months are the result of chromosomal abnormalities.

Of the children who survive the nine months in the womb despite genetic defects, many thousands each year are permanently handicapped by mental retardation or physical disorders, and a significant proportion of them will die in childhood. Also, for most cases of genetic disease, there is no cure or simple treatment.

Q: *I have read that some genetic diseases are aneuploidies. What does this mean?*
A: An aneuploidy is simply an abnormal number of chromosomes. The number may be 45, 47, 48, or even 49, instead of the normal 46. Individuals with an abnormal number of chromosomes are likely to be afflicted with a physical or mental disorder.

Q: *Do mongoloid children have an extra chromosome?*
A: Some mongoloid patients have only 46 chromosomes. However, these 46 chromosomes ac-

tually contain the genetic material that is the equivalent of 47 chromosomes. A chromosomal abnormality can involve having too many genes in one chromosome, in addition to the condition of extra chromosomes, missing parts of chromosomes, and so on.

Q: *Is an albino condition a genetic defect?*
A: There are at least two different genetic factors that can account for albinism. Both are amino acid metabolic disorders involving the absence of an enzyme needed to convert the amino acide tyrosine into melanin, the substance that produces pigmentation in the skin, hair, and eyes. The type that affects the eyes particularly is transmitted as a sex-linked recessive gene.

Q: *Are there other genetic diseases that involve vision?*
A: Yes, visual defects are not uncommon signs and symptoms of genetic disorders. A half-dozen inherited metabolic diseases are characterized by visual abnormalities, in addition to other effects. Retinitis pigmentosa, which is marked by night blindness and abnormal visual fields, is one of the more common genetic diseases. One of the early signs of mongolism is the appearance of grayish-white spots around the edge of the iris.

Q: *What is mosaicism?*
A: Some individuals have two different kinds of body cells, some with 46 chromosomes and some with 47, forming a mosaic pattern.

Q: *What does chorea mean, as in Huntington's chorea?*
A: Chorea, which is pronounced like Korea, is applied to any disorder marked by spasmodic or jerking movements of the arms and legs, or the facial muscles, over which the patient has no control. There are many different kinds and causes of these symptoms. In the case of Huntington's chorea, the cause is a genetic defect resulting in general mental deterioration that begins after the age of 30.

Q: *Are boys more likely to be affected by genetic disorders than girls?*

A: In sex-linked inherited traits, the male is almost always the affected sex. Premature baldness, for example, is a sex-linked trait that generally involves only men, although women may show signs of the defect after menopause. Since boys seem to be more susceptible to certain bacterial infections than girls, there is good reason to suspect that a gene defect favoring girls also may be involved. However, girls are not immune to genetic diseases as evidence of the familial data from breast cancer shows.

Q: *Will a woman with a triple X chromosome combination, instead of the normal XX sex chromosome pattern, be sterile?*
A: There is no consistent pattern to this effect. It was originally believed that girls with an XXX sex chromosome combination would be abnormal because the first cases were discovered among females in mental institutions. Later, it was discovered that apparently normal women had an extra X chromosome. Among those who were married, some were sterile and some bore normal children.

Q: *What about men who have an extra Y chromosome?*
A: This type of genetic anomaly followed a pattern similar to that of girls with an XXX chromosome. The first XYY boys, having a total of 47 chromosomes rather than the normal 46, were thought to be the victims of a genetic disorder since they were found in prisons and had low I.Q.'s. However, further study indicated the same sex chromosome pattern existed in men who were not retarded criminals.

Q: *If parents have one child with a genetic disease, what are the chances that others will be born to the same parents?*
A: With one exception, the chances of a man and wife having more than one child with a chromosomal anomaly are extremely rare. The exception is Down's syndrome, or mongolism. If the chromosomal translocation involved in this disorder—usually an extra chromosome 21 attached to another chromosome—exists in either parent, there is a chance that more than

one offspring will be a Down's syndrome patient.

Q: *How important is the environment in genetic diseases?*
A: It depends upon the disease. Down's syndrome, for example, is believed to be purely a hereditary effect in which environment would not alter the course of events. Some infections may have a large environmental role in cases where the inherited factor is simply an increased susceptibility. Xeroderma pigmentosum is a good example of an inherited susceptibility to the damaging effects of ultraviolet light. A patient with this genetic defect is literally at the mercy of the sunlight, a very obvious environmental factor, and can avoid skin cancer by staying out of the sun.

Q: *Is amniocentesis dangerous for either the mother or child?*
A: The only risks are from intra-abdominal bleeding or infection, which could result in complications for both the mother and child, but the chances of such a mishap are less than one in 100. There also is a possible adverse effect of overexposure of the fetus to the ultrasound vibrations that are used to locate the fetus and the placenta before the needle is inserted through the abdominal wall. But competent and experienced medical personnel are unlikely to endanger either the mother or child during an amniocentesis procedure.

Q: *What are my chances of having a baby with PKU?*
A: The random chance of anyone in North America becoming the parent of a child with PKU has been calculated at one in 16,000. However, if you are a member of certain ethnic groups, such as blacks or Ashkenazi Jews, your chances are even less since the disease is extremely rare in those population groups. On the other hand, if you have a cousin who becomes a mother of a PKU child, your chances of also having a PKU child are about 20 times higher than the random odds.

Q: *What is meant by a homozygous recessive trait?*

A: It is one that may be carried by both parents although neither the mother nor father show signs of the trait. An example might be a rare disease such as albinism, or lack of pigmentation. The genes might be carried for generations by ancestors of both parents, only to be expressed through the random mating of two unrelated individuals. When a child with that trait is born, everyone is quite surprised. But with the many thousands of genes carried on the chromosomes of both parents, there is always a possibility in any marriage that a child will be born with characteristics unlike those of either parent or their close relatives.

Q: *Do a pair of recessive genes always become dominant when one comes from the mother and one from the father?*
A: The statistical odds are that only one in four of their children will be affected.

21

ALLERGIES
MOST PEOPLE HAVE ONE

Allergies are so common that it's almost considered normal if you are allergic to one or more substances in the environment. Estimates of the number of people who experience identifiable allergic reactions run as high as 50 percent of the general population. Many other persons feel a mild reaction to something they eat, inhale, or come in contact with, but since they do not consult a doctor about the problem, there is no clinical record of the allergic effect that could be added to the statistics.

Allergy covers such a broad scope of reaction signs and symptoms that even medical professionals occasionally have difficulty in deciding how to classify or define the problems. Hay fever, for example, is an allergy; many doctors prefer to use the term, hypersensitivity reaction. A hay fever allergy is a hypersensitivity reaction to an exogenous antigen that produces symptoms of discomfort in the respiratory and ocular mucosal surfaces. This means that hay fever is an allergy characterized by the reaction of body tissues to a foreign substance, or an exogenous antigen, which usually is a plant pollen. The reaction causes respiratory discomfort in the form of sniffles, sneezes, and a runny nose, plus watery eyes and congested conjunctival membranes between the eyes and eyelids—the ocular mucosal surfaces. Although the type of arthritis sometimes identified as SLE, for systemic lupus erythematosus, also is considered a hypersensitivity reaction, SLE actually is an allergic reaction to one's own body tissues.

Some people are allergic to drugs given by injection, such as antibiotics, tetanus serum, liver extract, insulin, or hormones. Other people may be allergic to drugs given by mouth, including aspirin, antibiotics, tranquillizers, laxatives, or sedatives. Some individuals have hypersensitivity reactions to mold spores or dust. Others may have reactions to the skin or hair shed by cats, dogs, or other animals. Some are allergic to cosmetics or hair lotions. Feathers, tobacco, and chemicals used in industry can trigger allergic reactions.

Foods are among the most common causes of allergic reactions. Lobster, crab, fish, nuts, chocolate, eggs, meat, milk, fruits, vegetables, and spices are among the offenders. There are individuals who cannot take vitamin tablets until after the colored coating has been washed away because they are hypersensitive to a chemical dye used in its manufacture.

The list of allergens, as these allergy-producing substances are called, obviously is endless. Even certain plastics, metals, fabrics and fabric dyes, resins, plant leaves, viruses, and bacteria can produce hypersensitivity reactions in you or a friend or relative. But a hypersensitivity reaction to a substance generally is not normal. The substance that is an allergen usually is harmless to most people, even though many individuals are sensitive to the substance. The number of people sensitive to hay fever allergens is in the many millions. If there was a place in the world relatively free of plant pollens—the North and South Poles excluded—the hay fever sufferers of the world could move there and form one of the largest populations on the face of the earth.

How Allergies Develop

Allergies usually do not develop suddenly. In fact, a true allergy does not exist the first time a person comes in contact with an allergen. The patient may or may not show signs or symptoms of a hypersensitivity reaction the second time the offending substance enters his body cells. The reason an allergic reaction does not occur on initial contact is that the reaction involves a response by the antibodies produced by the patient's immune system, and the antibodies cannot be produced until after a particular allergen has made contact.

In some cases an allergic response develops early. That's why allergies often appear in small children. Other allergies can be insidious; the reaction antibodies may lie in wait for years while the patient continues exposing himself to the allergen.

An antibody is a sort of tailored protein molecule that is designed by the body's lymphatic system to attack and render harmless a foreign substance that is considered to be a threat to the individual's survival. If a patient's immune system decides that a particular substance should be added to its allergenic "hit" list, it manufactures great quantities of antibodies that are posted in vulnerable tissue areas, ready to pounce on any allergen that pays a return visit to the patient's body.

Our immune system is vastly complicated and capable of designing and manufacturing a wide array of antibody weapons. Some antibodies are designed to neutralize any toxin or poison that might be carried by an allergen. Others are designed to dissolve or liquefy an allergen. Antibodies can cause a foreign cell to rupture or to clump together with others of its type so that they become ineffective invaders. One remarkable type of antibody forms a coating over the allergen in order to make it appear appetizing to phagocytes, which are tiny cannibal-like cells that roam through the body ingesting stray microorganisms and other foreign material, as well as tissue cells that the body no longer needs.

Symptoms of Allergic Reactions

The symptoms produced by an allergic reaction generally result from interactions of the antibodies and the allergens. Cells may be ruptured or destroyed, releasing powerful chemical substances such as histamines that cause fluid accumulation in mucous membranes, spasms of respiratory muscles, and other symptoms that are identified as the allergic, or hypersensitivity, reactions.

Because antibodies and allergens, which also may be called antigens, tend to react in certain rather specific patterns, doctors can take a few shortcuts to diagnose a hypersensitivity reaction by observing the reaction pattern. When a potent substance such as histamine is released from cells, for example, the signs and symptoms of dilated blood vessels, contractions of smooth muscles, and spasms of respiratory muscles are similar, even though the source of the allergen might be from an insect sting, hay fever, a type of dust in the air, or a substance in a bowl of fish chowder. The allergens causing such a reaction might be quite diverse, but the reaction pattern helps pinpoint the type of cell chemistry being caused by the allergen. This information helps the doctor to decide what should be done to relieve the symptoms.

Another type of reaction, which could be due to an allergic reaction to penicillin, results in changes in the body's red blood cells—a response sometimes identified as a cytotoxic reaction. This category also includes the reactions observed when the wrong blood type might be used in a transfusion, in Rh blood factor problems of newborn infants, and possibly the SLE condition which involves hypersensitivity of multiple body systems. SLE also is suspected of being involved in still another type of hypersensitivity reaction that is characterized by the release of enzymes that break down protein molecules to produce acute inflammations. This type of reaction is associated with certain drug allergies, particularly medications prepared with serums of other animals.

Why Are Some People Hypersensitive?

Everyone, obviously, does not react to the same potential allergen as everybody else. Some people are sensitive to poison ivy or poison oak, but others fail to show the signs or symptoms of exposure to the toxic substance produced by plants of that species. Some individuals seem to be unaffected by insect bites or stings, while others may react quickly and severely in a condition known as anaphylactic shock. This is a potentially fatal reaction marked by edema, respiratory distress due to bronchial constriction, and circulatory changes that result in shock symptoms. Anaphylactic shock is perhaps the ultimate example of an acute allergic reaction.

What makes some people more sensitive than others is believed due in part at least to hereditary factors. Animal experiments show that some strains of a species display a highly active response to certain allergens, while other strains of the same species may respond poorly or not at all. Humans who are sensitive to plant pollens also tend to be sensitive to other substances that evoke a similar allergic response. This reaction indicates to medical scientists that those individuals have inherited a gene that is geared to produce a certain kind of antibody that will confront a particular class of antigens.

How does the body's immune system distinguish between its own molecules and those of a foreign substance? The answer is that sometimes it doesn't. Although this aspect of hypersensitivity reactions has provoked quite a bit of controversy over the years, the consensus is that the human body can develop a condition called autoimmunity. This condition is believed to occur in one or more of several possible ways, including a phenomenon that may occur when the individual is still a fetus and tissues developing in one part of the body become potential antigens to tissues developing in another body area. It is more likely, however, that the normal immune system simply loses its ability to distinguish its own molecules from those of substances produced outside the body. Some arthritic disease symptoms have been explained as possible autoimmune reactions.

Urticaria (Hives) and Angioedema

Hypersensitivity reactions often result in a symptom that doctors call urticaria, commonly called hives. The hives may occur as inflamed welts of varying sizes and colorations, either darker or paler than the surrounding skin, and accompanied by an itching sensation. The urticaria may occur on the face, lips, tongue, throat, eyelids, ears, or even internally, although the wheals most commonly appear on the skin. Small wheals sometimes merge to form larger ones.

A related symptom of allergy is called angioedema, which is an accumulation of fluid in the deep layers of the skin, including the subcutaneous tissues. Angioedema sometimes is called giant urticaria because the edema produces a wheal-like swelling in the skin. Urticaria and angioedema generally occur in the same areas at the same time in response to the same kind of allergen, but they actually are different types of skin reactions.

Urticaria may or may not be a true symptom of allergy since the effect also can be produced by infection, emotional stress, exposure to sunlight or cold, or mechanical irritation of the skin. But the skin effect as a hypersensitivity reaction can occur in response to inhaled allergens, such as plant pollens, mold spores, or animal dander. Foods that are known to produce the reaction in sensitive individuals include fresh fruits, nuts, shellfish, chocolate, tomatoes, and milk that is contaminated with penicillin. Penicillin and other drugs also can cause the hive effect.

The wheals of urticaria may last from one to several days and may appear in one area of the body while disappearing from another area. The symptom may appear rather suddenly but generally is self-limiting and leaves no permanent scar or discoloration of the skin.

While the urticaria may be the allergic symptom that attracts the attention of the patient because it is more highly visible, angioedema can be much more serious. The edema that causes the swelling in subcutaneous and deep skin layers also can occur in the mucous membranes of the respiratory and gastrointestinal tract. The angioedema of the G.I. tract may cause abdominal colic and perhaps nausea and vomiting. Angioedema of the upper respiratory tract may result in obstruction of the larynx and threaten suffocation of the patient.

Eczema (Allergic Dermatitis)

Another type of skin reaction associated with allergies is eczema, which also may be called allergic dermatitis. This type of skin eruption is marked by itching, swelling, blistering, oozing, and scaling. Eczema may begin in one skin area and spread over other parts of the body surface. Like other kinds of allergies, eczema seems to have many possible causes and appears to have a hereditary factor since it tends to occur in some families but not in others.

One type of eczema can affect children as young as three months of age and probably is related to an allergic reaction to foods being added to the diet as the infant begins to eat things other than mother's milk or an infant formula. The common offending foods associated with infantile eczema include milk, eggs, and wheat, although other factors also may be involved.

Allergic contact dermatitis is a type of hypersensitivity reaction to allergens in industrial chemicals, metals, cosmetics, deodorants, mouth washes, dyes, textiles, and medicines such as skin ointments containing antibiotics. Common plants causing allergic contact dermatitis include poison ivy, poison oak, and poison sumac. The symptoms include the appearance of a rash with or without fluid-filled blisters or vesicles, and itching. The skin area affected usually is limited to the surfaces that actually have been in contact with the contact allergen.

Among unexpected sources of contact dermatitis allergy are compounds of nickel, chrome, and mercury. Depilatories, nail polishes, and deodorants are common cosmetic sources. Clothing causes may include chemicals used to produce permanent-press finishes, tanning agents used in the manufacture of shoe leather, and antioxidants used in producing gloves, underpants, bras, and shoes.

Some allergens involved in contact dermatitis are triggered by exposure to sunlight and are known as photoallergic substances. These chemicals may include antibacterial agents used in the manufacture of soaps and cosmetics, perfumes, after-shave lotions, and sunscreens.

Skin Tests for Allergens

Because many allergens can produce skin symptoms, the patient's skin is a common testing place for possible causes of hypersensitivity reactions to various substances in the environment. Several kinds of skin tests are used by doctors in their search for possible allergens. In a patch test, a tiny amount of a suspected allergen is applied to the patient's skin in a small dressing held in place by an adhesive bandage. In a scratch test, a small amount of the potential allergen is applied over an area of the skin that has been scratched to break the surface of the epidermis, and the substance is injected under the skin. If the patient has antibodies to a particular allergen, a skin reaction similar to the usual allergic reaction, but generally much milder, will occur at the spot where the test was made.

The tests usually are made on the patient's arm, above or below the elbow, or on the back. Several substances may be tested at the same time for screening and comparison purposes. Several dozen suspected allergens may have to be tested in this manner before the real culprit is found.

Food Allergies

When the offending substance is believed to be a food, the patient may have to delete certain foods from his meals to see if their absence for a period of several days seems to clear up the allergy symptoms. This can be a time-consuming inconvenience for the patient, but if the procedure

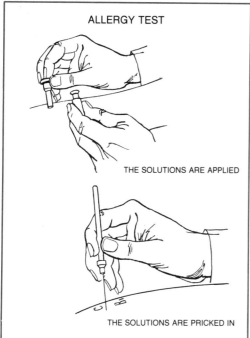

ALLERGY TEST

THE SOLUTIONS ARE APPLIED

THE SOLUTIONS ARE PRICKED IN

To determine whether a person may be allergic to a particular substance in the environment, the doctor can apply a few drops of a solution containing the substance to a small area of the skin. If the patient is sensitive to the substance, a skin reaction usually will appear within a few days where the allergen was applied. In some instances, a doctor may apply several different possible allergens and may prick the skin at the test sites to get the substances beneath the surface of the skin.

helps identify an allergen that may be the cause of a lifetime of discomfort, the food screening approach is worthwhile.

A fringe benefit of screening food items for the patient is that he may become more conscious than before of the substances used in most processed foods. If he is allergic to wheat, for example, he certainly will learn that many packages and cans of supermarket foods list wheat flour among the ingredients on the label.

Food allergies occasionally undergo remission—that is, the symptoms disappear for no apparent reason. After eliminating from the diet any foods that produce allergic reactions, a patient may discover later that a food that once was a cause of allergic reactions no longer produces its usual symptoms and can be restored to the diet.

Allergic Rhinitis

Another kind of hypersensitivity reaction that waxes and wanes at least slightly during a patient's life is allergic rhinitis, the disorder associated with inhalation of airborne pollens. The hay fever reaction of runny nose, sneezing, obstruction of swollen nasal passages, and watery, itching eyelids is probably the best example of an allergic rhinitis effect.

Allergic rhinitis tends to occur in persons with a family history of the same complaint, or a related allergy problem such as asthma or urticaria. The symptoms usually appear before the age of 30 and gradually diminish as the patient grows older.

Allergic rhinitis that is caused by plant pollens is a seasonal affair for patients who remain in one geographic area for most of the year. Only a relatively few plants propagate by producing a pollen that must be spread by air currents rather than by insects. The season of pollination is quite regular, but it may vary with different geographic areas, so that a patient who travels widely is likely to be exposed to airborne pollens in different climates or areas. Thus, he is subject to allergic rhinitis symptoms more often than one who is exposed to a single local pollinating season.

The seasonal allergic rhinitis symptoms can be extended by mold spores in the air.

Molds are more widespread than plants that depend upon the wind for distributing pollen, and the mold spore season may be different, starting earlier or later, and lasting longer.

When allergic rhinitis is a constant problem, regardless of the season, chances are the allergen is animal dander from hair and skin cells shed by wild or domestic animals in the area, by household or workplace dust, or by chemicals used regularly at work or at home. Dust often is infested with mites that are a cause of allergic reactions.

Why inhaled pollens and other allergens may affect the upper respiratory tract rather than the lungs can be explained in terms of the size of the allergen particles. The explanation is that the mucosal surfaces inside the nose are designed to trap foreign particles that otherwise would be drawn into the lungs with inhaled air. The smallest airborne particles, including some disease organisms, manage to slip through the respiratory screen. But pollen and other foreign substances, although too tiny to be noticed by most people, are at the same time too large to pass through the nasal mucosa trap. Enzymes in the nasal mucosa dissolve the outer coats of the pollen grains and release the protein molecules which are the actual allergens responsible for the symptoms.

Hay Fever

Hay fever is a good example of this allergy, but the name is somewhat misleading because the symptoms are not produced by hay and fever is not one of the symptoms. The allergic rhinitis that is called hay fever usually is caused by pollen grains of the ragweed types of plants.

With the exception of some sections of South America, ragweed pollen is present only in the atmosphere of North America, particularly the area east of the Great Divide.

The airborne pollens generally are those of plants that lack the colorful flowers or attractive odors that entice insects to them when the time comes to fertilize the species in order to produce seeds for next year's crop. These plants produce enormous amounts of pollen because survival of their species depends on a certain amount of luck. So they quite literally saturate the air with pollen, increasing the chance that at least part of the pollen will land on another plant of the same species somewhere downwind.

When the weather is sunny, hot, and windy, the pollen content of the air is likely to be high, and persons who suffer from hay fever can expect to experience severe allergic rhinitis symptoms. Cool, rainy days, when the air is relatively still, usually forecast a period of relief from hay fever symptoms. Ragweed hay fever days generally occur in late summer or early fall.

There are other hay fever seasons in North America that are not ragweed pollen seasons. During the spring months of April and May, some individuals experience a type of hay fever that actually is due to the pollen of trees such as maple, elm, poplar, birch, ash, and oak. During early summer another wave of airborne pollen begins, and the source usually is grass—bluegrass, timothy, Bermuda grass, Johnson grass, etc. In fact, grass pollens account for much of the hay fever symptoms experienced by sensitive persons who live outside the ragweed belt of the Americas.

Mold spores thrive during the warm

months of the year and account for the highest percentage of allergic rhinitis cases next to the pollen-caused cases. Molds grow profusely on vegetation, and grain crops of wheat, corn, barley, and oats are among favorite sites used by molds to manufacture the spores which are the mold equivalent of pollen grains. These spores carry the genetic material needed to help produce another generation of molds.

Farmers and others who live or work in areas where grains are stored or processed, such as in grain elevators, may experience a type of year-round allergic rhinitis because they are exposed continuously to mold spores spawned in stored grain or straw.

Still another kind of allergen that is associated with and may be confused with hay fever pollen is insect body parts. Although it is not a pleasant subject to contemplate, the fact is that the summer air quite frequently carries bits of insect bodies that are inhaled by humans. The scales, hairs, and particles of disintegrated insect bodies cause the same kind of allergen-antibody reaction as pollen grains or mold spores. Since there are more insects in warmer climates, the chance of developing a respiratory allergy, including asthma, is much greater in tropical or subtropical climates.

Asthma

Asthma is one of the most common allergic diseases, with many millions of victims in North America alone. Asthma is a disease characterized by obstructed breathing, or recurring spasmodic contractions of the bronchi which distribute air from the throat to the air sacs of the lungs. The disease can begin at any age, although the symptoms usually make their earliest appearance in childhood.

An asthma patient usually begins life in a family with a history of allergies. During early childhood the patient often develops juvenile eczema or an allergic rhinitis of the hay fever type. From hay fever to bronchial asthma may be a short step since about one-third of young hay fever patients eventually become asthma victims. It is not uncommon for a patient with hay fever, without asthma symptoms, to develop a bad cold and find that he has acquired asthma after the cold symptoms subside. An emotional upset also has been known to change a balanced case of allergy—one in which antibodies are present but there are no symptoms—into a case of asthma.

Asthma represents a severe case of chronic hypersensitivity reaction. The patient may suffer repeated attacks that require emergency treatment and hospitalization. The attacks are characterized by a narrowing of the airways because of spasmodic contractions of the muscles controlling the diameter of the bronchial tubes. Bronchial muscles are composed of smooth muscle tissue that gets signals from the autonomic nervous system. The attacks are marked by edema or swelling of the bronchial mucosal wall, inflammation of the tissues of the bronchi, and production of a thick mucus that is hard to expel.

All cases of bronchial asthma are not true allergies. Only those that are triggered by allergens are considered allergic asthma cases, usually designated as extrinsic asthma. Other cases, with the same or similar symptoms, are due to emotional causes, infections, or other factors that do not involve the antibody-allergen reaction.

At the same time, there are cases of intrinsic asthma, the nonallergenic kind, that apparently are triggered by allergen-type stimuli.

Allergy skin tests often are employed to determine if a case of asthma is extrinsic or intrinsic. Other tests that may be employed include one called the inhalational bronchial challenge, which requires the patient to inhale a suspected allergen to determine if it triggers an attack. A blood serum analysis that may be identified as RAST, for Radio-Allergo-Sorbent Test, involves the use of known allergens that are tagged with radioactive isotopes. If the patient's blood sample contains antibodies that have been sensitized against the test allergen, those antibodies will combine with the radioactive allergens. Laboratory personnel also can tell how strong the antibody response to a known allergen may be from the results of a RAST test.

GLOSSARY

ALLERGIES

The following entries define and describe the common and medical names of ailments, anatomical features, and other terms relating to allergies. Words in italics refer to separate entries in the list that provide further information on the subject.

allergen A substance that is capable of inducing hypersensitivity or an *allergy*. See *anaphylaxis*.

allergic dermatitis A disorder involving the skin, usually marked by redness, vesicles, and swelling that may extend beneath the dermis layer due to edema. The symptoms may result from a reaction between *antibodies* and *allergens* that may or may not be in response to direct contact between the skin and the allergen. The dermatitis symptoms may indicate an allergic response to a substance in food eaten by the patient.

allergist A doctor who specializes in the diagnosis and treatment of allergic disorders.

allergy An abnormal hypersensitive reaction by one's body tissues to a substance that is generally harmless to most people.

anaphylactic shock A serious state of shock resulting from a hypersensitive reaction to contact with an allergen. An anaphylactic shock may result from a bee sting in a person who is hypersensitive to bee venom. Symptoms may include breathing difficulties, falling blood pressure, cyanosis, convulsions, unconsciousness, and, if untreated, death.

anaphylaxis An exaggerated reaction of the body's vital systems to contact with an allergen to which the individual has become hypersensitized.

angioedema A swelling in the deep layers of the skin as a result of fluid accumulation. The effect is a symptom of *allergic dermatitis*. The condition also may be known as giant hives or giant urticaria.

antibodies Protein molecules that are designed and produced by the body's immune system for the purpose of participating in search and destroy missions against allergens that have entered the body.

antihistamines Drugs that are administered to counteract the effects of *histamines*, potent substances released from body cells as a result of antibody-allergen reactions. Antihistamines are intended to relieve the symptoms of histamine release, such as hay fever symptoms.

asthma A respiratory disorder characterized by bronchial muscle spasms that constrict the air passages to the lungs, plus accumulation of thick mucus in the air passages and other symptoms. Many but not all cases of asthma are associated with allergic reactions to substances in the environment.

contact dermatitis A form of *allergic dermatitis* that results from contact between the skin and an *allergen*. A skin rash resulting from touching poison ivy leaves would be an example of contact dermatitis.

dander Similar to dandruff; bits of skin cells and hairs from domesticated animals such as dogs and cats, or from wild animals, which produce allergic reactions in some humans.

desensitization The reduction or elimination of sensitivity of a person to a particular allergen.

eczema A general term covering most forms of dermatitis but involving mainly the epidermal layer of the skin. Symptoms may include redness, itching, scaling, oozing, etc., as a common allergic reaction. Eczema may begin in early infancy as a reaction to foods other than mother's milk and often signals the development of other allergies later in life.

elimination diet A procedure for defining the source of a food allergy by eliminating foods from the diet, then replacing them one by one to see if allergic symptoms disappear and reappear.

hapten A term used to identify an incomplete antigen. By itself a hapten is unable to elicit the formation of an antibody and must be combined with a protein in order to do so.

hay fever A common term for the symptoms of allergic rhinitis. The disorder actually has nothing to do with either hay or fever.

histamine A substance present in tissue cells throughout the body that has the ability to stimulate the autonomic nervous system and to act directly on the capillaries to increase their diameter. Histamine is released from the cells during antigen-antibody reactions.

hypoallergenic A substance that ordinarily may be an allergen but which has been treated or processed to reduce its allergic effect.

immune system A functional system of the body responsible for maintaining immunity or resistance to effects of disease organisms. Immunity is controlled in part by the lymphatic organs which produce antibodies. Active immunity can be produced by injection of a vaccine or serum containing the antigen of the disease, or by exposure to the disease itself. Passive immunity is acquired by an injection of antibodies from another person or animal.

mold spore A reproductive element of a mold. A number of species of fungi and other primitive plants reproduce by dispersing spores into the environment.

passive transfer A method of skin testing for allergens when it is not feasible to perform the skin tests directly on the patient. A sample of blood serum from the patient is injected into the skin of a subject who has shown no positive reaction to the suspected allergens. The allergen skin tests are performed several days later on the subject's skin sites where the serum was injected and where the patient's antibodies would be attached to the subject's skin cells.

patch test A technique for testing reaction of a patient to a possible allergen by treating an adhesive bandage with the substance and fastening it to the patient's skin for 24 to 48 hours. A skin reaction at the site is evidence that the patient is allergic to the substance.

scratch test A method of testing a patient's reaction to a potential allergen by scratching the skin on his arm or back and placing a small sample of the allergen in the scratches. If the patient is allergic to the substance, there will be a rash or other sign of dermatitis at the test site.

sensitization The initial exposure of a patient to an allergen, resulting in the production of antibodies resistant to the allergen.

tissue fluid A fluid with a composition similar to that of blood plasma which carries nutrients and metabolic products between the tissue cells and the blood in the capillaries.

toxin Any poisonous substance. A toxin may be carried by an allergen or produced in the body by an allergen. Antibodies sensitized to the allergen usually react by neutralizing the poison.

urticaria A medical term for hives, which are raised skin lesions surrounded by areas of inflammation. The swellings also may occur in mucous membranes. The lesions are accompanied by an intense itching sensation.

QUESTIONS AND ANSWERS
ALLERGIES

Q: *Is there any cure for allergies?*
A: A person whose immune system has developed antibodies for a particular allergen can be treated so that the symptoms are relieved. Or if the allergen can be identified, the patient can avoid the offending substance for the rest of his life. And there are remissions that occur in some cases regardless of treatment. But once the antibodies are established, they remain in the patient's tissues for many years, perhaps for life. They can be triggered to react by the mere exposure of the patient to the allergen at almost any time in the future.

Q: *My cousin develops hives just by being outdoors in cold weather. Is this the same as an allergy?*
A: The effect you describe is known as cold urticaria. Some people have a blood serum factor that is capable of transferring urticaria effects to the skin as a result of exposure to cold. While the cold temperature does not present itself as an allergen, it can trigger the same kind of physiological changes in people who are temperature sensitive. Blood samples taken of persons who are sensitive to the cold while they have an arm immersed in ice water usually will show the presence of histamines and other cell breakdown products that are the same as those caused by antibody-allergen reactions in the tissues.

Q: *Are there any places in North America where you can avoid ragweed pollen?*
A: Alaska probably would be the safest place to be if you really want to get away from hay fever. One survey of ragweed pollen showed no measurable pollen in Juneau, Fairbanks, or Nome, Alaska. There are a few places in New England that have a very low ragweed pollen index, but New England also has a few communities with a very high ragweed pollen in-

dex. These places range well over 40 on a scale that rates anything above 10 as "not recommended" for hay fever sufferers. The highest readings, those over 100, were recorded in the Middle West, with Omaha scoring a very sneezy 148.

Q: *Is alcohol something you should avoid if you are concerned about allergies?*
A: The answer might depend upon what form of alcohol you have in mind. Some people are allergic not to the alcohol itself but to the substances mixed with the alcohol in alcoholic beverages. A person who is allergic to grapes, for example, would be wise to avoid grape wines. But if the same person is not allergic to rum or vodka, there would be no reason to avoid such beverages on the basis of a possible allergic reaction. Some allergists might even recommend an occasional bit of alcohol to relax the patient, and the alcohol could be helpful by dilating arteries to improve the blood flow.

Q: *Is there anything an asthma patient can do to prevent an attack of the disease?*
A: Asthma attacks sometimes gain momentum once they start, so that it's important to try to get a head start on the attack once the patient becomes aware that an attack may begin. The patient must take his prescribed medication as soon as he gets the first signal of a forthcoming attack. The patient should keep the medication on hand at all times, even when going to bed at night. If it is important to take repeat doses of asthma medicines at specific times, the patient should keep that schedule even if it means setting an alarm clock as a reminder.

Q: *Will a room air conditioner help relieve the symptoms of a hay fever sufferer?*
A: An air conditioner can be quite beneficial to

a person afflicted with the effects of airborne allergens. But you must remember that air conditioners have filters that need to be changed or cleaned at regular intervals. The air ducts and other passages through which the air travels in an air-conditioning system also should be cleaned periodically. Otherwise, the irritants that can cause hay fever symptoms simply accumulate. And obstructed air passages in the system lower the efficiency of the air-conditioning equipment.

Q: *How do you find out if you really have an allergy or some other kind of medical problem?*
A: You can start by having a discussion about the subject with your doctor, who can then examine you for clues as to possible causes of allergies or other health problems. The doctor may refer you to a specialist in allergic diseases for a series of tests. The skin tests, blood tests, and inhalant tests of common allergens can produce rather conclusive results for most true allergy cases.

Q: *Suppose you find out you really are allergic to common things in the environment. What can you do about it?*
A: One of the first problems faced by many patients is simply one of adjusting to the fact that they may be allergy-prone. Discovering you have a health problem is not a reason to indulge in self-pity. Very few humans are perfect, and fewer still are able to live forever.

After recognizing the fact that you must accept some limitations to your desired lifestyle because of an allergy, you should make a detailed list of things to avoid. Avoiding allergens is perhaps the easiest way to cope with the problem. You may have to live without a cat or canary. You may have to stop sleeping with the windows open during the warm summer months. You may have to stop ordering lobster at restaurants. You may have to stop buying canned soups at the supermarket. You may have to stop putting chocolate sauce on your ice cream. These lifestyle changes are not tragedies, and the chances are that you won't have to give up all of your favorite goodies since individuals who are sensitive to many allergens are quite rare. But perhaps half the world's population may be allergic to one or a few substances in the environment.

Q: *How does a mother tell if her baby might have juvenile eczema?*
A: The signs of the eczema are one good clue, although they should be verified by a doctor. Heat rash, diaper rash, cradle cap, and other skin signs may or may not be indications of an allergy.

Other signs might be evidence of colic, vomiting, or diarrhea. When such signs and symptoms appear, the mother should try to keep notes, written or mental, about factors that might account for the health changes. For example, did the symptoms appear after a new kind of food was added to the child's diet, or did the child start wearing woolen garments? That sort of information can help the doctor determine whether the baby's symptoms might be an allergic reaction.

22

FACING EMOTIONAL PROBLEMS

Everybody has at least occasional days when nothing seems to go right. It is doubtful that anyone, no matter how wealthy or famous, is without a share of frustrations and disappointments, although the rich and powerful of the world often find help in coping with their problems that is not available to other people. It is the ways that various individuals cope with their emotional problems that can become the signs and symptoms of mental illness.

Emotional illness often is identified as a mild form of mental illness, a condition associated with purely emotional factors, while real mental illness suggests a disorder associated with a significant change in the anatomy or physiology of the brain. However, a mental illness can in fact appear in the form of abnormal behavior, regardless of whether the cause is psychological or physical. Doctors learn early in their training that diseases frequently involve a mixture of emotional and physical causes. Many patients' health problems are of a functional nature, that is, the pain is very real or there is a loss of hearing or some other disorder

for which X-rays, laboratory tests, and other diagnostic techniques cannot find a possible cause in the form of injury or disease. Functional illnesses are not the same as mental illnesses, but they fall in the gray area that fills the gap between organic diseases and psychological problems.

Doctors sometimes use the term "psychosomatic" to identify illnesses that seem to involve a greater emotional component than might appear to be warranted by the nature of the disease. It has been estimated that perhaps 50 percent of patients who visit a doctor's office have physical complaints that are at least tinged with some emotion. At least a small share of the doctor's time is spent in reassuring the patient that the future is not as gloomy as it might appear.

Emotional upsets, at the same time, can be the cause of a wide variety of physical illnesses. Asthma attacks, hives, peptic ulcers, high blood pressure, and certain diseases of the colon are among examples of disorders that are exacerbated by emotions.

The mind, of course, is difficult to find

or define with the usual medical research tools. Nobody has been able to catch an image of a mind on a piece of X-ray film or produce a piece of mind in a test tube. The best the scientists have been able to accomplish so far is a somewhat tangible record of the functioning of the mind on an electroencephalogram, or evidence of chemical changes that occur in brain cells during mental events such as dreaming. Most of the rest of our knowledge of the mind and its influence on health is based on circumstantial evidence from observing animal and human behavior, with and without stimuli or physical changes in the brain tissue.

It is simpler to define what is normal and what's not in terms of physical features of humans than in terms of mental health. What is considered normal mental health in a rural culture of an Asian country might not be accepted as normal in London or Kansas City, and vice versa.

What is Normal Mental Health?

For purposes of classifying mental health problems, doctors often begin by trying to define what is acceptable mental health for our own culture. The definitions might include an ability to give and accept love in relationships with other persons. Another definition might be an ability to withstand the usual stresses of everyday life without developing adverse physical or psychological effects. The latter definition does not exclude the possibility that any otherwise normal person might "crack up" under an unusual accumulation of stressful experiences such as those encountered by prisoners of war. Still another definition of normal mental health might be an ability to face reality and plan one's future activities in a realistic manner. Most definitions might be summed up as describing a practical and independent approach to survival without causing harm to one's self or to others.

Who Suffers from Mental Illness?

People who do not fit into such classifications include those who are mentally retarded because of brain damage caused by birth defects, accidents, or disease. A mentally retarded person usually has difficulties in learning and adapting to standard social behavior in addition to or because of below average intelligence. About three percent of the general population is mentally retarded because of genetic or chromosomal disorders such as Down's syndrome, complications resulting in premature birth or oxygen deprivation at the time of birth, infections during the fetal stage by such organisms as syphilis or rubella, viral and bacterial infections after birth, lead poisoning, and malnutrition before or after birth, in addition to dozens of other possible specific factors.

In addition to the definitely retarded, there is a much larger group of persons who are mentally handicapped because of below average intelligence that may interfere with normal social functioning. Sometimes identified as mildly retarded, they are able to attend school but have difficulty in learning, and they require supervision and support because they often are unable to function independently in a productive manner. They are employable and may marry, but their employment and marriage may be unstable. They may show poor judgment in situations involving the real world. These individuals cover a wide range of intellectual and social abilities, but many require custodial or supervisory care for most of their lives.

Loss of intellectual and emotional ability, by normal mental health standards, can occur as a result of aging processes, accidents resulting in injury to brain tissues, or abuse of drugs, including alcohol. Brain damage in later life usually is the result of arteriosclerosis of the arteries providing oxygenated blood to the brain tissues. The condition may be known as senile degeneration, or senility. This condition is likely to become more common in future years as the population of older persons increases—an ironical situation because they have been saved or protected from pneumonia, cancer, or cardiovascular accidents that previously were a threat to the aging person.

Types of Mental Illness

The traditional forms of mental illness have been the psychoses and psychoneuroses, disorders characterized by some loss of contact with reality. Persons suffering from a psychosis may have delusions, or hallucinations, or severe paranoid ideas. It is not necessarily abnormal to believe you hear voices or see things that are not actually present, or to feel "picked on" by others. But for a psychotic person such false or misleading mental inputs are real and vivid—a living nightmare from which he cannot escape. A psychotic patient may injure himself or others in an attempt to defend his life against imaginary enemies.

A psychoneurotic person might be described as one with an undefined sense of worry and apprehension associated with headaches, gastrointestinal upsets, and difficulty in sleeping. Again, most people experience occasional anxiety or tension that is strong enough to make sleeping difficult or cause indigestion. But when the anxiety is persistent and so intense that it results in a functional physical disability, such as hysterical paralysis, it reaches beyond the limits of normal mental health. Depression that is so deep and continuous that the person is unable to do productive work or has an obsession or compulsion, such as a fear of germs that requires the patient to bathe and wash his hands repeatedly, are examples of other forms of psychoneurosis.

However, there are other kinds of self-defeating behavior that are not in the same category as mental retardation, senility, psychosis, or psychoneurosis, but which are associated with ineffective ways of coping with reality. Those people, for example, who turn to alcohol, tranquilizers, or other drugs may feel anxious, tense, depressed, or otherwise insecure in their world. They retreat into a type of behavior which may or may not be acceptable to their peers, although it helps the person adjust temporarily to his problems. In some segments of society the individual may receive implied approval of his behavior because friends or relatives do not object to his excessive use of alcoholic beverages, tranquillizing drugs, or other drugs that are regarded as illicit.

Psychological Factors Causing Alcoholism

Public attitudes toward use of alcoholic beverages have always been paradoxical. Alcohol, or at least the ingredients for manufacturing alcoholic beverages—sugar, yeast, and water—have been on earth for perhaps 200 million years longer than humans have existed on this planet. Ancient Egyptian papyri, Chinese scrolls, and even the Old Testament discuss both the use and abuse of alcoholic beverages. The earliest American settlers in Virginia and Massachusetts encouraged the production of beer, wine, and distilled spirits, but at the same time they punished with jail, fines, and public whippings colonists who consumed too much of the products.

The attitude toward alcoholism then as now seemed to be that persons who drank more than their friends and neighbors were lacking in willpower and self-control. The modern mental health approach, however, is that how much a person drinks is far less important than when he drinks, how he drinks, and why he drinks.

The reasons may be physiological. While the possibility exists that there could be a genetic, physiological, or biochemical factor leading to alcoholism, no definitive data has been compiled to date to support this theory. If alcohol addiction were caused entirely by consumption of alcohol, one might expect that the heaviest drinkers would have the highest rate of alcoholism. But Americans and Swedes have a high rate of alcoholism and actually consume less per capita than people in France, Italy, and Greece. A number of psychological factors have been proposed to account for this situation, but efforts to identify the factors by various researchers have resulted in conflicting information as to traits or "unconscious instincts."

Sociological factors uncovered in various studies indicate that the incidence of alcoholism is low in cultures or subcultures in which all members agree to unwritten ground rules regarding the use of alcoholic beverages. There generally is an atmosphere in which the parents have established a pattern of moderate drinking. Drinking is not considered either a sin or a virtue, and one might decline a drink without offending any member of the group. No moral or social importance is associated with drinking; one doesn't have to drink to prove his manhood or adulthood. The beverages consumed usually are diluted or contain large amounts of nonalcoholic components, as in wine or beer, and the beverage is served with meals as a food. Finally, excessive drinking is not considered stylish, comical, or even tolerable. In families and communities that practice the foregoing rules, there may be moderate to high average rates of alcohol consumption, but the lowest incidence of alcoholism.

Determining where manageable drinking ends and abusive drinking begins for any individual is a difficult task. Familiar signs are job absenteeism, particularly on Monday morning, early-morning drinking, arguments about excessive drinking marked by insistence by the drinker that he is not an alcoholic, solitary drinking, an increasing intake of alcohol over a period of time, and the need to drink before facing a trying situation—like the individual who needs a couple of shots in order to feel comfortable at a party where alcohol will be served.

Despite jokes and cartoons depicting the typical alcoholic as a skid row bum or a patient in a state hospital, those categories of drinkers constitute only 10 to 15 percent of American alcoholics. The vast majority of alcoholics actually are married men and women who live at home with their families and hold responsible jobs while maintaining the respect of other members of their community. These alcoholics, however, have the best chance of kicking the habit, compared to the psychotic and skid row alcoholics whose prognosis for recovery is very poor.

Helping the Alcoholic

The married, home-owning, job-holding alcoholic can obtain effective therapy through his physician, his clergyman, professional therapists, and such groups as Alcoholics Anonymous (AA). Many doctors believe that AA can be an important adjunct to professional therapy because it is a voluntary fellowship of persons who are willing to admit their lack of control over alcohol and are dedicated to trying to keep each other from returning to the condition of alcoholism. Because of the AA emphasis on a nonsectarian spiritual direction in its programs—a member agrees to turn over his life and will to a "power greater than his own"—the AA therapy may not appeal to all alcoholics seeking help.

Psychotherapy may apply a similar approach but on an individual rather than a group basis. The alcoholic is taught to accept his condition as a form of sickness which requires the help of others to overcome. Details of the treatment vary with the therapist and the patient. Clergymen may offer a similar program that provides pastoral-psychiatric counseling for the patient.

Some physicians have offered treatment involving the substitution of tranquillizers or other drugs for alcohol. The obvious risk is that the tranquillizer might in itself become the basis for physical or psychological dependence.

There is a consensus that alcoholics are never cured. Surveys indicate that fewer than 20 percent of treated alcoholics maintain absolute abstinence for more than three to five years, although in some company-directed programs the rate of former alcoholics who have not returned to drinking may be as high as 50 percent. Whether a former alcoholic can learn to be a completely controlled moderate consumer of alcoholic beverages has been the subject of some controversy. Most doctors believe this theory not only is invalid but also dangerous to propose because it might lure former alcoholics back into alcoholism in the mistaken belief that they can control the problem.

Despite recent publicity about drug abuse, involving marihuana, cocaine, heroin, methadone, etc., the Drug Abuse Council maintains that alcohol still is the most widely consumed and abused drug. What is different is that more people are using alcoholic beverages *with* drugs, rather than instead of one or the other. Wine and methadone or alcohol and barbiturates became typical trends of the late 1970's among drug or alcohol abusers. The National Institute of Drug Abuse reported similar findings in its studies of the possibility that marihuana might "reduce the severity of the alcohol problem" by replacing in part the consumption of alcohol. "In reality," the government agency reported, "it now appears that alcohol use is a typical concomitant of cannabis use." Furthermore, the government cautioned, increasing use of marihuana seems to lead to an increasing use of alcohol.

Effects of Drug Abuse

Although marihuana apparently does not produce the type of physical dependence, or addiction, associated with alcohol, and there is little evidence to indicate long-term chronic effects of marihuana might be harmful, most doctors agree that there is no such thing as an entirely safe drug—and marihuana is no exception. Most of the scientific information about marihuana is based on clinical or anecdotal reports—studies with small groups or observations of patients by doctors. Lacking is the sort of long-term, broad-range research similar to the National Institutes of Health's famous Framingham Study, in which an entire community of 5,000 men, women, and children were examined, observed, and reexamined over a period of 20 years to see what effects food, exercise, smoking, and other daily habits might have on the development of cardiovascular diseases.

As a kind of rule of thumb, drugs that are sometimes called "uppers," or stimulants, amphetamines, cocaine, and most hallucinogenic drugs, cause only psychic dependence. Habit is the major reason for continued use of the substance. The use of an "upper" usually gives the person a sense of improved well-being or otherwise enhances his mental outlook.

Drugs that are "downers," like alcohol, narcotic drugs such as morphine and heroin, and barbiturates, cause physical dependence on and tolerance to the drug in addition to some psychic dependence. Also in that category are some nonbarbiturate sedatives and some minor tranquillizers. Physical dependence means that the body's tissues become dependent upon its regular, and often increasing, use; if the body's supply of the drug is interrupted, withdrawal symptoms develop. These symptoms vary somewhat according to the drug, the size of dose used, how long it has been used, and other factors, but the symptoms generally are the opposite of the effects produced by the drug. For heroin users, withdrawal may include lying in the fetal position on the floor and experiencing muscle twitches or tremors, hot and cold flashes, aching bones and muscles, anorexia, nausea and vomiting, diarrhea, fever, and spontaneous ejaculation or orgasm. Some patients develop muscle spasms that cause kicking movements. Fear of going through such withdrawal symptoms generally induces the heroin user to get another fix.

Tolerance means that the person addicted to the downer must gradually increase the size of the dose used because the drug's effectiveness at the previous dose is decreased.

Drug users also can develop a condition known as cross tolerance, or the development of tolerance to a drug that is chemically related to the one they have been using. Cross tolerance can develop within the basic narcotic family—opium, morphine, heroin, etc.—but not between narcotics and alcohol or between narcotics and barbiturates or minor tranquillizers. Cross tolerance does occur between barbiturates and minor tranquillizers or between those drugs and alcohol.

Information about cross tolerance, tolerance, and physical dependence can become seriously important to a patient or his family in the event of an emergency. A drug user may be relatively safe from the real world until he is injured and requires surgery. If the surgeons know what kind of drugs the patient has been using, they can manipulate their use of anesthetics to prevent complications. Otherwise, the patient may begin to experience withdrawal symptoms, and an anesthetic will not be administered in the proper dosage to compensate for the patient's drug dosage. A similar situation may face an alcoholic, or heavy alcohol user, whose body tissues have developed a tolerance for large doses of alcohol, requiring an adjustment in the amount of anesthetic administered to assure a lack of sensation during surgery.

Emotional Problems Causing Drug Abuse

The so-called hard drugs follow a usage pattern similar to that of alcohol. Generally, the behavior of the individual and the availability of the drug are important factors. Some medical experts in the field of mental health believe there may be an addictive personality who is attracted to this means of escaping from the reality of his frustrations and disappointments. His emotional distress is relieved by drug effects during early experimentation with the substance, and drug abuse behavior progresses from occasional use to tolerance and physical dependence.

While there may be no well-defined addictive personality, many patients who become physically dependent upon drugs exhibit personality traits that are contrary to those defined earlier in this chapter in the discussion of good mental health. The drug abuser often has a poor sense of self-esteem. He feels unable to cope with the stresses of his environment, particularly if he feels he is powerless to change the conditions. Drug users have difficulty in forming normal social relations with other people. They are dependent rather than independent. They are escapists who cannot face reality. Studies on drug users also indicate they may be self-destructive; they often have records of self-inflicted injuries and/or suicide attempts.

Like "good" alcoholics, some drug-dependent individuals are married, family-oriented, and otherwise successful, educated people who apparently developed addiction through the use of medications prescribed to control pain. As in the case of any "drug addict," the respected professional person who develops physical dependence upon a drug is likely to experience a certain amount of behavioral change, perhaps becoming a less responsible person. Eventually, he or she can expect to spend some time in hospitals undergoing treatment for withdrawal symptoms.

Preventing Mental Illness

As a result of the impact of drug abuse by young people in the 1960's, the attention of some public health workers was directed toward establishing areas of mental illness prevention. Just as preventive medicine was established as a method of controlling infectious disease, rather than trying to cure the effects of the disease after the damage was done, doctors specializing in mental health were asked to help define some of the specific factors associated with mental illness of the types in which retardation or brain damage was not the primary cause.

It was apparent that human behavior, whether bizarre, deviant, or normal, can be traced to a cause. The behavior of individuals does not depend upon random factors. Human behavior may be influenced by unconscious motivation and determined by emotional drives which sometimes compete with rational considerations.

Problem areas considered were specific behavior patterns that are self-defeating or harmful to others; role failures as students, parents, and employees; relationship breakdowns between husband and wife, parent and child, employee and employer; other interpersonal "games" that can become destructive; emotional over-reactions such as panic, escape, new situation anxiety, and temper tantrums; and personality decompensations, "going to pieces," or fits of depression.

Problem areas became "stress models" for identifying people or groups of people likely to be disabled or adversely affected by stressful situations, such as school children who could become dropouts or have behavior problems.

One study by the mental health workers took emotional development factors back to the birth of the child. Mothers of first-born infants were asked to rate their own babies at the age of one month compared with an average baby. Some mothers rated their infants as better than average while others did not. The results were concealed from a team of psychiatrists who interviewed the first-born children when they were four and a half years old, and again when the children were between 10 and 11 years of age. When the results of the psychiatric interviews were compared with the ratings the mothers gave the same children at the age of one month, it was found that offspring rated as better than average by their mothers had fewer emotional problems than children who had been rated as no better than average.

A follow-up study found that mothers of high-risk children, those expected to have emotional problems in later life, seemed less able to anticipate and fulfill the needs of the child. High-risk mothers had difficulty in perceiving danger or threats to their child and often were unable to protect the child adequately. The high-risk mothers seemed to use a limited variety of techniques for comforting the child, as compared to low-risk mothers.

They lacked confidence in themselves, were very vulnerable to criticism, and generally lacked self-esteem. The mother's attitude, therefore, appeared to set the stage for later emotional problems in the child.

One result of the study was a recommendation that the mother be encouraged to develop a new image of herself during the first weeks after the birth of her child. It was found that this is a period in which the mother's perception of her infant is still in a fluid state, but it also is a period in which there is little or no professional guidance given new parents. The new mothers need support and guidance, yet they usually do not see medical professionals again until four to six weeks after leaving the hospital, when they return to the doctor's office for a first checkup. The study group discovered that by providing the mother with background guidance, utilizing the help of other young mothers, the new mother could be given a positive attitude, making her feel valued and respected as a mother. This emotional support, in turn, makes the child feel valued and respected, and reduces the risk of emotional problems in later life.

Emotional Development of Children

The first months of a baby's life are seldom smooth, and the same might be said for the first years of a child's life. A great deal of patience is required of parents. By the time a second or third child has arrived on the scene, parents often are aware that each child is a different personality with his own pattern of growth and development. Stages in development more often than not occur earlier or later than the average predicted in many books on child development. Most children, in fact, tend to display a mixture of patterns, some typical of a preceding period and some typical of a later period of development.

During the developmental years the child encounters his first stresses, frustrations, and disappointments. Stressful situations that occur early in childhood usually have a greater impact than the same kind of event in later childhood. Stressful episodes for a young child can be feelings of isolation or abandonment. He also may develop emotional stress over feelings of deprived love. The sense of love deprivation may be interpreted from a child's fantasies that other children in the family get more toys, more food, more clothing, more attention, and so forth.

Other childhood concerns, which may be carried into adult life like the sense of deprivation, are death, disease, and disfigurement. Disfigurement fantasies may be expressed in concern about injuries or surgical operations that will change the appearance of a person's body or result in the removal of internal organs. Anxieties about physical capabilities may receive an added bit of stress as the child progresses in school and encounters other children who are bigger and stronger. The child also will have to contend with other children of his own age who will challenge his mental abilities. Then he can learn to be concerned about defeat or the loss of prestige among his peers.

Childhood emotional stresses often are not much different from the emotional challenges of adulthood. In later life, we also can be concerned about love deprivation, loss of prestige, the fear of death, disease, and disfigurement, and perhaps an inability to compete with the physical or mental capabilities of others. But the world is a world of stress and always has been. Emotional ills can begin when we feel overwhelmed by stresses that often are exaggerated in the mind.

Rules for Relieving Mental Stress

There are a number of rules that can be applied to help relieve stress when it threatens one's peace of mind. One is to laugh when you really want to cry. This obviously isn't easy, especially in the presence of a psychiatrist who may regard the reaction as an abnormal form of behavior. But actually it can help relieve tension just as easily as the sad approach.

When things go wrong, be as cheerful as you can under the circumstances. Keep yourself free of resentment or smoldering hate.

Recognize your abilities and weaknesses, and set realistic goals for yourself that can be attained with what you have to work with, including your hidden potentials that perhaps haven't been utilized so far.

Measure your success in long time periods, not by short, transient events. If you must compare your success with others', include *all* others—not just the competitors at the top of the heap.

Credit other people with having good motives. Try to see the good points in other peoples' characters even if they aren't your idea of good friends or neighbors.

Be willing to help those who need help. No matter what your own problems may be, there may be others with greater problems.

Keep as physically active as may be feasible. Physical exercise is a good tension reducer.

Do the best you can at whatever task you must perform. When you have done your best, don't worry about criticism from others.

Do not worry about the threat of death. It is the natural and inevitable end to life. Life is a gift that we are allowed to borrow for a brief while and then it must be returned.

Coping with the Death of a Loved One

Coping with grief after the death of a loved one can be a normal but stressful situation for any person. Yet attempting to cope with grief is regarded by some mental health experts as the wrong approach to the situation. Instead of treating natural grief as an illness and trying to help people recover from the emotional state, the bereaved should be helped to cope with death. As one psychiatrist explained, "We have forgotten how to mourn."

During the initial impact of death, the bereaved usually experience a sense of isolation and deprivation. The first few days after the death, close members of the family may be unable to grasp the reality of the situation and to accept the fact that the deceased person has gone from their

lives. They may need guidance at this time because they are confused.

The second phase of bereavement normally may last from a month to a year. This is a particularly critical period for a mourner who may be on the brink of mental illness because the bereaved person may create the false impression of adjusting nicely when actually he functions as if the deceased might be watching from the great beyond. The widow or widower may also feel angry and lonely.

The final, or recovery, phase of normal mourning usually doesn't begin until from three months to perhaps as much as two years after the death. Then the bereaved spouse or other close family members really begin to adjust to the reality of the loss and start to make plans for the future without the deceased.

Just as mothers often can help new mothers develop proper mental attitudes toward their role, widows or others who have made the transition from mourning back to reality can be helpful to those who have just lost a loved one by sharing their own experience in coping with death.

QUESTIONS AND ANSWERS
FACING EMOTIONAL PROBLEMS

Q: *What is the difference between a psychologist and a psychiatrist?*
A: The primary difference is that a psychiatrist, in addition to having special training in psychology, must have a license, either M.D. or D.O., to practice medicine. To be a certified psychiatrist, a doctor must complete three years of postgraduate studies in psychiatry and have two full years of experience in his field. He also must pass both a written examination and an oral examination which includes the examination of psychiatric patients while being observed by board-certified psychiatrists.

Doctors who specialize in child psychiatry may be required to complete a course of residency training in pediatrics, in addition to training and field experience in psychiatry and neurology.

Requirements for being a practicing psychologist vary with local regulations, but generally the person must have completed a minimum course of college education in psychology.

Q: *Is it possible to inherit a gene for emotional illness?*
A: There are certain types of mental illness that tend to occur more frequently in some families than in others. An example is a condition called primary depression which appears to occur in three different types of genetic patterns. The patient may have at least one close relative who suffers from depression and who may or may not also suffer from alcoholism, antisocial behavior, mania, etc. Because of inherited hormonal differences, patients in each of the three categories respond differently to medications.

Q: *Although my father died more than five years ago, my mother still talks about him once in a while, especially when she is troubled about something. Is this normal?*
A: It is not abnormal for a widow to display an attachment to a dead spouse after five years or more. The reaction depends in part on how deeply attached the man and woman were during their marriage. The behavior involving a dead loved one, particularly during life crises of pleasure as well as stress, is considered by experts as a means of "ego attachment" rather than a manifestation of mental illness. The condition, of course, might be considered pathological if the bereaved spouse was significantly involved with or totally devoted to remembrance of the loved one after the usual period of mourning.

Q: *Do hyperactive children develop into adults with mental health problems?*
A: Studies of adults who were classified in childhood as being hyperactive have found that some hyperactive behavior continued into adulthood, and that there was a higher incidence of alcoholism in formerly hyperactive individuals than in those with otherwise normal childhoods. However, the findings showed that hyperactive children were no more likely to develop psychotic disorders or to use drugs than were normal children.

Q: *I have read that tranquillizers can stunt the growth of children. Could this be true?*
A: Your information apparently is based on reports of animal experiments in which certain tranquillizing drugs were found to suppress the production of a hormone necessary for normal growth. However, studies of the use of tranquillizers in treating youngsters for periods as long as four years revealed no significant effect on the rate of growth as compared to children of the same age, sex, and mental disorder who did not receive the tranquillizer.

Q: *Are emotional problems the result of our modern lifestyles, or do people in primitive communities have the same kinds of mental illness?*

A: American mental health experts who have visited tribal villages in Third World nations have discovered that the people in those remote areas have similar psychotic and psychoneurotic disorders. What is different mainly is the explanation given for the condition of a person considered to be abnormal.

In villages of Laos, for example, a man considered by the other members of the community to be "insane" was found to be suffering from an organic brain disease; the villagers attributed the psychosis to an "abscess in the upper abdomen." Another person found to be psychotic was believed by the villagers to have "air going to the head." Cases that would be classified as psychoneurosis in America were attributed by Laotians to "exhausting the mind from worrying too much" or the fact that "her boyfriend treated her badly, then left her." Abnormal behavior also was blamed frequently on evil spirits acting independently or being manipulated by other humans through witchcraft or sorcery.

Q: *What effect can the behavior of parents have on the developing personality of a child?*

A: This subject has been rather thoroughly explored from the days of Dr. Sigmund Freud to the present, and there is an overwhelming amount of evidence that even unconscious communication between parent and child can result in various forms of psychoneurotic behavior. Unconscious communication can mean body language clues that may encourage antisocial behavior, depression, etc. A child's antisocial behavior, for example, may be encouraged simply by a lack of parental control, which is interpreted by the child as implied approval.

23

WHAT YOU SHOULD KNOW ABOUT PHYSICAL CONDITIONING

There are certain basic facts about physical fitness which, if applied conscientiously, can make almost any conditioning program work for you.

One is the fact that physical exercise helps to burn calories. If you burn more calories than you consume, you can expect to lose body weight.

Another fact of physical conditioning is that muscle strength can be increased up to an optimum level by gradually increasing the work load demanded of the muscle.

Still another fact is that heart and lung conditioning can be improved by performing exercises that cause the muscles to consume a greater amount of oxygen.

Muscles that are not used regularly will atrophy, lose strength, and grow smaller. Physical conditioning effects can be lost faster than they can be acquired.

There are no easy exercise routines. If an exercise seems easy to perform, you probably don't need it.

And there is no single exercise routine that will benefit all parts of the body. Physical conditioning requires a variety of exercises to be generally beneficial, just as good nutrition requires a careful balance of a number of different kinds of nutrients. Weight lifting is not likely to make you a better swimmer, and swimming is not likely to make you a better weight lifter. But a well-rounded physical conditioning program should include some swimming and some weight lifting, along with other types of exercises.

Will Exercise Get Rid of Calories?

Physical exercise may not be the best way to control calories; it's actually easier to avoid excess calories in one's meals. But exercise will help your body get rid of some of the fat deposit that represents an accumulation of excess calorie intake.

The rule of thumb for eating versus exercise is that one pound of body fat is approximately equivalent to 3,600 calories of food. A pound of fat can appear somewhat insidiously over a period of weeks or months. Just ten extra calories of food per day can add a pound of fat in one year.

One hundred calories of intake that exceeds your amount of calories burned each day can result in ten pounds of fat in one year.

Most people accumulate body weight during their young adult years. They may still have their teenage appetites, but they have acquired new lifestyles that demand more hours every week seated at steering wheels, desks, and TV sets. Just one pound of fat per year acquired in this manner can make a person at age 45 weigh 20 pounds more than he or she did at age 25.

A relatively simple form of exercise, walking, can help. But to burn the calories in one large gumdrop, a 125-pound woman has to walk for about 10 minutes. The same amount of walking will compensate for the calories in one medium-sized caramel. One piece of peanut brittle would provide enough calories to require a half-hour of walking.

Moving up the exercise effort scale a bit, a woman who consumed a 12-ounce chocolate milkshake would have to walk for two hours and 10 minutes to restore her caloric balance, or about three times the 40-plus minutes of walking required to burn off the food energy in one doughnut.

The notion that one "burns" calories of food energy by physical exercise really isn't hard to understand. When you exercise in the outdoors on a cold winter day, you may begin to feel pleasantly warm. At some time in your life you may have wondered why you could "work up a sweat" while working or playing vigorously in the snow. On a warm summer day the warmth of physical activity can become unpleasant, and it can be hazardous in the case of football players who fall unconscious during the first workouts of the season.

How Muscles Burn Up Calories

The body heat that produces such effects is evidence that the body is burning calories of energy that are released during the contractions of muscle cells. Each time a muscle cell contracts, the action requires a bit of energy. The energy comes from molecules of fats or carbohydrates that have been stored in the tissues. A molecule of a carbohydrate such as glucose, for example, contains atoms of carbon and hydrogen which combine with oxygen carried by the bloodstream from the lungs. The chemical reaction in the body cells produces molecules of carbon dioxide and water, and releases a tiny amount of heat which is dissipated from the body.

The energy released from the contraction of one muscle cell doesn't amount to much heat. But the human body contains a total of some 600 muscles, and each muscle contains an average of 10 million muscle fibers. A person playing football or tennis or chopping wood may be triggering the contractions of hundreds of millions of muscle fibers each minute. This activity results in the production of a significant amount of body heat.

During some sporting events the body heat produced by physical activity can literally limit the performance of the athlete, as in the example mentioned earlier of football players who collapse during early season practices when the weather may still be hot and humid. Distance runners, even though dressed much more lightly than football players, often complain about the effect of their own body heat as it affects their performances in competitive races.

When people are not physically active enough on a cold day, the body's own temperature control system sometimes takes over and produces body heat by automatic rapid muscle contractions that we know as shivering. This is another bit of physical evidence that calories are released by muscle activity. But it takes a lot of shivering on a cold day in January to balance the calories consumed in a piece of blueberry pie à la mode.

Developing Muscles Through Exercise

The fact that muscle tissue can be quickly lost when the muscle is not used is known to most people who have experienced a broken arm or leg. Some medical studies have found that a muscle can atrophy to about one-fourth its natural size within one year if it is not used regularly. Furthermore, the muscle fibers may be replaced by tough fibrous connective tissue. Occasionally, a doctor may find an elderly person who has lost the use of one or more of his limbs through muscle tissue atrophy that started from lack of regular use of the muscle.

Muscles that are exercised regularly and vigorously, however, gradually increase in size and strength. New muscle fibers may appear to meet the demand placed on the muscle group, and new capillaries will develop to supply the larger muscle with more oxygen and nutrients.

As muscle tissue is exercised, its operating efficiency improves so that less oxygen is required for a given amount of effort, but the improvement occurs only in muscles that are exercised regularly and strenuously. Professional or Olympic athletes sometimes show this effect in the larger than average muscles of their legs or arms, or on their left or right side, depending upon which part of the body carries the greatest work load for a particular athletic event.

Training Muscles For Strength or Endurance

Muscle tissue can be developed in one of two different basic patterns. Muscles can be trained for either strength or endurance, or for both strength and endurance. But strength and endurance development patterns are somewhat different. For endurance events, such as running in marathons, muscle tissue becomes adapted in a pattern that leads to more effective use of energy. Muscle tissue trained for greater strength acquires added amounts of protein in the parts of the muscle fibers involved in contraction.

If your objective is a conditioning program built around marathon running or jogging, exercises designed to increase muscle strength may not do much for your endurance performance. Championship weight lifters, on the other hand, may become quickly fatigued by a running event.

Natural body build may be a contributing factor to one's performance in physical conditioning. Marathon runners tend to evolve from the lean, wiry sort of people, while the "Mr. Muscle" type of physique may find greater satisfaction in fitness programs that emphasize development of muscular strength.

Nearly any serious physical conditioning program is better than none at all, regardless of body build. There are numerous activities that can combine the fitness effects of both strength and endurance training. Backpacking, for example, can be practiced in a manner that demands both endurance training by day-long cross-country hikes and strength training through carrying 40 pounds or so of food, clothing, and camping gear over every mile of the hiking trail.

As physical condition improves through regular workouts, the lungs and circulatory system become more efficient. The heart acquires a stronger stroke so that oxygen-enriched blood circulates more effectively through the muscle tissues and waste products are removed at a faster rate.

Avoid Muscle Overloading

Nature is very conservative about the use of bodily resources and will provide only as much muscle or bone tissue, or blood circulation, as the body demands in day-to-day action. When the body demands less, it gets less from nature, and the muscles do not develop but begin to atrophy. This is the underlying principle of conditioning sometimes called muscle overloading.

This means that in order for your muscles to improve or progress, you must try every day to demand more of them than they delivered the day before. There are some obvious limits to this approach; you are not expected to force yourself into a state of collapse, or suffer muscle strain or torn tendons. You will eventually reach a maximum or optimum plateau of physical performance. But to play the muscle overloading game, you must push a bit harder every day or every week toward a higher level of muscle development. Just one maximum effort each day is better than several less-than-maximum efforts.

How can you tell if you are overdoing the maximum efforts? If your body recovers overnight without signs or symptoms of muscle strains or soreness, you probably are not pushing yourself too hard.

But if you feel stiff, sore, and fatigued the morning after a big workout, drop back to a lower level of physical exertion and gradually work back up to a high level of maximum performance.

Establish Proper Exercise Routines

Don't be discouraged if you have days when you just don't feel like moving another step upward along the physical fitness climb. Keep in mind that your main objective is that of improving your own physical condition. You are competing only with your previous state of fitness. The program should never become tedious or boring, so if you really don't enjoy the exercise routines you have been using, try a different routine for a change. There probably are more different ways to exercise than any person is capable of mastering in a normal lifetime.

Any exercise routine should include a period of warmups before and after the main course of workouts. The warmups should include stretching and limbering exercises. Muscle and tendon damage often occur when a person plunges into a strenuous workout without first going through a warmup period of as much as 15 or 20 minutes. A similar period of stretching and limbering up exercises after a heavy round of physical activity can prevent a condition in which the muscles become shorter and lose some function as a result of repeated abrupt endings to strenuous workouts.

Stretching exercises for limbering up the muscles of the arms, legs, and trunk should be performed at a slow and easy stretching pace. At one time it was believed that warmups should be of the vigorous calisthenic type, but studies have found that they should instead begin like the slow limb-stretching exercises used by cats, dogs, and other animals getting ready for action after a nap.

The easier warmup exercises can be performed without an increased demand for oxygen by the body tissues. The body normally stores enough oxygen to carry a human through about four minutes of life without a fresh supply of the vital atmospheric gas. You can hold your breath under water for a few minutes, for example, without suffering permanent injury. And simple exercises such as walking can be performed without causing the normal person to develop the huffing and puffing associated with an oxygen debt that must be repaid.

Aerobic Exercises

Such easy exercises, because they do not exercise the heart and lungs sufficiently, are not the kind of activity that has become popularly known as "aerobic" exercises. Aerobic means simply "with oxygen," which is not to say that walking is "anaerobic" or "without oxygen," since any muscle activity requires the consumption of some oxygen. But endurance types of exercise require additional effort on the part of the heart and lungs because they consume the normal four-minute supply of oxygen in the tissues. Breathing and blood circulation must be increased to repay the oxygen borrowed from the four-minute supply in the tissues, and to supply a temporarily continuing demand for more oxygen than is normal.

Ideally, an endurance exercise should help the body achieve a steady state of aerobics—a condition in which breathing is heavier than normal but more than adequate to replace the body's reserve supply of oxygen. A runner who can keep up a rapid pace with little or no huffing and puffing—the sign of an oxygen debt—has achieved a steady state of aerobic conditioning. The heart and lungs work with the muscles in a well-coordinated pattern of oxygen intake, circulation, and calorie burning. The oxygen is used with increased efficiency and with less waste of energy than it would be in a person who is not physically fit.

Going back to the concept of the calorie burning aspect of exercise for a moment, it might be noted that a tremendous amount of breathing is required to burn a bit of fat or sugar. It takes about one quart of oxygen to burn one gram of carbohydrate. Since the atmosphere is about 20 percent oxygen, one has to inhale approximately five quarts of air to provide the body with enough oxygen to release the energy in one gram, or about 1/30th of an ounce, of sugar. A gram of fat requires more than twice as much oxygen for calorie burning than a gram of sugar, or perhaps 300 quarts of air for each ounce of fat.

Ordinarily, a human inhales enough oxygen every three seconds to sustain life in his body tissues. A vigorous aerobic exercise can increase the amount of oxygen needed by the body by 40 to 50 times the oxygen required by the same person while resting. After a very strenuous athletic event, an individual might require as much as ten minutes of heavy breathing in order to repay the body's oxygen debt. However, the carbon dioxide, water, and other waste products of calorie burning may take as long as one hour to be expelled from the body.

Most adults may not be able to achieve a level of physical conditioning that would permit such a tremendous demand on the heart and lungs, especially if they have dropped out of the fitness programs offered during high school or college years. Many young adults, those under the age of 35 and otherwise healthy, are able to reach an exercise performance level that increases by five times the heart and lung demand for the same individual who walks at a rate of about four miles per hour. This is equivalent to advancing a young adult man who is out of shape to a physically fit person who can run a mile in eight minutes.

The Air Force Exercise Plan

A program that can accomplish this feat requires progressive workouts over a period of about 16 weeks, and is similar to the plan developed by the U.S. Air Force for testing recruits.

The person begins by running, walking, jogging—or whatever can be done without discomfort—a measurable distance in 12 minutes. The only objective at first is to see how much distance can be covered in that time. If you can move at a pace of five miles an hour, you should be able to cover one mile in those 12 minutes.

Once you have established your beginning benchmark, you can try each day to either cover the same distance in less time than before, or travel a greater distance along the same route in the same amount of time. As you work toward either goal, you should gradually increase your heart and lung demand so that more oxygen is utilized more efficiently. A person who covers a distance of one mile at a jogging pace of six miles per hour utilizes from three to four times as much oxygen as when walking at a leisurely three miles per hour. A person who can run one mile in less than eight minutes uses between five and six times the oxygen consumed

by a moderately slow walker of the same age and body weight. At a pace of less than three miles per hour, a walker probably would not incur an oxygen debt.

Persons over 35 years of age generally are not expected to perform at the same level as younger persons. Most older, but not necessarily elderly, persons will cover less distance in the same amount of time, such as 12 minutes, and they will have a normally lower rate of oxygen consumption.

Isometric Exercises

Among the many exercise fads of past decades that may have some merit despite a few myths about the benefits was the wonderful world of isometrics. Isometric exercises can be useful for developing certain muscle groups and rehabilitating body areas that may have lost their total usefulness because of disease or injury. Unfortunately, isometric exercises have been identified as "easy" exercises that could be used to lose body weight and increase general physical fitness while the person is seated in an armchair with a cup of coffee in one hand. This, of course, is nonsense.

Actually, when properly performed, isometric exercises can be as physically demanding as almost any other strength-building exercise. The effort and energy that could be used to demonstrate certain isometric exercises at maximum performance levels might damage the muscles and tendons of the exerciser—as well as walls, doorways, furniture, or other objects used in the exercise test.

Most isometric exercise routines are of the "irresistible force against an immovable object" type of muscle-strength developers. They can be performed by busy people who do not have the time or space for weight-lifting or tennis. A businessman on a trip can perform some of the exercises in his hotel or motel room without disturbing guests in neighboring rooms. Isometrics can be performed by people who can't get away from home or the office because of bad weather, an expected telephone call, or other reasons.

In addition to the requirement that isometrics be performed forcefully, which is not always a convenient thing to do, the person seeking a new and different way to exercise should be aware that each isometric exercise is designed to enhance the quality of a single muscle group. In order to exercise the entire body with isometrics, one might need to run through quite a long list of different exercises, one for each muscle group of the body. However, to rehabilitate a weakened muscle or to develop strength in a muscle needed for a favorite sporting event, isometrics may be just the thing.

The theory behind isometrics is that the muscle exercised must be contracted with as much effort as possible without moving the part involved. It is a static exercise. A dynamic type of exercise, for purposes of comparison, is called an isotonic exercise. Examples of isotonic exercises are situps and pushups. Weight lifting is a type of exercise that incorporates both isometrics and isotonics—isometrics for grasping the weight on the floor and holding it overhead, and isotonics for lifting the weight from the floor to the overhead position.

A typical isometric exercise that can be done within a standard door frame, such as the doorway of a closet, is the arm press: stand in the doorway with the legs spread toward the sides, or door jambs. Keep the legs straight and the knee joints locked. From this starting position, extend the arms upward to the lower surface of the top of the door frame. Next, without actually moving the arms, begin pressing with as much power as possible against the door frame top. Gradually increase the pressure until maximum muscle contraction is reached, and hold the maximum contraction for five to ten seconds. Then relax the muscles for several seconds. Begin the muscle contraction pressure again and push it through maximum effort. Relax the muscles a second time. Then do a third arm press against the door frame top.

An isometric exercise should be done three times a day for the first week, with the number of repetitions gradually increasing until each exercise is repeated at least ten times a day. When maximum pressure is exerted, the person exercising may develop an oxygen debt, the door frame may give a bit, and the exerciser may be sweating after several maximum effort pushes.

A variation of the arm press is the leg press: stand with the arms extended to the top of the door frame as you did in the previous isometric exercise. The elbow joints should be locked but the knees may be bent slightly. Beginning with a gradual effort, press as hard as possible against the bottom edges of the door frame, pushing the leg muscles to maximum contraction. Hold the maximum contraction for five to ten seconds. Then relax the muscles for a few seconds. Start again and do at least three repetitions of the exercise.

The side press is performed as follows: standing in a doorway, extend both arms to the side of the door frame. The feet can be extended toward the sides but should not touch the door frame. Hold the palms of the hands outward against the sides of the door frame. Begin pressing with the palms against the sides of the door frame, gradually increasing the muscle contractions of both arms to a maximum effort. Hold the maximum muscle contraction for five to ten seconds. Relax the muscles for a few seconds. Then repeat the exercise. Do at least three repetitions of the exercise.

To do the lateral raise exercise, stand in a doorway and extend both arms to the side of the door frame. The feet may be extended toward the sides of the door frame but should not touch the frame. The backs of the hands should be placed against the sides of the door frame, the palms facing toward the body. Press the backs of the hands against the frame's sides with as much pressure as you can muster, increasing the pressure gradually toward a maximum contraction of the arm muscles. Hold the maximum effort for five to ten seconds. Relax the muscles for a few seconds. Then repeat the exercise and run through at least three repetitions.

Still another variation, one designed to strengthen the neck muscles, makes use of a door frame as the immovable object. The irresistible force is your forehead or the back of your head.

While isometric exercises generally are designed for persons who may be alone, there are several routines that allow two or more persons to do isometrics together.

One such routine requires two people and a length of rope or a stout cord. The two persons sit facing each other with the soles of their feet firmly planted against each other. Each person holds one end of the rope or cord. From this starting position, one of the team members lowers himself backward to the floor so he is in a supine position, while the other team member remains in a sitting position.

Each of the team members, presumably being of equivalent strength, exerts maximum effort in an attempt to overcome the effort of the partner and to change his position from supine to sitting, or vice versa. Like other isometric exercises, this one should go through several repetitions.

Some people like isometrics because the exercises require no expensive equipment. They can be performed almost anywhere one happens to be—alone or in the company of others. And they can be incorporated into other exercise programs, serving as warmups for other fitness routines.

Like other physical conditioning exercises, there always is a risk with isometrics of damaging the cardiovascular system, the muscles, or other body systems. Ligaments and joints can be injured by strenuous efforts to reach maximum muscle contractions. Therefore, a doctor should be consulted before one embarks on a strenuous physical conditioning program of isometrics or any similar effort. Doctors usually do not discourage patients from participating in fitness activities. But your physician might suggest an alternative approach better suited to your individual condition at the start. Dancing, for example, may provide as much exercise as several kinds of sports. Swimming or golf might not give the strength or endurance training your body actually needs. Certain sports are not suited for everybody, but for every person there is at least one suitable sport.

Exercise Equipment

When buying exercise equipment, the buyer should keep in mind that unless the equipment actually helps to improve physical health, it may be nothing more than an expensive toy. Exercising equipment is only as good as the effort one puts into its use in improving strength, endurance, and heart and lung fitness. A person who regularly lifts objects weighing 50 to 100 pounds might benefit from the purchase of a set of 10-pound dumbbells, but only if they are used to strengthen certain muscles.

Simple exercise equipment often is the best. An ordinary jumping rope, for example, can be helpful in developing both strength and endurance. Rope jumping can require good muscular coordination, breathing, and posture. Rapid body movement, muscular efficiency, and good timing are needed for long periods of high-speed rope jumping. Professional boxers have included rope jumping as a training exercise for decades, and some military combat units have adopted rope jumping as a fitness exercise.

Weight Lifting Weight lifting can be beneficial if it is part of a serious program of exercises directed toward a specific goal. Weight lifting should be used to increase the strength of certain muscle groups through a progressive pattern of muscle overloading. Muscles of the arms, legs, back, and shoulders are the most likely groups to benefit from weight lifting routines. Most traditional weight lifting exercise patterns are designed to help develop a specific set of body muscles. The weighted bar can be held on the shoulders while the person exercising goes through a series of alternate standing and squatting positions. The bar can be raised and lowered directly or moved from hip level to overhead, while swinging the weights through an arc in front of the body. The weighted bar can be held on

the shoulders while the upper part of the body is bent forward, then raised to an upright posture, and so on.

Exercises with weight-lifting equipment should be preceded by a series of warm-ups. The weights should be of moderately heavy size, perhaps 40 to 50 pounds. The weighted bar should be grasped with the hands held close to each other and the palms facing backward. The body should be in a squatting position when lifting the weights from the floor, and the back should remain straight through the lifting part of the exercise. Most experienced weight lifters inhale while raising the weighted bar and exhale while lowering it.

Dumbbells, like bar bells, are intended to be used to develop specific muscle groups, mainly of the arms, shoulders, and trunk. An upper arm exercise, for example, involves lifting the weights from hip level to shoulder level and back again while rotating the dumbbells in a curling movement. When done properly, the exercise requires strong alternate contractions of the biceps and triceps muscles. Because the biceps bends the arm and the triceps straightens the arm, a full contraction of one muscle produces a full extension of the opposing muscle.

Exercises with bar bells or dumbbells should be restricted to a few repetitions per exercise during the first week, gradually increasing the repetitions by perhaps two each week until a performance level of as many as 25 repetitions can be handled without stress or strain.

Bicycling Stationary bikes can provide an adequate amount of physical exercise for many people, if they are willing to work hard in a sitting position. Although stationary bikes that are equipped with speedometers and odometers may be more expensive than the simple basic models, the gauges can give you some guidelines as to your level of performance during a daily workout.

Ordinary bicycling, on a real two-wheeler, will help an average adult to burn about 4.5 calories per minute, or the equivalent of one ounce of body fat per hour. This level of activity is about the same as swimming, gardening, or hiking. But increasing the rate of bicycle speed, which

can be accomplished with most stationary bikes by adjusting the amount of resistance against the pedals, can hike the rate of calorie loss. Bicycling at ten miles per hour, for example, requires an average loss of seven calories per minute, compared with about four calories per minute at a speed of five miles per hour.

The same rule of progressively increasing the effort applies to the use of stationary bikes. Try to cover the equivalent of one or two miles a day for the first week,

STEP-UP

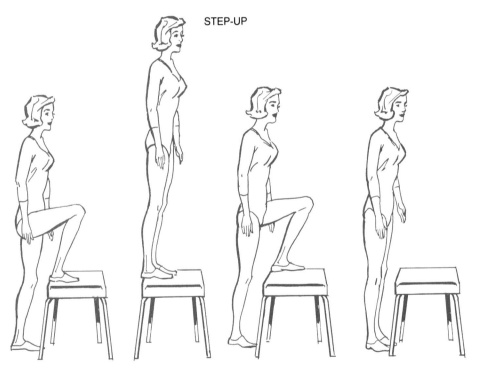

The President's Council on Physical Fitness recommends that a person embarking on a conditioning program use the "step-up" test to evaluate their physical ability to handle strenuous exercise and to check their conditioning progress from time to time. All that is required for the test is a sturdy bench, stool, or chair around 15 inches high and a watch or clock for checking the pulse. In a continuous four-count movement, the individual places the right foot on the bench (1), then the left foot so the body stands erect on the bench (2), followed by lowering the right foot to the floor again (3), and then placing the left foot on the floor again (4). The routine is repeated at a rate of 30 times a minute for two minutes. Next, the exerciser sits on the bench for two minutes after which his or her pulse is counted. The step-up test in itself can prove strenuous to a person who is not in good physical condition. But generally a person's pulse rate will become slower as the benefits of the exercise program tend to include improved muscular and heart-lung efficiency.

then gradually increase the distance logged to 15 or 20 miles a day.

Stationary bikes provide some benefits in the form of added muscle strength and endurance involving muscle groups from the shoulders to the ankles. A stationary bike can answer the fitness needs of many people who are unable to fit an hour of running or jogging into their daily routine, or who live in areas where it may be neither safe nor convenient to use a real bicycle. Also, a stationary bike in the bedroom can guarantee some vigorous exercise any day of the year regardless of the weather.

Step-bench Exercise An amazingly simple piece of indoor exercise equipment is a wooden bench about 15 inches tall and strong enough to support the weight of an adult standing on it. Doctors often use a bench of this sort to test the cardiovascular condition of patients. To use the step bench, as it is called, one steps up on the bench, one foot at a time, then back down to the floor, again one foot at a time.

To make a proper exercise routine of the step bench it is necessary to step up and down in a pattern and at a regulated pace. For example: (1) left foot up, (2) right foot up, (3) left foot down, (4) right foot down. After 10 repetitions of left foot first, change the pattern to right foot first. The pace should be at a rate of 90 steps per minute, which can be measured with a metronome if one is available. If there is no metronome to tick off the ideal rate of step movements, the exerciser can simply count from one through four and repeat the count.

The step bench exercise routine may appear easy. But anybody who has tried to maintain a steady pace of stepping up and back at a rate of 90 steps per minute over a period of five minutes knows this can be a very tough endurance test. And he will understand why doctors use this exercise test to determine the cardiovascular fitness of patients.

Physical Fitness Programs for Women

Modern women have demonstrated that they are capable of handling most, if not all, of the traditional male exercise routines. They also develop the same kinds of medical problems as men when they avoid physically demanding activities in favor of a sedentary lifestyle that can lead to obesity, heart disease, muscle atrophy, or disorders of weight-bearing joints.

Girls who plan to fill the traditional adult role of wife and mother rather than, or in addition to, that of a liberated career woman may have a greater need for optimum physical fitness than they may have expected. Some fitness experts have recommended that girls should learn weight-lifting exercises because they need strength in the arms, shoulders, and trunk for the duties associated with motherhood and home management.

A young mother who gives birth to a seven-pound infant can expect to be lifting a 20-pound child a year later. She may have to lift or carry a 30-pound youngster a dozen times a day before the child is old enough to walk. In addition to supporting the weight of one or more infants or toddlers, she may have to cope with loads of laundry, groceries, and other tasks that require great resources of energy, strength, and endurance. Marriage and motherhood thus can be more physically demanding than a job that requires operation of a fork-lift truck in a factory.

Every woman, particularly one who is old enough to have been a wife and mother, should consult a physician before embarking on a vigorous program of exercises and sports activities. While most women can adapt easily to a progressively active fitness program during their adult years, the doctor may want to make a careful examination to determine whether childbearing years or years of physical inactivity have resulted in bodily changes that might require a shift in fitness conditioning plans. Since each individual, male or female, is somewhat different from the next individual, the doctor might advise one person to be less physically active and also might recommend that another seek a more vigorous form of exercise. An overweight woman who told her doctor during a physical examination that she got plenty of exercise daily by walking her dog was advised by the physician, "Maybe you should get a bigger dog."

Although women obviously are different from men in certain ways, their heart, lungs, and muscles work in approximately the same manner, and they require the same sort of effort for improved strength, endurance, and energy efficiency. An exercise that does not develop better muscle, cardiovascular, or respiratory functions probably is not a good exercise.

In addition to exercises already mentioned, such as weight lifting and isometrics for developing muscle strength in the arms and shoulders, many women need exercise routines that help improve the musculature of the back and abdomen. Jogging or running in place, twisting and bending at the waist, touching the right hand to the left foot and the left hand to the right foot from a standing position, doing situps, and performing modified pushups are all recommended for women.

According to the President's Council on Physical Fitness, a mature young woman should be able to do five situps and run in place for two minutes at the *beginning* of a fitness program. Within two or three months she should be able to increase that ability to 25 situps and running in place for six minutes. Some women may require longer to advance from the lower level of performance to the maximum; others may be able to do maximum performance exercise on the first day of their conditioning program.

The modified pushup exercise is done as follows: from the starting position—lying prone, or face down, on the floor with the legs together but the knees bent and the feet raised above the floor—position the hands with the palms facing downward on the floor beneath the shoulders.

KNEE PUSHUP

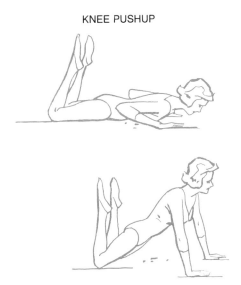

Knee pushups are sometimes recommended for women and others in the early stages of physical conditioning. The exerciser starts by lying on the floor, the legs together, knees bent and feet off the floor, but hands on the floor with palms down. At the count of one, the arms are extended to push the upper body off the floor in a straight line from head to knees. On the count of two, return to the starting position.

At the count of one, push the upper part of the body off the floor until the elbows are straight and the arms are fully extended. The body should form a straight line from the head to the knees. On the count of two, return to the starting position. This is a modification of a regular pushup, in which the knees are raised above the floor and the legs as well as the arms are straight. In the modified pushup recommended for women, the knees are allowed to remain in contact with the floor.

To perform the toe touch exercise, stand at attention. On the count of one, bend forward and down, keeping the knees straight, and touch the fingers to the ankles. On the count of two, bounce and touch the fingers to the tops of the feet. On the count of three, bounce again and touch the fingers to the toes. Then count four and return to the starting position.

During the first week of a fitness program, an otherwise healthy woman should be able to do eight modified pushups and five toe touches. She also should be able to do eight sprinters, according to the President's Council on Physical Fitness. A woman who is in very good physical condition can do 24 sprinters.

To do the sprinter, squat with the hands on the floor and the fingers pointed forward, with the right knee bent and the left leg extended fully to the rear. On the count of one, reverse the position of the feet in a single bouncing movement, bringing the left foot forward while extending the right leg backward. On the count of two, reverse the feet again in a bouncing movement, returning to the starting position.

There are several warmups that are particularly recommended for women as

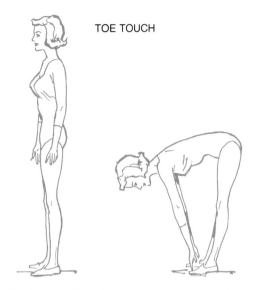

TOE TOUCH

The "toe touch" routine is a basic warmup exercise for both women and men. From a starting position of standing at attention, the exerciser bends forward and down at the count of one, touching the finger tips to the ankles. On the count of two, the exerciser bounces and moves the fingers down a bit to touch the top of the feet. On the count of three, the fingers move farther so they touch the toes. On the count of four, the exerciser returns to the starting position. Women should be able to begin with five "toe touch" exercises in a row and gradually progress to 20; men are expected to start with ten and progress to 30 as their level of conditioning improves.

muscle toners and stretchers. One is a make-believe bicycle movement performed while lying in a supine position, the hips and legs supported by the hands while the elbows rest on the floor. The legs are pumped vigorously for several minutes in a movement simulating the pedaling of a bicycle.

Another warmup favored by many women is the cheerleader exercise. The woman kneels on the floor with the back held straight and hands on the hips, like a high school cheerleader. Then she bends her body backward as far as it can be moved without discomfort while keeping the back straight and the knees on the floor. After returning to the starting position, the warmup is repeated several times.

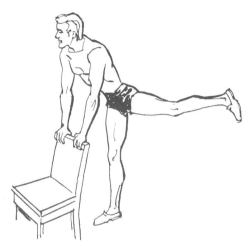

Some exercises, such as the back leg swing, are recommended by the President's Council on Physical Fitness as a conditioner for developing muscles in the lower part of the body. They should be included with every workout. The exercise is performed by starting from a standing position, with the feet together and the hands resting on the back of a chair for support. On the count of one, lift one leg back and up as far as it will go without straining the muscles. On the count of two, return to the starting position. The exercise should be repeated 20 times with each leg.

Ballet-type warmups to develop muscles in the lower part of the body can be done with a piece of furniture, such as the back of a straight chair, for support. With both hands on the chair back, the weight of the body is balanced on one leg while the other leg swings forward, backward, and sideways as far as the leg can be stretched without discomfort. After several repetitions, the weight of the body can be trans-ferred to the leg just exercised, and the same ballet stretches in three directions can be applied to the other leg.

Exercises for Children Because children generally give the impression of possessing limitless energy, adults often assume that youngsters are in good physical condition. Unfortunately, most children are expected to shift for themselves in obtaining proper physical fitness, even in schools that allow daily periods for recess or sports. When standard physical fitness tests are given children in some schools, nearly half can be expected to fail. A U.S. Air Force study found that two-thirds of its teenage recruits were unable to run a mile in less than eight minutes, although the recruits were considered fit for active military duty. An eight-minute mile is approximately equivalent to twice the speed of a brisk walk.

As with adults, children should receive a good medical examination before entering a vigorous physical conditioning program. Adults may need advice about activities that might cause complications in conditions such as heart disease, high blood pressure, or hernias. Children may have to contend with the effects of abnormalities that might have gone unnoticed, such as orthopedic defects involving development of bones and muscles, and vision or other perceptual difficulties which might interfere with the proper coordination required for many contact sports.

Parents should watch for signs or symptoms of abnormal effects following physical exertion by children. Breathlessness after exercise is not unusual; it may be assumed to represent the normal oxygen debt repayment associated with any aerobic activity. But huffing and puffing long after exercise, persistent weakness, shakiness or fatigue, pale or clammy skin, or cyanosis (bluish coloring) of the lips or fingernails could signal a serious medical problem requiring the attention of the family doctor or a specialist.

If a youngster fails to recover quickly from the effects of strenuous exercise, this does not necessarily mean that the child is destined to lead a life of physical restriction. The doctor may recommend corrective medical care for the problem. In some cases the condition may be corrected with a diet that assures a proper intake of essential nutrients. Parents should never assume that food consumed away from home, including school lunches, will some-

how guarantee good nutrition. The doctor may find that the child is trying to compete at a performance level beyond his current abilities and may recommend a more basic fitness conditioning program until the child is able to advance to a more demanding level of physical activity.

The President's Council on Physical Fitness has established several basic standards of physical fitness for boys and girls over the age of nine years. A ten-year-old boy should be able to do at least one pull-up as a test of arm and shoulder strength, 25 sit-ups as a test of abdominal muscle strength, and four squat-thrusts in ten seconds. A ten-year-old girl is expected to do one pull-up, 20 sit-ups, and three squat-thrusts in ten seconds.

The number of pull-ups required to pass the standard fitness test gradually in-

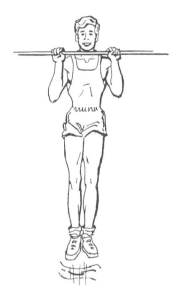

Boys are expected to be able to outperform girls in several areas of muscular fitness. While a ten-year-old girl, for example, needs only to hold her body in a pull-up position for three seconds in order to pass the arm and shoulder strength test, a boy of the same age must be able to pull his body up from the floor with his arms until his chin is higher than the bar. (A girl can be lifted to the pull-up position and thus does not have to be strong enough to pull up her body weight.) To complete the test, the boy must be able to lower his body until the arms are fully extended.

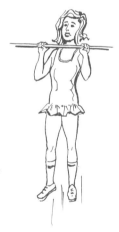

The President's Council on Physical Fitness has devised a number of tests and exercises for children. One test for girls between the ages of 10 to 17 helps evaluate the arm and shoulder muscle strength. Called the flexed arm hang, the youngster hangs with the chin above a bar, the elbows flexed but the legs straight and feet off the floor. Knees must not be raised and kicking is not permitted. The idea is to see how long the girl can hold herself in that position. The minimum amount of time required to pass the test is three seconds.

creases with age to a minimum of five for a 17-year-old boy. One pull-up is credited for each time the boy can raise his chin above a crossbar that is high enough for the youngster to grasp with the palms of his hands while his arms and legs are extended and his feet are off the floor. For girls, the pull-up is easier; she may be supported until she is in the position of hanging by her arms, with the elbows flexed and her chin above the bar. However, the girl is required to hold that position for at least three seconds without allowing her chin to touch the pull-up bar.

Sit-ups are the same for both boys and girls. The youngster must lie on his back with the knees flexed and the hands grasped behind the head, the fingers laced. Another person holds the ankles to make sure the heels remain in contact with the floor during each sit-up. Girls above nine years of age are expected to be able to do 20 sit-ups. For boys the number required by the standard test increases each year from 25 at age ten to 50 sit-ups at age 16.

The squat-thrust test for physical agility is a four-count exercise. The starting position requires the child to stand erect with hands at the sides. At the count of one, the youngster bends his knees and places his hands on the floor in a squatting position. At the count of two, he thrusts his legs backward so his body forms a straight line from shoulders to

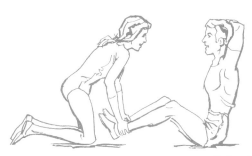

Both girls and boys should be able to pass a "sit-up" test for abdominal muscle strength. No equipment is required but a soft surface can be used rather than hard ground or floor. Boys and girls can test each other on sit-ups, one holding the heels of the partner to the floor while counting the number of sit-ups. The starting position is from a supine position, the knees flexed and the feet about 12 inches apart. The hands are grasped behind the head and held with fingers laced. On the count of one, the person being tested raises his, or her, trunk to a sitting position and turns the body to the left, touching the right elbow to the left knee. On the count of two the exerciser returns to the starting position. At the count of three, the body is raised again to a sitting position, but the trunk is turned to the right so that the left elbow touches the right knee. Then, on the count of four, the exerciser returns to the starting position.

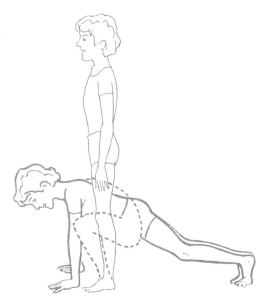

An agility test for children, is the "squat-thrust," an exercise useful for men and women as well. The exercise is started from a position of standing at attention. At the count of one, the youngster bends his knees and moves into a squatting position with both hands on the floor. On the count of two, he thrusts both legs backward so that the body forms a straight line from the shoulders to the feet. The position is the same at this point as that required in doing pushups. At the count of three, the youngster returns to the squat position and on the count of four resumes the starting position.

feet, with the arms extended and elbow joints locked. At the count of three, he returns from the pushup position to the squatting position. And at the count of four he resumes the starting position.

There are many conditioning exercises designed especially for children. Some are modifications of exercises used by adults. For example, a game known as "tortoise and hare" is little more than an adaptation of the adult exercise of jogging in place. For children the jogging pace goes slowly after the command of "tortoise," and at a double-time rate when the leader says "hare."

Other children's exercises are games youngsters are likely to play without adult supervision. Hopping on one foot in a large circle is something children often do for fun, little realizing that it is a recommended exercise for strengthening the leg extensor muscle. The wheelbarrow game, in which one child walks forward on his hands while a second child walks behind while holding his legs, is regarded as an excellent exercise for developing strength in the arm, shoulder, and abdominal muscles.

Cartwheels, forward rolls, backward rolls, shoulder rolls, and other tumbling exercises that seem to come naturally to

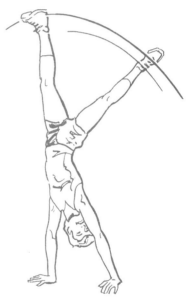

Cartwheels help a youngster develop coordination, agility, and control of the body in motion. A cartwheel should be practiced on a relatively soft surface, like a tumbling mat. It begins from a standing position. The child makes a quarter turn to the left, placing the right foot sideward with the right arm extended upward. Next, the weight is transferred to the right foot while the right hand is extended to the mat. Meanwhile, the exerciser swings the left leg upward while placing the left hand on the mat. Arms and legs are kept spread apart during the exercise. When the left foot touches the mat, the exerciser pushes off with the right hand to follow through to the original standing position.

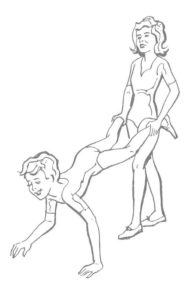

Wheelbarrow is a game children often play by themselves. However, it also is a good exercise for developing muscle strength in the arm, shoulder, and abdomen. One youngster takes the hands and knees position, the hands directly under the shoulders and the fingers pointing outward. The other child grasps the partner's ankles, raising the legs. The first youngster then walks forward on his hands, the feet and legs being supported by the partner walking behind.

children can help develop agility, coordination, and muscle tone.

As youngsters grow older, they become capable of mastering exercises designed to test strength and endurance, such as the fireman's carry that requires lifting and carrying the weight of another person of the same age group, or rope-climbing drills. Most individuals in their later teens are able to participate in nearly any exercise or sporting event offered to adult men and women. In some sports, teenagers today often turn in better performances than the adult champions of a generation ago.

Exercise Tests for Older People Some loss of strength and heart-lung efficiency can be expected in adults approaching the retirement years of life. There also is an almost predictable osteoarthritis condition in older persons that may be demonstrated by X-rays or other medical diagnostic techniques before the individual begins to experience the symptoms of the disorder.

The rate of decline of strength and endurance often can be slowed by older persons who maintain a regular program of fitness conditioning. The ability to move body joints through a normal range of motion tends to decline with advancing age, but moving the joints in proper exercise routines can delay this apparently natural process.

Another common problem of aging is a gradual loss of the sense of balance. The body's balance mechanism is particularly vital for older people who may suffer from visual disorders that require the wearing of bifocals or trifocals, the eyeglass lenses for near, far, or in-between focusing due to the loss of visual accommodation. People who must shift from one

visual focus to another while walking or climbing stairs are vulnerable to missteps and mishaps, and the risk increases greatly if the sense of balance has been lost. For this reason, the older persons should include in their fitness program exercises that help them maintain some agility and coordination.

The President's Council on Physical Fitness recommends a three-stage exercise test for older persons. The test may appear simple enough for young adults who are normal and healthy, but for a person beyond his prime the pre-exercise test may represent quite a challenge.

The first stage requires a brisk ten-minute walk on a level surface outdoors, although it can be done on a suitable indoor surface. The main thing is to walk briskly for ten minutes without interruption and discomfort.

Any adverse health effects experienced during the test are good reasons to interrupt the test. Some individuals may feel a throbbing in the head, pain in the chest or legs, nausea, tremors, or breathlessness. Any ill effects should be reported to the patient's doctor. If the older person can walk for only five minutes before the adverse effects begin, it doesn't mean he's out of the game. If he can walk at least three minutes at a brisk pace before the onset of the symptoms, it simply means the patient should not adopt the same exercise program as the fellow who can go the full ten minutes without problems.

The older person who passes the ten-minute walk test qualifies for the second stage, a walk-jog test. The walk-jog test requires 50 steps walking followed by 50 jogging steps, and repetitions of the series for a total of six minutes. The walking part of the test must be done at a pace of 120 steps per minute, a task that is accomplished by having the left foot touch the ground once every second. The jogging pace of 144 steps per minute is at a brisker rate that may require a little practice to master.

The third stage, an advanced walk-jog exercise that may be postponed until the following day, requires ten minutes of walking and jogging in alternate series of 100 walking steps and 100 jogging steps.

The pre-exercise tests are not competitive. Nobody wins a medal for doing ten minutes of walk-jogging, and few people ever flunk the three-minute minimum walk test. The purpose is merely to give the older person and his doctor a rough idea of where the patient should begin an exercise rehabilitation program. The program should not be too easy or too difficult.

Most of the recommended exercises for older persons are modified calisthenics. The warmup routine may consist of nothing more strenuous than walking briskly about a room, or outdoors, for two minutes. He begins with perhaps two repetitions of each of a series of calisthenics and works up to ten repetitions over a period of from one week to one month, working at his own pace.

A typical exercise might be the bend and stretch: start from a position of standing erect with the feet a shoulder-width apart. Bend forward at the waist and try to touch the toes. Bending the knees is permitted. Then return to the starting position.

Another exercise could be the head rotation: start from a position of standing erect, with the feet a shoulder-width apart, and hands on the hips. At the count of one, slowly rotate the head as far as possible from left to right. At the count of two, rotate the head in the opposite direction.

Still another exercise consists of walking a straight line ten feet long by means of heel-to-toe steps, with the arms held away from the body for balance. Then one turns and walks back in the same manner.

No matter how young or old, healthy or disabled a person is, there are physical conditioning exercises for people of all ages and stages of fitness.

QUESTIONS AND ANSWERS
PHYSICAL CONDITIONING

Q: *I have been hospitalized for coronary heart disease. Would isometric exercises be a suitable type of conditioning program for me?*

A: Probably not. Isometric exercises can have the effect of constricting your coronary arteries, according to University of Texas studies, at a time when your heart needs additional blood flow because of the physical effort. Ask your doctor to recommend a conditioning exercise that allows more total body motion, such as swimming.

Q: *I have read that golf is not a good way to exercise. What's wrong with the game as a form of exercise?*

A: The problem is not so much with the game of golf but the way some people go about it. For example, there's not much physical effort required to travel about a golf course in a motorized cart, or to have a caddy carry the clubs. A golfer who carries his own clubs and jogs along the fairways probably gets more benefit from the game than one who takes it easy. There's nothing in the rules that says you can't put some physical effort into your game.

Q: *How does walking compare with jogging in burning calories?*

A: When male college students were tested on a treadmill, it was found that jogging a mile required an average of 26 calories more than walking, although the walking speed was measured at five miles per hour compared with the usual pace of about three miles per hour for serious exercise walking.

Q: *Does jogging speed affect the rate of calories burned?*

A: Yes, if the speed exceeds about seven miles per hour. Slow jogging requires only slightly more energy than walking at that same speed.

Q: *Are there any health conditions that would make it dangerous for a person to participate in scuba diving?*

A: This is a difficult question to answer because there are a number of factors that need to be resolved, including the age of the person, his mental health, and any underlying conditions that might be affected by the effect of deep water pressures on the human body. Only your own doctor can tell you if you as an individual should take up scuba diving.

To summarize briefly the parameters of the health effects of scuba diving, nearly any chronic disease involving the respiratory system, the nervous system, and the cardiovascular system could provide a reason to avoid scuba diving. Asthma, a perforated eardrum, sinus problems, middle ear infection, essential hypertension or high blood pressure, arthritis, angina pectoris, congestive heart disease, abnormal heart rhythm, and juvenile onset diabetes are among the possible reasons a doctor might advise against scuba diving. The list also might include pregnancy, drug addiction, and certain psychotic and psychoneurotic disorders. A rather recent addition to health problems that might preclude scuba diving is obesity; at one time doctors assumed that a fat person would have an advantage in buoyancy and insulation, but it has been found from experience that obese scuba divers are particularly prone to decompression sickness.

Q: *Should a woman wear a brassiere when she exercises?*

A: There are special brassieres that have been developed in recent years to provide proper support for women who want to participate in vigorous exercise routines. The exercise bras were designed to overcome the complaints of university women who found that plastic and metal parts of ordinary brassieres caused chafing and soreness from the friction of body motion during jogging and similar exercises.

Q: *Will jogging protect you from a heart attack?*
A: No. It's unlikely that any particular exercise routine will protect anyone from a heart attack. Jogging, marathon running, and other forms of aerobic exercises can reduce your chances of developing coronary heart disease prematurely, provided you also watch your weight, avoid cigarette smoking, and, among other factors, choose the right parents. In fact, there have been cases of runners who died of heart disease while exercising, but in documenting the cause of death it was found the runners had a strong family history of heart disease.

Q: *Are there any conditioning exercises a skier should do during the warm weather months to keep the legs in shape?*
A: A number of different exercises can be performed to keep the hamstrings, quadriceps, and Achilles tendons in fairly good shape for winter skiing. They generally include leg stretches done by standing on your toes at the edge of a step, sitting on the floor so that the soles of the feet touch each other while the knees are pressed downward, plus running, bicycling, and rope skipping. But do a little of each exercise to balance the training effect, rather than concentrating on just one approach.

Q: *I do a lot of housework every day. Should I take up an exercise program in addition to the work I do around the house, which is plenty?*
A: Housework can use quite a few calories, but it's not the same as a regular exercise program, particularly one that can take perhaps an hour or less each day to get you away from the house and household chores. If you have children, take them along on walks, jogging, or runs. If they are too small to keep up with you, get a bicycle with a seat for the youngster, or youngsters—one company makes a bike trailer that will hold two children—and give them a bit of fresh air and sunshine, too.

24

HOW TO EAT WELL
WITHOUT GAINING WEIGHT

How many times have you heard the old saying, "You are what you eat"? And when you visit a doctor for a checkup, do you learn that you are literally too much—because you eat too much? The human body has a remarkable ability to adapt to whatever edibles are stuffed into it, and in most cases regardless of the quantity of edibles consumed. Families living in tropical regions seem able to subsist almost entirely on starchy plant foods and rarely have animal meat on the table. At the other extreme are families living near the Arctic Circle whose meals consist almost entirely of animal fats and proteins, and who seldom—if ever—include a starchy plant product.

Most people are acquainted with one or more individuals who seem to live almost entirely on animal protein—steaks, chops, bacon, ham, eggs, hamburger, etc.—and they appear to be healthy, strong, and perhaps even athletic. Yet, other individuals eat only plant foods—fruits, vegetables, and grains—and they also appear to be healthy, strong, and athletic. In fact, some vegetarian groups claim to have a lower incidence of cancer and heart disease than the husky beef eaters in the same geographic areas.

Basic Food Units

A fair question at this point might be a paraphrase of the above quotation, "If you are what you eat, why do vegetarians look like meat eaters?" At least part of the answer is in the fact that the body's nutritional chemistry works with basic food units such as carbohydrates, proteins, and fats, the subunits of which generally occur in plant foods as well as in animal food products. Also, if the body receives the right kinds of fats and proteins, or the subunits of molecules that form fats and proteins, it can fabricate whatever it needs to build, repair, and sustain the body.

All food products, from anchovies to zucchini—whether animal or vegetable—come from the same basic elements on our planet through the process of photosynthesis. In photosynthesis the green coloring matter of plants utilizes energy from the sun to convert carbon dioxide and water into glucose, a simple molecule of sugar. This is the starting point for the foods consumed by humans and also the form in which most food products finally are utilized by the human body, regardless of whether the bodily activity is running a marathon or simply thinking great thoughts. The energy used to permit physical or mental activity comes from the glucose molecule formed from carbon dioxide and water by the original solar energy factory, a green plant.

True, the description above is a bit simplistic. Photosynthesis can be performed by red or brown algae and purple bacteria, as well as by green plants; but the point is that the foods we eat, from the pickle and mustard to the hamburger and the bun, derive from carbon dioxide and water combined into a glucose molecule with the help of photosynthesis. Glucose molecules are converted into amino acid molecules to form proteins, or into fatty acids to become fats, or into carbohydrate combinations of starches and sugars. Some are blended with other elements, such as nitrogen in the formation of amino acids, or with important minerals like calcium and phosphorus—all of which can be found in a glass of milk.

There is no single food that satisfies all the nutritional needs of the body, and nearly all foods have something worthwhile to contribute. In general, some foods contain a greater proportion of essential nutrients than others, so that the secret of eating well without eating too much is to select food combinations that provide the energy you need along with the nutrients required for good health. This may be easier than you might think at first because nature has provided such a wide variety of good nutrient sources. Humans have survived for countless generations on whatever happened to be in season in whatever part of the world they lived.

Most people, regardless of their age, sex, and size, need the same nutrients for normal body health, although the amounts required can vary somewhat. Women require more iron during their reproductive years because their bodies lose iron through menstruation. A growing child may need more calcium, phosphorus, and protein than an adult in order to build tissues such as bone. A person who is physically active or who does hard physical work needs more energy-rich foods than an inactive person. And most adults need fewer calories than teenagers. In fact, the amount of food a person needs at 20 years of age generally is too much for a person who is 30 years old, while the energy demands from food of a 30-year-old person usually are greater than the requirements of somebody who is 40, and so on.

The Importance of Counting Calories

Food energy is measured in calories, the same kind used to measure physical activity. Calories in food can be balanced directly against the energy needed by an average person to perform a certain task. For example, one gram of carbohydrate, such as sugar, will provide about four calories; and one gram of protein also will supply approximately four calories of energy. Four calories of energy should be enough for the average person's muscles to saw wood for two minutes. The same four calories of energy are enough to keep the brain at work thinking great thoughts for a half hour. Obviously, one needs less energy for mental activity than for physical effort.

For those who think in terms of English measure, a gram is about 1/28th of an ounce. One ounce of sugar, as a carbohydrate, contains about 112 calories. Fats have more than twice as much energy per gram or ounce than either carbohydrates or proteins; the ratio is about 9 to 4. Alcohol contains around seven calories per gram. When counting calories, approximations and averages are used except in the scientific reports of nutrition research because the precise number of calories per gram of fat, for example, depends upon which molecules of fatty acids are found in the fat. Each type of fatty acid has a slightly different calorie value. Similarly, different proteins and carbohydrates may have different numbers of calories. So for practical purposes, the numbers are rounded off. Also, the foods we eat are complex mixtures of nutrients. A "pure" food on the table may be free of contaminants, but it is not a pure protein or pure carbohydrate if it came from a grocer's shelf.

Briefly, the energy in food is the energy that came originally from sunlight. It may be stored in the body, just as it was stored in the flesh of a steer before the steer became hamburger for a Big Mac. But eventually that energy will be released in order to provide body heat, mental activity, or the ability to climb a flight of stairs. As the body requires energy, it shuffles around the fats, carbohydrates, and proteins, and breaks them down into the simple glucose molecules formed originally in the plant. The glucose molecules are the fuel for the human body's chemical engine. When each molecule of glucose is burned in a muscle cell or elsewhere, the original molecules of carbon dioxide and water are released to return to the environment, perhaps to be joined again someday to form a new glucose molecule in another plant.

In calculating the amount of calories of energy you need for your daily routine, you might easily overlook the fact that a lot of calories are burned automatically by your body in order to keep its basic systems functioning normally. The medical profession sometimes refers to this calorie need as your basal metabolism. It includes such things as the energy required by the heart to pump the equivalent of some 4,000 gallons of blood every day through your 70,000 miles of blood vessels, plus the energy needed to expand and contract the lungs about 25,000 times a day. It supplies the energy needed to operate the digestive system and kidneys, and the fuel necessary to maintain the body temperature at around 37 degrees Celsius, or 98.6 degrees Fahrenheit. For all these basal metabolism activities, your body needs around 1,450 calories a day—even if you don't get out of bed to do anything!

For most activities, however, people today require few additional calories. For a small woman who works in an office, the requirements of her basal metabolism are met largely by the calories from her normal diet. Even for a rather active man, it's doubtful that his total calorie needs would be twice his basal metabolism requirement. However, proper calorie balancing can be the greatest trick you can perform during your lifetime.

As a rule of thumb, an average adult may need about 15 calories per day for every pound of body weight. Thus, a 100-pound woman needs only about 1,500 calories a day, unless she happens to be a very active person. A 150-pound man needs about 2,250 calories a day for a moderate level of activity. A 200-pound man needs around 3,000 calories a day. The 15-calories-per-pound rule doesn't apply across the board for all people, however, because there are normal variations in size and rates of activity. For some individuals, the need might only amount to 12 calories per pound of proper body weight. Also, the many different sizes and shapes of 100-pound women and 200-pound men will vary calorie requirements. But in most cases of calorie balancing, a target of 12 to 15 calories per pound of body weight is a reasonable one.

While it may seem simple enough to aim for a calories-per-pound target that should maintain a healthy body weight, you must keep in mind that it takes a miss of only a few calories a day to make a slim person fat. Unless they are exercised or dieted away rather vigorously, extra calories can stick like glue. For example, an extra ten calories a day may not seem like much, but they add up to 3,650 calories a year, or the equivalent of one pound of fat. Although that may not seem like the first step on the road to obesity, the total weight gained between the ages of 25 and 65 will amount to 40 pounds of fat—and all because of a mere ten calories a day!

What food has ten calories? One jellybean. Or one saltine cracker. Or one potato chip. Or five pretzel sticks. Or one-fourth cup of popcorn. Or one-half tablespoon of half-and-half in the coffee. Of course, the extra calories that put on weight must be blamed on the fun foods of life. But in reality all foods contain calories and one can just as easily gain an extra pound or two of fat every year by eating steak and potatoes or ham and eggs. But the steak and potatoes or ham and eggs, or for vegetarians the beans and corn, offer something else in addition to calories.

Proteins

Protein foods are among the nutrients to consider first when reviewing any kind of weight control program. One of the first things to understand is that some proteins are better than other proteins.

A protein is a food substance composed of building blocks called amino acids. There are 22 naturally occurring amino acids in food, and they differ from each other in size and chemical structure. A protein is formed by a combination of amino acids arranged in a pattern something like a long word made from a combination of letters. However, some protein "words" formed by amino acids are of tremendous size and use hundreds or thousands of amino acids in a particular pattern. A protein molecule also may contain mineral elements in its amino acid pattern. An example is hemoglobin, the red coloring factor of blood cells; hemoglobin is a protein made up of amino acids and iron atoms.

Of the 22 amino acids, nine are designated essential amino acids that must be included in your diet on a regular basis in order to maintain normal health. The 13 other amino acids are important, but they can be built by the body's chemical processes from other foods, whereas the body is unable to fabricate essential amino acids. Because the body cannot function normally without the essential amino acids in the daily diet, proteins that are sources of essential amino acids are considered better than proteins that lack them. A *complete* protein contains all nine of the essential amino acids—for example, milk and eggs. Gelatin, on the other hand, contains only seven of the essential amino acids, and while it is almost pure protein, gelatin is not a complete protein. If you are served milk or cream with your gelatin dessert, the flavor is enhanced and the food becomes a complete protein.

A complete protein can be lost if it isn't prepared for the table in a proper manner. Some amino acids are destroyed by high cooking temperatures, or they can be rendered indigestible by cooking them in oil rather than water. A complete protein food fried in fat at high temperatures can be a wasted food because the amino acid molecules are converted to chemical compounds that cannot be absorbed or utilized by the human body.

After milk and eggs, the best sources of proteins with a high proportion of essential amino acids are meats, fish, and poultry. Some vegetables and grains contain a few of the essential amino acids, but they have to be used in the diet in a skillful way if you are a vegan, that is, a person who subsists entirely on a vegetarian diet that is not supplemented by milk and eggs. For example, beans and corn each contain some of the essential amino acids, but neither beans nor corn contain all the essential amino acids found in some other plant foods. So vegetarian diets need a combination of corn and beans in order to provide most of them. However, even a good vegetarian combination may lack three of the essential amino acids—lysine, methionine, and tryptophan—in amounts adequate to insure normal nutritional health, unless some milk or eggs, or both, are added to the menu.

What happens if you don't get all the essential amino acids? One possible effect is cirrhosis of the liver, an ailment commonly associated with heavy drinking of alcoholic beverages. The liver is an organ that is particularly sensitive to a deficiency of essential amino acids. If they are lacking in the diet, normal liver functions may diminish and the liver cells may be replaced with fatty and fibrous tissues. In young children a lack of essential amino acids can be marked by retarded growth, digestive system problems, and changes in the skin and hair. In older persons a severe lack of essential amino acids can result in blood and hormonal disorders. Because of the abundance of protein foods in the industrialized nations, protein deficiency diseases are rarely seen there. But such diseases are relatively common in some developing nations where meat, milk, and eggs are missing from the daily diet. The effects of protein deficiency are possible whenever essential amino acids are not included in one's meal planning.

Fats

Like proteins, fats are composed of subunits, which are called fatty acids. Also like proteins, fats have important functions in building and maintaining body tissues that are above and beyond their usual role. Some fat molecules, for example, combine with phosphorus atoms to form phospholipids, which are important structural units of body tissues. Another type of fat, the well-publicized cholesterol molecule, serves as a starting material for vitamin D and certain sex hormones. In addition, cholesterol helps form a waterproof barrier in the human skin that keeps you from becoming waterlogged when you are swimming. Thus, despite the bad press that fats in the diet have received in recent years, we really couldn't live very well without them.

The *essential* fatty acids must be included in the human diet in order to insure normal health. Essential fatty acids are of the unsaturated linoleic variety produced from natural vegetable oils, such as corn, soybean, safflower, and wheat germ. Skin ailments similar to eczema develop in persons whose diets lack linoleic fatty acids. But the skin disorders disappear when linoleic acid foods are added to the diet.

An unsaturated fatty acid can be defined technically as a fatty acid that has room in its molecules to add more hydrogen atoms. A saturated fatty acid, by the same rules of the game, is one that has all the hydrogen atoms it can handle. In most cases an unsaturated fatty acid is a liquid at room temperature, and a saturated fatty acid is a solid at room temperature. An unsaturated fatty acid sometimes can be converted into a saturated fatty acid by adding hydrogen atoms. Liquid corn oil or cottonseed oil, for example, can be transformed into a semisolid margarine by a process in which hydrogen is added. The process is called hydrogenation.

Unsaturated fatty acids generally are found in nature in the form of plant oils, such as corn oil, olive oil, sesame oil, and so on. The fats from animal tissues generally are composed of saturated fatty acids. However, there are differences of hardness among animal fats. Fish oils, for example, are close to the consistency of the fatty acids of plants, while the fats of deer and sheep may be of a solid tallow composition, like hard wax.

The problem with fat as a food is that most people in the industrialized countries eat too much of it. North Americans, for example, consume about seven times as much fat as the peoples of the Third World countries. Many individuals could easily reduce their intake of fatty foods by 50 percent without suffering ill effects. As noted previously, a certain amount of fats are needed in the diet. Fatty foods take longer to digest and have the effect of delaying the onset of hunger following a meal. Some fatty foods are needed to help the body absorb and store the fat-soluble vitamins, A, D, E, and K. But fatty acid deficiency is not likely to occur unless the essential fatty acids in your diet comprise less than one or two percent of the total calories consumed by the body.

Excess calories, that is, calories consumed beyond the amount actually needed to maintain basal metabolism and to supply energy required for work and play, will be converted by your body's chemical factories into fat that can be stored for possible future use. This probably was a good idea of nature in the early days of human life when a feast was often followed by a famine. But today in much of the industrialized areas where every day can be a feast day, the fat merely accumulates instead of being consumed eventually during a famine or food shortage. Storing excess energy in the form of fat is a practical move on the part of nature. Fat provides about nine calories per gram, compared to four calories per gram of protein or carbohydrate. It's much easier to carry 3,500 or so calories of reserve energy under your belt as a pound of fat than as two and a fourth pounds of excess carbohydrate.

Most of your body fat is stored under the skin, in the cavity of the belly, and around such deep organs as the liver and kidneys, and it is packed into muscle layers. During periods of starvation or food deprivation because of illness or other factors, the stored fat gradually is transported from depots beneath the skin and elsewhere in the body, and is converted into glucose molecules. The body's chemistry processes are able to manipulate the carbon and hydrogen atoms in carbohydrates, fats, and proteins into fatty substances for storage in fat cells, or to change the fats into other molecules.

Carbohydrates

Carbohydrates include sugars, starches, and cellulose, which are almost exclusively produced in fruits, grains, and vegetables. The only significant carbohydrates of animal origin are glycogen, also known as animal starch, a quick-energy food stored in muscles as a fuel source; and lactose, a type of sugar found in milk.

The so-called high-protein vegetables and cereals actually contain more carbohydrate than protein. Wheat and dry beans, for example, are high-protein plant foods only by comparison with other vegetables and grains that contain less protein. At the same time, pure carbohydrates are virtually nonexistent in nature. With the possible exception of pure sugar, carbohydrates contain varying amounts of other substances.

Like proteins and fats, carbohydrates are formed from subunits. A basic subunit is a monosaccharide such as glucose, a molecule with six carbon atoms; this six-carbon atom sugar also may be called a hexose. Some other carbohydrates may be composed of from two to ten or more monosaccharides that are joined together somewhat like proteins are formed by combinations of amino acids. When carbohydrates are digested in the human body, they are broken down into monosaccharide-size chunks. An exception is cellulose, which the human body cannot digest be-

cause it lacks an enzyme needed to break up the huge cellulose molecules. Cellulose is not wasted in the human diet, however, because it provides the roughage popular in high-fiber diets. Cellulose is a natural component of most fruits, vegetables, and cereals, and special cellulose-rich diets seldom are needed by people who eat a wide variety of plant foods.

Carbohydrates sometimes are called "protein-sparing" foods because they provide a quick source of fuel for a variety of energy needs. While it would be possible, though difficult, to plan a diet without carbohydrates, the body would eventually convert the proteins of the body into the basic carbohydrate molecule, glucose, to satisfy the energy needs of the human mechanism. Fats also would be converted into glucose for fuel, as happens during starvation or in some cases of malnutrition. The proteins would have to be stripped from vital tissues of the body to provide fuel in much the same way as the crews of steamboats or steam trains strip their conveyances of furniture and flooring to stoke the boilers in old movies about riverboat or train races. The riverboats and train coaches, of course, can be refurbished after being stripped of their fuel sources, but when the protein in body tissues is sacrificed because of a lack of carbohydrate in the diet, the body often is permanently damaged. After the protein stripping reaches a critical point of organ damage, the tissues can never be restored to their original state of health.

The average proportions of carbohydrates in meals of peoples around the world range from about 20 percent in Arctic regions to 80 percent in tropical countries. North Americans take 11 percent less calories in the form of carbohydrates today than they did at the beginning of the 20th century. Because of a shift in eating habits from the use of potatoes, bread, and other starchy foods as sources of carbohydrates, more than half the carbohydrate calories today are consumed as sugar, whereas at the end of World War I only 30 percent of the carbohydrate calories consumed were sugar.

People in some parts of Europe still eat a high proportion of carbohydrate calories in the form of cereals and other starchy foods. In North America, on the other hand, the average person eats about two pounds of refined sugar, or sucrose, each week, and may consume as much as 600 calories a day in refined sugar.·Except for the possible effect of refined sugar on the teeth, some nutritionists contend that the use of large amounts of sugar in the diet may not be all bad. Since all carbohydrates are broken down into glucose in the digestive tract, they argue, what difference does it make if the carbohydrate enters the mouth as sugar or cereal starch? Also, some experts claim, a diet rich in sugar may be less risky than a diet rich in fats. For people on a fat-restricted diet, carbohydrates are an important source of energy.

Alcohol as a Source of Calories

One additional source of calories in the diet is alcohol. A gram of ethyl alcohol, the kind used in whiskey, beer, wine, and other alcoholic beverages, is about seven calories. This makes alcohol a richer source of calories than carbohydrates and proteins, on an ounce-per-ounce or gram-per-gram basis, but less rich than fats. People who are on weight-control diets frequently overlook the calories that may be accumulated on a daily basis from a couple of cans of beer or a cocktail. One

ounce of 100-proof whiskey, vodka, gin, or other distilled liquor contains about 82 calories. By a rough rule of thumb, 100 proof is equivalent to around 50 percent pure ethyl alcohol, although the precise ratio varies somewhat in different parts of the world according to local government standards. Distilled liquors of less than 100 proof, of course, have fewer calories per ounce. An 80-proof Scotch whiskey, for example, provides about 65 calories per ounce.

Distilled liquors, like refined sugar, offer little more than calories in the nutrient department. Beers and wines may contribute small amounts of vitamins and minerals in addition to carbohydrates and calories. A 12-ounce can of beer may contain anywhere from 95 to 165 calories, depending upon the alcohol content and other factors of manufacturing. Dry wines may provide 85 to 90 calories per three-ounce serving, while sweeter dessert wines may contain up to 125 calories for the same measure.

A person who has a glass of beer with lunch should be aware that the calorie intake from the beer is equivalent to the energy in a slice of bread with butter. A couple of martinis before dinner could add as many calories to the meal as two orders of salad with blue cheese dressing.

Water: Essential to the Diet

About the only thing you can consume with a meal that doesn't contribute calories is water. Water is an essential part of your daily meal pattern whether you drink it straight or as a water-based food item such as coffee, tea, milk, soft drinks, beer, etc. People who eat big meals usually need more water than those who have a small daily food intake. If there is such a thing as a recommended measure of daily water needs, it is something like one quart of water for every 1,000 calories of food. For example, if your average calories each day total about 2,500, your fluid intake should be around two and a half quarts.

The average human loses between two and two and a half quarts of water a day through urination, perspiration, and water vapor exhaled through the lungs, as well as some water excreted with feces. If too much fluid is consumed, the excess is simply excreted as part of the urine. If your water consumption falls below the needs of the body, the kidneys will try to conserve fluid by reducing the normal daily volume of urine. If you do not drink at least 90 percent of the water your body requires each day, you may become aware that your body efficiency falters and you become exhausted more easily than when you drink more fluid. When your body's water supply falls below 80 percent of its normal requirements, you can expect to become seriously ill.

The Essential Minerals

Most fats and carbohydrates are composed of three elements—carbon, hydrogen, and oxygen—in various arrangements. Proteins also contain these three elements plus nitrogen. With some exceptions, such as cellulose, the three basic categories of food can be digested by chemical processes of the body that break the larger molecules of carbohydrates, fats, and proteins into smaller, simpler units that are easily absorbed through the digestive tract.

When it comes to minerals, however, the human body frequently encounters difficulty in utilizing elements such as calcium, phosphorus, and magnesium be-

cause they may be bound in complex chemical compounds that are not easily digested or absorbed. On the other hand, calcium, phosphorus, and magnesium are easily excreted if the body accumulates too much of those minerals, provided that the kidneys are functioning normally. Some problems of mineral metabolism are worth noting because you can't assume that because a meal contains X milligrams of a mineral, which is your recommended daily intake, your body will actually absorb X milligrams of the nutrient. From certain minerals, such as iron, your body may get only a small fraction of the amount of the element present in your food.

An average human adult body may require about 700 milligrams of calcium each day. This is about the same amount that leaves and enters the skeleton on an average day. An adult human skeleton contains around two and a half pounds of calcium (1,200 grams), plus water, protein, fat, and other minerals. Although the skeleton is solid as iron, its matrix is in a constant state of chemical flux because it serves as a storehouse and supplier of calcium and phosphorus for the rest of the body. The blood and soft tissues, as well as the teeth, also consume calcium from the diet. Calcium helps the blood to clot and the nerves to function normally, and muscles lose tone when calcium is lacking. Laboratory experiments have shown that calcium is needed to make the heart beat, although there is no published proof of a person succumbing to heart failure because of a lack of calcium in the diet.

Growing children need calcium for growing bones and teeth. Nutrition experts recommend at least 800 milligrams of calcium a day for a child's diet. This is approximately the amount of calcium in three full glasses, or one and a half pints, of whole or skim milk.

For people who are allergic to the lactose in milk, or who have other reasons for avoiding this source of calcium, it is possible to obtain about 800 milligrams of calcium a day by eating four ounces of a cheese, such as brick cheese. Many nuts and some vegetables also are sources of calcium.

Teenagers and pregnant women need about 1,400 milligrams of calcium each day, or double the recommended level for otherwise normal adults. Nursing mothers are advised to increase their intake of calcium-rich foods because breast-feeding an infant takes about 300 milligrams of calcium per day from the mother's body stores.

Phosphorus is closely related to calcium in the structure of bones and teeth, and the recommended daily intake of phosphorus for most people is about the same as their daily needs for calcium. In fact, a well-balanced diet that is geared to satisfy calcium needs probably will take care of one's phosphorus quota. Calcium-rich foods often are good sources of phosphorus as well—milk, cheese, nuts, and legumes. Additional sources of phosphorus include meat, fish, poultry, and eggs.

Besides playing an important part in building bones and teeth, phosphorus helps to liberate the solar energy locked in proteins, fats, and carbohydrates. Phosphorus is vitally involved with blood and nervous tissue functions.

One must be careful about the use of foods or medications that contain iron or magnesium, however, because those minerals can interfere with the ability of the body to absorb phosphorus from the gastrointestinal tract.

Magnesium is one of the minerals that is linked with calcium in maintaining normal bone, muscle, and nervous tissue functions. When magnesium is missing from the diet, the human body tissues tend to lose calcium quite rapidly. In a case of severe magnesium deficiency, it may not be possible to prevent calcium loss even by consuming large quantities of calcium-rich foods such as milk and cheese.

Severe magnesium deficiency sometimes is marked by muscle tremor, convulsions, and delirium. The daily dietary needs for magnesium amount to around 250 to 300 milligrams a day, or about 1/100th of an ounce. An adult body needs about one ounce of magnesium for normal operations, half going into the bones and one-fourth to the muscles. As is the case with certain other nutrients, a balance should be maintained between a lack of magnesium and too much magnesium. Among good sources of magnesium are cocoa, soy flour, nuts, and grains.

Iron combines with a protein to form a substance, hemoglobin, that gives the color to red blood cells and, as a result, to oxygenated blood in general. It is the hemoglobin molecules that enable blood to transport tremendous amounts of oxygen from the lungs through the thousands of miles of blood vessels reaching into every bit of living tissue. The hemoglobin also carries the carbon dioxide waste material of energy release away from the tissue cells, giving the "used" blood its dark or "blue" coloration. An iron-rich substance in the muscles, similar in chemical structure to hemoglobin, is called myoglobin. Among other odd jobs performed by iron are the synthesis of certain enzymes that aid chemical reactions in the body cells.

Iron requirements can vary quite a bit among individuals, including members of a family sharing the same meal. A normal adult male, for example, may need only one milligram of iron a day to replace the amount lost through sweat, urine, and the shedding of skin cells. But a woman during her reproductive years requires about twice that amount of average iron intake because she can expect to lose from 15 to 30 milligrams of iron during each menstrual period. After menopause, however, her iron needs are the same as those of an adult male. Anybody who donates blood or experiences some loss of blood through surgery or injury also should have an increased daily intake of iron to make up for the loss. A pregnant woman should plan on a daily ration of two milligrams of iron; although she does not have to be concerned about replacing iron lost through menstruation, she must provide iron for the developing fetus from her own body stores.

Through one of the somewhat mysterious information feedback systems of the human body, there is some automatic control over the iron levels maintained for the blood and other tissues. When the red blood cells are discarded by the body after an average life of about four months, for example, most of the iron is salvaged so it can be used again. There also is some evidence that the body tries to avoid accumulating more iron than it actually needs. In some cases it is necessary to offer the body 10 milligrams of iron in order to get it to accept one milligram of additional iron.

Good natural food sources of iron include liver, liver sausage, heart, kidney, lean meats, shellfish, and egg yolks. Vegetarian sources are legumes such as dried beans, dried fruits, nuts, green leafy vegetables, and whole grain and enriched cereals. One of the poorest sources of iron is milk. Because of the lack of iron in milk, parents should make sure that infants and young children get adequate amounts of iron-rich foods such as iron-enriched cereals with the milk.

Copper is important as a mineral nutrient because without it the body has difficulty in absorbing iron from the digestive tract and helping it to combine with the protein molecules that form hemoglobin. However, copper deficiency is an unlikely problem because the element occurs naturally in meats, poultry, fish, vegetables, fruits, nuts, and grains. Milk is not a good source of copper; the few cases of copper deficiency that have been recorded have involved children who subsisted mainly on an all-milk diet. The average person's recommended intake of copper is about two milligrams a day, which is easy to achieve even on a vegetarian diet.

Zinc is one of the minerals that has become an important addition to the diets recommended for normal body functioning in recent years. A deficiency of zinc seems to cause some degree of disorder in nearly all of the body's physiologic systems, including that of reproduction. Zinc appears to be involved in the functioning of the body's enzymes and in obvious health defects such as hypertension; studies indicate an increased risk of the disease in a zinc-deficient diet.

Zinc is found in a wide variety of meats, vegetables, fruits, and grains, so that a diet lacking zinc is not likely to occur if well-balanced meals are planned on a regular basis. Zinc also is one of the minerals that should not be added to the diet in abundance, because an excess of zinc in the diet can result in gastrointestinal disorders. On the other hand, some nutrition experts claim that a zinc deficiency can result from a high-fiber diet. The explanation is that fiber tends to bind zinc in the digestive tract so it cannot be absorbed easily. Vegetarians who consume only plant food products are among individuals most likely to show symptoms of a zinc-deficient diet.

Iodine is a vital nutrient but most people get about twice as much as their daily requirement through the use of iodized salt on their food and by eating seafood and vegetables that have been grown in soil containing iodine. Iodine is needed to form the thyroid hormone that regulates the body's metabolism. During pregnancy the mother's iodine intake should be monitored rather carefully to insure normal mental and physical development of the fetus, which gets its iodine from the mother's own body stores of the mineral. A form of mental retardation called congenital cretinism can result in the offspring from an absence of iodine in the mother's diet. A lack of iodine in the diet of an otherwise normal person can cause a disease called hyperthyroidism, which is characterized in some cases by a goiter, or enlarged thyroid gland, protruding from the neck in the area of the Adam's apple.

Before the development of iodized salt, which is ordinary table salt with a bit of iodine added, the goiter problem was not uncommon in regions where people did not have easy access to seafood and their vegetables were grown in iodine-deficient soil. Today, because of a semidependence upon iodized salt to prevent hyperthyroidism, the people who must be alerted to watch their iodine intake are those on a salt-free or salt-restricted diet. Those individuals may require an additional source of iodine-rich foods or a mineral supplement to their diets.

Two minerals that should be mentioned among the nutrients essential for normal health are sodium and potassium. Sodium, as some nutrition experts have noted, is such a common part of the human diet that it usually is ignored in preparing lists of food items needed for your physical well-being. Sodium, of course, is one of the two elements in ordinary table salt, sodium chloride.

Sodium is the principal mineral of the body's extracellular fluids, which are simply those outside the body cells, such as blood. Sodium helps control the acid-base balance of the body's fluids and the amount of water in the body cells. During an intensely hot day the loss of sodium through perspiration can disrupt the balance of water in the body and the chemicals dissolved in it, causing cramps, headache, muscular weakness, and other symptoms. The symptoms usually are relieved by consuming increased amounts of salt. Additional salt is needed to help the body recover from prolonged diarrhea or vomiting.

People who consume abnormally large amounts of fluid should increase their salt intake in order to help maintain a normal balance of salt to water. The recommended ratio is about one extra gram of salt for each additional quart of water per day. There are wide individual variations in the use of salt, depending upon such factors as individual taste preferences and family habits; some people use about one ounce a day and others are satisfied with one-tenth of an ounce. Persons on sodium-restricted diets may learn to live on as little as one-fourth of a gram, or about 1/100th of an ounce, of sodium a day, and get their daily quota almost entirely from the sodium naturally present in foods.

Persons who are not concerned about hypertension, congestive heart disease, or other conditions that might warrant a salt-free or sodium-restricted diet, usually find a self-limiting level of salt use. In other words, they adjust their salt intake to their own liking and do not use so much that it causes either discomfort or loss of food flavor; any excess sodium received by an otherwise normal body is excreted in the urine.

While sodium is the primary mineral of the body's extracellular fluids, potassium plays a similar role as the controlling element of fluids within the body cells. Potassium affects the normal functioning of nervous tissue and the ability of all muscle tissue—skeletal, smooth, and cardiac— to contract. A potassium deficiency is marked by muscular weakness, nervous irritability, mental disorders, and irregularities of the heart. Too much potassium in the diet can also produce heart irregularities.

The Trace Elements

Some other minerals are needed in the diet in trace amounts, that is, amounts measured in thousandths or millionths of a gram (a gram represents less than four percent of an ounce). Fluorine is such an element needed in trace amounts to strengthen teeth and bones. In many parts of the world fluorine is added to drinking water or occurs naturally in it in amounts that meet the body's normal daily requirements. Where fluorine is not a part of the local drinking water supply, the element can be obtained from common food items such as meat, poultry, fish, fruits, vegetables, cereals, nuts, and dairy products.

Manganese, another trace nutrient, becomes part of an enzyme system that produces urea. Molybdenum is part of another enzyme system needed by the body tissues to pry loose the calories of energy locked in fatty acid molecules. Silicon appears to be related to the normal functioning of the body's connective tissues because several body organs are found to be silicon-deficient as the deterioration of aging affects them. Selenium seems to be associated with protein manufacture by the body's tissues; children who have abnormally low blood levels of selenium also show signs of protein deficiency.

There are some trace elements which may or may not be important in the human diet, but experiments with animals indicate they might be essential for normal human body functioning. They include nickel, which seems to be associated with membrane structure and reproductive ability; vanadium, an element that affects normal growth and bone development of animals; and tin, which also has been found to be essential for normal animal growth.

One trace element necessary for normal human health is acquired in an indirect manner. This is cobalt, which is a part of the structure of vitamin B12. Because humans do not have the proper physiology for synthesizing vitamin B12, the cobalt that is absorbed from the gastrointestinal tract apparently passes through the body and is excreted. Some animals, particularly those that are herbivores, or plant eaters, can manufacture vitamin B12 in their digestive tracts. But humans not only cannot synthesize the vitamin from cobalt in their diets, they generally are unable to get enough of the vitamin from plant products and in most cases must depend upon animal meat, eggs, and milk for their supply of cobalt in vitamin B12.

Vitamins

Vitamins are substances required by the body in trace amounts to make it possible for certain chemical reactions to take place so that normal body functions are possible. The different vitamins vary greatly in their own chemical structure and functions. The one thing they have in common is their jobs as catalysts for the metabolism of foods. In their functions the vitamins are similar to hormones, the main difference being that the body produces its own hormones while vitamins must be obtained from outside sources such as food.

One other fact to keep in mind is that just as no single food is the best source of proteins, fats, carbohydrates, and minerals, no single food is the best source of all the vitamins needed for normal human health. Therefore, it is necessary to eat a variety of foods that includes the best sources of the essential nutrients.

Vitamins generally are cataloged as either water-soluble or fat-soluble. Fat-soluble vitamins, identified by the letters A, D, E, and K, are absorbed with fatty foods and stored in fat deposits in the body. Because they are stored, it is not as essential to renew the body's supply on a day-to-day basis, as may be necessary with the water-soluble vitamins which, as a general rule, are not stored in the body in significant amounts but are excreted in the urine if not needed immediately. A further rule of the vitamin game states that a health problem that interferes with normal fatty acid metabolism also is likely to interfere with the absorption of fat-soluble vitamins.

The water-soluble vitamins include the B-complex vitamins and vitamin C, which deserves a special place among the vitamins because humans are among the few animals that do not manufacture their own ascorbic acid, the chemical name for vitamin C. In fact, because most of the animals used in laboratory studies of vitamins do not require vitamin C in their diets in order to function normally, the importance of this vitamin to human life has been gleaned mainly from studies of what happens to people deprived of vitamin C.

Long before vitamin C was identified, it was known that sailors on long sea voyages developed a disease called scurvy. The signs and symptoms included bleeding and sore gums, loose teeth, swollen and tender joints, a general feeling of weakness, and poor healing of wounds. When the sailors reached a port where they could obtain citrus fruits, oranges, lemons, or limes, the effects of scurvy gradually disappeared. The British Navy, on the advice of a doctor who had studied the disease, began a policy of providing lemons or limes to sailors on sea voyages. The British sailors thus became known as "limies," but more important, the availability of citrus fruit aboard ship reportedly improved the capability of the navy to dominate the seas for many years.

Later it was learned that not only citrus fruits but strawberries, cantaloupes, many green vegetables, and potatoes also are sources of vitamin C. Unfortunately, it was not learned until still later that storing the fruits and vegetables for long periods of time, or cooking them, destroyed vitamin C.

Today, the recommended minimum daily requirement of vitamin C for the average adult is 45 milligrams, about three times the level estimated as necessary to prevent scurvy. While the body technically does not store vitamin C, the tissues can become saturated with enough of the substance to postpone the onset of scurvy for several weeks or months of vitamin C deprivation. In addition to preventing the symptoms of scurvy, vitamin C increases the ability of the body to absorb iron from the diet and aids in the metabolism of protein.

The reported effect of vitamin C in preventing or controlling the symptoms of the common cold is somewhat controversial. Some experts advise against taking large doses of vitamin C because of the possibility of various side effects, ranging from diarrhea to kidney and reproductive system disorders.

Among the B vitamins, the first to be discovered and so numbered, B1, is required in the diet to prevent the symptoms of a disease known as beriberi. Characterized by fluid accumulation in the body cavities, beriberi is a form of nerve ailment that leads to loss of the use of the muscles.

Vitamin B1, also known as thiamine, is involved in the metabolism of carbohydrates. In fact, the daily requirement is linked to the number of calories in the form of carbohydrates consumed each day, at the rate of one-half milligram of vitamin B1 for each 1,000 calories of food consumed, but not less than four-fifths of a milligram per day for persons whose food intake amounts to less than 2,000 calories. While thiamine can be found in a wide variety of common foods, the ones that contain the vitamin in significant amounts are relatively few and include meats—lean meats as well as heart, kidney, and liver cuts—liver sausage, eggs, yeast; and for vegetarians, green leafy vegetables, whole or enriched cereals, legumes, nuts, and berries.

The next B vitamin on the list, B2, or riboflavin, is needed as a catalyst for the normal functioning of body cells, particularly those of the skin and eyes. A riboflavin deficiency may be marked by inflammation of the skin about the mouth area and nose, as well as the skin of the male genitalia. The eyes can develop an abnormally large number of capillaries about the cornea, and the patient may experience photophobia, or intolerance for bright light, as well as a symptom described as visual fatigue. The sources of vitamin B2 are generally the same as the best foods needed for vitamin B1 intake: lean and organ meats, liver sausage, eggs, milk and cheese, plus green leafy vegetables, whole grain cereals, and legumes.

Vitamin B6, or pyridoxine, is needed for a number of metabolic jobs in the human body. It is involved in many reactions of the body chemistry that relate to the use of amino acids, the building blocks of proteins. In fact, there is evidence that some amino acids are not absorbed from the digestive tract if the patient suffers from a vitamin B6 deficiency. Another role of pyridoxine is to metabolize certain fatty acids and carbohydrates. In addition to enhancing the absorption of amino acids from the digestive tract, vitamin B6 helps prevent a form of dermatitis that involves the sebaceous, or oil, glands in the skin, especially around the eyes, nose, mouth, and ears. The vitamin also seems to prevent the occurrence of nervous system disorders which have appeared in persons who inherit a requirement for above-average amounts of pyridoxine, and in infants who have been bottle-fed a formula deficient in vitamin B6.

Still another important function of vitamin B6 is its ability to transform an amino acid, tryptophan, into another B vitamin called niacin. As part of its job of metabolizing fatty acids, the B6 vitamin has been found to be able to create nonessential fatty acids from the essential fatty acid known as linoleic acid. Thus, a diet lacking adequate levels of pyridoxine can trigger a toppling domino effect of health problems.

The average adult's daily need for vitamin B6 is only one or two milligrams, but persons who have a congenital need for pyridoxine may require from five to ten times that average in order to stave off effects of a vitamin B6 deficiency. The best sources of the vitamin are blackstrap molasses, brewer's yeast, wheat germ or wheat bran, and soy beans—foods which may not be found in everybody's pantry. More commonly available sources of pyridoxine include lean and organ meats, rice, corn grits, peanuts, bananas, barley, potatoes, and dry peas.

Cyanocobalamin is an unlikely name for a B vitamin, so it has become better known as vitamin B12. The chemical name indicates that the vitamin contains the mineral cobalt. Since the most important function of vitamin B12 is the production of red blood cells, a lack of B12 in the diet eventually leads to a red blood cell deficiency and a type of anemia. The anemia, specifically pernicious anemia, not only leads to serious blood disorders but results in severe damage to the nervous system and, if untreated, causes death. Vitamin B12 also is involved in the formation of chemical molecules that become a part of DNA (deoxyribonucleic acid), a chemical keystone of life itself. Laboratory experiments with animals indicate that an absence of vitamin B12 may enhance the development of cirrhosis of the liver, a disease popularly associated with abuse of alcoholic beverages.

Only a very tiny amount of vitamin B12 is needed in a person's daily diet to prevent deficiency effects such as pernicious anemia. The suggested daily intake amounts to only about 1/30,000,000th of an ounce. As small as that requirement may be, however, there are only a handful of commonly available foods that provide that much vitamin B12 in an average serving: beef kidney, beef liver, lean beef, powdered whole milk, powdered skim milk, ham, and fresh filet of sole.

The lack of vitamin B12 in significant amounts in vegetables, fruits, and grains can be bad news for vegetarians. According to data from analysis of the vitamin B12 content of plant products, one might have to consume a pound of soybeans or a half-pound of oats to obtain one microgram of the vitamin. Other vegetarian foods contain even less of the vitamin per average serving. While some vegans claim they suffer no ill effects from eating vitamin B12-deficient foods, others consume milk or eggs, or both, to avoid pernicious anemia effects, and some take vitamin B12 tablets or vitamin B12 fortified yeast as a source of this vital nutrient.

Vitamin-like Substances

After a flying start by nutritionists at identifying vitamins by letters and numbers, so many chemical substances were found to have vitamin-like functions that the use of chemical names of the substances eventually gained respectability. Even when vitamins were identified by the name of the chemical molecule, researchers discovered that substances with similar chemical structures had similar effects on the body. As a result, instead of one specific chemical producing a vitamin effect, there might be several different chemicals that could be identified as a particular vitamin. An example among the B vitamins is niacin, or nicotinic acid, which may occur in plant tissues and animal tissues in different forms, but in either variation will have a similar effect on the human body.

One of the effects of niacin is that of a vasodilator; that is, it dilates the blood vessels and may increase the skin temperature with a flushing of the skin. Niacin also is known as the "antipellagra vitamin" because its lack in the diet produces a triad of health problems—diarrhea, skin disorders, and mental health deterioration. The niacin deficiency signs and symptoms include a red and inflamed tongue and a burning sensation in the mouth.

Pellagra was a common problem in some parts of North America in past years, and it still is a cause of concern in Third World countries, because families consumed meals that consisted largely of cornmeal, molasses, and ham fat—foods that are notoriously deficient in niacin. Since the amino acid tryptophan can be converted to niacin when vitamin B6 is present, pellagra symptoms are not likely to appear in persons whose meals include adequate amounts of the B6 vitamin and tryptophan. The latter is found in eggs, most muscle and organ meats of fish and animals, dried brewer's yeast, peanuts, soybeans, and wheat germ. Good niacin sources include fish and lean meats, whole-grain or enriched cereals and breads, peas, beans, and nuts, including peanuts.

Other chemicals now included in the family of water-soluble B-complex vitamins are biotin, folic acid, and pantothenic acid. Biotin is found in a wide range of foods, from cow's milk to chocolate, beef liver, and peanuts. It is required for an equally broad range of bodily functions, from protein building to carbohydrate breakdown. Insomnia, loss of appetite, and muscle pains are among the symptoms of insufficient biotin in the diet.

Folic acid is required for normal cell growth since it is involved in the development of each cell nucleus. Folic acid also supports the work of other water-soluble vitamins, particularly vitamin B12. When folic acid is missing from your meals, the vitamin B12-deficiency type of anemia results because new red blood cells cannot be produced. Good sources of folic acid include orange juice, dark green leafy vegetables, nuts, beans, whole-grain cereals, and liver.

Pantothenic acid becomes part of an enzyme system needed for the body's effective use of proteins, fats, and carbohydrates. A lack of pantothenic acid may be felt as abdominal pains, muscular weakness, and susceptibility to infections.

The Fat-Soluble Vitamins

The fat-soluble vitamins generally are more stable than the water-soluble vitamins. Since fat-soluble vitamins can withstand more cooking and storage time, they can be stored in the body as reserve supplies of the vital substances. On the minus side of the ledger, fat-soluble vitamins are dependent on the body's ability to handle fatty foods and problems that might interfere with normal fat intake. Also, faulty metabolism could disrupt the normal absorption of fat-soluble vitamins from an average diet.

Vitamin A, the first of the fat-soluble vitamins, conforms to the general pattern in that it has a chemical name, retinol, and occurs in nature in several molecular variations which have similar properties. There are about five precursors of vitamin A, sometimes identified as carotenoid provitamins, which means simply that five different chemicals occurring in yellow- and orange-colored fruits and vegetables can be converted into vitamin A by the body's chemistry.

There is an important need for vitamin A because it becomes a part of the system of rods and cones in the retina of the eye, the rods being the part of normal vision sensitive to low intensity light and the cones being the receptors for colors and bright light. The vitamin A molecules form part of a light-sensitive pigment that absorbs energy from light and converts it into nervous system signals that are transmitted to the brain, which forms visual images from the signals.

When vitamin A is lacking in the diet, a form of so-called night-blindness results. It is characterized by impaired vision in poorly lighted or darkened areas, particularly after exposure to bright lights. The affected person may become aware of this visual defect during night driving when it becomes necessary to focus his gaze on a darkened pavement immediately after facing the headlights of an oncoming automobile. This form of night-blindness usually is corrected by increasing one's consumption of fruits and vegetables containing the vitamin A precursors, such as apricots and carrots. Egg yolks, liver and liver sausage, butter, whole-milk cheese, and fortified margarine are among other sources of vitamin A.

In addition to its role in insuring normal vision, vitamin A is important for maintaining the normal growth and health of cells of the epithelium tissues, such as the mucous membranes that line the mouth and nasal cavity, lungs, and urinary tract.

And vitamin A is vitally involved in the development of bones and teeth so that a vitamin A-deficient diet can result in thin and poorly formed enamel surfaces on the teeth.

At the other end of the vitamin A range of effects is the hazard of consuming too much of the substance, which could occur by taking too many vitamin A tablets containing large doses. While a lack of vitamin A can interfere with normal bone development, too much vitamin A can cause the bones to become fragile and painful. The condition, sometimes called hypervitaminosis A, a medical term for too much vitamin A, may be associated with itching skin, hair falling out, an enlarged liver, headaches, and nausea.

Vitamin D, which has the chemical name of calciferol, has a chemical cousin with the more formidable chemical name of 7-dehydrocholesterol. Sometimes the two variations of vitamin D are identified as D2 and D3, but since both have the same general effects in human physiology, for practical purposes they are both referred to simply as vitamin D.

The main purpose of vitamin D is to help the body absorb, use, and retain the minerals calcium and phosphorus for bones and teeth. A deficiency of vitamin D in children results in a condition known as rickets, which is characterized by teeth that are late in erupting, poorly formed, and more susceptible to decay. Rickets has possibly more serious effects in delaying the formation and closure of skull bones and long bones. Chest and pelvis deformities, curvature of the spine, and legs with the deformities commonly called knock-knees or bowlegs also can result from vitamin D deficiency in children. In adults the lack of vitamin D results in a bone disease known as osteomalacia, which is similar in effects to rickets because of the loss of bone minerals. A couple of specific results of osteomalacia include compression of the pelvis and spinal column, with degeneration of the vertebrae.

One of the most commonly available sources of vitamin D is fortified milk. Fish-liver oils are the best source of the vitamin, and for those who shun cod-liver oil as a direct method of acquiring vitamin D, eating canned salmon and canned sardines may be a suitable alternative. Exposure to sunlight helps the body form vitamin D in the skin from precursor cholesterol molecules.

Infants and growing children need the vitamin D equivalent of a quart of vitamin D-fortified milk each day and/or plenty of exposure to sunlight. Children who live in Sun Belt regions are more likely to avoid vitamin D deficiency than those who live in colder, cloudier areas where opportunities for exposing the skin to the sun may be more difficult. An alternative is the administration of regular doses of vitamin D supplements.

A word of caution is in order regarding overdosing with vitamin D. Too much vitamin D, or hypervitaminosis D, can be hazardous to one's health, causing symptoms of diarrhea and vomiting, headache, fatigue, and loss of appetite. Hypervitaminosis D also can result in disorders of the urinary system and the development of calcium deposits in the heart and other organs.

Vitamin E, which bears the chemical name of tocopherol, comes in four molecular variations and occurs in such a wide variety of common foods that a vitamin E deficiency in humans is extremely rare. This vitamin's importance was discovered largely through experiments with animals, which can be fed such rigidly controlled diets that almost any substance can be added or subtracted from their meals so that the effects can be observed. In experiments it was found that when the animals were deprived of vitamin E they developed degeneration and paralysis of skeletal muscles, as well as reproductive failure. In humans vitamin E is believed to protect the integrity of vitamin A and, in turn, the red blood cells.

Adequate amounts of vitamin E are present in most meats, poultry, fish, vegetables, fruits, and cereal grains, with the highest levels occurring in corn, cottonseed, soybean, and peanut oils, and in margarines manufactured from those oils. One whole egg or an average serving of oatmeal provides at least twice the estimated daily human needs for vitamin E, as does a serving of sweet potatoes or turnip greens.

Vitamin K, the last on the list but not the least important of the fat-soluble vitamins, is a vital factor in normal clotting of the blood. In fact, it is so important that pregnant women and newborn infants sometimes are administered extra doses of vitamin K to help prevent hemorrhaging at the time of childbirth.

Green leafy vegetables are recommended as a prime source for vitamin K, although pork liver provides more of the substance per average serving than any green vegetables. The best vegetarian sources of vitamin K include spinach, cauliflower, and cabbage. One form of vitamin K is produced by friendly bacteria in the human intestinal tract.

On the problem side of vitamin K utilization, it is not easily stored in the human body, and in case of disease or injury involving the liver it may not be stored at all. Also, the use of sulfa drugs and antibiotics can interfere with vitamin K availability. A wide variety of digestive tract disorders may prevent absorption of vitamin K from the digestive tract, and so will the ingestion of mineral oil. Any of these factors that interfere with normal absorption and storage of vitamin K can result in an increased risk of hemorrhage from disease or injury.

Calculating Calories for Your Energy Needs

There is no way the average person can calculate precisely the amounts of calories or nutrients that may be contained in a single food, a single meal, or a single week's accumulation of meals and snacks. A nutrition scientist probably would be the last person to try to guarantee that a 100-gram tomato contains one gram of protein and 23 milligrams of vitamin C, which are the figures listed in a typical table of food values. Because of the individual variability factor in food values, the nutrition expert might agree only that among all the tomatoes on a supermarket counter one could expect that each would contain some protein and some vitamin C. But the exact nutrient values of fruits, vegetables, and meats of all kinds vary from one plant or animal product to the next. Two tomatoes from the same vine probably would not have the same nutrient values. So the numbers used in tables of calories and nutrients are usually averages based on analysis of a large number of samples of the food product.

Humans vary considerably in their anatomy and physiology, so the way in which your body handles calories or specific foods or nutrients probably is different from all the other members of your family. Age, sex, and genetic factors, as well as individual physical condition, can affect how each person's body will handle a fat, protein, carbohydrate, mineral, or vitamin. Thus, tables of height and weight for males and females, and of calories and nutrients recommended for the average human being, are only estimates or averages based on samples of large numbers of humans. The data for some averages, for example, may be based on information obtained by examining women who applied for insurance policies or men who had been conscripted for military duty. The information obtained may or may not be truly representative of the entire population and it certainly should not be interpreted as an ideal model for your own body. The numbers used for height, weight, calories, milligrams, or other units of nutrients should be regarded only as general guidelines or targets. If you are not average, don't worry; a truly average human may not exist.

Once you understand that for an effective weight-control program you need to plan meals containing adequate amounts of the various minerals, vitamins, carbohydrates, and essential fatty acids and amino acids, you can adjust your eating habits to achieve a satisfactory body weight without sacrificing the quality of your food intake.

Begin your own calorie count by calculating approximately the amount of energy your body needs for basal metabolism; that is, the calories needed for such basic functions as maintaining a normal body temperature, respiration, heartbeat, and so on. For a moderately active adult, the basal metabolic calorie need should be around one-half of a calorie for each hour of the day for every pound of body weight. In terms of the metric system,

Desirable Body Weights

The desirable body weight for an adult is approximately what a person weighs around the age of 21 years—assuming that one is not seriously overweight or underweight at that age. The U.S. government has found that men and women in their 20's are likely to have the body weights shown on the following tables. Ideally, these are the body weights that should be maintained throughout adult life.

The numbers in the left column indicate body height without shoes. Body weights are measured without clothing. The columns marked "low," "average," and "high" allow for body weight variations due to differences in bone structure, or body frame.

WEIGHTS OF PERSONS 20 TO 30 YEARS OLD

Height (without shoes)	Weight (without clothing)		
	Low	Average	High
	Pounds	Pounds	Pounds
MEN			
5 feet 3 inches	118	129	141
5 feet 4 inches	122	133	145
5 feet 5 inches	126	137	149
5 feet 6 inches	130	142	155
5 feet 7 inches	134	147	161
5 feet 8 inches	139	151	166
5 feet 9 inches	143	155	170
5 feet 10 inches	147	159	174
5 feet 11 inches	150	163	178
6 feet	154	167	183
6 feet 1 inch	158	171	188
6 feet 2 inches	162	175	192
6 feet 3 inches	165	178	195
WOMEN			
5 feet	100	109	118
5 feet 1 inch	104	112	121
5 feet 2 inches	107	115	125
5 feet 3 inches	110	118	128
5 feet 4 inches	113	122	132
5 feet 5 inches	116	125	135
5 feet 6 inches	120	129	139
5 feet 7 inches	123	132	142
5 feet 8 inches	126	136	146
5 feet 9 inches	130	140	151
5 feet 10 inches	133	144	156
5 feet 11 inches	137	148	161
6 feet	141	152	166

with a kilogram equivalent to 2.2 pounds of weight, and using an example that provides a simple calculation, a 60-kilogram (132-pound) woman needs 60 calories per hour, 24 hours a day, for a total of 1,440 calories a day. Her work and play activities might require an additional 1,000 to 1,200 calories a day.

Many people forget to include the basal metabolic calorie demand when figuring their food intake and think only in terms of the amount of calories needed for work and play. To simplify the calorie counting process and spare the reader the risk of damaging his body tissues by offering energy expenditure data that fails to include basal metabolism, the calorie information in this chapter is given as one combined number, including energy needs for basic body functions and the additional energy requirement for a specific physical activity. A range of calorie values is offered to allow for differences in body size and the degree of exertion involved. Some people are very efficient in body actions; others expend a lot of energy to accomplish a small amount of work.

Sedentary activities require little more energy than simply lying in bed. Playing cards increases the body's calorie needs by only a fraction of a calorie per minute. Operating an old-fashioned manual typewriter requires only about one more calorie every five minutes than operating an electric typewriter. Translated into terms of the amount of food required for the actual physical effort, above and beyond basal metabolic needs, very few extra calories are demanded for sedentary activities. In fact, a 12-ounce can of ginger ale should provide all the calories required to operate a typewriter for an eight-hour day.

Driving an automobile may require

APPROXIMATE CALORIE COUNT PER TYPE OF ACTIVITY

Calories per hour: 80 to 100 calories
Sedentary activities: reading, writing, watching television, eating, listening to radio or record player, sewing, or simple office duties that can be done while seated, such as typing or filing.

110 and 160 calories
Light activities: Activities that can be performed while seated or standing but which require some arm movement, such as rapid typing, preparing a meal, washing dishes, hand washing small articles of clothing, ironing, or walking slowly.

170 to 240 calories
Moderate activities: Activities that may be performed while seated that require vigorous arm movement, or activities while standing that require moderate arm movement, such as sweeping, mopping, and scrubbing floors, polishing and waxing, light gardening or carpentry, or walking moderately fast.

250 to 350 calories
Vigorous activities: Heavy scrubbing and waxing, hand washing large articles of clothing, hanging clothing on a clothes line, stripping and making beds, fast walking, bowling, active gardening, or playing golf.

350 or more calories per hour
Strenuous activities: Swimming, tennis, bicycling, dancing, skiing, or playing football.

twice as many calories per hour as typing, depending upon whether the car is equipped with such features as power steering and an automatic transmission. And all the energy required to do easy housework chores, such as dusting or washing dishes for an hour, should be contained in only 10 or 12 potato chips.

A leg of fried chicken or a hamburger patty without the bun would give you enough calories of energy to walk for an hour at a moderate pace. An ice cream cone or a slice of fruit pie could provide enough fuel for an hour of gardening or golfing, give or take a few calories because of variations in body size.

In most types of body activities the actual amount of calories needed to perform simple work or play tasks is much less than most people imagine. Putting mayonnaise on a luncheon sandwich can add 100 calories, which is enough to carry on general office work for one hour—including the calories needed for basal metabolism. But if the additional 100 calories is not balanced by an equivalent amount of muscular activity, an extra 100 calories a day will add up to almost an extra pound of fat each month, or about ten pounds of unwanted body weight in one year.

Advancing into the higher stages of extra food calories, a delicious luncheon dessert such as pie à la mode or chocolate layer cake can add 400 to 500 calories to one's energy inventory. Of course, it is possible to work off or walk off the extra 450 calories, but this would take a lot of working or walking. Roughly one hour of jogging or marathon running, or playing football or tennis, would just about wipe out the dessert calories. But most humans wouldn't be able to walk off 450 calories in less than two hours, even if they could step off at a moderately fast pace. Burning off excess calories at a rate of 10 to 20 per minute requires something even more strenuous, like skiing or backpacking up a steep slope, cross-country running, or hiking through loose snow with a 44-pound pack on your back.

Calorie-expenditure figures represent averages with peaks and valleys of exertion evened out. A tennis player, for example, may burn calories at a rate of as much as 100 per minute in brief spurts of match play. This is as much energy used in one minute that a sedentary person might spend over a period of one hour by sewing or playing cards. But tennis players also spend a lot of time doing little more than standing around. Similarly, a football player burns calories at rates that vary from three to more than 23 per minute, depending upon whether he is waiting for a play to start or if he is in the middle of a play moving down the field. But he may average only nine or so calories per minute for an entire game.

Some people consume enormous amounts of food without gaining weight, but they also work or play at activities that burn enormous amounts of calories. Soldiers on duty in the bitterly cold weather near the Arctic Circle may consume 4,500 calories in food each day without gaining weight. Finnish lumberjacks may burn more than 5,000 calories per day in cutting timber. And some Olympic athletes have been found to consume as much as 8,000 calories a day without gaining an ounce of flab. These people are living proof that is possible to eat large quantities of food without getting fat. Their bodies are attuned to an activity pace that literally burns away the calories as rapidly as they are acquired; they have achieved a healthy balance between calorie intake and calorie expenditure. In other words they have literally learned to eat their chocolate cake and have it, too.

Planning Diets to Cut Calories

If you want to lose or gain weight by controlling your food intake while not changing your work or play activities, your rate of loss or gain should depend upon the number of calories you add to or subtract from your diet each day. Unless you are under the direct supervision of a doctor, you should not try to cut down on your food intake to reduce body weight at a pace that is faster than perhaps 500 calories a day or 3,500 calories a week, the equivalent of a pound of fat. This rule ap-

FIRST DAY

1,200 Calories	3,000 Calories
BREAKFAST	
Grapefruit, 1/2 medium.	Grapefruit, 1/2 medium.
Wheat flakes, 1 ounce.	Wheat flakes, 1 ounce.
Skim milk, 1 1/2 cups.	Banana, 1 medium.
Coffee (black), if desired.	Whole milk, 1 1/2 cups.
	Toast, enriched, 2 slices.
	Jelly, 1 tablespoon.
	Butter or margarine,
	1 1/2 teaspoons.
	Coffee, 1 cup.
	Cream, 1 tablespoon.
	Sugar, 1 teaspoon.
LUNCH	
Chef's salad:	Chef's salad:
Julienne chicken,	Julienne chicken,
1 ounce.	2 ounces
Cheddar cheese,	Cheddar cheese,
1/2 ounce.	1 ounce.
Hard-cooked egg,	Hard-cooked egg,
1/2 egg.	1/2 egg.
Tomato, 1 large.	Tomato, 1 large.
Cucumber, 6 slices.	Cucumber, 6 slices.
Endive, 1/2 ounce.	Endive, 1/2 ounce.
Lettuce, 1/8 head.	Lettuce, 1/8 head.
French dressing,	French dressing,
2 tablespoons.	2 tablespoons.
Rye wafers, 4 wafers.	Rye wafers, 4 wafers.
Skim milk, 1 cup.	Gingerbread, 2 3/4-inch-
	square piece.
	Lemon sauce, 1/4 cup.
	Whole milk, 1 cup.
DINNER	
Beef pot roast, 3 ounces.	Beef pot roast, 3 ounces.
Mashed potatoes, 1/3 cup.	Gravy, 1/4 cup.
Green peas, 1/2 cup.	Mashed potatoes, 2/3 cup.
Whole-wheat bread,	Rolls, enriched, 2 small.
1 slice	Butter or margarine,
Butter or margarine,	1 teaspoon.
1/2 teaspoon.	Fruit cup:
Fruit cup	Orange, 1/2 small.
Orange, 1/2 small.	Apple, 1/2 small.
Apple, 1/2 small.	Banana, 1/2 medium.
Banana, 1/2 medium.	Sandwich cookies, 2
BETWEEN-MEAL SNACK	
Banana, 1/2 medium.	Sandwich:
	Enriched bread, 2 slices.
	Beef pot roast, 2 ounces.
	Mayonnaise
	Lettuce, 1 large leaf.
	Whole milk, 1 cup.

SECOND DAY

1,200 Calories	3,000 Calories
BREAKFAST	
Orange juice, $\frac{1}{2}$ cup. Soft-cooked egg, 1 egg. Whole-wheat toast, 1 slice. Butter or margarine, 1 teaspoon. Skim milk, 1 cup. Coffee (black), if desired.	Orange juice, $\frac{1}{2}$ cup. Soft-cooked egg, 1 egg. Bacon, 2 medium strips. Whole-wheat toast, 2 slices. Butter or margarine, 2 teaspoons. Whole milk, 1 cup. Coffee, 1 cup. Cream, 1 tablespoon. Sugar, 1 teaspoon.
LUNCH	
Sandwich: Enriched bread, 2 slices. Boiled ham, $1\frac{1}{2}$ ounces. Mayonnaise, 2 teaspoons. Mustard Lettuce, 1 large leaf. Celery, 1 small stalk. Radishes, 4 radishes. Dill pickle, $\frac{1}{2}$ large. Skim milk, 1 cup.	Tomato soup, with milk, 1 cup. Sandwich: Enriched bread, 3 slices. Boiled ham, 3 ounces. Mayonnaise, $2\frac{1}{2}$ teaspoons. Mustard Lettuce, 2 large leaves. Celery, 1 small stalk. Radishes, 4 radishes. Dill pickle, $\frac{1}{2}$ large. Apple, 1 medium. Whole milk, 1 cup.
DINNER	
Roast lamb, 3 ounces. Rice, converted, $\frac{1}{2}$ cup. Spinach, $\frac{3}{4}$ cup. Lemon, $\frac{1}{4}$ medium. Salad: Peaches, canned, 1 half peach. Cottage cheese, 2 tablespoons. Lettuce, 1 large leaf.	Roast lamb, 4 ounces. Rice, converted, $\frac{2}{3}$ cup. Spinach, buttered, $\frac{2}{3}$ cup. Lemon, $\frac{1}{4}$ medium. Salad: Peaches, canned, 2 halves. Cottage cheese, 2 tablespoons. Lettuce, 1 large leaf. Rolls, enriched, 2 small. Butter or margarine, 1 teaspoon. Plain cake, iced, 1 piece, 3 by 3 by 2 inches.
BETWEEN-MEAL SNACK	
Apple, 1 medium.	Saltines, 4 crackers. Peanut butter, 2 tablespoons. Whole milk, 1 cup.

THIRD DAY

1,200 Calories	3,000 Calories
BREAKFAST	
Tomato juice, $\frac{1}{2}$ cup. French toast: Enriched bread, 1 slice. Egg, $\frac{1}{2}$ egg. Milk Butter or margarine, 1 teaspoon. Jelly, $1\frac{1}{2}$ teaspoons. Skim milk, 1 cup. Coffee (black), if desired.	Tomato juice, $\frac{1}{2}$ cup. French toast: Enriched bread, 2 slices. Egg, $\frac{1}{2}$ egg. Milk Butter or margarine, $1\frac{1}{2}$ teaspoons. Syrup, 3 tablespoons. Whole milk, 1 cup. Coffee, 1 cup. Cream, 1 tablespoon. Sugar, 1 teaspoon.
LUNCH	
Tunafish salad: Tunafish, 2 ounces. Hard-cooked egg, $\frac{1}{2}$ egg. Celery, 1 small stalk. Lemon juice, 1 teaspoon. Salad dressing, $1\frac{1}{2}$ tablespoons. Lettuce, 1 large leaf. Whole-wheat bread, 2 slices. Butter or margarine, 1 teaspoon. Carrot sticks, $\frac{1}{2}$ carrot. Skim milk, 1 cup.	Tunafish salad: Tunafish, 3 ounces. Hard-cooked egg, $\frac{1}{2}$ egg. Celery, 1 small stalk. Lemon juice, 1 teaspoon. Salad dressing, $2\frac{1}{2}$ tablespoons. Lettuce, 1 large leaf. Whole-wheat bread, 2 slices. Butter or margarine, 1 teaspoon. Carrot sticks, $\frac{1}{2}$ carrot. Grapes, 1 large bunch. Whole milk, 1 cup.
DINNER	
Beef liver, 2 ounces. Green snap beans, $\frac{2}{3}$ cup. Shredded cabbage with vinegar dressing, $\frac{2}{3}$ cup. Roll, enriched, 1 small. Butter or margarine, $\frac{1}{2}$ teaspoon. Grapes, 1 small bunch.	Beef liver, 4 ounces. Bacon, 2 medium strips. Mashed potatoes, $\frac{2}{3}$ cup. Green snap beans, buttered, $\frac{2}{3}$ cup. Coleslaw, $\frac{2}{3}$ cup. Rolls, enriched, 2 small. Butter or margarine, 1 teaspoon. Cherry pie, $3\frac{1}{2}$-inch piece.
BETWEEN-MEAL SNACK	
Orange, 1 medium.	Orange, 1 medium. Iced cupcake, 1 medium. Whole milk, 1 cup.

plies particularly to individuals who already are of short stature or have low body weight.

A person who already has an intake of only 2,000 calories a day, for example, would drop to 1,500 calories by cutting 500 calories a day from his average food consumption. This figure borders on the number of calories needed for basal metabolic functions for a person weighing around 60 kilograms or 132 pounds. Some nutritionists doubt that a person can obtain well-balanced meals with all the essential nutrients on calorie-intakes much lower than 1,400 calories per day, unless they are in a hospital where minerals, vitamins, essential amino acids, and other nutrients can be measured into every meal by a professional dietitian.

To calculate the amount of calories you now consume, check the table of representative food values on pages 634-36. Make a list of the foods you usually eat each day or week and estimate the number of calories you probably consume. If the number is significantly larger or smaller than you might have guessed, you should consider which items can be reduced or increased to bring your own calorie count into line with the body weight you would like to have.

The menus on pages 628-29 suggest ways in which a member of a family can control his or her intake of calories by carefully selecting foods from the meals eaten by other members of the family who require greater amounts of food energy.

The menus on the preceding pages were developed by the U.S. Department of Agriculture to help families or individuals plan meals that contain the essential nutrients. One menu provides 1,200 calories a day while the other offers 3,000 calories a day. The idea behind the parallel meal

plans is that a person can gain or lose weight by selecting items from the same basic food list. Also, if one person in a family wants to lose weight while another wishes to gain or maintain a certain body weight, the calorie juggling can be done with the same foods available to all members of the family.

By checking back against the table of calories per food item, you can make individual adjustments for calorie counts somewhere between 1,200 and 3,000 per day. By adding the extra foods listed in the breakfast menu for the first day, for example—that is, the banana, toast and butter, or margarine, jelly, and sugar and cream in the coffee—the 1,200-calorie day can be increased to around 1,650 calories. Or by subtracting those foods from the 3,000-calorie day, the larger meal can be reduced to 2,550 calories. Almost any other number of calories per day can be planned by adding or subtracting individual food items.

People on weight-control programs should avoid fudging on the calorie counts. The content of each meal of the day is important in gaining, losing, or maintaining a desirable body weight. Skipping meals or eating token meals in order to reduce food intake can lead to snacking, and snack foods usually contribute more calories with fewer essential nutrients. At least half of the day's total calories should be accounted for during the first two meals of the day, ideally with one-fourth of the calories consumed at breakfast and at least one-fourth during a lunch break. Each of the three main meals should provide essential amino acid proteins, which is an easier task for people who are not vegans because essential amino acids are most conveniently available in meat, poultry, fish, eggs, milk, and cheese.

If you find that it is important to re-strict calorie intake, there are several food preparation traps to avoid. On the other hand, if your objective is to gain weight or help a member of the family gain weight, the same calorie catches can be used in re-verse to add calories to the day's meals. For instance, adding fats or sugar in cook-ing or at the table will increase the calorie content of a food. Sauces, gravies, salad dressings, and cream or whipped cream will add more calories to a food than were present in the first place. For example, one-half cup of boiled potato, diced, should contain about 55 calories, but the same amount of potato mashed with milk and fat added has about 100 calories. Served as hash-browned, one-half cup of potato has 175 calories, and one-half cup of pan-fried potato will provide around 230 calo-ries. Thus, starting with one-half cup of raw potatoes, the calorie count can be dou-bled, tripled, or quadrupled simply by changing the manner in which the vegeta-ble is cooked and served.

Another example is that one-half cup of sliced fresh peaches should offer only about 30 calories, but with two teaspoons of sugar added, the calorie count doubles up to 60. Adding one-fourth cup of half-and-half milk and cream mixture would bring the number of calories per serving up to 140, or more than four times the calorie value of the fruit without sugar and half-and-half. A simple salad made with one tomato and two leaves of lettuce would provide approximately 25 calories if served without dressing, but served with one tablespoon of French dressing, the salad would contain about 90 calories. Or by substituting one tablespoon of mayon-naise for the French dressing, the calorie count would be closer to 125, or five times the energy value of the original salad.

Measuring Food Portions and Body Weight

The calorie values listed in the tables in this chapter are based on the average sizes of typical servings of food, or in terms of 100-gram portions (three to four ounces). A quarter-pound of hamburger, for example, is approximately equivalent to a 100-gram portion of hamburger. When servings are prepared in larger amounts, it is obvious that the amount of calories per serving also will be larger.

To estimate serving sizes, a small diet scale usually can be purchased in models that are calibrated in both English and metric weight systems. An inexpensive diet scale may not be precise in measur-ing the weights of food to the nearest gram, but it will be accurate enough to help estimate the number of calories per serving of the foods you select from the dieting menu. A small plastic cup or simi-lar lightweight container should be used to place the food in while weighing it, and the weight of the food container should be subtracted from the total weight so that you don't shortchange yourself on food measurements. For solid foods such as meat cuts, a small sheet of waxed paper placed under the food will protect both the scale surface and the food to be consumed from possible contamination. In lieu of a regular diet scale, a postal scale can be used for weighing food. If the postal scale is calibrated in the English system of weights and measures, the reading in ounces can be converted to grams by mul-tiplying the ounces by 28—or 28.34 if you want to be exact. However, it is unlikely that either the scale or the calorie count of the food will be accurate to the first or second decimal place, so there's really not much point in trying to be so precise.

A bathroom scale to measure your total weight probably is as important in weight control as the diet scale. Bathroom scales also are available in both metric and English systems of measurements. It is best to weigh yourself in the nude and at the same time each day, usually in the morning before getting dressed. You should keep a record of your body weight on a day to day basis. If you fail to check your weight regularly, it can easily drift away from the target weight that you may have established as your goal.

Because of various subtle metabolic factors, you can expect to observe fluctuations that you won't be able to relate to anything you have eaten or have not eaten. In fact, you may not observe any significant weight change for the first couple of weeks or so after starting a weight-control diet. In some cases of quick weight-loss dieting, the weight change you observe—or do not observe—may be accounted for by shifts of body fluid. The loss may be due to water depletion from the body tissues, or fat may be consumed as body fuel and the fat cell spaces occupied by fluid. Other physiological factors can disrupt your careful weight control plans, as in the case of hormonal cycles that result in fluid accumulation in the tissues of some individuals.

However, faith and persistence usually win out in any weight-control program. You may cut your calorie count by a considerable amount for several days and discover you haven't lost an ounce of body weight. Then you may have other periods when you top double servings of main dishes with pie à la mode, yet find when you step on the bathroom scale the next day that your body weight has suddenly dropped a pound or two. But if you work conscientiously at consuming an average of only enough calories per day to achieve a certain body weight, your body will gradually adjust to that objective and you will reach your goal.

Overeating is a common problem in a society where food is plentiful and strenuous physical effort is not required to earn a living. However, some individuals for various reasons may not have an appetite or hunger drive that is strong enough to direct them toward regular full meals. A condition called anorexia, or absence of appetite, is associated with a number of different organic diseases as well as certain psychological problems. In addition, there are some individuals who seem unable to obtain enough food to meet the demands of their bodily energy requirements.

A skinny person may have no more desire to be underweight than an overweight person may enjoy being obese. In fact, the anorexia patient can be so dangerously underweight that vital organ tissues may become permanently damaged. Seriously underweight individuals can adjust their calorie intake upward, using the same calorie counting and body weight information used for reducing diets, in order to provide a healthful nutritional margin above the basal metabolic requirements of the body.

The Value and Danger of Snack Foods

In some cases snack foods can be used to supply the extra calories needed, keeping in mind that snack foods should be of the type that furnish vitamins, minerals, and essential amino acids and fatty acids as well as calories. An extra glass of milk as a snack food could serve that purpose. Snacks that are very low in calories and sometimes low in nutrients as well include some of the beverages. A bottle of club soda, for example, contains no more calories than a glass of water because it is only water that has been charged with carbon dioxide bubbles. A cup of coffee or tea will contain about two or three calories, with trace amounts of a few vitamins and minerals. A stalk of celery weighing about 100 grams will provide between 15 and 20 calories, and a three-ounce sour pickle could contain approximately a dozen calories. Carbonated beverages, such as cola drinks, may contain around 100 calories if sweetened with sugar, but very few if manufactured with artificial sweeteners.

Coffee or tea has hardly any calories if consumed in the "black" or unsweetened condition, but it takes on a significant amount of calorie value if sugar and cream are added. Each teaspoonful of sugar contributes about 15 calories, and a tablespoon of light cream about 30 calories. Sugar and cream therefore can raise the number of calories in a cup of coffee from two or three to more than 60. If a half-and-half mixture of milk and cream is used instead of light cream, the calorie portion of the dairy additive can be trimmed from 30 to about 20.

Snacks that contain chocolate generally can add calories quite rapidly. One piece of chocolate cream or mint chocolate will contain about 35 calories; one piece of chocolate fudge or a one-ounce bar of milk chocolate is worth from 115 to 150 of your day's ration of calories. But a chocolate milk shake can contain around 515 calories, or the equivalent of an entire meal for a person on a weight-reducing diet.

Planning Nutritious Meals

You may have to change some of your past eating habits in order to establish a pattern of effective weight control and healthful balance of essential nutrients. However, you should not deprive yourself of a favorite food if doing that will make proper eating seem like some form of torture. If you have an inherent craving for chocolate milk shakes or milk chocolate candy bars, for example, try to find a way to work them into your personal diet. Although such foods may cost you a big pack of calories from your energy budget, they will provide some of the nutrients you need for normal health. Just be sure you select enough straight foods to make up any deficits in vitamins, minerals, and other nutrients that may be lacking in the foods you can't diet without.

If your food selections lack some of the essential nutrients, your body has no other way to get them. Your body has its own ideas about what it needs to function properly, but it has to make its selections from the foods you make available to the digestive system. If your meals do not include enough calcium, the body's chemical foragers will steal calcium from your bones. If the stolen calcium is not replaced, the entire body eventually will be in big trouble. Nutrient deficiencies, like certain other diseases, can go unnoticed for a long period of time. But when the disorder makes itself felt you may find yourself in for a long and expensive program of normal health restoration, which could be the good news. The bad news would be that the deficiency had reached a point of permanent tissue damage that could not be corrected at any price.

One way to increase your chances of

FOODS WITH CALORIE VALUES

The following table shows approximate calorie values of commonly used foods within the major food groups. Not included are fats, sugars, or other substances that might alter a food's calorie content (unless specified).

Calories
MILK, CHEESE, AND ICE CREAM

Milk, fluid

Whole	1 cup or glass	160
Skim	1 cup or glass	90
Buttermilk	1 cup or glass	145
Evaporated	$\frac{1}{2}$ cup	175
Condensed	$\frac{1}{2}$ cup	490

Cream

Half-and-half (milk and cream)	1 tablespoon	20
Light, coffee or table	1 tablespoon	30
Sour	1 tablespoon	25
Whipped (pressurized)	1 tablespoon	10
Whipping (unwhipped)	1 tablespoon	50

Imitation Dairy Products
(made with vegetable fat)

Creamers, powdered	1 teaspoon	10
Creamers, liquid	1 tablespoon	20
Whipped topping	1 tablespoon	10

Cheese

Natural:

Blue/Roquefort	1 ounce	105
Camembert	4 ounces	115
Cheddar	1 ounce	115
Parmesan	1 ounce	130
Swiss	1 ounce	105

Pasteurized processed:

American	1 ounce	105
Swiss	1 ounce	100

Cottage cheese:

Creamed	2 tablespoons	30
Uncreamed	2 tablespoons	20

Cream cheese	1 ounce	105

Yogurt

Skimmed milk	1 cup	125
Whole milk	1 cup	150

Milk desserts

Chocolate milk	1 cup	200
Chocolate milk shake	12 ounces	515
Custard	1 cup	305
Ice Cream (10% fat)	1 cup	255
Ice Cream (16% fat)	1 cup	330

MEAT, POULTRY, FISH, EGGS

Beef

Roast, lean and fat	3 ounces	245
Roast, lean only	3 ounces	165
Steak, lean, broiled	3 ounces	175
Ground, hamburger patty	3 ounces	245
Ground, lean only	3 ounces	185
Corned beef, canned	3 ounces	155
Dried beef, chipped	2 ounces	115
Veal cutlet, broiled	3 ounces	185

Lamb

Loin chop, lean and fat	$3\frac{1}{2}$ ounces	355
Loin chop, lean only	$2\frac{1}{3}$ ounces	120
Leg, roasted, lean	3 ounces	160
Shoulder, roasted, lean	3 ounces	175

Pork

Chop, lean and fat	$2\frac{2}{3}$ ounces	305
Chop, lean only	2 ounces	150
Roast, loin, lean	3 ounces	215
Ham, cured, lean and fat	3 ounces	245
Ham, cured, lean only	3 ounces	160
Bacon, broiled	2 thin slices	60
Canadian (back) bacon	$1\frac{3}{16}$-inch slice	60
Pork sausage	4 ounces	255

Miscellaneous

Frankfurter	2 ounces	170
Bologna	2 ounces	170
Braunschweiger	2 ounces	180
Salami	2 ounces	175
Beef liver	3 ounces	195
Beef heart	3 ounces	160
Beef tongue	3 ounces	210

Poultry, without bones

Broiled chicken (skinless)	3 ounces	115
Fried chicken	$2\frac{4}{5}$ ounces	160
Roasted turkey, dark	3 ounces	175
Roasted turkey, light	3 ounces	150

Fish and Shellfish

Bluefish, baked with fat	3 ounces	135
Clams, raw, meat only	3 ounces	65
Crabmeat, cooked	3 ounces	80
Fish sticks, breaded	3 ounces	150
Haddock, breaded	3 ounces	140
Mackerel, broiled with fat	3 ounces	200
Ocean perch	3 ounces	195
Oysters, raw	$\frac{1}{2}$ cup	80
Salmon, fresh, baked	4 ounces	205
Salmon, canned	3 ounces	120
Sardines, canned	3 ounces	170
Shrimp, canned	3 ounces	100
Tuna, canned	3 ounces	170

Eggs

Fried	1 large	100
Boiled, hard or soft	1 large	80
Scrambled or omelet	1 large	110
Poached	1 large	80

DRY BEANS AND NUTS

Baked beans, cooked, with pork	½ cup	155
Lima beans	½ cup	130
Red kidney beans	½ cup	110
Almonds, shelled	2 tablespoons	105
Brazil nuts, shelled	2 tablespoons	115
Cashew nuts, roasted	2 tablespoons	100
Coconut, shredded	2 tablespoons	55
Peanuts, roasted, shelled	2 tablespoons	105
Pecans, shelled	2 tablespoons	95
Walnuts, English, halves	2 tablespoons	100

VEGETABLES

Fresh and Cooked Vegetables

Asparagus, cooked	½ cup spears	20
Beans, snap, green or yellow	½ cup	15
Beets, cooked	½ cup	30
Beet greens	½ cup	15
Broccoli, cooked	½ cup	25
Cabbage, raw	½ cup	10
Cabbage, cooked	½ cup	15
Cabbage, coleslaw with mayonnaise	½ cup	60
Carrots, raw, grated	½ cup	25
Carrots, cooked	½ cup	25
Cauliflower, cooked	½ cup flower buds	15
Celery, raw	3 5-inch stalks	10
Corn, on cob, cooked	1 5-inch ear	70
Corn, kernels, cooked	½ cup	70
Corn, cooked cream-style	½ cup	105
Cucumbers, raw	6 center slices	5
Lettuce, raw	½ cup or 2 large leaves	5
Onions, green	2 medium size	15
Onions, mature, cooked	½ cup	30
Peas, cooked or canned	½ cup	65
Potatoes, baked	1 large size	145
Potatoes, boiled	1 medium size	90
Potatoes, hash browned	½ cup	175
Potatoes, French-fried	10 pieces	215
Potatoes, mashed with milk	½ cup	70
Potatoes, salad with mayonnaise	½ cup	180
Potatoes, scalloped	½ cup	125
Pumpkin, canned	½ cup	40
Sauerkraut, canned	½ cup	20
Spinach, cooked or canned	½ cup	25
Squash, summer, cooked	½ cup	15
Squash, winter, baked	½ cup	65
Sweet potatoes, baked in skin	1 potato	160
Sweet potatoes, canned	½ cup	140

Tomatoes, raw	1 tomato	20
Tomatoes, cooked	½ cup	30
Tomato juice	½ cup	25
Turnips, cooked	½ cup	20
Turnip greens, cooked	½ cup	15

FRUITS

Fruits and Fruit Juices

Apples	1 medium apple	80
Apple juice	½ cup	60
Applesauce, sweetened	½ cup	115
Apricots, raw	3	55
Apricots, canned in syrup	½ cup	110
Avocados, California	5 ounces	190
Avocados, Florida	8 ounces	205
Bananas, raw	1 7-ounce banana	100
Berries:		
Blackberries, raw	½ cup	40
Blueberries, raw	½ cup	45
Raspberries, raw	½ cup	35
Strawberries, raw	½ cup	30
Cantaloupe, raw	½ melon	80
Cherries, sour, raw	½ cup	30
Cherries, sweet, raw	½ cup	40
Dates, fresh	½ cup	245
Figs, raw	3 small	95
Fruit cocktail, canned	½ cup	95
Grapefruit, raw	½ grapefruit	45
Grapefruit juice	½ cup	50
Grapes, American varieties	½ cup	35
Grapes, European varieties	½ cup	55
Grape juice	½ cup	85
Honeydew melon	1 wedge	50
Lemon juice, raw	½ cup	30
Oranges, raw	1 orange	65
Orange juice, raw	½ cup	55
Peaches, raw	1 medium	40
Peaches, canned, syrup	½ cup	100
Pears, raw	1 pear	100
Pears, canned, syrup	½ cup	95
Pineapple, raw	½ cup	40
Pineapple, canned, syrup	½ cup	95
Pineapple juice	½ cup	70
Plums, raw, Damson	5 1-inch plums	35
Plums, raw, Japanese	1 plum	30
Plums, canned, syrup	½ cup	105
Prunes, cooked, sweetened	½ cup	205
Prune juice	½ cup	100
Raisins, dried	½ cup	240
Rhubarb, cooked	½ cup	190
Tangerine, raw	1 tangerine	40
Watermelon, raw	1 4- by 8-inch wedge	110

BREAD AND CEREALS

Bread

Cracked wheat	1 slice	65
Raisin	1 slice	65
Rye	1 slice	60
White	1 slice	70
Whole wheat	1 slice	65

Miscellaneous

Graham crackers	4 crackers	55
Saltine crackers	4 crackers	50
Muffins, plain	1 muffin	120
Muffins, bran	1 muffin	105
Pancakes, wheat	1 4-inch cake	60
Pancakes, buckwheat	1 4-inch cake	55
Pizza, cheese	1 5-inch wedge	155
Pastry, Danish	1 pastry	275
Waffles	1 7-inch waffle	210

Cereals

Bran flakes with raisins	1 ounce	80
Corn flakes	1 ounce	110
Hominy grits	¾ cup	95
Oats, rolled, cooked	¾ cup	100
Rice flakes	1 ounce	110
Wheat flakes	1 ounce	100

Pasta

Macaroni, cooked	¾ cup	115
Spaghetti, cooked	¾ cup	115
Noodles, cooked	¾ cup	115
Wheat germ	1 tablespoon	25

getting a proper balance of essential nutrients is to follow a daily meal plan that provides items from each of the four major food groups—milk, meat, vegetables and fruits, and breads and cereals. The milk group includes dairy products in general, such as yogurt, cheese, ice cream, and cottage cheese. Adults should include in their daily meals two or more cups of milk or the equivalent in other dairy products; growing children need about twice the adult requirement because of their developing bones and teeth. One cup of milk in dairy product equivalents would amount to one and a half ounces of cheese, or one and a half cups of cottage cheese or ice cream.

While milk is a prime source of complete protein as well as of calcium and phosphorus, it also is a good example of the rule that no single food is the best source of all nutrients. Cow's milk is a poor source of iron and vitamin C, and it also is somewhat unreliable as a source of vitamins A and D unless it has been fortified. Vegans and individuals who are allergic to cow's milk can obtain the same essential amino acids from other foods, but for most of the population dairy products are a convenient source of proteins and minerals.

The meat group may be a bit misleading in its identity because it includes vegetarian foods that obviously are not animal protein sources as such. The meat group basically consists of beef, veal, pork, lamb, poultry, eggs, fish, and shellfish. But the proteins in animal meats also can be obtained from dry beans, dry peas, lentils, nuts, and peanuts or peanut butter.

An average serving of food from the meat group provides about three ounces of lean cooked meat, poultry, or fish, without the bones and fat which would of course not be protein sources. Alternative equivalents to three ounces of cooked lean meat might include servings of two eggs; one cup of cooked dry beans, peas, or lentils; or four tablespoons of peanut butter.

Vegetarians who shun the use of any animal products in their meals learn to balance their diets of legumes and other vegetables so as to make the most effective use of essential amino acids in those foods. While plants generally are deficient in essential amino acids, vegetarians have learned to combine in their meals the plant foods that contribute what are called complementary proteins, or amino acids. For example, corn is deficient in the amino acid called lysine, but it is a good source of amino acids containing sulfur. Beans, on the other hand, may be deficient in sulfur-containing amino acids but serve as a good source of lysine. By eating beans and corn together, vegetarians obtain the essential amino acids that meat-eaters receive from animal food products. Peas and rice offer another example of complementary amino acids. Such meatless meals form the basis of traditional diets in many countries of the world.

Vegans also are able to obtain most of the essential amino acids from whole cooked soybeans. Soybeans can be processed into a vegetable beverage quite similar to milk, lacking only the essential amino acid methionine for which cow's milk is a better source. Cottonseed meal, peanuts, oats, and rice are among the plant seeds, besides soybeans, which are sources for most if not all of the essential amino acids. Thus, vegetarian meals can be sources of all the basic food elements needed for healthful living. However, they lack much of the versatility and convenience of foods derived from both plant and animal sources. Vegetarian meal planning requires an adequate knowledge of nutrition so that proper levels of essential amino acids, fatty acids, minerals, and vitamins are accounted for in the daily diet.

People in the meat-and-potatoes category of meal planning frequently neglect the food items in the vegetables and fruit group, which are good natural sources of vitamins and minerals. The daily selections from this group should include a source of vitamin C, such as citrus fruits, cantaloupe or muskmelon, strawberries, broccoli, brussels sprouts, or green pepper. Broccoli is one of the members of the vegetable-fruit group that is a valuable source of vitamin A as well as vitamin C. Carrots, pumpkin, winter squash, sweet potatoes, turnip greens, spinach, and collards are other sources of vitamin A.

Food items from the vegetable-fruit group should be provided in at least four servings each day. A serving should be one-half cup of a vegetable or fruit, or one regular portion such as an orange or apple, or one-half cantaloupe or grapefruit.

To make the most effective use of vegetables in the diet it is important to remember that part of the protein and other nutrients is in the skins or peelings, so that if possible the peelings should be cooked with the inner portion of the vegetables. This is especially true of potatoes. Also, it is helpful to know that more of the nutrients can be retained if vegetables are steamed rather than boiled. Nutrients that may be lost in the cooking of vegetables may be found in the cooking water, which is frequently saved for use in making soups by people who are vitamin-wise.

Breads and cereals should be whole-grain, enriched, or restored. Included in this group are such items as breads, cereals that are to be cooked or are ready to eat, crackers, cornmeal, flours made from grains, grits, rice, rolled oats, macaroni, spaghetti, noodles and other pasta products, and baked goods in general. Most commercially baked breads and other products will state on their labels that they are made with whole-grain flours or are otherwise enriched.

Breads and cereals are sources of B vitamins, iron, protein, and carbohydrates. Four or more servings from this group should be included in the day's meal plan. A typical serving would be one slice of bread, one ounce of ready-to-eat cereal, or one-half to three-fourths of a cup of rice or macaroni. Servings of one food can be substituted for most other items in this category: for example, if no cereal is eaten, the quota can be met by having an extra slice of bread.

There are additional foods not listed in the categories above that are consumed daily by almost everyone to round out meals. These include sugar, butter and margarine, cooking oils or fats. They frequently are included in commercially prepared food products, such as breads and convenience foods, or they may be added in your own kitchen during meal preparation. The fact that they were not mentioned should not indicate they are to be avoided. Indeed, such things as spices, herbs, vinegars, and fruit and wine flavorings, as well as fats and sweeteners, will enhance the palatability of some essential foods. With the possible exception of fats and oils, however, the additional foods are not necessary. They may be important in helping to move food from the plate to the stomach, but the body's chemical factories are interested only in the basic foods in the four main groups.

Exceptions to the Dieting Rules

There are certain periods in the lives of most people when the general formulae for proper eating have to be altered to accommodate changes in anatomy and physiology. Childhood, pregnancy, and old age are among the factors that can call for reshaping the requirements for those who may not fit into the large category sometimes identified as otherwise normal healthy adults.

If pregnancy occurs before a woman has reached full physical maturity, the mother-to-be must have foods that provide for her own growth and development as well as those of the unborn baby. Pregnancy for an older woman can require special meal planning if her body stores of essential nutrients have been reduced by demands of earlier pregnancies. However, a mature woman who has maintained good eating habits over the years will not have to alter her gastronomic lifestyle except for minor changes needed to insure the nutritional health of her unborn child. A woman can expect to gain weight during pregnancy; a range of from 20 to 25 pounds of weight gain is considered normal. If a proper pregnancy diet is followed, this amount of weight change will permit normal development of the child while also allowing for support and protective changes in the body of the mother.

Pregnancy is not the time to begin a weight reduction program without direct supervision of a doctor even if the pregnant woman is overweight. A woman who is underweight at the start of a pregnancy, however, may be able to gain enough poundage during the period of gestation to be closer to an average weight for her height and body build following the birth of the child. A woman of normal weight at the beginning of a pregnancy probably will return to her original weight within a few weeks after giving birth.

The rate of weight gain during pregnancy will amount to only about one pound per month during the first three months. After the first trimester, the pregnant woman can expect to gain about three-fourths of a pound a week, or close to that average, until the baby has been delivered.

The nutrients needed for successful fetal development are about the same as those required before and after pregnancy. Since the daily energy requirement will increase by about 300 calories a day, the pregnant woman should anticipate that need. The extra calories should come from the four food groups: milk and milk products, meat or meat substitutes, vegetables and fruits, and breads and cereals. But the pregnant woman should not attempt to "eat for two people" because this might lead to calorie overloading. Overloading the stomach, especially during the last three months of pregnancy, can be a cause of discomfort. Some doctors recommend that food intake for a pregnant woman be divided into a series of a half-dozen or so mini-meals instead of the traditional three square meals every day. A minimeal routine will not result in missing get-togethers with other members of the family during mealtimes; the mother-to-be simply should eat less at the regular meals and make up the difference with midmorning, midafternoon, and late evening meals.

The first food for the infant is milk, and whether the milk comes from humans or cows, the choice should be made with care because this food will be the main source of nutrients for about the first two years of life. Human, or mother's milk, will supply nearly all essential nutrients for the first few months. Even mother's milk is not always a perfect food, however, and the infant may need supplements of iron, fluoride, and vitamin D.

If the infant is bottle-fed, the parents should make sure the milk used in the formula has vitamin D added. If the milk is not vitamin-fortified, vitamin D supplements will be needed. A bottle formula also may lack vitamin C, which can be provided in liquid vitamin drops or in a fruit juice rich in vitamin C. Iron and fluoride also should be part of the infant's menu, although fluoride may be present in the drinking water, and medicinal iron, iron-fortified infant cereal, or an infant milk formula fortified with iron could be sources of that mineral.

By four months of age the baby may be eating cereals, strained fruits, and vegetables, and then advance slowly to eggs and strained meats. By the age of about eight months, the baby probably will be eating mashed, chopped, or ground "table foods" prepared from the regular family meals. As the child becomes more dependent upon adult foods, the parents should continue to make sure that the foods given the youngster contain the essential amino acids, fatty acids, minerals, and vitamins. Even if commercial baby foods are used, the parents should check the ingredients because there are wide variations in the food values of various commercial baby foods, just as there are many differences in the food values of various home-cooked meals.

Older people have special eating problems because of the tendency of people past middle age to be overweight and bothered by problems of the digestive system. All people do not age at the same rate; some will claim they are as healthy at 65 as they were at 35. But by the age of 55, humans in general can reduce their food intake by about 200 calories a day. They need the same essential nutrients but can get along with fewer calories. The goal for people in this age group is to change their eating habits so that they select foods with all the essential nutrients that are packaged with less energy per ounce. The foods should emphasize animal protein sources, calcium, and vitamins C and D. Animal protein is a better source of amino acids needed by older persons. The calcium and vitamins are helpful in preventing the loss of bone tissue.

QUESTIONS AND ANSWERS
NUTRITION

Q: *I have to watch my potassium intake because of a diuretic medication I am taking, but I don't like bananas as a source of potassium. Are there any other foods that are better-than-average sources of potassium?*
A: One advantage of bananas as a potassium source is that they also are relatively low in sodium, and most people who are on diuretics also have to avoid sodium-rich foods. However, on an ounce-for-ounce basis, nuts—unsalted, of course—are a pretty good dietary source of potassium. Raw or canned apricots, avocados, boiled and drained lima beans, okra, oranges, and squash are high in potassium and low in sodium as long as table salt is not added in the preparation. A couple of frequently overlooked foods that are high in potassium and low in sodium are dates and bitter chocolate. Dates have almost twice as much potassium as bananas for the same amount of sodium per gram or ounce. Cocoa and bitter chocolate are very good sources of potassium, but only if they are unprocessed as in Dutch chocolate or chocolate-flavored beverage powders. Alkali-processed cocoa averages more than 100 times as much sodium and has less than half as much potassium as the unprocessed variety.

Q: *Are there any particular foods a nursing mother should eat in order to improve milk production?*
A: Nothing in a typical modern mother's diet is likely to influence milk production. However, this is not the same as saying that a mother's diet will not affect the quality of milk produced. A nursing mother needs approximately the same nutrients—minerals and vitamins—as a pregnant woman, plus about 20 grams more of protein per day than the usual adult requirement, and more than the usual amounts of fluids in the form of milk, water, fruit juices, coffee, tea, etc.

Q: *If your child is allergic to milk, can he get along without it?*
A: Yes, if he is provided with other foods that contain the minerals and other nutrients contained in milk. One of the advantages of milk is that it contains so many important food elements in a beverage form. But virtually all the nutrients in milk can be obtained from cheese, for example. Calcium is one of the important minerals contained in milk and a very essential component of the bones of growing children, but it can be obtained from calcium tablets.

Q: *My husband has an intestinal disorder and is not allowed to eat fruits or vegetables that have seeds and peelings. But he gets violent abdominal cramps from one of his favorite desserts, strawberry cheesecake. Is there something in strawberries that could cause this reaction?*
A: Strawberries have very tiny seeds that can prove very irritating to patients with sensitive gastrointestinal tracts.

Q: *A person on a gluten-free diet is allowed to have coffee made from regular ground roast coffee, but instant coffee is not allowed. What does instant coffee contain that would interfere with a gluten-free diet?*
A: Some instant coffees, as well as certain coffee-substitute beverages, are made with various amounts of grains such as wheat, rye, oats, buckwheat, and barley. These grains can produce the malabsorption symptoms of celiac disease or nontropical sprue, disorders that require an absence of gluten. Gluten is a protein that occurs naturally in many common cereals. However, it should be noted that gluten-free wheat starch can be obtained from firms that manufacture dietetic food products. And some cereal grains such as corn and rice do not contain gluten. So a patient of nontropical sprue or

celiac disease does not have to go through life without his corn flakes, rice puffs, or hominy grits for breakfast. But he should read the label on the container of coffee before making a cup of the beverage.

Q: *Are there fruits and vegetables besides the citrus fruits that contain vitamin C?*
A: Yes. There are quite a few food sources of ascorbic acid, or vitamin C, other than oranges, lemons, and grapefruit. The acerolo, for example, also known as the West Indian cherry or Barbados cherry, contains more than 20 times as much vitamin C per equal weight as the orange. But oranges are more easily available and a better source of vitamin C than, say, apples. An average orange contains about 50 milligrams of vitamin C per 100 grams (about three and a half ounces), compared to about 10 milligrams of vitamin C for a freshly harvested summer apple of the same weight. Some green vegetables, such as broccoli, brussels sprouts, and cauliflower, on the other hand, provide twice as much vitamin C per 100 grams as an orange. But to put the whole story into a proper perspective, the vitamin C values of fruits and vegetables vary considerably with the variety, the season, and other factors. Chopping, shredding, cutting, capping, and storing fresh fruits and vegetables can reduce the vitamin C content by as much as 50 percent from its freshly picked value. Cooking or otherwise processing the fruit or vegetable can eliminate the vitamin C altogether.

Q: *If a doctor told you to avoid exogenous cholesterol, would he mean cholesterol that is in butter, milk, meat, etc.?*
A: Yes. Exogenous cholesterol is a term sometimes used to identify the cholesterol supplied by foods in the diet. The human body produces a certain amount of cholesterol during normal metabolic processes. It is the same chemically as the cholesterol in a pork chop or a pat of butter. For some patients, adding exogenous cholesterol to the cholesterol produced by the body's own tissues may be supplying more cholesterol than the body can handle without increasing the risk of cardiovascular disease.

Q: *My brother claims that veal has a greater percentage of cholesterol than beef. I say he is wrong. Can you settle the argument?*
A: If the U.S. Department of Agriculture can be the judge of the argument, young animals of each species tend to have a greater concentration of cholesterol than mature animals. Therefore, veal does have more cholesterol than beef, lamb contains more cholesterol than mutton, and so on.

Q: *Is it true that milk is the only animal food that contains carbohydrates?*
A: That is generally but not completely accurate. About one-third of the solid matter in milk is lactose, a carbohydrate sometimes called milk sugar. Eggs and shellfish contain small amounts of carbohydrates. Blood contains small amounts of glucose, the basic sugar molecule. And liver contains glycogen, a carbohydrate that is broken down to glucose after an animal is slaughtered. But only a few foods of animal origin contain carbohydrates, and milk is the only significant animal source of carbohydrates.

Q: *I have been reading about nitrate and nitrite preservatives being added to foods and the chance that they can cause cancer. What did people use to cure meats and other foods before they had nitrites and nitrates?*
A: Food processors have been using nitrates and/or nitrites as food preservatives for centuries. The nitrate used for curing meats and pickles was a preservative commonly known as saltpeter. Around the end of the 19th century, food chemists discovered that some of the nitrate used actually was nitrite, perhaps as a result of bacterial action on the nitrate molecules. It also was found that nitrites improved the color of meats by giving them a reddish complexion. So, nitrates and nitrites have been used for the same purpose for hundreds of years as food preservatives. But it was not until the 1970's that modern scientists discovered that the nitrites could combine with certain amino acids to form a substance known as nitrosamine, which might be a cause of cancer in humans.

25

EMERGENCY FIRST AID

First aid means literally the aid that should be given first to the victim of an accident to prevent death or disability. An accident could be an automobile collision, a fall from a ladder or down a flight of stairs, a fire, a tornado, an earthquake, a drowning, contact with an electric wire, and so on. An accident also might be a sudden stroke, heart attack, or a choking spell.

Accidents are relatively common but seldom occur at places and times that are convenient for either the victim or the nearest available doctor.

Heart attacks, strokes, and accidents involving autos or mechanical devices are among the leading causes of death and disability. When the toll of the various separate types of mishaps is combined, the total number of victims in any year will be far greater than the number of cases of cancer or any other dreaded disease. The statistics warn that you, a close friend, or a member of your family will quite likely be the victim of an accident in which the chances of survival with or without disability may depend upon the quality of emergency first aid that can be delivered, and the speed with which both emergency and professional care can be provided.

What To Do First at the Scene of an Accident

If you happen to be first at the scene of an accident, there are four rules that will help you to decide the order in which first aid should be administered: (1) stop any serious bleeding; (2) maintain normal breathing; (3) prevent further injury to the victim; and (4) take whatever action may be indicated to prevent shock.

A few corollary rules for rendering first aid are: (1) don't panic; (2) summon a doctor, ambulance, police, firemen, or anyone who can provide trained assistance as quickly as possible; (3) don't do any more than is necessary to prevent the situation from getting worse; and (4) show confidence even if you're not inwardly confident, because it's good for the morale of the patient and bystanders.

Accidents often are quickly followed by an accumulation of "rubber-neckers," that is, people with a morbid curiosity in disasters. Try to recruit some of the rubber-neckers who may be willing to assist but need to be told what to do. Have them telephone the nearest police or hospital, and send them to get blankets, coffee, or whatever may be needed. If nobody is taking charge at the scene of a mishap, your role may be to organize the crowd to help. Most of those who would not be helpful may leave the scene quickly to avoid being recruited.

The reader should bear in mind also that if he should happen upon an accident scene where rescue efforts seem to be going as smoothly as possible, his best move may be simply to keep moving unless he can contribute some needed assistance.

How to Control Bleeding

The control of bleeding is extremely important in most emergency first aid situations. Blood is the vehicle that carries oxygen and nutrients to the brain and other vital organs. Lost blood is not easily replaced since transfusions seldom are available at accident sites. Therefore, immediate steps should be taken to stop the flow of blood.

The method used to control the loss of blood should be appropriate for the type and degree of bleeding. Simple pressure over the bleeding point often is sufficient if the blood is oozing from a capillary or vein. Bleeding from small arteries also can be controlled in many cases by applying pressure between the wound and the source of the blood flow; pressure on the artery beyond the wound probably would not stop the flow of blood.

Wounds in the extremities often can be treated in an emergency by elevating the limb above the level of the heart while applying pressure. Blood flow below the lev-

el of the heart can be exacerbated by the pull of gravity. But don't raise the limb if a bone is broken.

Pressure can be applied in serious bleeding cases directly over the wound. If a dressing is quickly available from a first aid kit, the dressing can be placed over the wound and pressure applied on the dressing. If a sterile dressing is not available, a clean handkerchief or clean cloth can be applied. If a dressing or cloth pad of any kind is not immediately available, close the wound with the hand or fingers.

Locating the Body's
Arterial Pressure Points

Know the location of the half-dozen pressure points where bleeding from an artery usually can be stopped or reduced considerably by compressing the artery against a bone that the artery crosses. The main pressure points are located in the area of the groin, where the femoral artery

BLEEDING FROM FOOT, LEG, THIGH

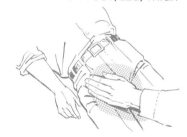

The main artery supplying blood to the lower limb, all the way from the thigh to the foot, passes over one of the bones of the pelvis at a point just below the groin. Pressure applied here by pressing the artery against the bone should stop the flow of blood to any point along the length of the leg. Do not continue to apply pressure after bleeding stops, but resume the use of pressure if the bleeding starts again while awaiting professional medical care. Avoid use of a tourniquet on an arm or leg unless the loss of blood is so severe that the patient is likely to bleed to death otherwise.

PRESSURE POINT FOR NECK, MOUTH, OR THROAT

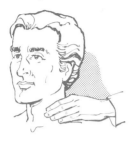

One of the first actions that can be taken to save the life of an accident victim is to control any loss of blood. In many cases, in the absence of professional medical help, you can stop bleeding at least temporarily by applying finger pressure at certain points on the body where a main artery passes near the skin. To stop bleeding from the neck, mouth, or throat area, for example, apply pressure at a point on the neck where an artery passes alongside the trachea, or windpipe. Place the thumb of the hand against the back of the victim's neck and the fingers on the neck just below the larynx, or Adam's apple. Then push the fingers against the artery. If the blood flow slackens or stops, you can assume you have found the pressure point.

STOP BLEEDING FROM TWO-THIRDS OF ARM

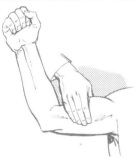

An artery supplying the arm passes close to the bone of the upper arm about halfway along the length of the upper arm. By applying pressure at that point, pressing the artery against the arm bone, bleeding from nearly any point beyond can be stopped. It should be remembered when using the pressure point technique to control bleeding that interrupting the blood flow means that tissues along the path of the artery will be deprived of blood. Therefore, the pressure should be released at intervals to permit some blood to reach the tissues normally supplied by the damaged artery.

PRESSURE POINT IN UPPER ARM

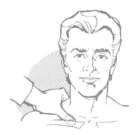

A pressure point for controlling the loss of blood in the area of the upper arm, shoulder, or arm pit, should be found where an artery passes over the outer surface of the top rib. Place the thumb in the position shown (the top rib is indicated in the drawing), and the fingers over the shoulder so they press against the area behind the collarbone. Apply pressure to the artery crossing the top rib.

BLEEDING BELOW EYE AND ABOVE JAWBONE

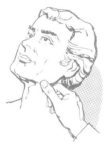

Bleeding from an artery supplying the area of the face below the level of the eye usually can be controlled by finding the pressure point that is located along the edge of the jawbone.

BLEEDING FROM HEAD ABOVE EYE LEVEL

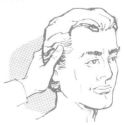

For bleeding above the level of the eye, the rescuer should be able to find a pressure point where an artery passes over one of the skull bones in front of the upper portion of the ear, as shown in the drawing.

crosses the pelvic bone on the way from the abdomen to the inner side of the upper leg; on the inner side of the upper arm, where the brachial artery passes close to the humerus, or upper arm bone; behind the collarbone, where the main artery supplying the arm and shoulder area, the subclavian artery, passes; the neck, where the carotid artery passes on the way to the head; the edge of the jaw, where the external maxillary artery crosses to supply the facial area between the chin and the bridge of the nose; and the temple area on the side of the head, where the temporal artery passes close to the skull.

The pressure points sometimes are called digital pressure points since the blood flow of arteries at those locations presumably can be controlled by finger, or digital, pressure. In most persons the pressure can be applied with the thumb or the heel of the hand to control blood flow. The body build of the patient is one of several factors that can make digital control of bleeding more or less effective.

In addition to the usual pressure points, which cover the blood flow to most of the human body, there are several other points that may be used by doctors in special cases. There is a point in the lower abdomen, for example, where pressure can be applied to the aorta to control hemorrhage in an emergency. Smaller areas of bleeding can also be controlled by pressure points in the ankle.

Controlling the flow of blood at a pressure point can be difficult for one person to manage over a long period of time. If the arrival of professional medical care is delayed, another person may be needed to apply pressure for a part of the time. If another person is not available to help, a tourniquet might be required.

Applying a Tourniquet

A tourniquet should be applied only as a last resort to save the life of the victim. A tourniquet can be very dangerous and its use may be equivalent to physiological amputation since the prolonged interruption of blood flow by the tourniquet will result in the death of tissues beyond the point of interruption. In fact, some doctors advise the use of a tourniquet only to stop the loss of blood from a limb that probably would have to be amputated anyway because it had been crushed, mangled, or severed.

The tourniquet should be made, if possible, from a wide strip of strong cloth tied about the arm or leg above the wound. The cloth should be tied in a manner that will permit the insertion of a stick that can be used to tighten or loosen the pressure on the bleeding artery. This can be accomplished by first tying a half-knot, then placing a stick across the half-knot and tying a full knot above the stick. The stick thus becomes a sort of control valve that can be used to stop and start the blood flow. The valve should be opened for a few seconds every 15 minutes to permit the flow of some blood to the tissues beyond.

If a tourniquet is applied, its presence should be well advertised. If possible, it should not be covered even though the victim might require a blanket or other covering to prevent chilling. Write a message on the forehead of the victim, or some other obvious place, so that medical personnel in the emergency room will know about the tourniquet. Use a pen, lipstick, or whatever to write simply the letters "TK" if there is not a better way to alert the medical professionals. One should never assume that interns and doctors in a hospital some miles away will understand the intentions of a person who applied first aid at an accident scene. In addition to the confusion surrounding an accident, ambulance attendants may fail to get the message or to pass it along to the doctors at the hospital. That is why it is imperative that information about a tourniquet or other unique first aid measures be conveyed to the medical professionals in a way that will not be missed.

Do's and Don'ts For Rendering First Aid

The person applying first aid should never touch an open wound except to apply pressure when a sterile pad or similar dressing is not available. Never explore the wound with the fingers in an effort to locate fragments of glass, metal, or other substances that may have caused the wound.

If the victim is conscious and does not appear to have suffered internal injuries, offer him plenty of fluids in the form of water, tea, coffee, soup, etc. But do not give the victim alcoholic beverages.

If there is more than one accident victim with serious bleeding, try to attend to the bleeding problems of each of the victims before attending to other needs such as the warmth or thirst of any injured individual.

If a victim is bleeding and has ceased breathing, it may be necessary to attempt to correct both problems at the same time. The combination of life-threatening conditions obviously forms a dire emergency. If attention is directed toward control of the bleeding, there may be no oxygen entering the blood. Or if the first aid activity is concentrated in first restoring normal breathing, the blood carrying the oxygen will be lost. If more than one person is

available, one should take charge of the breathing problem while the other first aider tries to stop the loss of blood.

How To Restore Normal Breathing

The most frequent reasons for the cessation of breathing are: (1) face or neck injuries that result in blockage of the upper air passages; (2) choking; (3) drowning; (4) compression of the chest; (5) inflammation and spasm of the upper air passages from exposure to smoke or flame; and (6) lack of oxygen in the environment.

Signs of interrupted breathing include cyanosis, or bluish coloration, of the fingernail beds, lips, or tongue, in addition to gasping, wheezing, or other more obvious signs of breathing difficulty.

The most important thing you can do when breathing has been interrupted is to restore normal breathing as quickly as possible. But first there must be an unobstructed airway between the mouth and the trachea. If the airway is blocked, artificial respiration will not be effective. Assuming there are no other complications, such as face or neck injuries, you should insure the presence of an open airway by quickly exploring the mouth with a finger to remove any foreign object and to be sure the tongue does not interfere with the passage of air.

The victim should be placed on his back with the shoulders elevated so the neck is extended in a straight line. The head should be held slightly back and the lower jaw held well forward. For mouth-to-mouth resuscitation, the most effective method of artificial respiration in most cases of interrupted breathing, the person administering first aid can manage the position of the patient's forehead, neck, and jaw with his hands, while holding the head and pinching the nose shut. During the actual resuscitation procedure, the first aider places his mouth over that of the victim and exhales. If the airway is open, the victim's chest and abdomen should expand.

The mouth of the person administering the mouth-to-mouth resuscitation and that of the victim should form a tight seal so that air blown into the victim will not escape along the edges of the lips. When the technique is applied to children, the mouth of the first aider usually will cover both the mouth and nose of the child so the nose of the young victim will not have to be held closed. At the same time, the hand of the rescuer that is not needed to hold the nose closed can be placed on the chest of the victim to help the lungs exhale.

Exhalation ordinarily occurs passively—that is, without any additional effort on the part of the rescuer. The breathing rate should be paced at about 15 times per minute, or once every four seconds. The first aider removes the lips and takes a deep breath, then blows into the mouth of the victim, then takes another deep breath while the air previously forced into the victim's lungs is exhaled.

Like applying finger pressure to a pressure point of a bleeding artery, mouth-to-mouth resuscitation for a lengthy period requires a considerable amount of endurance, and it is best if more than one person is available for the task, each taking a turn of several minutes. There is a chance that the person applying mouth-to-mouth artificial respiration may "overbreathe," or hyperventilate. This means that taking too many deep breaths can deplete the body's normal level of carbon dioxide, a factor that controls the need for oxygen intake. When this happens, the person who overbreathes usually faints and does

not regain consciousness until after the normal level of carbon dioxide in his body has been restored.

Efforts to restore breathing should continue as long as possible until professional medical help arrives. It may even be necessary to continue artificial respiration after a doctor has reached the scene and examined the victim. As long as there is any sign of life, the resuscitation efforts should continue.

Mouth-to-mouth resuscitation is recommended for drowning victims and should be started as soon as the patient has been recovered from the water. If the victim is pulled into a boat, resuscitation should be started in the boat.

If the cessation of breathing is caused by lack of oxygen or an excess of carbon monoxide or another noxious gas in the environment, the victim should be moved as quickly as possible to an area of fresh air before starting mouth-to-mouth resuscitation. The rescuer should not enter the oxygen-depleted area alone or without a gas mask or other appropriate respiratory gear.

Some first aid kits contain a plastic tube that is designed to aid in mouth-to-mouth resuscitation. One end of the plastic tube is inserted into the mouth of the victim, and the rescuer blows through the other end.

What Not to Do to an Accident Victim

Preventing further injury often can be accomplished by following the rule that the first aider should do no more than necessary. Also, knowing what not to do in an emergency can be helpful. For example, an injured person should not be moved from the accident site before a doctor, ambulance crew, or other experienced paramedical people arrive, unless there is a probability that further injury might result.

If there is an injury to the neck or spinal column, the victim should not be moved until a stretcher or other carrying device is available to provide proper firm support. A physician should supervise the removal of a patient with neck or spinal injuries. Improper movement of the patient's body could cause a broken or dislocated bone to pinch or sever the spinal cord or a spinal nerve root, resulting in death or disability that might otherwise be avoided.

If the victim appears to have a head injury, he should not be moved until after examination by a doctor, and then only under the supervision of a doctor. Any person who is found unconscious may be assumed to have a head injury. Do not move the head or any other part of the body if there are signs of bleeding from the nose, mouth, or ears.

A rescuer should not assume that an unconscious person who appears to have been drinking alcoholic beverages is merely drunk. He might have injured his head in a fall or suffered a head injury during a robbery or other physical assault. A rescuer should never give alcoholic beverages to any accident victim. And fluids of any kind should never be offered to a patient who is unconscious or semiconscious, or who has internal injuries.

How to Treat Shock

Shock of some form accompanies all serious injuries. It is a natural reaction of the body to any physical or emotional insult. In theory, shock is a circulatory change that is intended by nature to assure an adequate supply of blood to vital organs when the body's survival has been threatened. Unfortunately, the changes in blood flow can get out of hand and progress to circulatory collapse. Circulatory failure in turn can result in death of the victim. Because of the high risk of shock and death, all persons who are victims of accident injuries should be treated for possible shock effects.

The usual signs of shock may include a weak but rapid pulse, and skin that is pale, cold, and moist with "cold sweat." The victim's eyes appear vacant, with dilated pupils, and his behavior indicates restlessness, fright, and anxiety. The patient may complain of nausea and thirst as well as feelings of dizziness or faintness and weakness. As the shock deepens, the patient becomes quiet and slips into unconsciousness.

The person administering first aid should not wait for signs and symptoms of shock. Although control of bleeding and restoration of breathing take top priority, prevention of shock is not far behind, and whenever possible it should be managed along with treatment of the specific injury.

A prime consideration in the prevention of shock is the body position of the victim. There are two possible courses of action: either the victim has a head injury, or he does not have a head injury. If he has a head injury, the body should be kept flat on the back with the head slightly raised. If the victim does not have a head injury, the body should be arranged so that the head is lower than the rest of the body, a position that permits gravity to help maintain an adequate flow of blood to the brain.

The injury victim should be kept warm and protected from bad weather. But too much warmth can be dangerous. Too much heat causes a loss of vital body fluid through sweating, and excessive warmth draws the blood circulation to the surface of the body when the blood should be concentrated in the deep, vital organs.

The matter of providing fluids to potential shock victims is one that may require a bit of first aid intuition to resolve. If the accident site is close to a community where professional medical services may be a few minutes away, fluids should not be given to the victim. Among other reasons, fluid intake might interfere with the use of anesthetics to be administered by the medical professionals. But if the accident site is somewhere in the boondocks and professional medical aid may be hours away, small amounts of warm water or tea might be offered the victim if he is conscious, can swallow, and has no internal injuries.

Fluids may be more beneficial in the early stages since they may not be absorbed from the intestine in later stages of shock. Victims of burns may have a special need for fluids while awaiting rescue. The doctor who is summoned to the accident site should be consulted for a final verdict on the administration of fluids to injury victims.

Emotional shock can produce similar signs and symptoms in some individuals during an emergency. These patients may be persons who escaped a serious accident or disaster without injury or with only minor cuts or bruises. But they should be watched carefully, as time and manpower permits, to prevent their condition from progressing into an advanced stage of shock that would require greater attention from the first aid personnel.

When possible, persons who are helping at the scene of a mishap should compile some basic information about the situation while the facts are available. The information should include the names and addresses of victims, the names of relatives and of members of the clergy who should be notified, and the cause of the accident or other data relating to the situation. Note also any pre-existing disease or injury that the medical professional should know about, any medications the victims might have been taking—which might interact with drugs administered by the doctors—and a record of whatever type of first aid has been administered, including fluids given the victims, application of a tourniquet, and so on. If the victim happens to wear a Medic-Alert type of bracelet or pendant, the jewelry usually will contain some data of interest to the medical professionals. That fact should be noted in the information compiled since the identification jewelry may provide a clue to the source of detailed medical information stored in a computer data bank or a medical records library.

Stocking a First Aid Kit

Most families have a first aid kit at home or in the car. It may be a commercially packaged kit or a do-it-yourself collection of assorted adhesive bandages and containers of over-the-counter medications.

Below is a suggested list of items that should be in every family's first aid kit, but may be absent from most commercially packaged as well as most do-it-yourself kits:

12 10 cm x 10 cm sterile dressings in sealed envelopes
12 5 cm x 5 cm sterile dressings in sealed envelopes
2 2.5 cm x 5 m roller bandages
2 5 cm x 5 m roller bandages

1   roll of adhesive tape
4   triangular bandages with safety
    pins
1   clean bed sheet
2   small bath towels
2   large bath towels
1   pair blunt nose scissors
1   pair tweezers
1   eye dropper
1   set of measuring spoons
12 wooden tongue blades
12 12 to 18 inch lengths of ¼ inch x 4
    inch wood splints
1   bar of antiseptic soap
1   package of salt
1   package of baking soda
1   package of antihistamine tablets
1   package of aspirin tablets
1   package of antimotion sickness
    tablets
1   large package adhesive bandages
And personal prescription medications

Each family member may have a personal preference for one or more additional items. Some ex-servicemen like to include a pair of needle-nosed pliers with wire cutting jaws, which can be used for such minor home surgery tasks as removing splinters or fish hooks from the skin.

Adhesive tape and safety pins help an untrained first aider apply dressings and bandages more effectively. A dozen safety pins—small, medium, and large sizes in an assortment—would add very little to the size and weight of a home first aid kit.

Wooden tongue blades, which can be obtained at many hobby supply stores as well as at pharmacies, can be used to stir solutions of salt and soda water or other medications. For families on the road, a package of paper cups should be included. Wooden tongue blades also can be used as

temporary splints for fingers. The dozen pieces of wood are intended for splints for possible injuries to arms or legs.

Measuring spoons should provide a precise measure of teaspoon size since there are as many different sizes of teaspoons as of coffee cups. A medical dose of one teaspoon should be a dose that is precisely five milliliters.

Towels and sheets are for emergency bandages or dressings. They should be laundered and ironed before being stored in the first aid kit, which when fully equipped is likely to fill a grocery carton. The various items should be organized for easy access as needed, perhaps with the real emergency materials on the bottom and the aspirin and antimotion sickness tablets near the top. Some items may be separated and protected in plastic bags. Any personal prescription medications certainly should be stored in a separate container and marked with a label or tag.

When traveling on a vacation or camping trip, a few additional items should be added to the kit. They should include one or more jugs of clean water, either water from the kitchen tap at home or the water sold in plastic gallon jugs at supermarkets, and a small stack of clean newspapers. Clean newspapers are remarkably useful in emergencies to place on the ground under an accident victim or to cover a patient when blankets or other covering materials may not be available.

If the family is likely to be in a remote area where snakes may be encountered, a snakebite kit should be included. Snakebite treatments by amateur first aid personnel, like the use of tourniquets, have the potential for doing more harm than good. But in a true snakebite emergency, it probably is better to do something than to do nothing.

The traditional approach to snakebite first aid has recommended slashing the flesh on the leg or arm, or wherever, so that the venom can be drained or sucked out. But there is often a risk that blood vessels, muscles, tendons, or other tissues will be slashed in a frantic effort to save a life. The damage to the limb from the amateur emergency surgery can result in permanent disabling effects for the snakebite victim, so any cutting of the patient's flesh must be done with extreme caution.

GLOSSARY

EMERGENCY FIRST AID

The following entries define and describe the common and medical terms relating to first aid. Words in italics refer to separate entries in the list that provide further information on the subject.

abdominal perforation Abdominal wounds may be caused by gunshot, stabbing, or flying glass or metal. There may be little or no external bleeding, but considerable internal bleeding. Cover the wound with a large, clean dressing, but avoid touching the wound area inside or outside with the fingers. Do not give the victim anything, including fluids, by mouth. Keep the victim on his back with the knees flexed to reduce tension on the abdominal wall. He should be transported to a hospital or doctor's office on a stretcher that has been slipped under the body.

abrasion A break in the skin caused by rubbing or scraping, such as a skinned knee. The wound should be washed and a mild antiseptic such as hydrogen peroxide can be applied. The abrasion should then be covered with a sterile gauze dressing held in place by a cloth bandage or adhesive tape.

acid burns Contact by the skin with acids, such as hydrochloric, nitric, or sulfuric acid, does not result in a true thermal, or heat, burn, although heat is released by chemical destruction of body tissues. To give first aid, flush away the acid with great amounts of water; if a shower bath is handy put the victim in it and turn the water on full force. If the patient is outside, turn a garden hose on the victim. Don't waste time removing clothing unless the victim's clothes are soaked with the chemical; once flooding with water has begun, the clothing can be stripped off or cut away with a scissors. Dry the burn area with sterile dressings,

treat the victim for shock, and summon professional medical help.

Chemical burns of the eye should be treated in a similar manner, by flushing the eye with copious amounts of cool, clean water. Water should be applied so it flows from the inside edge—near the nose—to the outer edge of the eye. After the acid has been washed away, both eyes should be covered with sterile dressings held in place with a bandage. Whenever one eye is injured, it is best to keep both eyes covered until professional medical care becomes available.

aerosol sprays Chemicals used in some aerosol sprays can be toxic if inhaled accidentally, or even deliberately in the case of persons who experiment with mind-altering substances. Some aerosol spray chemicals can damage the liver and heart, as well as produce mind effects ranging from intoxication to unconsciousness. A person suffering from aerosol spray effects should receive professional medical care immediately. Mouth-to-mouth resuscitation should be started if the victim's breathing has stopped.

alcohol abuse Alcohol is a depressant drug, despite misleading references to its stimulating effects. Taken in large doses, the drug acts as an anesthetic, causing reduced respiration and loss of consciousness. The intoxication associated with smaller doses is due to changes in reasoning areas of the brain and a disruption of normal motor skills and coordination.

If a person has consumed an overdose of alcohol, the pulse and breathing may be abnormal and the skin cold and clammy. Attempts should be made to determine whether the victim may be in shock and/or unconscious. If he cannot be aroused, emergency medical aid should be summoned. Meanwhile, efforts should be directed toward restoration of normal breathing, using mouth-to-mouth resuscitation if necessary. Sometimes all that is needed is to place the victim on his side, with the head resting on one arm and the mouth opened so that air can enter the lungs without obstruction.

alkali burns Alkali burns should be treated in the same manner as acid burns: flood the burn area with water; remove the victim's clothing, using care not to damage the skin or other tissues; continue washing until danger of chemical action has ended; dry the burn area with sterile dressings; and summon professional medical help.

altitude sickness A rapid change in altitude above sea level can cause a variety of symptoms to persons not used to the differences in air pressure and oxygen content of the higher altitude. The patient may experience cyanosis, or bluish coloring of the lips and fingernails, weakness, chills, headaches, loss of appetite, nausea, dizziness, or ringing in the ears. Difficult breathing and a pounding heart can result from physical effort. Normally, such effects last only a day or two as the body becomes acclimated to the new environment. If the effects persist, the patient should be returned to a lower altitude. Altitude sickness often can be avoided by ascending into higher altitudes gradually.

animal bites Bites by animals can result in a puncture, laceration, or avulsion—which means a part of the flesh is torn away. The bite should be treated initially as an open wound by controlling the bleeding and protecting against infection until it can be examined by a medical professional.

If the bite is caused by a rabid pet or wild animal, the victim will require special serum injections to help the body develop immunity to the rabies virus transmitted by the bite. There is no known cure for rabies in humans after the infection becomes established.

In addition to rabies, bites of pets and wild animals can transmit a variety of disease organisms. Tetanus, for example, can be acquired through an animal bite. Any animal bite that breaks the skin should be reported to a doctor; if rabies is a possible factor, local health authorities also should be notified. The bite area should be washed with soap and water, and covered with a sterile dressing before taking the victim to a doctor's office or hospital emergency room.

appendicitis Inflammation of the fingerlike appendix at the beginning of the large intestine. The patient should not be given anything to eat or drink while waiting for a doctor. If a doctor is not immediately available, take the patient to the emergency room of a nearby hospital.

aspirin overdose Aspirin is a generally safe and effective drug for the relief of minor aches, pains, fevers, and inflammations. A usual adult dose is two five-grain tablets every four hours; for children the dose is one-fourth to one-half the adult dosage. First aid for an overdose requires emptying the stomach as quickly as possible. If the victim is conscious, give ipecac syrup. Fluids to dilute the drug and help flush it through the body should be given every hour for the first 24 hours; the fluids can include nonalcoholic beverages. Symptoms of aspirin overdosage may include rapid breathing, headaches, and ringing in the ears.

back injury A back-injury victim should be treated as a patient who may have a damaged spinal cord or compressed nerve root: avoid moving the victim until he has been examined by a doctor. Any unnecessary motion of the victim's body can result in severe pain, paralysis, or death. Protect the victim from heat, cold, or weather while awaiting medical help.

bandage A term often used to describe any wound covering. Technically, a bandage is a strip of muslin, gauze, or other material used to hold a dressing or compress in place. A roller bandage is a long strip of cloth rolled into a cylinder for use as a dressing or compress. Triangular bandages, cut from a square of cloth along a diagonal line, can be shaped, like roller bandages, with adhesive tape and safety pins into a variety of patterns for emergency uses.

black eye A black eye is a closed wound in which blood lost by injury to soft tissues beneath the skin becomes trapped under the skin. First aid treatment can include use of cold packs to reduce swelling and the rate of internal bleeding.

blister A small, fluid-filled lump on the skin surface.

boil A pus-filled swelling, or furuncle, on the skin.

bruise A closed wound, like a black eye.

burns Burns cause damage to the skin and underlying tissues by exposure to excessive heat, chemicals, or electricity. Shock, fluid loss, and infection are common complications. Excessive heat can occur from open flame, exposure to sunlight, scalding liquids, steam or hot air, or nuclear radiation.

Burns often are classified as first, second, or third degree, depending upon the extent of tissue damage. First-degree burns are marked by redness, or other skin discoloration, accompanied by pain and swelling, such as a severe sunburn. Second-degree burns may be quite painful and associated with damage to tissues beneath the skin. There may be extensive swelling and the skin usually acquires a reddish mottled appearance, due to loss of body fluid through the damaged skin. Second-degree burns can result from exposure to flame, scalding liquids, or a very deep sunburn. Third-degree burns can be caused by contact with high-voltage electricity, very hot water, napalm or other war weapons, or by clothing that catches fire. All layers of skin are destroyed and there is damage to tissues beneath the skin. The effects may appear at first as second-degree burn damage but quickly progress to a whitish or charred coloration.

Emergency first aid calls for application of cold water to areas affected by first-degree

burns. Usually a dry dressing can be applied to the burn, which normally will heal without further treatment. Second-degree burns also should be treated with cold water for at least one hour and as long as two hours. After carefully drying the burn area, cover it with a sterile dressing. Do not touch the blistered skin or apply any ointment, antiseptic, or other remedy. If arms or legs are burned, keep them elevated while awaiting professional medical care. If large areas of the body are involved, the doctor may advise hospitalization.

Third-degree burns are a true medical emergency requiring professional care as quickly as possible. Do not apply cold water, ice, ointments, or any medication to the burned areas. Do not remove clothing from burn areas. Cold packs may be applied to the hands, feet, or head if they are not likely to increase shock symptoms. But do cover the burned areas with thick sterile dressings; otherwise, use clean sheets or other clean household linens, or even plastic bags from dry cleaners—but do not put plastic bags over burns of the face. Elevate the arms and legs if they are involved, and try to maintain normal breathing by keeping the victim's airways open. If professional medical help cannot reach the scene quickly, and the victim is conscious and not vomiting, small amounts of fluids can be offered a third-degree burn victim. The preferred fluid is a solution of one teaspoon of table salt and one-half teaspoon of baking soda dissolved in one quart of lukewarm water, to be sipped at a rate of one ounce every four or five minutes while waiting for the arrival of a doctor or paramedic.

carbon monoxide poisoning Preliminary symptoms include headache, yawning, dizziness, faintness, ringing in the ears, nausea, or heart palpitations. The victim soon becomes unconscious with a distinctive sign—the mucous membranes become a bright cherry red. A similar coloration occurs in the skin of persons with a naturally light complexion. Fresh air and mouth-to-mouth resuscitation are first aid measures until an ambulance crew with oxygen tanks can give professional treatment.

cardiac arrest Heart stoppage can result from a number of factors, ranging from a blocked blood vessel of the heart to a drug overdose. The victim will be unconscious, the pupils dilated, lips and fingernails turning blue, and breathing and pulse will be absent. Death can occur within a few minutes if immediate action is not taken.

Roll the victim onto his back and check his mouth and throat for any breathing obstruction. Then administer mouth-to-mouth resuscitation for about five puffs. If the patient does not respond, press the heel of the hand on the lower half of the breastbone and depress it quickly about 15 times at the rate of once each second. Then give two more mouth-to-mouth puffs, followed by 15 breastbone presses, repeating each series until professional medical help arrives.

choking Obstruction of the air passage by food or other objects can be relieved by one of two accepted methods. One involves delivering firm blows over the spinal column between the shoulder blades. The second, the Heimlich maneuver, is performed by the rescuer putting his arms around the torso of the victim from behind so that his hands can be clasped to form a fist at the bottom of the victim's breastbone. Then, by suddenly pushing the fist upward into the victim's chest, lung pressure is increased to help push the obstruction out of the trachea. A person whose windpipe becomes obstructed cannot talk and should use whatever sign language or other message is needed to advise others of the problem so that rescue efforts can begin immediately. Otherwise, death can occur within a few minutes.

cold applications Cold temperatures are used to cool local body areas by causing blood vessels near the surface to contract, thereby reducing inflammation, relieving pain, and controlling blood loss. Cracked ice in ice bags or other containers, or cold, moist compresses prepared by soaking a cloth in ice water and wringing it out, are commonly used methods of applying cold. Ice or cold water usually are not applied directly to the skin, which should be protected by a dry waterproof barrier.

compress A square of fabric used to apply heat, cold, or medications. Soft wool or flannel are preferred fabrics for compresses.

concussion A head injury that causes a brief or prolonged loss of consciousness. The victim also may experience headaches, blurred vision, or lapse into a coma. He should be treated as an unconscious person, with body warmth and breathing maintained until professional medical help arrives.

convulsion A nerve and muscle disturbance marked by involuntary muscle contractions; muscles may twitch or become rigid. The victim should be protected from self-injury by placing pillows, cushions, or rolled blankets around the head and body while awaiting the arrival of a doctor.

demulcent Any soothing, bland substance given a poisoning patient in addition to fluids administered to dilute or neutralize the chemical. Demulcents such as milk, egg white, or olive oil coat the lining of the digestive tract to retard absorption of the poison.

dressing Any material placed over an open wound to control bleeding, absorb blood or wound secretions, and prevent infectious agents from entering the wound. A dressing ideally is made of sterile gauze, but in an emergency any clean woven material, light clear plastic, or even clean paper can be used as dressing material. Fluffy cotton, or cotton wool, should not be used as a dressing because the fibers come loose and stick to body tissues. Dressings are held in place by bandages.

drowning Drowning victims usually suffocate from lack of oxygen. Thus, first aid efforts must be directed toward restoring normal breathing by mouth-to-mouth resuscitation. Once breathing is restored, shock prevention should begin. Meanwhile, professional medical care should be summoned.

Only an expert swimmer trained in Red Cross rescue techniques should attempt to recover a drowning victim from deep water. Otherwise, a ring buoy, fishing rod, a long stick, or a boat should be used to reach the victim. If a boat is used, resuscitation can begin as soon as the victim has been pulled aboard.

electrocution Severe electric shock can be caused by contact with ordinary electric lines in a home, office, or factory, as well as high-voltage lines or lightning. Electric shock causes muscular contractions or seizures, producing paralysis of the lungs or abnormal heart function, as well as bone fractures, thermal heat burns, changes in blood chemistry, and death of muscle tissue.

The electrocution victim must first be separated from the electricity by breaking contact—throwing a switch, removing the wire or appliance with an insulated tool such as a dry stick, or throwing a loop of rope or cloth around a limb of the victim in order to drag him away from the electricity. If the victim is alive but unconscious, send for medical help. If breathing has stopped, treat the victim for *cardiac arrest.*

eye injury Any eye injury that causes bleeding or apparent damage to the eyeball should be treated immediately by a physician, preferably by an ophthalmologist. Cover both eyes with sterile dressings and rush the victim to an eye specialist or hospital emergency room.

A minor eye problem caused by a foreign object under the eyelid sometimes can be treated by carefully pulling down the upper eyelid and examining its inner surface. If the irritating object can be found, try removing it gently with the corner of a clean handkerchief or facial tissue. Sometimes it can be flushed out with water or tears. If the foreign object cannot be located or removed, cover the eye with a dry sterile dressing and take the patient to a doctor's office for professional care.

fainting A person faints because of a disruption in normal blood flow to the brain. A fainting victim may experience nausea, dizziness, a tingling sensation in the hands and feet, sweating, or have a pale and cold skin. A person who feels faint should lie down before he falls down. Unless the victim faints in a dangerous location, such as the middle of the street, it's better to let him lie where he falls. Loosen any tight clothing that may interfere with adequate breathing. The face may be bathed with cold water, but water should never be poured onto the head of an unconscious or semiconscious person.

If a fainting victim is injured in falling or is not easily revived, a doctor should be called. Fainting often is a sign of a serious illness. If a fainting victim vomits, roll him over on his side so the vomitus can drain without gagging the patient, and wipe out his mouth with a handkerchief or facial tissue. Do not offer fluids to an unconscious or semiconscious person.

food poisoning Most cases of food poisoning result from eating foods containing an enterotoxin, or poison, produced by germs which may or may not still be in the food. The enterotoxin induces a secretion of fluid in the intestinal tract. Symptoms that may not appear until several hours after eating the food may include headache, fever, nausea, vomiting, cramps, and diarrhea. First aid includes bed rest, close to a bathroom or bedpan, and nothing given by mouth until vomiting has ceased. Then soft drinks, sweetened tea, and strained broth or bouillon with salt added may be given. Severe cases, marked by shock or by blood or mucus in the stools, should be reported to a doctor.

One of the most serious forms of food poisoning, botulism, usually does not cause vomiting or diarrhea, and the symptoms may not occur until more than a day or two after the contaminated food was eaten. Botulinum toxins affect the nervous system, so the first symptoms include double vision or loss of normal vision, drooping eyelids, and difficulty in swallowing. Hospitalization is required; the effects of the toxin can be fatal in some cases.

foot and leg injuries Injured lower limbs should be elevated with pillows, cushions, or rolled blankets or coats. The victim should not be allowed to walk on an injured leg or foot. Shoes and stockings should be removed if they interfere with examination of the injury. Any open wound should be washed with clean water and soap, blotted dry with a sterile dressing, and covered with another sterile dressing. Serious foot or leg injuries should be given professional medical care.

frostbite Frostbite is the most common of cold weather injuries and is caused by inadequate blood circulation in the affected body tissues resulting from cold constriction of the blood vessels. The victim may feel an uncomfortable coldness in the exposed area, followed by a loss of feeling. The skin appears flushed or red at first, then turns white or a grayish-yellow color. The victim may not be aware of the injury until the skin discoloration is observed by himself or another person.

The victim must be taken to a warm environment immediately, and all tight or wet clothing in the affected area must be removed. The limb or other affected body part should be immersed in a warm bath of approximately 104 degrees Fahrenheit. Hot coffee, tea, chocolate, or similar warm fluids should be offered. Smoking should be prohibited because it further constricts the blood vessels. The damaged tissues should not be rubbed. If bleeding, fluid accumulation, or other adverse effects follow thawing, a doctor should be notified.

hand and arm injuries If the hand is severely injured, it should be elevated above the level of the heart (unless the injury is caused by snakebite), and the fingers separated with sterile dressings or gauze pads. Place a roller *bandage* in the palm of the hand and have the victim close his fingers around it, if possible. Then cover the entire hand with a towel or cloth, or enclose it in a plastic bag. An injured hand or arm should be supported in a sling until the injury can be examined by a doctor. A minor wound may be washed with clean soap and water, but do not try to clean a major wound before getting the victim to a doctor.

head injuries Treatment of head injuries depends upon whether the injury involves the scalp, skull, face, or brain. Open wounds of the scalp can be treated by the use of firm pressure dressings that help control bleeding. Facial injuries carry the risk of blood or body tissues obstructing air passages, so the mouth and throat must be swept clear of any obstructive material, using a finger wrapped in sterile gauze.

Skull fractures or brain damage may be indicated by the oozing of blood or blood-tinged cerebrospinal fluid draining from the nose or ears, loss of consciousness, or signs of paralysis. The patient should be treated as an unconscious person while professional medical help is summoned to the site: prevent shock, control bleeding, and maintain normal breathing.

insect bites Bites or stings of ants, bees, hornets, wasps, or yellow jackets may contain a venom that causes a reaction known as anaphylactic shock, the result of a foreign protein being injected into the human body. The reaction may be marked by respiratory edema and circulatory failure, and in certain sensitive individuals, collapse and death can occur within minutes after an insect bite or sting. Such sensitive individuals should carry medications prescribed by a doctor to prevent a severe reaction when they expect to be in areas frequented by venomous insects.

If an insect sting occurs, the stinger—which may look like a tiny wood splinter—should be removed carefully; it usually has the venom sac attached so it should not be squeezed. Ice or a cold compress should be applied to the area of the sting to slow the rate of venom absorption into the body tissues.

nosebleeds Nosebleeds usually start from small arteries in soft tissues near the tip of the nose, as a result of injury, high blood pressure, strenuous physical activity, or a change in altitude. First aid requires keeping the patient quiet and, if possible, in a sitting position with the head leaning forward. Press the outside of the bleeding nostril against the midline of the nose, but if that doesn't work, insert a small gauze pad in one or both nostrils and squeeze the outer sides of the nose toward the midline. Cold compresses also can be applied to the nose and surrounding areas of the face. But if the nosebleed is profuse or continues, call a doctor.

plant poisons The only safe way to avoid contact with plant poisons is to touch only those you know are safe and not eat any plant materials unless you are certain they can be ingested without adverse aftereffects. The three major contact poison plants in North America are poison ivy, poison oak, and poison sumac.

The tell-tale sign of poison ivy is that leaves always grow in clusters of three shiny leaflets. Poison oak, which may be found either as a shrub or vine, also has leaves that occur in clusters of three leaflets. These two and poison sumac are members of a family of plants that secrete an extremely irritating oil resin that causes a severe dermatitis.

Signs and symptoms of contacts with these plants include itching, swelling, and the appearance of blisters on affected parts of the skin. Persons who chew the leaves or inhale the smoke of burning poison ivy experience swelling and edema of the pharynx and larynx, along with fever and weakness. The symptoms may continue for as long as two or three weeks after contact with the plants.

First aid treatment begins with diluting and removing the resin from the skin by washing with strong laundry soap and water. A special solution of ferric chloride and alcohol sometimes helps dissolve the irritating resin. Follow-up treatments with mild wet dressings or with starch or oatmeal baths may be needed to help relieve the itching. If there is oozing and crusting from the blisters, exposure to warm dry air may be helpful.

snakebites The first step in handling a snakebite is to determine if the bite actually was caused by a poisonous snake. A severe bite by a nonpoisonous snake is not truly harmless since it will probably be a painful wound that will require the same kind of first aid treatment as a bite from a nonrabid wild animal. The bite from a poisonous snake often will result in an immediate, intense pain followed by a feeling of numbness in the area of the bite. Other symptoms will vary somewhat with the type of snake and its particular brand of venom.

A viper bite usually results in immediate swelling. A cobra bite, on the other hand, may cause no symptoms in the area of the wound except for an intense burning sensation. Coral snakes, like cobras, will produce a distinctive wound as a result of a chewing action on the flesh, whereas a viper bite is not a typical bite but rather a pair of fang punctures about one-half inch apart. Still other snakebites may appear as a semicircle of teethmark punctures with or without fang marks.

In general, the person who has been bitten by a snake should be kept quiet since any movement will tend to increase the flow of snake venom in the circulatory system. The victim should be transported as quickly as possible to a doctor's office or hospital emergency room. If the victim must walk any distance, he should walk very slowly.

If an arm or leg is the site of the wound, it should be immobilized and kept below the level of the heart. A constriction band should be tied around the arm or leg a few inches above the bite and between the bite and the blood vessels leading to the heart. A snakebite kit usually will contain some basic equipment for emergency treatment, including a sterile knife or razor blade, a constriction band, a suction cup, etc. The knife blade should be sterilized by holding it over a flame. Then small cuts should be made in the skin of the victim at the fang or bite marks and a bit beyond, since the venom often is deposited below the fang marks. The cuts should be only skin deep and run in the same axis as the limb treated. The venom should be sucked out of the cuts and spat on the ground. The mouth should be rinsed after this procedure.

Finally, the snakebite wound should be treated like any other animal bite; that is, it should be washed with soap and water, dried with a sterile dressing, and covered with a second sterile dressing held in place with a *bandage*. A cold *compress* can be applied but ice should not touch the wound directly. As in any other serious injury, the patient should be treated for shock even if signs or symptoms of shock do not appear right away.

QUESTIONS AND ANSWERS
EMERGENCY FIRST AID

Q: *What is a sucking wound of the chest?*
A: A sucking wound is a chest wound that penetrates the lung area so that it makes a sucking noise when the victim breathes. It is a very serious type of injury because it allows air to enter the chest cavity and usually is accompanied by a collapsed lung. In an emergency situation when doctors or paramedical personnel are unlikely to arrive immediately, the wound should be covered with a large thick dressing that is held firmly in place to prevent further entry of air into the chest cavity through the wound.

Sucking wounds may be caused by jagged fragments hurled through the air, by an explosion, or by a knife or gunshot.

Q: *Is there any kind of "shot" you can take to prevent a poison ivy reaction?*
A: Medical researchers have developed a way of treating red blood cells with molecules of urushiol, the chemical that causes an allergic reaction to poison ivy, poison oak, and poison sumac, so that the body will develop an immunity to the plants. However, it has not been cleared for use in humans so far and probably will not be available for several years.

Q: *What is a normal pulse rate that can be used as a benchmark for telling whether an injured or sick person's pulse is fast or slow?*
A: For young children, a normal pulse rate can range all the way from around 80 to 180 beats per minute. An adult woman generally has a faster pulse, 75 to 80 per minute, than an average adult male, at 55 to 70. To establish your own family's benchmarks for pulse rates, practice testing them when the individuals are in good health. An average of several "normal" pulse counts could give you a sound basis for comparison purposes in the event of illness or injury. In some diseases accompanied by a fe-ver, the pulse rate may increase by perhaps ten beats per minute for each degree of fever, but that rule is not always exact for every person.

Q: *I have read that you shouldn't make a child vomit if he has swallowed kerosene or any other petroleum product. Is this true?*
A: Yes. While the proper thing to do in the case of certain types of poisoning is to make the victim vomit, in order to get the poison out of the stomach as quickly as possible, this procedure can cause complications if the poison is a petroleum product. For example, kerosene can be inhaled into the lungs and cause a toxic form of pneumonia.

People who accidentally swallow a petroleum product often vomit as a result of the poison. If this happens, the victim should be held so that the head is lower than the rest of the body to prevent the poison from being sucked into the lungs.

Rather than waste time administering first aid to a child who has swallowed kerosene or a similar petroleum product, the victim should be carried as quickly as possible to the nearest hospital emergency room.

Q: *Are tarantula bites poisonous?*
A: Tarantula bites are seldom fatal but they can be equivalent to the bite of a black widow spider, and the bite can be particularly serious if the victim is a small child.

Q: *First aid advice almost always includes a recommendation that an injured person be covered with a blanket. Since most people don't carry blankets, wouldn't other covering materials, like canvas or plastic, do just as well?*
A: Yes. Most clean covering materials can be adapted in a serious emergency to protect the

body of an injured person. A blanket, obviously, is rather ideal since blankets are designed to cover people and thereby protect them from the outside environment.

Experienced outdoorsmen often carry a folded sheet of plastic and a length of nylon cord which can be used to fashion a barrier against the elements and help conserve body heat in an emergency. Protecting the body against heat loss is particularly important in cool, breezy weather, when each mile-per-hour of wind speed can be the equivalent of one degree of temperature Fahrenheit in its chilling effect on the body.

Q: *Is there one way to move an injured person that is better than simply carrying the patient from an accident site?*
A: The answer depends in part on the type of injury and the size of the victim. A small child might be carried safely to a car or doctor's office without using a stretcher if the injury does not involve a back or neck fracture, or a similar kind of problem that could be exacerbated by that technique of moving the victim.

An adult might be carried without a stretcher from a burning building or car. But the heroic rescue techniques sometimes portrayed in movies and TV shows actually can result in more harm to an accident victim than any other kind of amateur first aid measure.

When it is necessary to move an injured person from an accident site without the help of professional medical personnel, at least four healthy persons should be enlisted for the project. Three persons are needed to lift the injured person carefully and to roll the body of the victim toward them, while the fourth person positions the stretcher so that the victim can be rolled back onto it. The stretcher always should be carried to the victim rather than carrying the victim to the stretcher.

If the rescuer is unable to find other people to help move the injured person, the victim sometimes can be moved to an area where greater protection or assistance is available by getting the injured person onto some sort of emergency stretcher—which can be a sleeping bag, a door removed from its hinges, a blanket, or a coat. The victim should be pulled in the direction of the long axis of the body, that is, head or feet first, but not sideways.

INDEX

of breast, 292–94, 307, 458, 460–61
blood, *see* Leukemia
bone, 322–23, 460, 475–76
cervical, 281, 290, 462
of colon, 232, **243–44**, 466
development of cancer cells, 456–57
diet and, 475
of digestive tract, 465–66
drugs for treatment of, 390
of esophagus, 465
of female reproductive organs, 290–91
of intestines, 231–32
of kidneys, 457, 463–64
of larynx, 458, 465
of lungs, 458, 467
metastasis of cancer cells, 458–59
of mouth, 458, 465
nitrites and, 641
of ovaries, 290–91
of pancreas, 212–13, 466–67
of penis, 273–75
of placenta, 474
possible causes of, 455–56
of prostate, 278–79, 462–63
of rectum, 457, 466
risk of, 457
squamous cell, **473**
of stomach, 222, 457, 465–66
of testes, 462–63
thyroid, 467
of uterus, 290, 458, 461–62, 474
warning signs of, 457–58
Candidiasis, **39,** 50
  intestinal, 265
  during pregnancy, 283
  vaginal, 280
Canker sore, **105**
Cannulation, **105**
Capillaries, 155, **172, 494**
Carbohydrates, 612–13, 641
Carbon dioxide, **494**
Carbon dioxide depletion, 164–65
Carbon monoxide poisoning, **654**
Carbonic anhydrase inhibitors, 390
Carbuncle, **39**
Carcinogen, **296**
Carcinoma, **105, 296, 469**

alveolar cell, **167**
Cardiac arrest, **172, 494, 655**
Cardiac catheterization, **172**
Cardiac cycle, **494**
Cardiac heave, **172**
Cardiac output, **494**
Cardiac reserve, **494**
Cardiomyopathy, **494**
Carditis, **494**
Cardiovascular disease, *see* Heart disease
Carina, **172**
Carotenoderma, **328**
Carotid arteries, **494, 519**
Carotid arteritis, **105–6**
Carotid body, **494**
Carotid sinus, **172, 494**
Carpal tunnel syndrome, **328, 537**
Carpometacarpal joint, **328**
Carrier, **554**
Carrier tests, 549
Cartilage, **106, 328, 537**
Casts, **244**
CAT scanner, **106,** 513, 514
Cataract, **106**
Cat-cry syndrome, 549
Cat-eye syndrome, 549–50
Cathartic, **244**
Cathartic colon, 266
Catheter, **244**
Cauliflower ear, **106,** 144
Causalgia, **537**
Cavernositis, **296–97**
CCU, **172,** 486
Cecum, **244**
Celiac artery, **244**
Celiac disease, **244**
Cellulitis, **39, 106,** 444
Central tendon, **172–73**
Cereals, 637–38
  calories in, 636
Cerebellar system test, **106**
Cerebellopontine angle tumor, **106**
Cerebral hemorrhage, **106–7, 519**
Cerebrospinal fluid, **519**
Cerebrovascular, definition of, **519**
Cerebrovascular accident (CVA), *see* Stroke

Cerebrum, **519**
Certification, **13**
Cerumen, **107**
Cervical, definition of, **329**
Cervical caps, 400–2
Cervical rib syndrome, **173**
Cervical spondylosis, **329**
Cervix, 280–81, **297**
  cancer of, 281, 290, 462
  surgical removal of, 289–90
Chalazion, **107**
CHAMPUS, **379–80**
Chancre, **39, 107, 297**
  on penis, 274
  vaginal, 280
Chancroid, **39–40, 297**
  on penis, 274
Chaplaincy service, **380**
Chapping, 24
Charcot's joints, **537**
Charleyhorse, 340
Cheilitis, **107**
Chemonucleolysis, 339
Chemosis, **107**
Chemotherapy, **107, 297, 469**
  for bone cancer, 323
  for breast cancer, 294
  for cancer of female reproductive organs, 290
  drugs for, **173**
Chest, 147–99
  muscular movements in, 149
  organs of, *illus.* 148
  sources of pain in, 149–50, 163
  sucking wound of, 660
  See also Heart; Lungs
Chest aspiration, **173**
Cheyne-Stokes breathing, **173**
Chicken pox, **40,** 445
Chigger bites, **40**
Chilblains, **40,** 51
Childbirth, 422
  emergency, 422–24
  hospitalization for, 376
  labor and, 421–22
Children
  diabetic, 211
  eczema of, 564, 572
  emotional development of, 580–81, 584
  exercises for, 598–602, *illus.* 599–601

Mediastinum, **184**
Medicaid, **16**, 377
Medical College Admissions Test, 4
Medical colleges, 4–5
  admission to, 19
Medical history, 544
Medicare, **16**, 377
Medication
  administering, 366, 368
  See also Drugs
Melanin, 29–30
Melanocytes, **49**
Melanoma, **49, 472**
Melanosis, **49**
Melasma, **49**
Melena, **256**
Menarche, 287–88, **302**
Meniere's disease, **125**
Meningitis, aseptic, 446, 447
Meniscus, **334, 539**
Menopause, 288, **302**
  changes in breasts during, 292
Menorrhagia, 284
Menstrual cycle, 286–88, **302**
  disorders in, 283–84
  IUDs and, 309–10
Mental illness, 574–75
  genetic factors in, 583
  prevention of, 579–80
  in primitive cultures, 584
  types of, 575
Mental retardation, 574
Mercury fever thermometers, 348–49
Mesenteric artery, **256**
Mesenteric thrombosis, **256–57**
Mesentery, **257**
Metabolic diseases, 550–53
  amino acid, 551–52
  diabetes, 550–51
  storage, 552
Metals, allergies to, 60
Metaphase, **554**
Metastasis of cancer cells, 458–59
Metatarsalgia, **334**
Methotrexate, 390
Metrorrhagia, 284
Micturition, **257**
Middle ear, **125**

Midwives, 425
Migraine, **125**, 140
Miliaria, **49**
  types of, *illus.* 33
Miliary tuberculosis, **184**
Milk, 636
  allergy to, 640
  calories in, 634
  carbohydrates in, 641
Milk-alkali syndrome, **257**
Mineral corticoids, **302**
Minerals
  essential, 614–18
  trace, 618
Mirror examination, **125**
Mitosis, **554**
Mitral stenosis, **184, 498**
Mittelschmerz, **257**
Mold spore, **570**
Mole, **49–50**
Molybdenum, 618
Monaural loudness balance test, **125**
Mongolism, *see* Down's syndrome
Moniliasis, **50**
Mononucleosis, 447
Monozygotic twins, **555**
Morphea, **50**
Motor nerves, 319–20
Motor neuron, **334**
Motor system, **522**
Mourning, 582
Mouth, 85–92
  cancer of, 458, 465
  digestion and, 214–15
  internal structure of, *illus.* 86
  lines at corners of, 142–43
Mouth-to-mouth resuscitation, 647
Mucin, **257**
Mucocele, **125**
Mucopurulent chronic bronchitis, **184–85**
Mucous membrane, **257**
Mucoviscidosis, **185, 257**
Multifactorial inheritance, 546–47, **555**
Multiple coverage, 381
Multiple myeloma, 322, **472**
Mumps, 87, 447
  immunization against, 434
  inner ear symptoms in, 98

orchitis resulting from, 276
Murmur, **498**
Muscles
  of arm, *illus.* 316
  calories burned up by, 586–87
  of chest, 149
  dangerous symptoms of, 355
  deltoid, **329**
  disorders of, 318–19
  exercise to develop, 587
  of eyes, **114**
  of face, 521
  hamstring, **331**
  of head and neck, 67–71
  intercostal, **182**
  of legs, *illus.* 317
  overloading of, 588
  papillary, **498**
  pulled or torn, 341
  sensory and motor nerves and, 319–20
  skeletal, 316–18
  trained for strength and endurance, 587–88
Muscular dystrophy, **334, 420**
Musculoskeletal system, 311–41
  disorders of, 321–25
  nervous system and, 319–20
  sources of pain in, 320–21
  See also Bones; Muscles
Mutation, **555**
Mutism, akinetic, 518
Myalgia, **334**
Myasthenia gravis, **334**
Mycoplasmal infections, **185**
Mycosis fungoides, **50**
Mycotic aorta disease, **185**
Myelocytic leukemia, **472**
Myelomas, 322
  multiple, 322, **472**
Myocardial infarction, 151–52, **185, 485–86, 498,** *illus.* 486
Myocardiopathy, 501
Myocarditis, **185, 498**
Myocardium, **185**
Myoclonic jerks, **334**
Myomas, uterine, 282
Myopia, 78, **125**, *illus.* 94
Myringitis, **125–26**
  bacterial, **104**
  bullous, **105**

Rupture, **260**
of appendix, 228
RUQ, **260**

S

Saccular aneurysm, **522**
Saddle nose, **133**
Saline abortion, 408, 410
Saliva, hypersecretion of, 143
Salivary duct calculus, **133**
Salivary glands, 87–88
digestion and, 214–15
tumors of, **133**
Salmonellosis, **260**, 451
Salpingitis, **133, 260**
Salt-free diet, 511
Sarcoidosis, **54, 189**
Sarcoma, **472**
Ewing's, **470**
Scab, **54**
Scabies, **54, 59, 304**
Scalene node, **189**
Scar, **54**
Scarlet fever, **54**, 447
Schistosomal dermatitis, **54–55**
Sciatic nerve, **336**
Sciatica, 325
chemonucleolysis for treatment
of, 339
Scintillating scotoma, **133**
Scleritis, **133**
Scleroderma, **55**
Sclerosis, **499**
Scoliosis, **189–90, 336**, 340
Scratch test, **570**
Scrotum, 271, 275–77
disorders of, 278
hernia penetration of, 309
Scuba diving, 604
Scurvy, **55**
Seawater itch, **55**
Sebaceous adenoma, 37
Seborrheic dermatitis, **55**
Seborrheic keratosis, **55**
Secondary hypertension, **499**
Selenium, 618
Self-pay patients, **382**
Seminoma, **472**
Senile arthritis, 324
Sense of smell, 83, **133**, 198
Sensitization, **570**
Sensory nerves, 319–20, **336–37**

Septoplasty, **133**
Septum
interventricular, **183, 497**
nasal, *see* Nasal septum
Seven-year itch, 59
Sex determination, mechanism
of, 544, *illus.* 545
Sex hormones, 288
Sex organs, 270–306
cancer of, 290–91
female, 279–90
fetal development of, 270–71
male, 271–79
Sex-linked gene, **555**
Shaft, fracture of, **299**
Shaving, effect on hair growth of,
59
Shigellosis, **260**
Shin splints, 340
Shingles, **55**, 445
chest pain due to, 150
Shock
first aid for, 648–49
insulin, **260–61**
Shortness of breath, **190**
Shoulder, frozen, **331, 538**
Shunt, **499**
Sialadenitis, **133–34**
Sialorrhea, 143
Sickle-cell anemia, 543, 553, 556
Sickroom
controlling odors in, 369
selection and equipping of,
355–56
Sigmoid colon, **261**
Silent heart disorders, 502
Silicon, 618
Silicosis, **190**
Simmonds test, **337**
Single-gene defects, 546
Singultus, **522**
Sino-atrial block, **190**
Sino-atrial node, **190**
Sinus rhythm, **499**
Sinuses, 85, **134**
examination of, 98–99
signs of infection in, 95
Siphonage, **261**
Sippy diet, **261**
Sitz bath, 369
Skiing, 605
Skin, 20–62

allergic reactions of, 563–64
arthritic diseases involving,
535–36
cancer of, 59, 457, 459, *illus.*
458, 459
color of, 29–30, 59
disorders of, 35; *See also*
specific conditions and
diseases
distinctive patterns of, 30–31
effects of stress and allergies
on, 34–35
fatty deposits in, 32
healthy, aspects of, 22
inner layer of, 31–32
outer layer of, 23–26
permeability of, 26
route of penetration into, *illus.*
25
specialized types of, 26–29
structure of, *illus.* 22
sweat glands in, 32–34
wrinkles of, 60
"Skin writing," 61
Skull
bones of, 315–16, *illus.* 66
hot cross bun, **119**
or newborn, *illus.* 65
normal growth of, 64
position of brain in, *illus.* 72
SLE (systemic lupus
erythematosus), **48, 55, 191,**
535
Sleeping sickness, 451
Small intestine, 224–26
Smallpox, **55–56**, 444
vaccination against, 434
Smell, sense of, 83, **133**
adverse effect of disease on,
198
Smoking, *see* Cigarette smoking
Snack foods, 632–33
Snakebites, **658–59**
first aid for, 650–51
Sneezing, cause of, 141
Snellen test, **134**
Snuff box, 339–40
Sodium bicarbonate, 391
Specialists, training of, 4
Speculum, **134**
Speech
esophageal, 113